Molecular Pathology Protocols

METHODS IN MOLECULAR MEDICINE™

John M. Walker, *Series Editor*

60. Interleukin Protocols, edited by *Luke A. J. O'Neill and Andrew Bowie,* 2001

59. Molecular Pathology of the Prions, edited by *Harry F. Baker,* 2001

58. Metastasis Research Protocols: *Volume 2, Cell Behavior In Vitro and In Vivo,* edited by *Susan A. Brooks and Udo Schumacher,* 2001

57. Metastasis Research Protocols: *Volume 1, Analysis of Cells and Tissues,* edited by *Susan A. Brooks andUdo Schumacher,* 2001

56. Human Airway Inflammation: *Sampling Techniques and Analytical Protocols,* edited by *Duncan F. Rogers and Louise E. Donnelly,* 2001

55. **Hematologic Malignancies:** *Methods and Protocols,* edited by *Guy B. Faguet,* 2001

54. **Mycobacterium Tuberculosis Protocols,** edited by *Tanya Parish and Neil G. Stoker, 2001*

53. **Renal Cancer:** *Methods and Protocols,* edited by *Jack H. Mydlo,* 2001

52. **Atherosclerosis Methods and Protocols,** edited by *Angela F. Drew,* 2001

51. **Angiotensin Protocols,** edited by *Donna H. Wang,* 2001

50. **Colorectal Cancer: *Methods and Protocols*,** edited by *Steven M. Powell,* 2001

49. **Molecular Pathology Protocols,** edited by *Anthony A. Killeen,* 2001

48. **Antibiotic Resistance Methods and Protocols,** edited by *Stephen H. Gillespie,* 2001

47. **Vision Research Protocols,** edited by *P. Elizabeth Rakoczy,* 2000

46. **Angiogenesis: *Reviews and Protocols*,** edited by *J. Clifford Murray,* 2000

45. **Hepatocellular Carcinoma: *Methods and Protocols*, edited by** *Nagy A. Habib,* 2000

44. **Asthma: *Mechanisms and Protocols*, edited by** *K. Fan Chung and Ian Adcock,* 2000

43. **Muscular Dystrophy: *Methods and Protocols,* edited by** *Katherine B. Bushby and Louise Anderson,* 2000

42. **Vaccine Adjuvants: *Preparation Methods and Research Protocols*,** edited by *Derek T. O'Hagan,* 2000

41. **Celiac Disease: *Methods and Protocols*,** edited by *Michael N. Marsh,* 2000

40. **Diagnostic and Therapeutic Antibodies,** edited by *Andrew J. T. George and Catherine E. Urch,* 2000

39. **Ovarian Cancer: *Methods and Protocols*,** edited by *John M. S. Bartlett,* 2000

38. **Aging Methods and Protocols,** edited by *Yvonne A. Barnett and Christopher R. Barnett,* 2000

37. **Electrochemotherapy, Electrogenetherapy, and Transdermal Drug Delivery:** *Electrically Mediated Delivery of Molecules to Cells,* edited by *Mark J. Jaroszeski, Richard Heller, and Richard Gilbert,* 2000

36. **Septic Shock Methods and Protocols,** edited by *Thomas J. Evans,* 2000

METHODS IN MOLECULAR MEDICINE™

Molecular Pathology Protocols

Edited by

Anthony A. Killeen

MB, BCh, PhD, FFPathRCPI

Department of Pathology, University of Michigan, Ann Arbor, MI

Humana Press **Totowa, New Jersey**

999 Riverview Drive, Suite 208
Totowa, New Jersey 07512

This publication is printed on acid-free paper. ∞
ANSI Z39.48-1984 (American Standards Institute) Permanence of Paper for Printed Library Materials.

Cover illustration taken from Fig. 1, Chapter 9, by Susan Sheldon.

Cover design by Patricia F. Cleary.

For additional copies, pricing for bulk purchases, and/or information about other Humana titles, contact Humana at the above address or at any of the following numbers: Tel.: 973-256-1699; Fax: 973-256-8341; E-mail: humana@humanapr.com; Website: http://humanapress.com

Printed in the United States of America. 10 9 8 7 6 5 4 3 2 1

Library of Congress Cataloging in Publication Data

Main entry under title:

Methods in molecular medicine™.

Molecular pathology protocols / edited by Anthony A. Killeen.
p. cm. — (Methods in molecular medicine™ ; 49)
Includes bibliographical references and index.
ISBN 0-89603-681-2 (alk. paper).
1. Molecular diagnosis—Laboratory manuals 2. Pathology, Molecular—Laboratory manuals.
I. Killeen, Anthony A. II. Series.
[DNLM: 1. Pathology, Clinical—methods—Laboratory Manuals. 2. Genetic Techniques—Laboratory Manuals. 3. Immunologic Tests—Laboratory Manuals.
QY 25M7183 2001]
RB43.7.M646 2001
616.07'5--dc21 00-024928

Preface

The era of molecular pathology has arrived. From its promising beginnings in research laboratories, the field has grown, and continues to grow, to become a vital part of the care of an ever-increasing number of patients.

Because of its recent emergence from the research laboratory, many molecular pathology protocols are still to be found in the primary literature, and have not appeared in a text. *Molecular Pathology Protocols* contains laboratory protocols that have been developed by many of the authors for use in clinical molecular pathology laboratories and describe in detail how to perform these assays. This book is therefore intended for clinical laboratory use by medical technologists and pathologists. It will also be of interest to research workers who are performing these assays.

In its broadest meaning, pathology is the study of disease, and therefore it follows that any disease for which the molecular basis is understood would be suitable as a topic for inclusion in this work. When selecting protocols, it was necessary to place limits on the number of chapters that could be feasibly presented in a single work. Those protocols that were selected are performed more frequently, or have achieved recognition as having important diagnostic utility in contemporary practice. A decision was made to exclude inherited genetic diseases with certain exceptions, such as those diseases that are associated with thrombotic states and are part of the traditional domain of pathology. Undoubtedly their etiology would have been of much interest to the great pathologists of the past. A small number of chapters describe methods that are available as commercial assays. These chapters, particularly in certain methodological details described in the notes, offer much fuller description of the methods than is often available.

As will be apparent, many of the protocols described have been developed as in-house methods by the authors. This point highlights a characteristic of the field of molecular pathology: the lack of standardization of most assays, even those in reasonably wide clinical practice. Unlike some other areas of clinical laboratory analysis, there are no definitive methods available for molecular pathology. It would be of advantage to the field, if only to provide consistency among laboratories, if there were to be agreement on analytical issues such as probes and primer sets for various assays. These protocols offer methods that the authors have found to work in their laboratories. As with all clinical laboratory testing, the results should be interpreted in conjunction with other laboratory data and clinical findings.

Anthony A. Killeen
MB, BCh, PhD, FFPathRCPI

Contents

Contributors

NAHIDA AKEL • *Department of Pathology, University of Michigan, Ann Arbor, MI*

XIN BAI • *Department of Pathology and Laboratory of Molecular Pathology, University of Texas Southwestern Medical Center, Dallas, TX*

ALLEN E. BALE • *Departments of Human Genetics and Internal Medicine, Yale University, New Haven, CT*

DANIEL B. BELLISSIMO • *Diagnostic Laboratories, The Blood Center of Southeastern Wisconsin, Milwaukee, WI*

KARIN D. BERG • *Department of Pathology, Johns Hopkins School of Medicine, Baltimore, MD*

MICHAEL R. BLEAVINS • *Departments of Pathology and Experimental Toxicology, Parke-Davis Pharmaceutical Research, Warner-Lambert Co., Ann Arbor, MI*

KATARIINA CASTRÉN • *Department of Pharmacology and Toxicology, University of Oulu, Oulu, Finland*

ETHEL CESARMAN • *Department of Pathology and the Center for Lymphoma and Myeloma, Weill Medical College of Cornell University, and New York Presbyterian Hospital, New York, NY*

FELIX A. DE LA IGLESIA • *Departments of Pathology and Experimental Toxicology, Parke-Davis Pharmaceutical Research, Warner-Lambert Co., Ann Arbor, MI*

JAMES G. DONNELLY • *Department of Laboratory Medicine, Ottawa Hospital Civic Campus, Ottawa, Ontario, Canada*

JAMES R. ESHLEMAN • *Department of Pathology, Johns Hopkins School of Medicine, Baltimore, MD*

HONGXIN FAN • *Department of Pathology, University of Texas Health Science Center, San Antonio, TX*

JONATHAN A. FLETCHER • *Department of Pathology, Brigham and Women's Hospital, Harvard Medical School, Boston, MA*

THOMAS J. GIORDANO • *Department of Pathology, University of Michigan, Ann Arbor, MI*

MICHAEL GLYNN • *Department of Human Genetics, University of Michigan, Ann Arbor, MI*

CONSTANCE A. GRIFFIN • *Department of Pathology, Johns Hopkins School of Medicine, Baltimore, MD*

STEPHEN B. GRUBER • *Division of Molecular Genetics, Departments of Internal Medicine and Epidemiology, University of Michigan, Ann Arbor, MI*

MARGARET L. GULLEY • *Department of Pathology, University of Texas Health Science Center at San Antonio and Audie L. Murphy Memorial Veteran's Hospital, San Antonio, TX*

LAURA HEISLER • *Orton Scientific Consulting, Madison, WI*

STEVEN HERMAN • *Roche Molecular Systems, Alameda, CA*

MARTIN J. HESSNER • *Diagnostic Laboratories, The Blood Center of Southeastern Wisconsin, Milwaukee, WI*

SHAWN E. HOLT • *Departments of Pathology and Human Genetics, Medical College of Virginia/Virginia Commonwealth University, Richmond, VA*

SUZANNE HUBER • *Department of Pathology and Laboratory Medicine, Clinical Science Center, University of Wisconsin School of Medicine, Madison, WI*

KAREN L. KAUL • *Department of Pathology, Evanston Hospital, Evanston, IL*

ANTHONY A. KILLEEN • *Department of Pathology, University of Michigan, Ann Arbor, MI*

CHAO-HUNG LEE • *Department of Pathology and Laboratory Medicine, Indiana University School of Medicine, Indianapolis, IN*

SCOTT LUKE • *Department of Pathology, Evanston Hospital, Evanston, IL*

RONALD C. MCGLENNEN • *Department of Laboratory Medicine and Pathology, University of Minnesota Medical School, Minneapolis, MN*

NAHEED MITHA • *Department of Laboratory Medicine and Pathology, University of Minnesota Medical School, Minneapolis, MN*

DIANA MOHL • *Department of Pathology, University of Michigan, Ann Arbor, MI*

CARMELA P. MORALES • *Department of Internal Medicine, University of Texas Southwestern Medical Center and The Dallas VA Medical Center, Dallas, TX*

Scott P. Myrand • *Departments of Pathology and Experimental Toxicology, Parke-Davis Pharmaceutical Research, Warner-Lambert Co., Ann Arbor, MI*

Frederick S. Nolte • *Department of Pathology and Laboratory Medicine, Emory University School of Medicine, Atlanta, GA*

James Novotny • *Roche Molecular Systems, Pleasanton, CA*

I. Cetin Ozturk • *Department of Pathology, University of Michigan, Ann Arbor, MI*

Langxing Pan • *Department of Pathology, Weill Medical College of Cornell University, New York, NY*

Huaizheng Peng • *Department of Histopathology, University College London Medical School, London, UK*

Elizabeth M. Petty • *Departments of Internal Medicine and Human Genetics, Division of Medical Genetics, University of Michigan, Ann Arbor, MI*

Maurice Rosenstraus • *Roche Molecular Systems, Branchburg, NJ*

Jeffrey S. Ross • *Department of Pathology and Laboratory Medicine, Albany Medical College, Albany, NY*

Edward H. Rowsell • *Department of Laboratory Medicine and Pathology, University of Minnesota, Minneapolis, MN*

Richard H. Scheuermann • *Laboratory of Molecular Pathology, Department of Pathology, University of Texas Southwestern Medical Center, Dallas, TX*

Christine E. Sheehan • *Department of Pathology and Laboratory Medicine, Albany Medical College, Albany, NY*

Susan Sheldon • *Department of Pathology, University of Michigan, Ann Arbor, MI*

Michael M. Shi • *Departments of Pathology and Experimental Toxicology, Parke-Davis Pharmaceutical Research, Warner-Lambert Co., Ann Arbor, MI*

Yi-Wei Tang • *Division of Infectious Diseases, Departments of Medicine and Pathology, Vanderbilt University School of Medicine, Nashville, TN*

Elizabeth R. Unger • *Centers for Disease Control and Prevention, Atlanta, GA*

KIRSI H. VÄHÄKANGAS • *Department of Pharmacology and Toxicology, University of Oulu, Oulu, Finland*

SUZANNE D. VERNON • *Centers for Disease Control and Prevention, Atlanta, GA*

DAVID S. VISWANATHA • *Department of Pathology, University of New Mexico Health Science Center, Albuquerque, NM*

KARL V. VOELKERDING • *Department of Pathology and Laboratory Medicine, Clinical Science Center, Madison, WI*

LINDA M. WASSERMAN • *Division of Medical Genetics, Department of Medicine, University of California, San Diego, La Jolla, CA*

JUDITH A. WELSH • *Laboratory of Human Carcinogenesis, National Cancer Institute, National Institutes of Health, Bethesda, MD*

MYRA J. WICK • *Department of Laboratory Medicine and Pathology, University of Minnesota, Minneapolis, MN*

KRISTINE P. WORONZOFF-DASHKOFF • *Department of Laboratory Medicine and Pathology, University of Minnesota Medical School, Minneapolis, MN*

1

DNA Extraction from Paraffin-Embedded Tissues

Hongxin Fan and Margaret L. Gulley

1. Introduction

In routine histopathology, most tissues are fixed in formalin and embedded in paraffin for long-term preservation. DNA can be extracted from these tissues for subsequent molecular analysis by amplification methods. We describe herein a protocol for DNA preparation from paraffin-embedded tissues based on published procedures *(1–3)*. In brief, tissue sections are placed into microfuge tubes, then deparaffinized with xylene. The xylene is removed with ethanol washes, and the tissue is treated with proteinase K to make DNA available for amplification.

This protocol is simple, but there are several factors that influence the success of subsequent DNA amplification assays, including the type of fixative that is used, the duration of fixation, the age of the paraffin block, and the length of the DNA segment to be amplified (*see* **Note 1**). Ethanol fixation preserves DNA much better than does formalin. Formalin fixation randomly chops DNA in a duration-dependent manner, resulting in partial degradation. Even more severe DNA degradation occurs in bone samples subjected to acid decalcification. Because of this degradation, formalin-fixed tissue is not suitable for Southern blot analysis or for amplification of large DNA segments. Nevertheless, polymerase chain reaction (PCR) amplification of segments ranging up to 1300 bp has been reported *(2)*, and consistent amplification of segments up to 300 bp is commonly achieved from archival fixed tissues. Be aware that partial degradation of DNA may result in sampling bias, and therefore results should be interpreted with caution. For example, amplification of DNA from one cell may produce a PCR product that is not representative of the entire population of cells in the tissue. For this reason, it is wise to run tests in duplicate and always with appropriate controls.

From: *Methods in Molecular Medicine, vol. 49: Molecular Pathology Protocols*
Edited by: A. A. Killeen © Humana Press Inc., Totowa, NJ

2. Materials

2.1. Reagents

1. Xylene.
2. 100% Ethanol.
3. Proteinase K stock solution (20 mg/mL).
4. TEN buffer: 10 m*M* Tris-HCl, pH 8.0, 1 m*M* EDTA, pH 8.0, 20 m*M* NaCl.

2.2. Equipment

1. Microcentrifuge.
2. Heating block or water bath to hold 1.5-mL Eppendorf tubes.
3. Microtome.

3. Methods

Preparation of paraffin-embedded tissue for DNA amplification involves several manual manipulations; therefore precautions should be taken to avoid contamination, such as changing gloves frequently. When opening and closing microfuge tubes, do not touch the rim or inside of the cap. (Many laboratory scientists place a fresh gauze square over their thumb when opening a tube, or use a cap-opener device or screw-top lids.) Appropriate negative controls must be used to alert for contamination.

3.1. Cutting and Deparaffinizing Sections

1. Use a microtome to cut five sections, 5–20 µm thick, from a paraffin block, and place these directly into a 1.5-mL microfuge tube. The thickness of the sections depends on the size of the biopsy. For a small biopsy (up to 3 mm), 20-µm thick sections may be required, whereas a large biopsy requires only 5-µm thick sections. Although multiple thin sections can be placed in a single tube, fewer thick sections are more practical for processing. *See* **Note 2** for special precautions against contamination.
2. Add 800 µL of xylene to each tube, close, mix by gentle vortexing, and then incubate at room temperature for 10 min. Pellet the tissue by centrifugation for 3 min in a microfuge at full speed. Carefully remove and discard the supernatant using a pipet; do not disturb the tissue. If any translucent white paraffin remains, repeat the xylene wash one to two more times.
3. Add 800 µL of 100% ethanol to each tube, close the lid, and mix by inverting. Pellet the tissue by centrifugation for 3 min in a microfuge at full speed, and carefully remove and discard the supernatant with a pipet. Repeat the ethanol wash one more time, and remove as much supernatant as possible.
4. Open the tubes and let the residual ethanol evaporate by incubating in a dry heat block at 55°C for 15–30 min or until the sample is completely dry. (Speed-vacuum drying is not recommended because of the risk of contamination.)

3.2. Proteinase K Digestion

1. To the dried tissue samples add 100 μL of TEN buffer containing 200 μg/mL of proteinase K (prepared by mixing 1 μL of proteinase K stock solution in 100 μL of TEN buffer). Large tissue samples should be resuspended in 200 μL or more of this solution.
2. Close the tubes and incubate at 55°C for 3 h. (Large tissues should be incubated overnight.)
3. Spin briefly to remove any liquid from the cap. Cover the caps tightly with cap locks (PGC Scientifics, Gaithersburg, MD) to prevent them from popping open during high-temperature incubation. Incubate in a 95°C heat block for exactly 10 min to inactivate the proteinase K (*see* **Note 3**). Pellet the tissue in a microfuge at full speed for 10 min, and then transfer the supernatant to a clean tube and discard the pellet. Promptly proceed with PCR amplification.
4. Quantitation of DNA is not recommended; rather, the amount of supernatant required for subsequent DNA amplification is determined empirically. Try 1- and 10-μL vol of the supernatant as a template for a 100-μL PCR amplification. If PCR products are not generated, then different volumes can be tried (*see* **Note 4**). A positive control reaction (e.g., β-globin) should be run to ensure that amplifiable DNA of similar length to the target DNA is present in the sample. (*See* **Note 5** for modification of thermocycling parameters.)
5. Store DNA at –20°C, and avoid thawing and refreezing. (Freshly prepared samples are more efficiently amplified than those stored frozen, perhaps because the freeze-thaw cycle damages DNA.)

4. Notes

1. The most important factor affecting DNA quality is the type of fixative employed and the duration of fixation. Tissues fixed between 12 and 24 h in ethanol, acetone, Omnifix, or 10% buffered formalin usually yield good-quality DNA; but B-5, Zenker's, or Bouin's solutions, or duration of fixation longer than 5 d, are poor prognostic factors for PCR productivity ***(2,4)***. Prior studies showed that when the length of β-globin amplification product increased (175, 324, and 676 bp), the percentage of fixed tissues containing amplifiable DNA decreased (100, 69, and 45%) ***(5)***. And when the age of a block increased, PCR productivity decreased ***(6,7)***, although some blocks stored for more than 40 yr were successfully studied ***(8)***.
2. It is important that no tissue be carried over from one case to the next during microtomy. Between each block, shift to a fresh part of the blade. Use smooth-edge rather than toothed forceps for transporting sections into tubes. Do not allow bleach to come in contact with the tissue or the DNA will be destroyed. Ice cubes used to cool a block should be discarded between cases.
3. Longer incubation at 95°C may damage DNA, whereas shorter incubation may not fully inactivate proteinase K. Additional time is needed for volumes >500 μL.

4. The optimal amount of template for an amplification reaction depends on numerous factors specific to each sample, such as DNA concentration and presence of inhibitors. It is useful to test several concentrations of each template (e.g., 1 and 10 µL of template per 100-µL PCR). Large tissues may necessitate the use of a smaller fraction of the template (e.g., 0.1 µL). The amount of template that is "tolerated" in a PCR may be affected by residual fixation chemicals or paraffin, excessive tissue debris, and other factors. If the first attempt fails, a 10-fold dilution will often reduce inhibitors while still retaining enough DNA to allow amplification.
5. Amplification of DNA prepared from paraffin-embedded tissue is less efficient than amplification of DNA from fresh or frozen tissues. To compensate for this reduced efficiency, consider modifying the thermocycling parameters by increasing the number of cycles and lengthening the duration at each temperature within the cycle ***(1)***.

References

1. Wright, D. K. and Manos, M. M. (1990) Sample preparation from paraffin-embedded tissues, in *PCR Protocols: A Guide to Methods and Applications* (Innis, M. A., Glefand, D. H., and Sninsky, J. J., eds.), Academic, San Diego, pp. 153–158.
2. Greer, C. E., Wheeler, C. M., and Manos, M. M. (1994) Sample preparation and PCR amplification from paraffin-embedded tissues. *PCR Methods Appl.* **3,** S113–S122.
3. Rolfs, A., Schuller, I., Finckh, U., and Weber-Rolfs, I. (1992) *PCR: Clinical Diagnostics and Research*, Springer-Verlag, Berlin, pp. 85–87.
4. Shibata, D. (1994) Extraction of DNA from paraffin-embedded tissue for analysis by polymerase chain reaction: new tricks from an old friend. *Hum. Pathol.* **25,** 561–563.
5. Liu, J., Johnson, R. M., and Traweek, S. T. (1993) Rearrangement of the BCL-2 gene in follicular lymphoma: detection by PCR in both fresh and fixed tissue samples. *Diagn. Mol. Pathol.* **2,** 241–247.
6. Limpens, J., Beelen, M., Stad, R., Haverkort, M., van Krieken, J. H., van Ommen, G. J., and Kluin, P. M. (1993) Detection of the t(14;18) translocation in frozen and formalin-fixed tissue. *Diagn. Mol. Pathol.* **2,** 99–107.
7. Goelz, S. E., Hamilton, S. R., and Vogelstein, B. (1985) Purification of DNA from formaldehyde fixed and paraffin embedded human tissue. *Biochem. Biophys. Res. Commun.* **130,** 118–126.
8. Shibata, D., Martin, W. J., and Arnheim, N. (1988) Analysis of DNA sequences in forty-year-old paraffin-embedded thin-tissue sections: a bridge between molecular biology and classical histology. *Cancer Res.* **48,** 4564–4566.

2

DNA Extraction from Fresh or Frozen Tissues

Hongxin Fan and Margaret L. Gulley

1. Introduction

The first step in molecular analysis of patient tissues is preparation of purified, high molecular weight DNA. A number of methods and commercial kits are available for DNA isolation. Traditional organic extraction protocols *(1,2)* are based on the fact that DNA is soluble in water whereas lipids are soluble in phenol. In these protocols, tissues are disaggregated and then treated with detergent to lyse cell membranes followed by proteinase to digest proteins. Phenol, an organic solvent, is added to help separate the lipids and protein remnants from the DNA. Chloroform is then used to facilitate the removal of phenol. DNA is subsequently concentrated and further purified by precipitation in a cold mixture of salt and ethanol. Finally, DNA is resolubilized in Tris-EDTA buffer.

The traditional organic extraction procedure presented herein is used by many laboratories to obtain abundant high molecular weight DNA. However, in recent years, there has been a trend toward adoption of commercial non-organic protocols that are faster and avoid the toxicity inherent with phenol exposure. A popular nonorganic extraction kit that works particularly well on blood and marrow samples is the Puregene DNA Extraction Kit (Gentra Systems, Minneapolis, MN). This kit can also be adapted for use on solid tissue samples for subsequent polymerase chain reaction (PCR) analysis.

2. Materials

2.1. Reagents

1. Lymphocyte Separation Media (ICN Biomedicals Inc., Aurora, OH).
2. 1X phosphate buffered saline (PBS): 137 m*M* NaCl, 2.7 m*M* KCl, 4.3 m*M* Na_2HPO_4, 1.4 m*M* KH_2PO_4.

From: *Methods in Molecular Medicine, vol. 49: Molecular Pathology Protocols*
Edited by: A. A. Killeen © Humana Press Inc., Totowa, NJ

3. Liquid nitrogen.
4. DNA extraction buffer: 10 m*M* NaCl, 20 m*M* Tris-HCl, pH 8.0, 1 m*M* EDTA.
5. 10% sodium dodecyl sulfate (SDS).
6. Proteinase K solution: 10 mg/mL of proteinase K in 50 m*M* Tris-HCl, pH 7.5; store at 4°C.
7. Phenol equilibrated with 0.1 *M* Tris-HCl, pH 8.0.
8. Chloroform: isoamyl alcohol (24:1).
9. 3 *M* Sodium acetate, pH 5.2.
10. 100% Ethanol.
11. 70% Ethanol.
12. TE buffer: 10 m*M* Tris-HCl, pH 8.0, 0.1 m*M* EDTA.
13. Agarose.
14. 1X TAE buffer: 40 m*M* Tris-acetate, 1 m*M* EDTA.
15. Ethidium bromide (10 mg/mL).
16. 10X Gel loading buffer: 0.25% bromophenol blue, 0.25% xylene cyanol, 15% Ficoll (type 400) in 10X TAE buffer.
17. DNA molecular weight marker.

2.2. Equipment

1. Mortar and pestle.
2. Water baths at 37, 50, and 55°C.
3. Centrifuge.
4. Spectrophotometer.
5. Horizontal gel electrophoresis apparatus.
6. DC power supply.

3. Methods

3.1. Sample Preparation

3.1.1. Tissue Specimen

1. Mince fresh, solid tissue up to 3 mm^3 into small pieces (1–2 mm) with a sterile scalpel blade. Process the tissue within 2 h of collection, or freeze at –20°C or colder until the time of DNA extraction (*see* **Note 1**).
2. Place the tissue in a clean mortar filled with liquid nitrogen. (*See* **Note 2** for cleaning instructions.)
3. Using a clean pestle, grind the frozen tissue to a powder while it is submerged in liquid nitrogen. While grinding, cover the mortar with a paper towel to keep tissue fragments inside the mortar, and work under a hood to protect yourself from aerosolized powder.
4. Allow the liquid nitrogen to evaporate, leaving a dry frozen tissue powder in the mortar.

3.1.2. Ficoll Separation of Mononuclear Cells from Blood and Marrow Aspirates

Prior to DNA extraction, mononuclear cells are isolated from anticoagulated blood or bone marrow aspirates by Ficoll centrifugation. (*See* **Note 3** for information about sample stability.) About 10^7 nucleated cells yield 40 µg of DNA for Southern blot analysis, and 3×10^6 cells yield sufficient DNA for amplification testing.

1. To a 15-mL conical tube, add 4.5 mL of blood and an equal volume of PBS. For bone marrow aspirates, use 1 mL of marrow and 8 mL of PBS. If less sample volume is available, use all of it. If greater sample volume is desired, split the sample evenly among two or more tubes so that all of it is processed, and then recombine the samples on collection of the mononuclear cell layer.
2. Using a Pasteur pipet, underlay the diluted blood or marrow with 3 mL of Ficoll solution (Lymphocyte Separation Media).
3. Cap the tube and centrifuge at 400*g* for 30 min at room temperature in a swinging bucket rotor.
4. Use a plastic Pasteur pipet to aspirate the mononuclear cell layer, which is the fuzzy white layer located between the plasma and the separation medium, into a clean 15-mL conical tube. Avoid the red cell layer at the bottom of the tube. (If no mononuclear cell layer is visible, *see* **Note 4**.)
5. Resuspend the mononuclear cells in PBS to 12 mL total volume.
6. Centrifuge for 10 min at 1700*g* at room temperature. Remove and discard the supernatant by pouring it off.
7. Store the cell pellet at –20°C temporarily or at –70°C long term, or proceed directly to DNA or RNA extraction.

3.2. DNA Extraction

3.2.1. Cell Lysis and Digestion

The procedure for solid tissue differs from that of blood or marrow mononuclear cells only in the first step.

1. For solid tissue, add 920 µL of DNA extraction buffer to the tissue powder in the mortar, and gently mix with the pestle. If the buffer freezes, wait until it thaws before proceeding. Then transfer the fluid to a 15-mL conical tube or microfuge tube by gentle pipeting. For a mononuclear cell pellet (about 10^7 cells), resuspend the cells in 920 µL of DNA extraction buffer and mix well by gentle pipeting.
2. Add 50 µL of 10% SDS to the mixture and mix well; the solution should become viscous.
3. Add 30 µL of proteinase K solution to the viscous mixture. Close the cap tightly and mix vigorously by repeated forceful inversion or vortex.
4. Incubate in a 37°C water bath for at least 6 h or as long as 2 d, or at 55°C for 3 h; gently invert the tube a few times during incubation.

5. The lysed sample should be viscous and relatively clear. This sample may be stored at 4°C for up to 1 wk before subjecting it to phenol/chloroform extraction as described in **Subheading 3.2.2.**, or before proceeding with nonorganic extraction as described in **Note 5**.

3.2.2. Phenol/Chloroform Extraction of DNA

1. Add an equal volume of equilibrated phenol, close the cap tightly, and mix gently by inversion for 1 min.
2. Spin the tube at 1700*g* in a swinging bucket rotor at room temperature for 10 min.
3. With a plastic pipet, aspirate the upper clear aqueous layer and transfer it to another clean labeled tube. This should be done carefully to avoid carrying over phenol or white proteinaceous material from the interface.
4. Repeat the phenol extraction (**steps 1–3**) one more time.
5. Next, extract with an equal volume of chloroform instead of phenol, and save the supernatant to another clean tube after centrifugation.
6. Repeat the chloroform extraction; this helps eliminate all of the phenol from the DNA sample.

3.2.3. Purification and Precipitation of DNA

1. To the aqueous DNA solution add 0.1 vol of 3 *M* sodium acetate (pH 5.2), and mix well by vortexing.
2. Add 2 vol of ice-cold 100% ethanol to the tube. Close the cap tightly and mix by inversion. A white cotton-like precipitate should form.
3. Use a sterile plastic rod to spool the precipitated DNA. (If no precipitate is visible, then microfuge at full speed for 10 min, rinse the pellet with 70% ethanol, air-dry for about 10–15 min, and proceed with **step 6**.)
4. Rinse the spooled DNA thoroughly in 1 mL of cold 70% ethanol by dipping.
5. Remove the DNA-coated plastic rod and allow the precipitate to air-dry until the white precipitate becomes clear, usually about 5–10 min.
6. Dissolve the precipitate in an appropriate volume of TE buffer (typically about 100–500 µL; targeting an optimal DNA concentration 1 µg/µL), scraping the rod along the wall of the microfuge tube to help detach the viscous DNA.
7. Allow the DNA to dissolve in the TE buffer for at least 4 h at 50°C, gently shaking periodically during incubation. Failure to adequately resolubilize the DNA will result in uneven distribution of DNA within the solution.
8. The purified DNA sample may be stored for 4 wk at 4°C prior to analysis, or indefinitely at –20°C.

3.3. DNA Quantitation by Spectrophotometry

1. Mix the DNA sample by gentle vortexing and inversion.
2. Add 5 µL of the DNA sample to 495 µL of sterile water and mix well.
3. Place the diluted sample in a quartz microcuvet and measure the absorbance at 260 and 280 nm against a water blank. (Nucleic acids absorb light maximally at 260 nm whereas proteins absorb strongly at 280 nm.)

4. Compute the DNA concentration based on the concept that an OD_{260} of 1 corresponds to 50 µg/mL of double-stranded DNA, and adjusting for the 100-fold dilution factor, according to the following formula:

$$\text{DNA concentration } (\mu g/\mu L) = OD_{260} \times 5$$

5. The $OD_{260}:OD_{280}$ ratio should be between 1.7 and 2.0. Lower values indicate protein contamination, in which case the DNA can be further purified by additional phenol/chloroform extractions followed by ethanol precipitation.

3.4. Gel Electrophoresis to Analyze DNA Quality

Agarose gel electrophoresis can be used to assess the intactness of purified DNA. High molecular weight DNA is needed for Southern blot analysis, whereas partially degraded DNA might be suitable for amplification procedures.

1. Prepare a 0.7% agarose gel in 1X TAE buffer containing 0.5 µg/mL of ethidium bromide.
2. Mix an aliquot of the extracted DNA sample with loading buffer, and load into a submerged well. Control samples representing intact and degraded DNA should be loaded into adjacent wells.
3. Electrophorese in 1X TAE buffer with 0.5 µg/mL ethidium bromide at 2 V/cm, until the dye front reaches the end of the gel.
4. View the gel under UV light. High molecular weight DNA is too large to migrate well under these conditions, whereas degraded DNA contains a spectrum of smaller fragment sizes that appear as a smear across the lane.

4. Notes

1. Solid tissue samples should be processed immediately or else frozen to minimize the activity of endogenous nucleases. If frozen tissue immunohistochemistry is planned, then slice the tissue into pieces no more than 5 mm thick and snap-freeze in liquid nitrogen or in a cryostat. If morphologic preservation is not needed, then place the tissue in a –70°C freezer indefinitely, or at –20°C for up to 3 d until DNA or RNA isolation.
2. After washing with detergent and rinsing well, soak the mortar and pestle in 50% nitric acid or 10% bleach to prevent carryover of DNA to the next case, then rinse well.
3. Peripheral blood or bone marrow aspirate anticoagulated with EDTA or acid citrate dextrose should be stored at room temperature and processed as soon as possible. EDTA beneficially chelates ions to inhibit nucleases from degrading nucleic acid, and consequently DNA and RNA are often stable for up to 48 h at room temperature. Heparin anticoagulant is not recommended because residual heparin may interfere with subsequent restriction enzyme or DNA polymerase activity.

4. If no mononuclear cell layer is visible, follow these steps to recover mononuclear cells from the red cell pellet. (This procedure may be particularly helpful if the blood has been previously refrigerated, thus causing the white cells to clump and sediment with the red cells at the bottom of the tube. For this reason, refrigeration of samples is not recommended prior to Ficoll centrifugation.) Carefully remove and discard the supernatant with a Pasteur pipet. Avoid disturbing the red cell pellet. Add 3 vol of Puregene RBC Lysis Solution (Gentra Systems) to the pellet. Invert to mix several times, and incubate for 10 min at room temperature. Invert again once during the incubation. Centrifuge at 2000*g* for 10 min, remove the supernatant with a Pasteur pipet, and discard it. The mononuclear cell pellet is not always visible at this step, and if not, you may use half-volumes of the extraction reagents in the subsequent steps of extraction.
5. To avoid the use of organic solvents, numerous nonorganic extraction protocols have been developed. We recommend the Puregene DNA Extraction Kit (Gentra Systems) for blood and marrow aspirates. To adapt this kit for PCR analysis of solid tissues, follow the protocol in this chapter through SDS and proteinase K digestion. Then apply the Puregene kit according to the manufacturer's instructions, skipping the red blood cell lysis and cell lysis steps.

References

1. Strauss, W. M. (1995) Preparation of genomic DNA from mammalian tissue, in *Current Protocols in Molecular Biology* (Ausubel, F. M., Brent, R., Kingston, R. E., et al., eds.), John Wiley & Sons, New York, pp. 2.2.1–2.2.3.
2. Sambrook, J., Fritsch, E. F., and Maniatis, T. (1989) *Molecular Cloning: A Laboratory Manual*, 2nd ed., Cold Spring Harbor Laboratory Press, Cold Spring Harbor, NY, pp. 9.14–9.23.

3

RNA Extraction from Fresh or Frozen Tissues

Hongxin Fan and Margaret L. Gulley

1. Introduction

RNA can be isolated from fresh or frozen tissue, then purified and quantified for subsequent molecular analysis. RNA is quite labile compared to DNA for good reason: RNA is the transient message that transmits information from activated genes. Once gene transcription is turned off, no more RNA is produced, and preexisting RNA is rapidly degraded to prevent continued translation of proteins. Because RNA is so labile, special care is required at all steps of RNA extraction to prevent RNA degradation.

Total RNA can be extracted from cells by treating them with guanidine isothiocyanate, a chemical that disrupts cellular membranes and also inhibits endogenous RNase activity *(1,2)*. This reagent forms the basis for several commercial kits that are available for total RNA isolation. In the protocol described herein, we use the TRIzol™ reagent (Gibco-BRL, Gaithersburg, MD), which combines phenol and guanidine isothiocyanate in a single solution to produce high yields of RNA in a rapid isolation procedure. This method is applicable to fresh or frozen tissue including blood or bone marrow samples.

2. Materials

2.1. Reagents

1. TRIzol reagent (Gibco-BRL); store at 4°C.
2. Chloroform.
3. Isopropanol.
4. Diethylpyrocarbonate (DEPC)-treated H_2O (*see* **Note 1**).
5. 75% ethanol made with DEPC-H_2O.
6. Ribonuclease inhibitor (40 U/µL) (Promega, Madison, WI).

From: *Methods in Molecular Medicine, vol. 49: Molecular Pathology Protocols*
Edited by: A. A. Killeen © Humana Press Inc., Totowa NJ

7. 10X DNase I buffer (Gibco-BRL)
8. DNase I, amplification grade (Gibco-BRL).
9. 20 m*M* EDTA.
10. Phenol : chloroform : isoamyl alcohol (25 : 24 : 1).
11. Chloroform : isoamyl alcohol (24 : 1).
12. 2 *M* Sodium acetate made with DEPC-H_2O, pH 4.5.
13. 100% Ethanol.

2.2. Equipment

1. Mortar and pestle.
2. Centrifuge.
3. Spectrophotometer.

3. Methods

3.1. Sample Preparation

Fresh and frozen tissues including blood and bone marrow aspirates are initially prepared in the same way as for DNA extraction. For example, solid tissues are frozen and ground into a powder under the liquid nitrogen, whereas blood and marrow mononuclear cells are isolated by Ficoll centrifugation as described elsewhere in this volume. Once the tissue powder or mononuclear cell pellet is obtained, instead of adding DNA lysis buffer, proceed with the following RNA extraction procedure.

3.2. RNA Extraction

Total RNA is isolated using TRIzol reagent according to the manufacturer's directions (Gibco-BRL). The procedure for solid tissues differs from that of blood or marrow mononuclear cells only in the first step. All of the following procedures must be carried out using RNase-free solutions and labware (*see* **Notes 1–3**).

1. Cell lysis: For solid tissue samples that have been ground to a powder, add 1 mL of TRIzol reagent per 50–100 mg of tissue (up to 3 mm^3). Gently mix with a pestle and then transfer to a microfuge tube by pipetting. Pipet up and down three to five times until tissue clumps are dispersed. If desired, this sample can now be stored at –70°C for at least 1 mo. Prior to use, the mortar and pestle should be baked at 150°C for 4 h to remove RNases (*see* **Note 3**). For mononuclear cells obtained from blood or bone marrow, add 1 mL of TRIzol reagent per 10^6–10^7 cells and then lyse the cells by pipetting up and down three to five times until clumps are dispersed. This sample can now be stored at –70°C for at least 1 mo.
2. Phase separation: Incubate the sample for 5 min at room temperature. Add 0.2 mL of chloroform, shake the tube vigorously by hand for 15 s, and incubate at room temperature for 3 min. Centrifuge the sample at no more than 12,000*g* at 4°C for 15 min.

3. RNA precipitation: Transfer the upper colorless aqueous phase to a fresh labeled microfuge tube; the lower chloroform phase can be discarded. Precipitate the RNA by adding 0.5 mL of isopropanol. Incubate at room temperature for 10 min. Recover the RNA pellet by centrifugation at no more than 12,000*g* at 4°C for 10 min.
4. RNA wash: Remove and discard the supernatant by pipetting. Wash the RNA pellet with 1 mL of cold 75% ethanol, mix by vortexing, and centrifuge at no more than 7500*g* at 4°C for 5 min. Then remove as much ethanol supernatant as possible.
5. Redissolving of RNA: Air-dry the RNA pellet by opening the cap for about 30–60 min, but do not dry it completely because this will greatly decrease its solubility. Dissolve RNA in about 50 µL of DEPC-H_2O (targeting an optimal RNA concentration of 1 µg/µL) by pipetting up and down a few times and then incubating at 37°C for 10 min. This RNA sample may be stored temporarily at –20°C, or add 1 µL of RNasin and store long term at –70°C.

3.3. DNase Treatment

Contaminating DNA in the RNA sample could potentially interfere with subsequent RNA analysis. For example, genomic DNA might compete with cDNA in reverse transcriptase polymerase chain reaction if the two primers do not span an intronic splice. In this case, treatment of the isolated RNA with DNase is recommended as follows:

1. Add 5 µL of 10X DNase I reaction buffer and 2 µL of 1 U/µL of amplification grade DNase I (Gibco-BRL) into 43 µL of the RNA sample. Incubate at room temperature for 30 min.
2. Stop the DNase reaction by adding 5 µL of 20 m*M* EDTA.
3. Add 45 µL of DEPC-H_2O per tube to bring the sample volume to 100 µL, and mix with 100 µL of 25:24:1 Phenol:chloroform:isoamyl alcohol. Spin in a microfuge at 12,000*g* for 5 min at 4°C, and then transfer the upper aqueous layer to a fresh labeled tube.
4. Add 100 µL of 24:1 chloroform:isoamyl alcohol, mix well, spin for 5 min at 4°C, and transfer the upper aqueous layer to a fresh labeled tube.
5. Add 15 µL of 2 *M* sodium acetate (pH 4.5) and mix well Add 2.5 vol of cold 100% ethanol and precipitate at –70°C for at least 30 min.
6. Recover the RNA by centrifuging in a microfuge at 12,000*g* for 15 min at 4°C. Wash the pellet with 75% ethanol one time.
7. Air-dry the pellet and dissolve RNA in about 10 µL of DEPC-H_2O (optimal RNA concentration is about 1 µg/µL), add 1 µL of RNasin, and store at –70°C.

3.4. Spectrophotometric RNA Quantitation

1. Add 2 µL of the RNA sample to 398 µL of DEPC-H_2O.
2. Place the diluted sample in a quartz microcuvet and measure the absorbance at 260 and 280 nm against a DEPC-H_2O blank.

3. Compute the RNA concentration using the following formula based on the concept that an OD_{260} of 1 corresponds to 40 μg/mL of RNA, and adjusting for the 200-fold dilution factor:

$$\text{RNA concentration } (\mu g/\mu L) = OD_{260} \times 8.$$

4. Notes

1. All solutions used in RNA preparation should be treated with DEPC. DEPC inactivates RNases by covalent modification. Add 0.1% DEPC to each solution, mix well, and incubate at 37°C overnight (or stir vigorously for at least 2 h), and then autoclave for 20 min. Unfortunately, DEPC cannot be used to treat solutions containing Tris because Tris inactivates DEPC. Therefore, it is recommended that an RNase-free spatula be used to retrieve Tris crystals from a fresh stock, and these crystals should be dissolved in H_2O previously treated with DEPC.
2. The main factor influencing the success of RNA extraction is inhibition of endogenous RNase activity and prevention of exogenous RNase contamination. RNases are ubiquitous, stable enzymes that generally require no cofactors to function. Human skin is a primary source of external RNase contamination, so gloves should be worn during all steps of the extraction procedure. All solutions, glassware, and plastic containers must be RNase free. When feasible, disposable plasticware should be used and then discarded.
3. Glassware should be baked at 150°C for 4 h to reduce RNase activity. Plastic items can be soaked in 0.5 *M* NaOH for 10 min, rinsed thoroughly with water, and autoclaved. Plasticware taken straight out of the original manufacturer's package is generally considered to be free from RNase contamination.
4. The TRIzol manufacturer's protocol recommends a power homogenizer to disperse solid tissues, but we have found it easier to manually grind the tissue to a powder under liquid nitrogen prior to addition of TRIzol reagent.

References

1. Chomczynski, P. and Sacchi, N. (1987) Single-step method of RNA isolation by acid guanidinium thiocyanate-phenol-chloroform extraction. *Analyt. Biochem.* **162,** 156–159.
2. Kingston, R. E., Chomczynski, P., and Sacchi, N. (1995) Guanidine methods for total RNA preparation, in *Current Protocols in Molecular Biology* (Ausubel, F. M., Brent, R., Kingston, R. E., et al., eds.), John Wiley & Sons, New York, pp. 4.2.1–4.2.9.

4

Single-Strand Conformation Polymorphism Analysis of Mutations in Exons 4–8 of the *TP53* Gene

Kirsi H. Vähäkangas, Katariina Castrén, and Judith A. Welsh

1. Introduction

The *TP53* tumor suppressor gene coding for a nuclear phosphoprotein involved in cellular stress responses is the most frequently mutated gene in human cancers described so far *(1–4)*. Mutations are found throughout the gene but most frequently within the highly conserved middle region (exons 5–8) that encodes for the DNA-binding central region of the gene critical for the major function of TP53 protein as a transcriptional activator *(5)*. The mutation spectrum of the *TP53* gene varies from one tumor type to another with typical hot-spot codons for mutations *(1–2,6)*. For instance, codons 157, 248, and 273 are frequently mutated in cigarette smoking–associated lung cancer, whereas mutations in codon 175 are rare. This codon, on the other hand, is often mutated in breast and colon cancer. In some cases, typical mutations can be linked with environmental exposures, such as CC→TT double mutation with UV radiation *(7)* and codon 249 AGG→AGT mutation with aflatoxin B1 and hepatitis B virus *(8)*. These findings, in connection with the fact that one of the main functions of TP53 protein is putatively the protection of the genome *(9,10)*, implicate the mutations of the *TP53* gene in environmentally induced carcinogenesis in humans and the possible use of *TP53*-related markers in molecular epidemiology *(11–13)*.

Mutations of the p53 gene with the loss of wild-type function also seem to have clinical importance. The reported tumor types, in which either a *TP53* gene mutation or aberrant expression of p53 protein indicates a worse prognosis, include breast cancer *(14–16)* and bladder cancer *(17,18)*. Furthermore, the known polymorphisms of the p53 gene may be involved in the susceptibility to cancers and prognosis of the disease *(19,20)*. Proallele carriers of exon 4 codon

From: *Methods in Molecular Medicine, vol. 49: Molecular Pathology Protocols*
Edited by: A. A. Killeen © Humana Press Inc., Totowa, NJ

72 polymorphism (CGC^{Arg} or CCC^{Pro}) were found to be overrepresented among patients who smoke and also among those affected at a younger age ***(21)***, and an excess of Arg/Arg homozygotes was found in nonsmoking patients with lung cancers ***(22)***. p53^{Arg} allele displays several differences in comparison to p53^{Pro}. For instance, it is more susceptible to degradation by human papilloma virus (HPV) E6 protein ***(23,24)***. There are indications that this translates to higher susceptibility to HPV-associated cervical cancer ***(23,25)***, although studies contradicting these findings also exist ***(26–30)***.

Among the most frequently used methods for the detection of mutation of the p53 gene are sequencing and single-strand conformation polymorphism (SSCP) analysis. Although originally SSCP was developed as a radioactive method ***(31)***, currently nonradioactive applications are available and, for obvious reasons, gaining more popularity. Further reasons for the increasing popularity are that SSCP has also been shown to be more sensitive than manual sequencing ***(32–34)*** and because of the introduction of smaller, more manageable gels and temperature-controlled equipment ***(35–39)***.

2. Materials

As a negative control, lymphocyte DNA from a healthy volunteer determined to be wild type by sequencing can be used. For positive controls, wild-type lymphocyte DNA is amplified using modified primers to integrate a change in the sequence. A positive and a negative control are included in each gel, because slight variation in the performance of the assay may occur from one piece of equipment to another.

2.1. Purification of DNA

DNA purified for any other purpose serves well as a starting material for this protocol. However, for those who want to use paraffin-embedded tissue blocks, we provide a method that has worked well for us:

1. 100 mg of proteinase K in 20 mL of 10% sodium dodecyl sulfate (SDS).
2. Phenol buffered with Tris-HCl, pH 7.5–7.8 (cat. no. 15513-039; Life Technologies).
3. Chloroform : isoamyl alcohol (24 : 1).
4. 0.5 *M* ammonium acetate.
5. Glycogen suspension (20 mg/mL) (cat. no. 901 393; Boehringer Mannheim).
6. 100% Ethanol.
7. TE buffer: 10 m*M* Tris-HCl, 1 m*M* EDTA, pH 8.0.

2.2. Amplification of p53 Exons 4–8

1. Primers (*see* **Table 1**).
2. dNTPs (100 m*M*) (Pharmacia).
3. Dynazyme (Finnzymes) or AmpliTaq (Perkin-Elmer).
4. 10X Dynazyme or AmpliTaq buffer.
5. Sterile water.

Table 1
Intronic Primers Used in Nonradioactive SSCP for *TP53* Exons 4–8[a]

Exon	Location	Primers with orientation 5′ to 3′
Outer primers		
X4	Left	ACG TGA ATT CTG AGG ACC TGG TCC TCT GAC
	Right	ACG TGG ATC CAG AGG AAT CCC AAA GTT CCA
X5	Left	ACG TGA ATT CGT TTC TTT GCT GCC GTG TTC
	Right	ACG TGG ATC CAG GCC TGG GGA CCC TGG GCA
X6	Left	ACG TGA ATT CTG GTT GCC CAG GGT CCC CAG
	Right	ACG TGG ATC CTG GAG GGC CAC TGA CAA CCA
X7	Left	ACG TGA ATT CAC CAT CCT GGC TAA CGG TGA
	Right	ACG TGG ATC CAG GGG TCA GCG GCA AGC AGA
X8	Left	ACG TGA ATT CTT GGG AGT ACA TGG AGC CT
	Right	AGG CAT AAC TGC ACC CTT GG
Inner primers		
X4	Left	TGC TCT TTT CAC CCA TCT AC
X4A1	Left	TGC TCT TTT CAC CC**<u>G</u>** TCT AC
	Right	ATA CGG CCA GGC ATT GAA GT
X5	Left	TTC AAC TCT GTC TCC TTC CT
X5A5	Left	TT**<u>G</u>** AAC T**<u>G</u>**T GTC TC**<u>G</u>** TTC CT
	Right	CAG CCC TGT CGT CTC TCC AG
X6	Left	GCC TCT GAT TCC TCA CTG AT
X6A6	Left	GCC TCT GAT TCC TC**<u>G</u>** CTG AT
	Right	TTA ACC CCT CCT CCC AGA GA
X7	Left	CTT GCC ACA GGT CTC CCC AA
X7A2	Left	CTT GCC ACA G**<u>C</u>**T CTC CCC AA
	Right	TGT GCA GGG TGG CAA GTG GC
X8	Left	TTC CTT ACT GCC TCT TGC TT
X8A1	Left	TTC CTT ACT GCC TC**<u>G</u>** TGC TT
	Right	CGC TTC TTG TCC TGC TTG CT

[a]The artificial mutations introduced to positive controls in the second amplification are underlined and set in boldface. In the second amplification, the left primer is either wild type regular primer or a changed one ("A" within the code means artificial). The right primer is according to the unchanged sequence in each case.

2.3. Minigel Analysis and Gel Purification of Amplified Products

1. NuSieve 3:1 agarose (FMC BioProducts, Rockland, ME).
2. 10X Tris-borate EDTA (TBE) buffer: 108 g/L Tris base, 55 g/L boric acid, 4 mL/L 0.5 *M* EDTA, pH 8.0.
3. Ethidium bromide solution (10 mg/mL) (Research Genetics).
4. DNA size marker (e.g., GelMarker-I, Research Genetics).
5. Bromophenol blue (0.2 mg/50 mL) in 25% Ficoll 400.
6. 0.5 *M* Ammonium acetate.

For minigels, the Hoefer HE 33 Mini Submarine (Pharmacia Biotech) has proved quick and practical. For gel purification, the Model 850 gel apparatus with 8 × 2.5 mm lucite combs from Aquebogue Machine and Repair Shop (Aquebogue, NY) is used.

2.4. Single-Strand Conformation Polymorphism

1. Pharmacia PhastSystem® equipment.
2. Stop buffer from a Sequenase kit (Sequenase 2.0 from Amersham).
3. Pharmacia reagents for PhastSystem: homogeneous 20% polyacrylamide gels, PhastGel Native Buffer Strips, PhastGel DNA Silver Staining Kit.
4. Gel-Drying Kit (Promega, Madison, WI).

2.5. Preservation of Gels

1. Clear cellulose film (e.g., gel-drying film; Promega).
2. Gel-drying frames. These are provided by several companies (e.g., Gel-Drying Kit; Promega).

3. Methods

3.1. Purification of DNA from Paraffin-Embedded Tissue

1. Scrape the tumor tissue into a 1.5-mL conical screw-cap microfuge tube. Add 50 µL of sterile water or TE buffer and break up pieces with a pipet tip.
2. Add 220 µL of water or TE buffer and 30 µL of proteinase K in SDS. Vortex and incubate in a 37°C heat block for 2 d. After 2 d add another 30 µL of proteinase solution. If not totally digested after 4 d, another 30 µL can be added for another day.
3. Boil the samples at 100°C for 10 min to inactivate proteinase K.
4. Add 300 µL of phenol, vortex for 20 s, and centrifuge for 2 min. Transfer the upper (aqueous) layer to a new tube.
5. Add 300 µL of chloroform:isoamyl alcohol, vortex for 15 s, and centrifuge for 1 min. Transfer the upper (aqueous) layer to a new tube.
6. Add 100 µL (one-third of volume) of 10 *M* ammonium acetate, 2 µL of freshly vortexed glycogen, and 900 µL of cold ethanol (2.5 vol). Vortex and precipitate DNA at –20°C overnight or at –80°C for at least 6 h.
7. Centrifuge for at least 30 min at high speed (12,800*g*) in the cold (4°C), wash pellets once with 70% ethanol for 10–15 min, centrifuge for 2 min, and decant the supernatant carefully.
8. Dry the pellets in a 42°C heat block for 10 min and dissolve the pellet in 50–100 µL of water.

3.2. Amplification of TP53 Exons

This method is only specific for the primers in **Table 1**. For a new strand, new standards must be developed and the experimental conditons optimized.

All reagents should be sterile and reactions done under a laminar flow hood to avoid contamination. Dedicated pipets for this purpose should be used for amplification reagents and a different pipet used for the template. Also, pipet tips containing an aerosol barrier are important to reduce contamination. A negative control without a template will confirm the purity of reagents and the procedure. Regarding polymerase, we have found that Dynazyme and AmpliTaq work well for us. Two consecutive amplifications are carried out, first with outer primers and then with inner (nested) primers (*[40]*; primer sequences in **Table 1**).

1. Dilute the dNTPs by adding 250 µL of each into 12.33 mL of sterile water. Divide into about 1-mL portions and store at –20°C.
2. Prepare a mixture of all the reagents for the first polymerase chain reaction (PCR) (without the enzyme or template). The following mixture is for one reaction: 10 µL of the 10X enzyme buffer (according to the enzyme used), 15 µL of dNTPs (final concentration 300 µ*M*), 20 pmol of each of the outer primers, H_2O to give 100 µL.
3. Prepare at the same time a mixture (with the enzyme this time) for the second PCR. The following mixture is for one reaction: 20 µL of 10X enzyme buffer, 32 µL of dNTPs, 40 pmol of each of the inner primers, 1 µL of enzyme, H_2O to give 200 µL. Aliquot 200 µL in each tube and store refrigerated until the first-round reactions are completed.
4. Divide 100 µL of the mixture for the first PCR into the amplification tubes.
5. Add 2–5 µL of template.
6. Heat at 100°C for 10 min and keep at 85°C in a heat block until placed into the thermocycler.
7. Add 0.5 µL of enzyme.
8. Place tubes in a preheated 95°C thermocycler.
9. Amplify for 35 cycles (94°C for 1 min, 60°C for 1 min, 78°C for 30 s).
10. Add 5 µL from the first reaction tubes to the second tubes as templates. There should be two controls: one with 5 µL from the control from the first reaction series as a template, and another with no template to control for the reagents in the second series (*see* **Note 1**).
11. Amplify for another 35 cycles as in **step 9**.

3.3. Minigel Analysis of Amplified DNA

Prepare a 4% gel (NuSieve 3:1 agarose) with 0.1% ethidium bromide in 1X TBE buffer and run 5 µL of samples + 3 µL bromophenol blue, and 10 µL of controls + 4 µL of bromophenol blue, and run with DNA size markers (a marker with a band at 100–200 is needed) for about 30 min at 150–180 V. **Table 2** gives the sizes of the amplified products.

3.4. Gel Purification of Amplified Exons

1. Prepare a 4% gel, about 1 cm thick, with deep wells to hold the 200-µL amplified product.
2. Add 25 µL of bromophenol blue to the sample.
3. Run the samples for about 2 h at 125 V.
4. View the gel in long-wave UV light to visualize the bands.

Table 2
Amplification Products and Their Running Conditions in SSCP of *TP53* Exons 4–8

		Running times at different temperatures[a]		
TP53 exon	Size of product	4°C	15°C	20°C
Exon 4	353	800 AVh	700 AVh	
Exon 5	247	600 AVh		500 AVh
Exon 6	180	400 AVh		300 AVh
Exon 7	195	500 AVh		400 AVh
Exon 8	200	600 AVh		500 AVh

[a]AVh, average V-h.

5. Using a sterile, disposable scalpel, cut the bands very closely according to known controls. Cutting closely is critical, because any extra material will show as extra bands in SSCP.
6. Cut the gel piece into smaller pieces, place in an Eppendorf tube, and add 500 μL of ammonium acetate.
7. Let the tube rock at 37°C overnight.
8. The next morning carefully pipet the buffer into another tube, add 1 mL of 95% ethanol, and precipitate at –20°C for about 24 h.
9. Centrifuge at 4°C for 30 min at 12,800*g* and carefully decant the ethanol.
10. Wash DNA once; gently add 1 μL of cold 70% ethanol to each tube, let sit at room temperature for 5 min, centrifuge at 12,800*g* for 3 min, and carefully decant the ethanol.
11. Let the tube stand open at room temperature (for about 30 min) to evaporate any remaining ethanol.
12. Dissolve the pellet in 20–50 μL of H_2O, depending on the intensity of the DNA band in the minigel.
13. Store refrigerated, or at –20°C for long-term storage.

3.5. Separation of DNA Strands in PhastSystem

Two temperatures are used for each exon. The lower temperature is 4°C for all exons and the higher is 20°C for exons 5–8. However, the higher running temperature for exon 4 is 15°C for the best detection of the codon 72 polymorphism. This polymorphism is not detectable at 4°C ***(41)***.

1. Program the machine. Select a different method number for each of the temperatures (4°C, 15°C, and 20°C) and program according to the following conditions:
   a. Prerun: 400 V, 10 mA, 1 W, and 100 average volt-hours (AVh).
   b. Sample application: 25 V, 10 mA, 1 W, and 2 AVh.
   c. Run: 200 V, 5 mA, 1 W, and 800 AVh.
2. Mix 3 μL of sample and 3 μL of stop buffer from a Sequenase kit (*see* **Note 3**).

3. Set the temperature in the PhastSystem and let it settle.
4. Prepare the gels by bending one corner of the tab (for later removal of the gel), and cutting one corner from one gel (to distinguish left and right gels). Clean the gel bed with distilled water and pipet about 0.5 mL of water onto the gel area to keep the gel properly positioned during the run. Carefully position the gel along the lines on the gel bed and blot (do not wipe) excess water with a paper towel. Be sure that no air bubbles remain under the gel. Correct the position if needed.
5. Remove the cellophane covering the gel and save it for later use.
6. Replace the buffer strip holder carefully, so as not to disturb the gel. After the buffer strip holder is in place, insert the two buffer strips. Ensure the even contact between the buffer and the gel by applying light pressure over the strips.
7. Lower the sample applicator arm. Ensure an even contact between the electrode and the buffer strip again by applying light pressure over the electrodes. Close the chamber.
8. Prerun the gels for buffer equilibration.
9. When the AVh reaches 80 (about 5 min before the sample applicator drops on the gel), boil the samples at 100°C for 4 min and put on ice. Apply 1 µL of each sample in the grooves of the eight-well comb (note that the ends of the comb do not have grooves).
10. Place the comb carefully in its place immediately after the sample applicator has dropped. This has to be done between 100 and 101 AVh (about 4 min) before the sample applicator rises up again.
11. Stop the run by pressing the button "SEP start/stop" and then "DO" at the AVh according to the exon and temperature (**Table 2**) (*see* **Note 3**).

3.6. Silver Staining of Gels in PhastSystem

Program and store the developing method prepared according to the method optimized for native-polyacrylamide gel electrophoresis with PhastGel gradient media. (See table 3 in the PhastGel™ Silver Kit Instruction Manual. Steps 1 and 16, however, are not needed for this protocol.) Prepare the reagents for silver staining while running the gels (*see* **Note 4**).

1. For step 2, make up 100 mL of 50% ethanol + 10% acetic acid in deionized water.
2. For steps 3, 4, 6, and 7, make up a total of 500 mL of 10% ethanol + 5% acetic acid.
3. For steps 8, 9, 11, and 12, set aside 1000 mL of deionized water.
4. For steps 13 and 14 (developer), pipet one ampoule of 2% formaldehyde into one bottle of sodium carbonate (both of these are provided in the kit). Mix thoroughly.
5. For step 15, prepare the background reducer by adding one packet of sodium thiosulfate into 100 mL of deionized water. When dissolved, adjust the pH to 5.0–6.0 by adding about one drop of 10% acetic acid.
6. For step 5 the 5% glutaraldehyde and for step 10 the silver stain are ready to use.
7. Place tubes into correct solutions (as defined in table 3 in the instruction manual).
8. For the run, place the two gels, facing each other, in the developing chamber in the gel holders. Close the lid tightly and start the developing program. The pro-

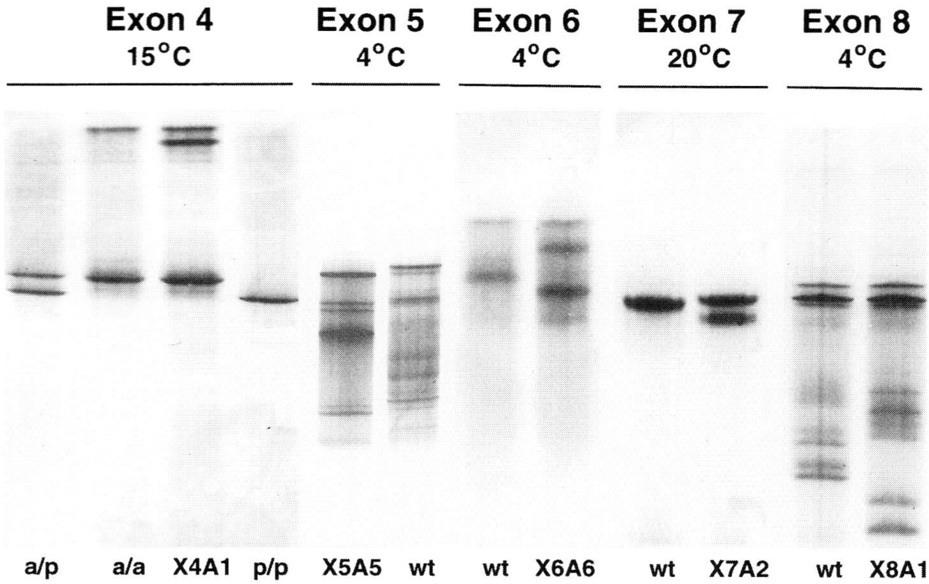

Fig. 1. Band patterns of p53 exons in SSCP. In exon 4, the band patterns for codon 72 polymorphism are shown: a, arginine; p, proline; a/p, heterozygote. The codes for mutated bands refer to strands amplified using exons listed in **Table 1**; wt, wild-type sequence.

gram takes about 1 h to run. For easier handling, when staining is finished, remove the gel and replace the cellophane on the gel.

3.7. Documentation and Preservation of Gels

Documentation of the gels is essential for later analysis, because silver stain fades with time. This may happen within a few days in daylight. We recommend both immediate photography and preservation of the gels (*see* **Note 5**).

1. For preservation of the gels, remove the cellophane and soak the gel in deionized water for 1–2 min.
2. Prewet the clear cellulose film with deionized water.
3. Place the gel in between the wet cellulose sheets and press out any air bubbles.
4. Secure the films tightly in the frame using clamps or bulldog clips.
5. Allow to dry completely at room temperature overnight. If properly done, the film is sealed and can be cut out with about a 0.5-cm frame for storage.

3.8. Interpretation of Results

To interpret results, the bands of the samples are compared with those of wild-type controls along the whole gel (**Fig. 1**). Double-stranded DNA runs off from the bottom of the gel and does not interfere with the interpretation of these conditions. Positive results in the analysis can result from a sample with a mutation, an amplified product with a polymerase error, or misinterpretation of SSCP owing to, e.g., an incompletely purified amplified sample. Very faint bands are usually owing to differences in the purification procedure from one time to another. If positive or suspicious, it is necessary to analyze another amplified product from the same sample.

4. Notes

1. Because there can be a slight variation among different machines, it is important to include both negative and positive controls on each gel. Each new set of controls must be confirmed to be wild type, either by comparison in the same SSCP gel with older known controls or by sequencing. This must be done for two reasons: (1) in each reaction there is a possibility of a polymerase error, and (2) apparently healthy people may carry a germline p53 mutation.
2. It is not necessary to know the DNA concentration exactly. However, note that as with sequencing, more is not necessarily better. The optimal concentration of DNA in the final sample, according to our experience, is 1–10 ng/µL.
3. After every use of the PhastSystem (which includes the separation by electrophoresis and silver staining), it is essential to run a cleaning program in the developing chamber. This is best done immediately after each run to avoid reagents drying in the tubes. Do not forget to place a blank plastic gel support (which is usually provided with the machine; if not, dedicate one of the unused gels for this purpose) in the gel holder in the chamber during the cleaning run to avoid overflowing of the chamber. The PhastSystem will not run without the blank gel support. After the cleaning program, careful manual cleaning of the staining chamber with soft paper including the level sensor (by cotton tip applicators) is still necessary. The electrodes should be cleaned with a soft brush. Without these cleaning procedures, dark background in the gels is inevitable and the problem grows worse with time. The tubing should be changed at least twice a year if the system is used regularly, and more frequently for heavier use.
4. Although the shelf life of the reagents is usually long (6 mo), it is better not to store them for a long time at the laboratory, but rather to use fresh reagents.
5. A practical way of storing the gels after drying is to use a plastic pocket sheet for slides. The dried gels within the cellophane sheets can be cut out to fit the pockets. Although the bands will stay visible for at least 1 yr if stored properly, it is advisable to photograph at least the key experiments. Dried gels break easily and careful handling is necessary.

Acknowledgments

We thank Mohammed Aslam Khan and Anna-Kaisa Lappi for critical reading of the manuscript.

References

1. Hollstein, M., Sidransky, D., Vogelstein, B., and Harris, C. C. (1991) p53 mutations in human cancers. *Science* **253,** 49–53.
2. Greenblatt, M. S., Bennett, W. P., Hollstein, M., and Harris, C. C. (1994) Mutations in the p53 tumor suppressor gene: clues to cancer etiology and molecular pathogenesis. *Cancer Res.* **54,** 4855–4878.
3. Hainaut, P., Soussi, T., Shomer, B., Hollstein, M., Greenblatt, M., Hovig, E., Harris, C. C., and Montesano, R. (1997) Database of p53 gene somatic mutations in human tumors and cell lines: updated compilation and future prospects. *Nucleic Acids Res.* **25,** 151–157.
4. Hussain, S. P. and Harris, C. C. (1998) Molecular epidemiology of human cancer: contribution of mutation spectra studies of tumor suppressor genes. *Cancer Res.* **58,** 4023–4037.
5. Gottlieb, T. M. and Oren, M. (1996) p53 in growth control and neoplasia. *Biochim. Biophys. Acta* **1287,** 77–102.
6. Hernandez-Boussard, T. M. and Hainaut, P. (1998) A specific spectrum of p53 mutations in lung cancer from smokers: review of mutations compiled in the IARC p53 database. *Environ. Health Perspect.* **106,** 385–391.
7. Brash, D. E., Rudolph, J. A., Simon, J. A., Lin, A., McKenna, G. J., Baden, H. P., Halperin, A. J., and Ponten, J. (1991) A role for sunlight in skin cancer: UV-induced p53 mutations in squamous cell carcinoma. *Proc. Natl. Acad. Sci. USA* **88,** 10,124–10,128.
8. Ozturk, M. (1991) p53 mutation in hepatocellular carcinoma after aflatoxin exposure. *Lancet* **338,** 1356–1359.
9. Kastan, M. B., Onyekwere, O., Sidransky, D., Vogelstein, B., and Craig, R. W. (1991) Participation of p53 protein in the cellular response to DNA damage. *Cancer Res.* **51,** 6304–6311.
10. Lane, D. P. (1992) p53, guardian of the genome. *Nature* **358,** 15,16.
11. Harris, C. C. (1996) The 1995 Walter Hubert Lecture—molecular epidemiology of human cancer: insights from the mutational analysis of the p53 tumour-suppressor gene. *Br. J. Cancer* **73,** 261–269.
12. Perera, F. P., Whyatt, R. M., Jedrychowski, W., Rauh, V., Manchester, D., Santella, R. M., and Ottman, R. (1998) Recent developments in molecular epidemiology: a study of the effects of environmental polycyclic aromatic hydrocarbons on birth outcomes in Poland. *Am. J. Epidemiol.* **147,** 309–314.
13. Hainaut, P. and Vähäkangas, K. (1997) p53 as a sensor of carcinogenic exposures: mechanisms of p53 protein induction and lessons from p53 gene mutations. *Pathologie-Biologie* **45,** 833–844.
14. Bergh, J., Norberg, T., Sjögren, S., Lindgren, A., and Holmberg, L. (1995) Complete sequencing of the p53 gene provides prognostic information in breast cancer patients, particularly in relation to adjuvant systemic therapy and radiotherapy. *Nat. Med.* **1,** 1029–1034.
15. Borresen, A.-L., Anderson, T. I., Eyfjörd, J. E., Cornelis, R. S., Thorlacius, S., Borg, Å., Johansson, U., Theillet, C., Scherneck, S., Hartman, S., Cornelisse, C. J.,

Hovig, E., and Devilee, P. (1995) TP53 mutations and breast cancer prognosis: particularly poor survival rates for cases with mutations in the zinc-binding domains. *Genes Chromosomes Cancer* **14,** 71–75.
16. Valgardsdottir, R., Tryggvadottir, L., Steinarsdottir, M., Olafsdottir, K., Jonasdottir, S., Jonasson, J. G., Ögmundsdottir, H. M., and Eyfjörd, J. E. (1997) Genomic instability and poor prognosis associated with abnormal TP53 in breast carcinomas: molecular and immunohistochemical analysis. *APMIS* **105,** 121–130.
17. Soini, Y., Turpeenniemi-Hujanen, T., Kamel, D., Autio-Harmainen, H., Risteli, J., Risteli, L., Nuorva, K., Pääkkö, P., and Vähäkangas, K. (1993) p53 Immunohistochemistry in transitional cell carcinoma and dysplasia of the urinary bladder correlates with disease progression. *Br. J. Cancer* **68,** 1029–1035.
18. Uchida, T., Wada, C., Ishida, H., Wang, C., Egawa, S., Yokoyama, E., Kameya, T., and Koshiba, K. (1999) p53 mutations and prognosis in bladder tumors. *J. Urol.* **153,** 1097–1104.
19. Peller, S., Halperin, R., Schneider, D., Kopilova, Y., and Rotter, V. (1999) Polymorphisms of the p53 gene in women with ovarian or endometrial carcinoma. *Oncol. Rep.* **6,** 193–197.
20. Wang, Y. C., Chen, C. Y., Chen, S. K., Chang, Y. Y., and Lin, P. (1999) p53 codon 72 polymorphism in Taiwanese lung cancer patients: association with lung cancer susceptibility and prognosis. *Clin. Cancer Res.* **5,** 129–134.
21. Murata, M., Tagawa, M., Kimura, H., Kakisawa, K., Shirasawa, H., and Fujisawa, T. (1998) Correlation of the mutation of p53 gene and the polymorphism at codon 72 in smoking-related non-small cell lung cancer patients. *Int. J. Oncol.* **12,** 577–581.
22. Murata, M., Tagawa, M., Kimura, M., Kimura, H., Watanabe, S., and Saisho, H. (1996) Analysis of a germ line polymorphism of the p53 gene in lung cancer patients: discrete results with smoking history. *Carcinogenesis* **17,** 261–264.
23. Storey, A., Thomas, M., Kalita, A., Harwood, C., Gardiol, D., Mantovani, F., Breuer, J., Leigh, I. M., Matlashewski, G., and Banks, L. (1998) Role of a p53 polymorphism in the development of human papillomavirus-associated cancer. *Nature* **393,** 229–234.
24. Thomas, M., Kalita, A., Labreque, S., Pim, D., Banks, L., and Matlashewski, G. (1999) Two polymorphic variants of wild-type p53 differ biochemically and biologically. *Mol. Cell Biol.* **19,** 1092–1100.
25. Storey, A., Thomas, M., Kalita, A., Harwood, C., Gardiol, D., Mantovani, F., Breuer, J., Leigh, I. M., Matlashewski, G., and Banks, L. (1998) p53 polymorphism and risk of cervical cancer. *Nature* **396,** 532.
26. Rosenthal, A. N., Ryan, A., Al-Jehani, R. M., Storey, A., Harwood, C. A., and Jacobs, I. J. (1998) p53 codon 72 polymorphism and risk of cervical cancer in UK. *Lancet* **352,** 871, 872.
27. Helland, A., Langerod, A., Johnsen, H., Olsen, A. O., Skovlund, E., and Borresen-Dale, A.-L. (1998) p53 polymorphism and risk of cervical cancer. *Nature* **396,** 530,531.

28. Josefsson, A. M., Magnusson, P. K. E., Ylitalo, N., Quarforth-Tubbin, P., Ponten, J., Adami, H. O., and Gyllensten, U. B. (1998) p53 polymorphism and risk of cervical cancer. *Nature* **396,** 531.
29. Hildesheim, A., Schiffman, M., Brinton, L. A., Fraumeni, J. F. Jr., Herrero, R., Bratti, M. C., Schwartz, P., Mortel, R., Barnes, W., Greenberg, M., McGowan, L., Scott, D. R., Martin, M., Herrera, J. E., and Carrington, M. (1998) p53 polymorphism and risk of cervical cancer. *Nature* **396,** 531,532.
30. Minaguchi, T., Kanamori, Y., Matsushima, M., Yoshikawa, H., Taketani, Y., and Nakamura, Y. (1998) No evidence of correlation between polymorphism at codon 72 of p53 and risk of cervical cancer in Japanese patients with human papillomavirus 16/18 infection. *Cancer Res.* **58,** 4585,4586.
31. Orita, M., Iwahana, H., Kanazawa, H., Hayashi, K., and Sekiya, T. (1989) Detection of polymorphisms of human DNA by gel electrophoresis as single strand conformation polymorphisms. *Proc. Natl. Acad. Sci. USA* **86,** 2766–2770.
32. Chaubert, P., Beautista, D., and Benhattar J. (1993) An improved method for rapid screening of DNA mutations by nonradioactive single-strand conformation polymorphism procedure. *BioTechniques* **15,** 586.
33. Cheng, J. and Haas, M. (1992) Sensitivity of detection of heterozygous point mutations in p53 cDNAs by direct PCR sequencing. *PCR Methods Appl.* **1,** 199–201.
34. Wu, J. K., Ye, Z., and Darras, B. T. (1993) Sensitivity of single-strand conformation polymorphism (SSCP) analysis in detecting p53 point mutations in tumors with mixed cell populations. *Am. J. Hum. Genet.* **52,** 1273–1275.
35. Mohabeer, A. J., Hiti, A. L., and Martin, W. J. (1991) Non-radioactive single-strand conformation polymorphism (SSCP) using the Pharmacia 'PhastSystem'. *Nucleic Acid Res.* **19,** 3154.
36. Neubauer, A., Brendel, C., Vogel, D., Schmidt, C. A., Heide, I., and Huhn, D. (1993) Detection of p53 mutations using nonradioactive SSCP analysis: p53 is not frequently mutated in myelodysplastic syndromes (MDS). *Ann. Hematol.* **67,** 223–226.
37. Bosari, S., Marchetti, A., Buttitta, F., Graziani, D., Borsani, G., Loda, M., Bevilacqua, G., and Coggi, G. (1995) Detection of p53 mutations by single-strand conformation polymorphisms (SSCP) gel electrophoresis. *Diagn. Mol. Pathol.* **4,** 249–255.
38. Kurvinen, K., Hietanen, S., Syrjänen, K., and Syrjänen, S. (1995) Rapid and effective detection of mutations in the p53 gene using nonradioactive single-strand conformation polymorphism (SSCP) technique applied on PhastSystem™. *J. Virol. Methods* **51,** 43–54.
39. Welsh, J.A., Castrén, K., and Vähäkangas, K. (1997) Single-strand conformation polymorphism analysis to detect p53 mutations: characterization and development of controls. *Clin. Chem.* **43,** 2251–2255.
40. Lehman, T. A., Bennett, W. P., Metcalf, R. A., Welsh, J. A., Ecker, J., Modali, R. V., Ullrich, S., Romano, J. W., Appella, E., Testa, J. R., Gerwin, B. I., Vogelstein, B.,

and Harris, C. C. (1991) p53 mutations, ras mutations, and p53-heat shock 70 protein complexes in human lung carcinoma cell lines. *Cancer Res.* **51,** 4090–4096.

41. Castrén, K., Vähäkangas, K., Heikkinen, E., and Ranki, A. (1998) Absence of p53 mutations in benign and pre-malignant male genital lesions with overexpressed p53 protein. *Int. J. Cancer* **77,** 674–678.

5

Cleavase® Fragment Length Polymorphism Analysis for Genotyping and Mutation Detection

Laura Heisler and Chao-Hung Lee

1. Introduction

DNA sequencing is the gold standard in DNA diagnostics and is the only absolute means of establishing the identity of a new mutation. However, the clinical cost of obtaining this information is often prohibitive, particularly when large DNA fragments are interrogated for the presence of any of a number of either known or previously undescribed genetic alterations *(1)*. Instead, several mutation scanning methods have been developed to eliminate the need to sequence every nucleotide when it is only the precise identity of one or a few nucleotides that is clinically significant. Until now such methods have provided only a "yes" or "no" answer in determining whether a test sample differs from a known reference. Relatively few methods have been proven capable of unambiguously identifying unique nucleic acid variants, particularly when multiple sequence changes occur *(2)*. Consequently, the majority of existing mutation scanning methods are unsuitable for PCR-based genotyping applications in which regions of sequence variability are used to categorize isolates for their similarities to known variants.

Third Wave Technologies has pioneered a novel mutation and polymorphism screening method that accurately and precisely distinguishes nucleic acid variants *(3)*. This approach relies on enzymatic cleavage of characteristic structures formed by single-stranded nucleic acids. On sequential denaturation and renaturation, both single-stranded DNA and RNA molecules assume three-dimensional conformations that are a precise reflection of their nucleic acid sequences *(4)*. This principle is the foundation of several mutation scanning techniques, such as single-strand conformation polymorphism (SSCP) and dideoxy fingerprinting *(5,6)*. Instead of relying on direct observation of these

From: *Methods in Molecular Medicine, vol. 49: Molecular Pathology Protocols*
Edited by: A. A. Killeen © Humana Press Inc., Totowa, NJ

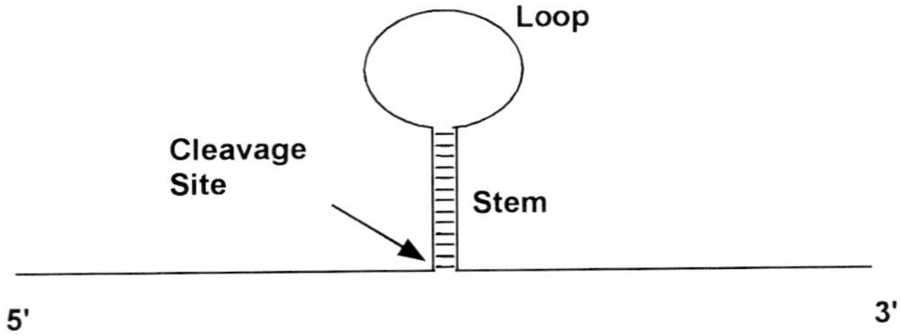

Fig. 1. Structures recognized by the Cleavase I enzyme. The Cleavase I enzyme is a structure-specific nuclease that recognizes the junctions between single- and double-stranded regions of nucleic acids, i.e., so-called hairpins or stem loops. Cleavage occurs on the 5′ side of such structures (*see* arrow). These intrastrand structures are formed when nucleic acid molecules are denatured and then allowed to cool.

structures, e.g., by noting subtle differences in how different DNA strands migrate through nondenaturing gels, the Third Wave Technologies' enzyme-based approach uses a structure-specific endonuclease engineered from the 5′ nuclease domain of *Taq* DNA polymerase, dubbed the Cleavase® I enzyme, to cut DNA strands wherever these structures occur *(3)* (**Fig. 1**). By analogy to restriction fragment length polymorphism analysis, Third Wave has named their method Cleavase Fragment Length Polymorphism (CFLP®) analysis.

The Cleavase I enzyme rapidly and specifically cleaves these structures, many of which are formed on a given DNA fragment, albeit transiently, in equilibrium with alternative, mutually exclusive structures. The CFLP method is thus able to elucidate a considerable amount of information about the sequence content of a DNA fragment without relying on cumbersome high-resolution analysis of each base. Each unique DNA sequence produces a distinctive collection of structures that, in turn, results in the generation of a singular fingerprint for that sequence. This capability makes the CFLP technology suitable for diverse mutation scanning applications, including genotyping *(1,3,7–14)*. Furthermore, the CFLP reaction is unaffected by the length of the DNA fragment and can be used to analyze far longer stretches of DNA than is currently possible with other methods, up to at least 2.7 kb (unpublished data).

1.2. Visualizing Sequence Differences in CFLP Fingerprints

The CFLP method comprises the steps of separation of DNA strands by heating, formation of intrastrand structures on cooling with rapid enzymatic cleavage of these structures before they are disrupted by reannealing of the complementary strands, and separation and visualization of the resulting "structural fingerprint" (**Fig. 2**). When closely related DNA fragments, such as a

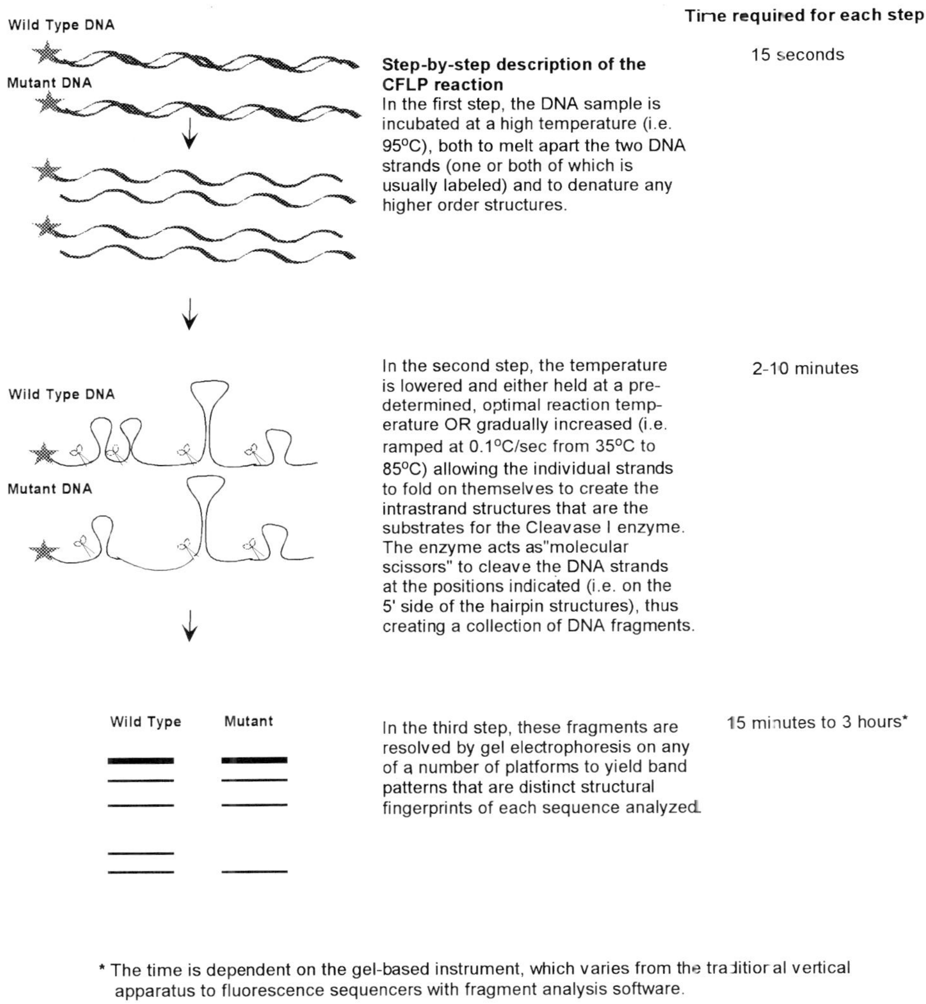

Fig. 2. CFLP reaction. The CFLP reaction itself is a simple three-step procedure that relies on the use of temperature to change some of the physical characteristics of DNA molecules.

wild-type and a mutant version of a gene, are compared, the CFLP fingerprints exhibit strong familial resemblance to one another such that they share the majority of bands produced. The sequence differences are revealed as changes in one or several bands. These unique band changes are manifest as mobility shifts, the appearance or disappearance of bands, and/or significant differences in band intensity (**Fig. 3**).

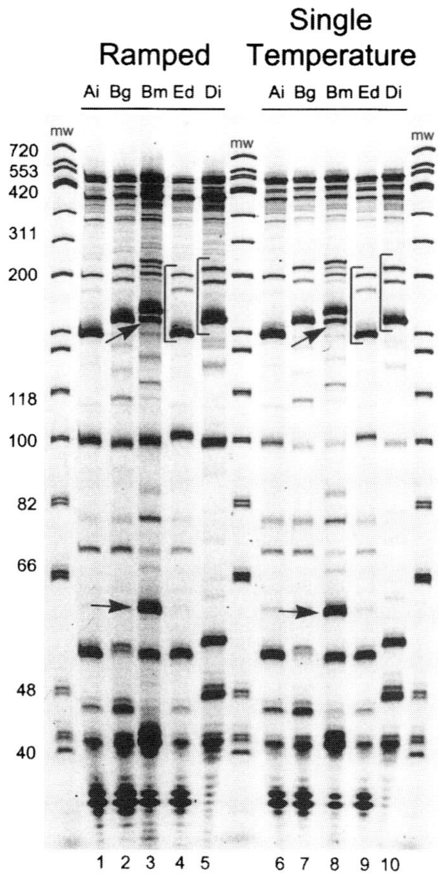

Fig. 3. CFLP analysis of the ITS regions of *P. carinii*. PCR products spanning the ITS1 and ITS2 regions of *P. carinii*, 534 bp long and labeled on the 5′ ends of both strands with TET, were subjected to CFLP analysis. Approximately 250 fmol of labeled PCR product was analyzed in the "ramped" reactions and approx 150 fmol in the single temperature reactions. The DNA aliquots were supplemented with DNA dilution buffer. The ramping assay was performed as described in **Subheading 3.2.** The genotypes of the samples from which the DNA was amplified are indicated above the lanes. Lanes marked "mw" contain molecular weight markets with fragment sizes as indicated. The gel was electrophoresed at constant wattage (20 W) until a bromophenol blue market dye, loaded in a far lane (not shown), reached the bottom of the gel. The gel cassette was scanned on a Hitachi FMBIO-100 fluorescence imager with a 585-nm emission filter.

CFLP analysis is exquisitely sensitive to the presence of minor sequence variations and can detect changes involving one or more bases, including missense mutations, with >95% sensitivity and 100% specificity. Because the CFLP method results in an easily examined pattern, rather than base-by-base analysis of each sequence, the value of this approach may be even more pronounced in genotyping applications. In these cases, what is sought is the rapid identification of compound sequence variations occurring throughout an amplified fragment. Rapid inspection of the patterns generated by CFLP analysis of fragments containing multiple, dispersed base changes has proven to be an effective approach to classifying bacterial and viral sequences according to genotype ***(1,3,11)***.

Pneumocystis carinii f. sp. *hominis* is the leading cause of pneumonia and the most commonly transmitted life-threatening opportunistic infection among AIDS patients ***(15)***. To establish the origin of particular infections, verify localized outbreaks, and determine whether an individual has sustained multiple, coincident infections, researchers have attempted to classify individual *P. carinii* strains based on sequence variability among isolates ***(16)***. Sequence variation in the internal transcribed spacer (ITS) regions of the rRNA genes of *P. carinii* can be used for such genotypic identification ***(17)***. The region located between the 18S and 5.8S rRNA genes is called ITS1, and that between the 5.8S and 26S rRNA genes is ITS2. Among the two regions, approx 60 different ITS sequences have been characterized by direct DNA sequencing ***(18)***. Sequence variation occurs throughout these 161- and 192-bp regions, respectively, and the majority of sequence changes within each ITS have been determined to be significant in establishing type ***(18)***.

The suitability of the CFLP scanning method for differentiating sequences in the ITS region of five cloned *P. carinii* sequences belonging to different types was investigated. The ITS region was amplified by polymerase chain reaction (PCR), and the 5′ ends of both strands were labeled by using tetrachlorofluorescein (TET) sense strand labeled primers (*see* **Note 1**). The amplified products were purified and then partially digested with the Cleavase I enzyme. The samples were analyzed in duplicate sets, one of which was subjected to CFLP digestion at a predetermined, optimized reaction temperature, whereas the other was digested under conditions in which the temperature was continually increased, or "ramped" (*see* **Subheading 3.2.** and **Note 2**).

The results indicate that the CFLP method is highly effective in reproducibly distinguishing different *P. carinii* types (**Fig. 3**). An inspection of the fingerprints generated from these samples reveals a high degree of similarity overall, indicative of the fact that only a few bases are altered in the variants, with some marked differences that reflect those base changes. In **Fig. 3**, there are several examples of bands that appear in some lanes but that are absent in others, as well as bands that appear shifted in some lanes relative to others. Unique bands, indicated by arrows, are apparent, e.g., in lanes Bm. In other cases, the most notable difference is a composite shifting downward of a substantial portion of the pattern, indicative of a small deletion, such that the fragments are shortened relative to the labeled 5′ ends (e.g., lanes Ed and Di, as indicated by brackets).

Note that the patterns generated by the ramping procedure appear to be enhanced relative to the single temperature procedure in several places. In particular, note the appearance of additional bands between 82 and 118 bp. This improvement in the richness of the patterns is likely due to the fact that certain substrate structures may not be as favored at a single temperature, as is used in the conventional approach, but rather emerge as the temperature changes over the course of the ramping reaction. In some cases the ramping approach not only eliminates the need for preliminary optimization steps but may also serve to improve the sensitivity of the CFLP method.

2. Materials

2.1. Preparation of End-Labeled PCR-Amplified Fragments

2.1.1. PCR Reagents

1. Sterile double-distilled H_2O.
2. 10X PCR buffer: 500 m*M* KCl, 100 m*M* Tris-HCl, pH 9.0, 15 m*M* $MgCl_2$.
3. dNTP (deoxynucleotide) mix: 0.2 m*M* each dNTP in sterile double-distilled H_2O.
4. Mineral oil or wax overlay.
5. Oligonucleotide primers at a concentration of 10 µ*M*, at least one of which is labeled with a fluorescent dye (e.g., tetrachlorofluorescein, fluorescein) or a moiety detectable by chemiluminescence (e.g., biotin, digoxyigenin).

2.1.2. Post-PCR Fragment Purification

1. Exonuclease I: Available at 10 U/µL from Amersham Pharmacia Biotech (Arlington Heights, IL), cat. no. E70073Z, or at 20 U/µL from Epicentre Technologies (Madison, WI), cat. no. X40505K.
2. High Pure PCR Product Purification Kit (HPPPPK), available from Roche Boehringer Mannheim Biochemical (Indianapolis, IN), cat. no. 1732668.
3. Sterile double-distilled H_2O or $T_{10}E_{0.1}$: 10 m*M* Tris-HCl, pH 8.0; 0.1 m*M* EDTA, pH 8.0.

2.2. CFLP Analysis

1. Cleavase I enzyme (25 U/µL) in Cleavase enzyme dilution buffer: 20 m*M* Tris-HCl, pH 8.0, 50 m*M* KCl, 0.05% Tween®-20, 0.05% Nonidet™ P-40, 100 µg/mL of bovine serum albumin, and 50% (v/v) glycerol.
2. DNA dilution buffer: 5 m*M* MOPS, pH 7.5.

3. 10X CFLP buffer: 100 m*M* MOPS, pH 7.5, 0.5% Tween-20, 0.5% Nonidet P-40.
4. 2 m*M* $MnCl_2$.
5. 10 m*M* $MgCl_2$.
6. Stop solution (for nonfluorescent gel-based detection): 95% formamide, 10 m*M* EDTA, pH 8.0, 0.05% xylene cylanol, 0.05% bromophenol blue (*see* **Note 3**).
7. Stop solution (for fluorescent gel-based detection): 95% formamide, 10 m*M* EDTA, pH 8.0, 0.05% crystal violet (*see* **Note 3**).
8. Sterile double-distilled H_2O.
9. Thin-walled reaction tubes (200 or 500 µL).

2.3. Gel Electrophoresis

1. Gel solution: 6–10% acrylamide:bis (19:1) solution, 7 *M* urea, 0.5X Tris-borate EDTA (TBE) buffer.
2. 0.5X TBE gel running buffer (pH 8.3): 44.5 m*M* Tris, 44.5 m*M* borate, 1 m*M* EDTA, pH 8.0.
3. Ammonium persulfate (10% [w/v]).
4. TEMED.
5. Teflon flat-bottomed combs and spacers (0.5 m*M* thick) ***(2)***
6. Glass plates (20 × 20 cm), nonfluorescing for use with fluorescence imager or standard for chemiluminescence detection.
7. Gel electrophoresis support.
8. Power supply capable of supplying up to 2000 V.

2.4. Visualization of CFLP Patterns

2.4.1. Fluorescence Detection

1. Hitachi FMBIO®-100 Fluorescent Method Bio-Image Analyzer (Hitachi Software, San Bruno, CA) or Molecular Dynamics 595 FluorImager™ (Molecular Dynamics, Sunnyvale, CA).
2. Lint-free laboratory wipes.
3. Lens paper.
4. Nonfluorescing detergent, e.g., RBS 35 Detergent Concentrate (Pierce, Rockford, IL).

2.4.2. Chemiluminescence Detection

1. 10X SAAP: 1 *M* NaCl, 0.5 *M* Tris-base, pH 10.0.
2. 1X SAAP, 0.1% sodium dodecyl sulfate (SDS): 100 m*M* NaCl, 50 m*M* Tris-Base, pH 10.0, 0.1% SDS (w/v).
3. 1X SAAP, 1 m*M* $MgCl_2$: 100 m*M* NaCl, 50 m*M* Tris-base, pH 10.0, 1 m*M* $MgCl_2$.
4. Sequenase Images™ 5X Blocking Buffer (cat. no. US75354; Amersham Pharmacia Biotech).
5. Streptavidin-Alkaline-Phosphatase Conjugate (cat. no. US11687; Amersham Pharmacia Biotech).

6. CDP-*Star*™ substrate (cat. no. MS250R; Tropix, Bedford, MA).
7. Isopropanol.
8. Latex gloves (powder free).
9. X-ray film.
10. Positively charged nylon membrane, pore size 0.2 μm (e.g., Nytran® Plus Membrane, Schleicher and Schuell, Keene, NH).
11. Blotting paper (20 × 20 cm) (cat. no. 28303-100; VWR Scientific).
12. Sealable plastic bags.
13. Forceps.
14. Small plastic containers for processing membranes.
15. Darkroom/film-developing facilities.
16. Permanent laboratory marker.

3. Methods

3.1. Purification of PCR-Generated Fragments (see Note 1*)*

PCR amplification should be performed according to established protocols for the particular locus in question. When PCR products are visualized by gel electrophoresis followed by sensitive detection of the label to be used to visualize CFLP products, contamination by labeled primers and prematurely truncated single-stranded PCR products is evident. These contaminating DNA species are effectively removed by the procedures noted. In particular, the HPPPPK procedure has been proven effective for eliminating lower molecular weight (i.e., >100 bp) DNA species, whereas Exonuclease I digestion is effective for removing larger DNA species. An alternative to the HPPPPK columns in conjunction with Exonuclease I digestion is to precipitate with 1 vol of isopropanol following Exonuclease I digestion.

If a single, labeled product is detected following PCR and HPPPPK and Exonuclease I digestion, then proceed with CFLP analysis. If more than one product is detected, then optimization of the PCR reaction or gel isolation of the desired product is necessary. The following protocol describes the method for Exonuclease I digestion:

1. Following PCR amplification, incubate the reaction mixture at 70°C for 10 min.
2. Bring the reaction mixture to 37°C.
3. Add 1 U of Exonuclease I/μL of original PCR reaction mixture (e.g., 100 U to a 100-μL reaction mixture).
4. Incubate for 30 min at 37°C.
5. Inactivate the reaction by heating at 70°C for 30 min.
6. Following Exonuclease I digestion, apply the reaction mixtures to the HPPPPK spin columns according to the manufacturer's suggested procedures. The supplied elution buffer should be replaced with either sterile double-distilled H_2O or $T_{10}E_{0.1}$, pH 8.0.

3.2. Preparation and Performance of CFLP Reactions

Prior to performing CFLP analysis, it is strongly recommended that the quality and quantity of the PCR-generated fragments following purification be checked. This can be done by visualizing the label used (i.e., by fluorescence analysis or chemiluminescence detection) on an aliquot of the DNA in a small denaturing polyacrylamide gel.

As seen in **Fig. 3**, there are two alternative approaches to be taken in configuring the CFLP reaction. The initial configuration of the assay involves performing the reaction under an abbreviated matrix of reaction times and temperatures in order to identify the optimal conditions for generation of a pattern with a broad spectrum of evenly distributed bands (temperature/time optimization). Alternatively, recent studies have demonstrated that the use of a programmable thermal cycler enables informative patterns to be generated by increasing the reaction temperature throughout the course of the reaction, specifically from 25 to 85°C at a rate of 0.1°C/s for a total ramping time of 10 min. In some genetic systems, such as *P. carinii*, the ramping approach appears to generate somewhat more even distributions of fragments and has improved mutation detection sensitivity. Furthermore, provided suitable thermal cyclers are available, the ramping approach is simpler and requires less DNA, since optimization reactions need not be run prior to analysis of test samples. The following protocol describes the method of performing CFLP analysis utilizing either the single temperature or ramping procedure:

1. Aliquot the desired amount of end-labeled DNA (approx 100–200 fmol) into a thin-walled reaction tube (200 or 500 µL, depending on the capacity of the thermal cycler). Bring the DNA to a final volume of 13 µL with DNA dilution buffer, if necessary.
2. In a separate tube, prepare an enzyme master mix that contains the following for each reaction: 2 µL of 10X CFLP buffer, 2 µL 2 m*M* $MnCl_2$, 1 µL of Cleavase I enzyme, 2 µL of 10 m*M* $MgCl_2$ (optional, *see* **Note 4**), and DNA dilution buffer to a final volume of 7 µL (if needed).
3. To denature samples, place tubes containing DNA in a programmable thermal cycler (or heat block) and incubate at 95°C for 15 s. If the single temperature method is used proceed to **step 4**. If the ramping method is to be used proceed to **step 5**.
4. Temperature/time optimization: After the 15-s denaturation step, set the thermal cycler to the desired reaction temperature (or place the tubes in a heat block held at reaction temperature if no thermal cycler is available). Optimal times and temperatures can be determined by examining matrices of different reaction times (e.g., 1, 3, and 5 min) and temperatures (40, 50, and 55°C). Choose the conditions that yield the richest and most even pattern (*see* **Note 5**). Incubate the CFLP reactions for the amount of time determined to be optimal, holding the temperature constant. After the incubation period, stop the reactions with 16 µL of stop solution. Proceed to **Subheading 3.3.**

5. Ramping: After the 15-s denaturation step, set the thermal cycler to 35°C. As soon as the thermal cycler reaches 35°C, add 7 µL of the enzyme/buffer mixture. Mix well by pipetting up and down several times. Incubate the CFLP reactions for 15 s at 35°C. Program the thermal cycler to increase in temperature at a rate of 0.1°C/s to 85°C, or set to ramp for an 8-min period from 35 to 85°C. On reaching 85°C, stop the reactions with 16 µL stop solution (*see* **Note 3**).

3.3. Separation of CFLP Fragments

1. Prepare a denaturing polyacrylamide gel, choosing a percentage of acrylamide (19 : 1) appropriate for the size of the fragment being analyzed (*see* **Note 6**).
2. Prerun the gel for approx 30 min before loading the samples at sufficient wattage to warm the gel (e.g., 18–20 W).
3. Heat denature the CFLP reactions at 80°C for 2 min immediately prior to loading onto the gel. The best resolution is achieved when the samples are fully denatured.
4. Load 5–10 µL of the appropriate CFLP reaction per well. The remainder of the reactions can be stored at 4°C or –20°C for later analysis.
5. Continue electrophoresis until sufficient separation of the CFLP fragments is achieved (the time will depend on the fragment size and the percentage of acrylamide used).

3.4. Visualization of CFLP Patterns

3.4.1. Fluorescence Imaging of CFLP Patterns

1. Following gel electrophoresis, thoroughly wash the outside of the gel plates using nonfluorescent soap.
2. Dry and wipe clear with lens paper to remove residual debris.
3. Place the gel carefully in the fluorescence scanning unit (Hitachi FMBIO-100 or Molecular Dynamics 595).
4. Scan using the correct wavelength or filter for the fluorescent group to be detected.

3.4.2. Chemiluminescence Detection of CFLP Patterns

1. After electrophoresis, wearing powder-free latex gloves that have been washed with isopropanol (*see* **Note 7**), carefully separate the glass plates to expose the acrylamide gel.
2. Cut a piece of Nytran Plus membrane (Schleicher and Schuell) to fit the gel size and moisten by applying 5–10 mL of 0.5X TBE.
3. Carefully place the moistened membrane onto the gel, avoiding lifting and repositioning the membrane, and smooth out air bubbles with a clean pipet. Transfer starts immediately, so the membrane should not be picked up and repositioned once it has come into contact with the gel.
4. Cover the membrane with two pieces of precut blotting paper, cover with a glass plate, and place a binder clip on each side of the sandwiched gel. Alternatively, for large gels (i.e., 20 × 20 cm or larger), place an approx 2-kg weight on top of the sandwich.
5. Allow the DNA to transfer onto the membrane for 4–16 h (e.g., overnight, if convenient) at room temperature.

6. After the transfer, disassemble the sandwiched gel and remove the membrane by carefully moistening it with distilled water. Mark the DNA side (i.e., the side touching the gel during transfer) using a permanent laboratory marker.
7. Rinse a dish thoroughly with isopropanol (*see* **Note 7**) and fill with 0.2 mL/cm^2 of 1X blocking buffer (e.g., 100 mL for a 20 × 20 cm membrane).
8. Transfer the membrane to the dish containing the blocking buffer and allow to rock gently for 15 min.
9. Repeat the 15-min wash with fresh blocking buffer and discard the buffer.
10. Add 2 µL of Streptavidin-Alkaline-Phosphatase Conjugate to 50 mL of fresh blocking buffer (or add conjugate to the blocking buffer at a volume ratio of 1:4000).
11. Pour the conjugate/blocking buffer mixture onto the blocked membrane and rock gently for 15 min.
12. Remove the conjugate and rinse for 5 min with 0.1% SDS/1X SAAP buffer, 0.5 mL/cm^2 each (200 mL for a 20 × 20 cm membrane). Repeat twice, for a total of three washes.
13. Remove the SDS and rinse 5 min with 0.5 mL/cm^2 1 m*M* $MgCl_2$/1X SAAP buffer. Repeat twice, for a total of three washes.
14. Place the membrane in a sealable bag and add 4 mL of CDP-*Star* (or 0.01 mL/cm^2).
15. Seal the bag and spread the CDP-*Star* gently over the membrane for 3–5 min.
16. Completely remove the CDP-*Star* and any air bubbles. Transfer the membrane while still in the bag to a film exposure cassette.
17. In the darkroom, expose the membrane to X-ray film. Initially expose for 30 min. For subsequent exposures, adjust the time for clarity and intensity (*see* **Note 8**).
18. Develop the film.

4. Notes

1. Depending on the objective of the analysis in question, the DNA can be labeled on either strand or on both strands using this approach. Single end labeling, i.e., of the sense or the antisense strand, permits some degree of localization of the base change(s) corresponding to the observed pattern changes *(3)*. The sensitivity of the CFLP method is approx 90% for single-stranded analysis and >95% for two-strand analysis. While double end labeling precludes this localization, it affords more sensitive mutational analysis.
2. It has been determined empirically that samples analyzed according to the ramping procedure require approximately twofold more DNA than do those analyzed by the conventional method. This is likely because in the ramping procedure, digestion occurs throughout the course of the temperature increase and optimally cleaves different hairpins at different temperatures.
3. The choice of dyes used in the stop solution depends on the system used to visualize the CFLP patterns. If chemiluminescence detection is used, then the stop solution should include 0.05% bromophenol blue and 0.05% xylene cyanol (**Subheading 2.2., item 6**). If fluorescent scanning is used, then a dye that migrates

with opposite polarity, such as crystal violet (0.05%), is preferable, because dyes that migrate into the gel fluoresce at the wavelengths used to detect the fluorescent dyes, thereby obscuring a portion of the CFLP pattern. Note that when a dye with opposite polarity is used, it is advisable to load 3–5 μL of stop solution containing bromophenol blue and xylene cyanol in a lane that does not contain CFLP reactions in order to monitor the progress of gel electrophoresis.

4. $MgCl_2$ dramatically reduces the rate of cleavage in the CFLP reaction. When $MgCl_2$ is added to a final concentration of 1 m*M* in the presence of standard $MnCl_2$ concentrations of 0.2 m*M*, the rate of cleavage is slowed by as much as 10-fold. This reduced reaction rate can be useful for analysis of DNA fragments that assume highly favored secondary structures that are rapidly cleaved in the CFLP reaction. The presence of such structures is readily identified by the appearance of a structural fingerprint comprising one or two prominent bands. When 1 m*M* $MgCl_2$ is added, the optimal time and temperature of digestion should be reevaluated to reflect the reduced rate of cleavage (*see* **Note 5**).
5. The structural fingerprint produced by CFLP digestion is a collection of fragments resulting from partial digestion, usually of 5′ end labeled fragments. Because the CFLP reaction is a partial digestion and because the formation of the substrate secondary structures depends on reaction temperature, it is possible to modulate the extent of digestion through variations in the duration and temperature of the reaction. Specifically, lower temperatures stabilize secondary structure formation whereas higher temperatures reduce the number of structures formed by a given molecule. Similarly, longer reaction times lead to increased accumulation of smaller cleavage products. The most informative fingerprints are those that contain a relatively even distribution of low and high molecular weight products, including a fraction of full-length, uncut DNA. Ensuring that the entire size distribution of cleavage products is visible increases the likelihood of detecting the products that reflect the presence of a polymorphism.
6. The percentage of polyacrylimide to be used is dictated by the size of the PCR fragment being analyzed. Appropriate percentages of polyacrylamide for various size ranges are well established ***(19)***.
7. The objective of this step is to minimize carryover of alkaline phosphatase from previous reactions and from exogenous sources (e.g., skin). Throughout this procedure, it is of paramount importance to minimize contamination by this ubiquitous enzyme.
8. An alkaline phosphatase reaction with the chemiluminescence substrate produces a long-lived signal, especially on membranes. Light emission increases of >300-fold are seen in the first 2 h on application of the substrate onto nylon membranes, with the chemiluminescence signal persisting up to several days. Because film exposure times range from minutes to several hours, multiple images may be acquired. Varying film exposure times enables the user to optimize signal to noise.

Acknowledgments

We wish to acknowledge the efforts of Mary Oldenburg, Senior Technical Scientist, Third Wave Technologies, in performing much of the CFLP reaction optimization as well as in providing critical commentary on the manuscript.

References

1. Sreevatsan, S., Bookout, J. B., Ringpis, F. M., Pottathil, M. R , Marshall, D. J., de Arruda, M., Murvine, C., Fors, L., Pottathil, R. M., and Barathur, R. R. (1998) Algorithmic approach to high-throughput molecular screening for alpha interferon-resistant genotypes in hepatitis C patients. *J. Clin. Microbiol.* **36,** 1895–1901.
2. Cotton, R. G. H. (1997) Slowly but surely towards better scanning for mutations. *Trends Genet.* **13,** 43–46.
3. Brow, M. A., Oldenberg, M., Lyamichev, V., Heisler, L., Lyamicheva, N., Hall, J., Eagan, N., Olive, D. M., Smith, L., Fors, L., and Dahlberg, J. (1996) Differentiation of bacterial 16S rRNA genes and intergenic regions and Mycobacterium tuberculosis katG genes by structure-specific endonuclease cleavage. *J. Clin. Microbiol.* **34,** 3129–3137.
4. Orita, M., Suzuki, Y., Sekiya, T., and Hayashi, K. (1989) Rapid and sensitive detection of point mutations and DNA polymorphisms using the polymerase chain reaction. *Genomics* **5,** 874–879.
5. Hayashi, K. (1991) PCR-SSCP: a simple and sensitive method for detection of mutations in the genomic DNA. *PCR Methods Applica.* **1,** 34–38.
6. Sarkar, G., Yoon, H., and Sommer, S. S. (1992) Dideoxy fingerprinting (ddE): a rapid and efficient screen for the presence of mutations. *Genomics* **13,** 441–443.
7. Sreevatsan, S., Bookout, J. B., Ringpis, F. M., Mogazeh, S. L., Kreiswirth, B. N., Pottathil, R. R., and Barathur, R. R. (1998) Comparative evaluation of cleavase fragment length polymorphism with PCR-SSCP and PCR-RFLP to detect antimicrobial agent resistance in Mycobacterium tuberculosis. *Mol. Diagn.* **3,** 81–91.
8. Tahar, R. and Basco, L. K. (1997) Analysis of Plasmodium falciparum multidrug-resistance (pfmdr1) gene mutation by hairpin-dependent cleavage fragment length polymorphism. *Mol. Biochem. Parasitol.* **88,** 243–247.
9. Wartiovaara, K., Hytonen, M., Vuori, M., Paulin, L., Rinne, J., and Sariola, H. (1998) Mutation analysis of the glial cell line-derived neurotrophic factor gene in Parkinson's disease. *Exp. Neurol.* **152,** 307–309.
10. Schlamp, C., Poulsen, G. L., Nork, M., and Nickells, R. W. (1997) Nuclear exclusion of wild-type p53 in immortalized human retinoblastoma cells. *J. Natl. Cancer Inst.* **89,** 1530–1536.
11. Marshall, D. J., Heisler, L. M., Lyamichev, V., Murvine, C., Olive, D. M., Ehrlich, G. D., Neri, B. P., and de Arruda, M. (1997) Determination of hepatitis C virus genotypes in the United States by Cleavase Fragment Length Polymorphism analysis. *J. Clin. Microbiol.* **35,** 3156–3162.

12. Rainaldi, G., Marchetti, S., Capecchi, B., Meneveri, R., Piras, A., and Leuzzi, R. (1998) Absence of mutations in the highest mutability region of the p53 gene in tumour-derived CHEF18 Chinese hamster cells. *Mutagenesis* **13,** 153–155.
13. Rossetti, S., Englisch, S., Bresin, E., Pignatti, P. F., and Turco, A. E. (1997) Detection of mutations in human genes by a new rapid method: cleavage fragment length polymorphism analysis (CFLPA). *Mol. Cell. Probes* **11,** 155–160.
14. Eisinger, F., Jacquemier, J., Charpin, C., Stoppa-Lyonnet, D., Bressac-de Paillerets, B., Peyrat, J.-P., Longy, M., Guinebretiere, J.-M., Sauvan, R., Noguichi, T., Birnbaum, D., and Sobol, H. (1998) Mutations at BRCA1: the medullary breast carcinoma revisited. *Cancer Res.* **58,** 1588–1592.
15. Centers for Disease Control and Prevention (1989) AIDS Weekly Surveillance Report, Centers for Disease Control and Prevention, Atlanta, GA.
16. Latouche, S., Ortona, E., Masers, E., Margutti, P., Tamburrini, E., Siracusano, A., Guyot, K., Nigou, M., and Roux, P. (1997) Biodiversity of Pneumocystis carinii hominis: typing with different DNA regions. *J. Clin. Microbiol.* **35,** 383–387.
17. Lu, J.-J., Bartlett, M. S., Shaw, M. M., Queener, S. F., Smith, J. W., Ortiz-Rivera, M., Leibowitz, M. J., and Lee, C.-H. (1994) Typing of Pneumocystis carinii strains that infect humans based on nucleotide sequence variations of internal transcribed spacers of rRNA genes. *J. Clin. Microbiol.* **32,** 2904–2912.
18. Lee, C.-H., Tang, X., Jin, S., Li, B., Bartlett, M. S., Helweg-Larsen, J., Olsson, M., Lucas, S. B., Roux, P., Cargnel, A., Atzori, C., Matos, O., and Smith, J. W. (1998) Update on Pneumocystis carinii f. sp. hominis typing based on nucleotide sequence variations in internal transcribed spacer regions of rRNA genes. *J. Clin. Microbiol.* **36,** 734–741.
19. Sambrook, J., Fritsch, E. F., and Maniatis, T. (eds.) (1989) *Molecular Cloning: A Laboratory Manual*, Cold Spring Harbor Laboratory Press, Cold Spring Harbor, NY.

6

Detection of Telomerase by *In Situ* Hybridization and by Polymerase Chain Reaction-Based Telomerase Activity Assay

Carmela P. Morales and Shawn E. Holt

1. Introduction

The onset of human cancer typically requires numerous genetic mutations, generally specific for the tissue type from which the cancer originates. Thus, it has been difficult to screen all tumor types for a single mutation. In recent years, telomerase activity has been associated with at least 85% of human malignancies as well as with some lesions considered preneoplastic by traditional cytology *(1,2)*. Telomerase appears to be ubiquitously associated with a wide array of human cancers from a variety of tissue sources. Therefore, detection of telomerase activity relative to human cancer development is likely to be an important and novel method, in combination with cytology, for cancer diagnosis.

Telomerase is a ribonucleoprotein, minimally composed of both an RNA component (hTR) and a catalytic protein component (hTERT) *(3)*. Most normal somatic cells and tissues express hTR at low levels but not hTERT, and are devoid of telomerase activity. Without a mechanism to ensure telomeric integrity and stability, telomeric repeats are lost with successive cellular divisions owing to the inability of conventional DNA polymerases to replicate the ends of linear chromosomes *(4,5)*. This loss of telomeric DNA signals a DNA damage response mechanism, requiring the tumor suppressor molecules p53 and pRB, which triggers an irreversible growth-arrested phenotype known as cellular senescence *(6–8)*. Those cells that are capable of bypassing senescence by blocking the normal functions of p53 and pRB continue telomere shortening until the cells reach a period of crisis *(9–11)*. During crisis, cells either die or in

From: *Methods in Molecular Medicine, vol. 49: Molecular Pathology Protocols*
Edited by: A. A. Killeen © Humana Press Inc., Totowa, NJ

rare instances, immortalize, and this immortalization event is almost always concomitant with activation of telomerase activity *(2)*. Telomerase is necessary for the continued proliferation of immortal and tumor cells, as inhibition results in reprogramming of the cellular senescence program *(12)*. Telomerase activation requires a significant increase in the expression of the integral RNA component (hTR) and the activation of the catalytic subunit (hTERT). Thus, determination of telomerase activity in human cancer can be accomplished by detecting either the upregulation of hTR or activity using a polymerase chain reaction (PCR)-based assay. In this chapter, we describe both the *in situ* hybridization technique and the PCR-based telomeric repeat amplification protocol (TRAP) assay.

1.1. In Situ *Hybridization for RNA Component of Telomerase*

The utility of *in situ* hybridization for the RNA component of human telomerase (hTR) for cancer diagnosis has been recently evaluated *(13,14)*. Whereas the detection of telomerase activity using the TRAP assay requires fresh or fresh-frozen tumor biopsies, analysis of hTR can be accomplished using archival, formalin-fixed, paraffin-embedded specimens, as well as frozen sections and cultured cells *(15–17)*. In lung cancer, an excellent correlation between *in situ* hybridization for telomerase RNA and relative telomerase activity levels has been demonstrated *(18)*. The excellent morphologic preservation of tissue with this technique makes it a useful alternative to the PCR-based TRAP assay.

1.2. Telomerase Activity Detection Using the TRAP Assay

The TRAP assay is a highly sensitive, PCR-based method for accurately determining levels of telomerase activity in a sample from fresh or frozen tissue or from cultured cells (**Fig. 1**) *(2,19,20)*. This technique has been used to detect telomerase activity in a wide variety of human tumors from varied tissue sources (for a review, *see* **ref.** *1*).

2. Materials

2.1. Telomerase Detection Using In Situ *hTR Assay*

2.1.1. General Reagents

1. Distilled, deionized autoclaved water.
2. Diethylpyrocarbonate (DEPC)-treated water: distilled, deionized water treated with 0.1% DEPC.
3. 10X Phosphate-buffered saline (PBS).
4. 100% Ethanol, room temperature and –20°C.
5. 1 *M* Tris-HCl, pH 7.8.

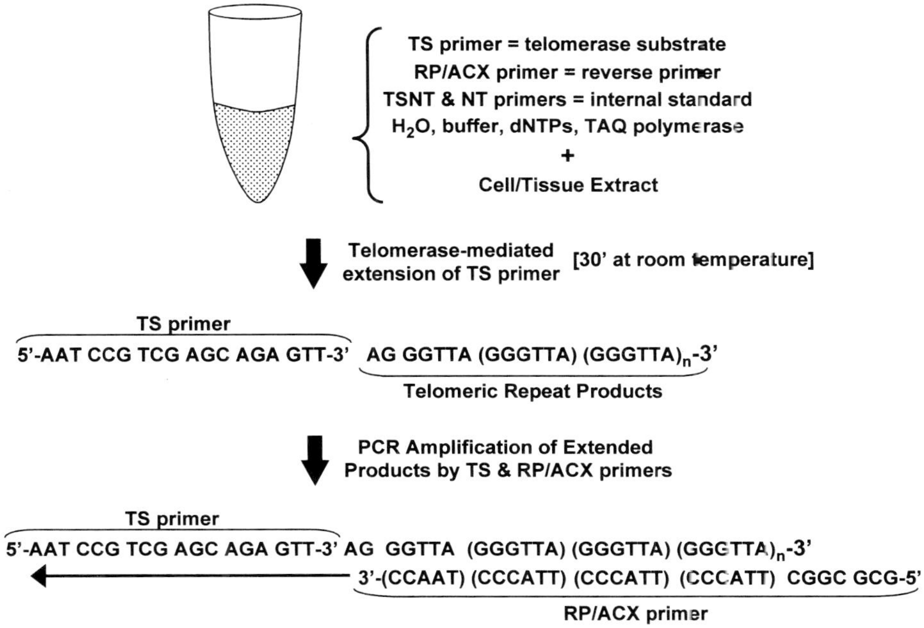

Fig.1. Schematic representing the TRAP assay. Telomerase samples are processed by mild detergent lysis. A nontelomeric primer that serves as the telomerase substrate (TS primer) is combined with water, buffer, dNTPs, *Taq* polymerase, the reverse primer (RP/ACX), and two primers that serve to amplify an internal control (TSNT and NT). After this cocktail is made, the tissue or cell extract is added and incubated at room temperature for 30 min for telomerase to extend the TS primer. Telomerase-mediated extension occurs in six base increments, corresponding to the integral RNA component of telomerase (hTR) and the telomeric repeat sequences (TTAGGG). PCR amplification of the telomerase products and the internal standard utilizes both the TS and RP/ACX primers. The internal control primer (TSNT) utilizes both the NT and the TS primers, hence a competition for TS primer in the amplification of both telomerase products and TSNT. The internal control measures 36 bp after amplification and serves as a quantitative standard to normalize sample-to-sample variation.

6. 0.5 *M* EDTA, pH 8.0.
7. 10 *N* Sodium hydroxide.
8. Phenol : chloroform (1 : 1).
9. 1 *M* Dithiothreitol (DTT).
10. 3 *M* Sodium acetate, pH 6.0.
11. 20X Saline sodium citrate (SSC): 3 *M* NaCl, 0.3 *M* sodium citrate.
12. 70% Ethanol.

2.1.2. Pretreatment of Paraffin-Embedded Sections

1. Fresh, filtered 4% paraformaldehyde, pH 7.5. **(Note: paraformaldehyde is highly toxic and should be made fresh for each use in a fume hood.)**
2. 0.85% NaCl.
3. Xylene.
4. Proteinase K (20 mg/mL).
5. TE buffer: 100 m*M* Tris-HCl, pH 7.5, 50 m*M* EDTA.
6. 1 *M* Triethanolamine.
7. 98% Acetic anhydride.

2.1.3. Pretreatment of Cultured Cells

1. Same as paraffin-embedded sections (except xylene).
2. Triton X-100.
3. 2 *N* HCl.
4. 1 *M* glycine.

2.1.4. Preparation of Antisense hTR DNA Template

1. *Eco*RV and *Nae*I restriction enzymes.
2. TE buffer (*see* **Subheading 2.1.2.**).

2.1.5. Preparation and Labeling of Probe

1. SP6 RNA polymerase (5 U/µL).
2. ATP, CTP, and GTP (10 m*M*).
3. ^{35}S-UTP (20 mCi/mL and 1000 Ci/mmol).
4. 10X SP6 RNA polymerase transcription buffer.
5. Hydrolysis solution: 0.01 *M* DTT, 0.08 *M* sodium bicarbonate, and 0.12 *M* sodium carbonate.
6. Neutralization solution: 0.2 *M* sodium acetate, pH 6.0, 1% glacial acetic acid, and 0.01 *M* DTT.
7. RNase inhibitor (5 U/µL).
8. DNase I (2 U/µL).
9. Quick Spin™ columns, G50 Sephadex columns for radiolabeled RNA (Boehringer Mannheim).
10. Yeast tRNA (20 mg/mL).

2.1.6. In Situ *Hybridization*

1. Cocktail solution: 3 *M* NaCl, 0.2 *M* sodium acetate, pH 6.0, 50 m*M* EDTA, pH 8.0, 50% deionized formamide, 1X Denhardt's, 10% dextran sulfate, 0.1 *M* DTT.
2. Clean glass cover slips.

2.1.7. Washing and Detection

1. Formamide solution: 2X SSC, 50% formamide, 10 m*M* DTT.
2. 5X SSC solution: 5X SSC, 10 m*M* DTT.

3. 10X Wash solution: 0.4 *M* NaCl, 10 m*M* Tris-HCl, pH 7.8, 5 m*M* EDTA.
4. Pancreatic RNase A (10 mg/mL).
5. Kodak emulsion type NTB-2 (cat. no. 165 4433).

2.1.8. Developing of Sections

1. Kodak Dektol developer (cat. no. 146 4700).
2. Kodak fixer (cat. no. 197 1720).
3. Hematoxylin.
4. Permount™ mounting medium.

2.1.9. Equipment

1. Glass slide chambers, 250-mL capacity.
2. Scintillation counter.
3. Tissue-Tek™ slide staining set (VWR Scientific).
4. Dip Miser (Electron Microscopy Services).

2.2. Telomerase Activity Using TRAP Assay

2.2.1. General Items and Reagents

1. DEPC-treated water: distilled, deionized water treated with 0.1% DEPC.
2. TRAP-eze™ Telomerase Detection Kit (Intergen).
3. Aerosol-resistant tips (USA/Scientific).
4. Beta-shield for protection from radioisotope.
5. Acrylic tube racks (24 place; USA/Scientific).

2.2.2. Preparation of Cell Extracts from Cultured Cells and Clinical Material

1. 3-[(3-cholamidopropyl)dimethylammonio]-1-propanesulfonate (CHAPS) lysis buffer: 10 m*M* Tris-HCl, pH 7.5, 1 m*M* EGTA, 1 m*M* $MgCl_2$, 5 m*M* β-mercaptoethanol, 0.5% CHAPS, 10% glycerol, 1 m*M* 4-(2-aminoethyl)-benzenesulfonyl fluoride hydrochloride (AEBSF), 0.5 U/μL of RNase inhibitor (Boehringer Mannheim).
2. NP-40 Lysis buffer: 10 m*M* Tris-HCl, pH 7.5, 1 m*M* EGTA, 1 m*M* $MgCl_2$, 5 m*M* β-mercaptoethanol, 1% NP-40 (renamed IPGAL), 0.25 m*M* sodium deoxycholate, 150 m*M* NaCl, 10% glycerol, 1 m*M* AEBSF.
3. 1.5-mL Microfuge tubes, RNase/DNase free.
4. Microfuge for speeds to 6000*g* (Eppendorf).
5. Refrigerated centrifuge for speeds to 14,000*g* (Eppendorf).
6. Kontes homogenization tubes with matching pestles (VWR Scientific).
7. Rechargeable, low-speed drill (CD1000; Black and Decker).
8. BCA assay for protein concentration (Pierce).
9. Liquid nitrogen.
10. Ice buckets.

2.2.3. Primer Labeling

1. TS primer (high-performance liquid chromatography [HPLC] purified), sequence 5′-AAT CCG TCG AGC AGA GTT-3′.
2. Redivue™ [γ-^{32}P]ATP (6000 Ci/mmol) (Amersham).
3. T4 polynucleotide kinase (10 U/µL) (Life Technologies).
4. 5X Kinase buffer (Life Technologies).

2.2.4. Telomerase Reactions Using TRAP Assay

1. Reverse primer (RP or ACX) (HPLC purified), sequence 5′-GCG CGG CTT ACC CTT ACC CTT ACC CTA ACC-3′.
2. 36-bp Internal standard primers (HPLC purified): 36-bp template sequence (TSNT) 5′-AAT CCG TCG AGC AGA GTT AAA AGG CCG AGA AGC GAT-3′; return primer (NT) sequence 5′-ATC GCT TCT CGG CCT TTT-3′.
3. 10X TRAP reaction buffer: 200 m*M* Tris-HCl, pH 8.3, 10 m*M* EGTA, 15 m*M* $MgCl_2$, 630 m*M* KCl, 0.5% Tween-20.
4. 50X dNTPs: 2.5 m*M* dATP, TTP, dGTP, dCTP each.
5. Labeled TS primer.
6. *Taq* DNA polymerase (5 U/µL) (Life Technologies).
7. 0.5-mL Microfuge tubes (USA/Scientific).
8. MJ Research PCR machine with heated lid (PTC-100).

2.2.5. Gel Electrophoresis and Detection

1. TRAP loading buffer: 50 m*M* EDTA, 50% glycerol, 0.25% bromophenol blue, 0.25% xylene cyanol.
2. 40% Acrylamide (19:1, acrylamide:bisacrylamide ratio) (Bio-Rad).
3. 10% Ammonium persulfate.
4. TEMED.
5. 10X TBE running buffer: 50 m*M* Tris-borate, 1 m*M* EDTA, pH 8.3.
6. Vertical Gel Electrophoresis System (Life Technologies).
7. Plastic disposable transfer pipet.
8. Power supply to 300 V with timer (power pac 3000; Bio-Rad).
9. Fix solution: 0.5 *M* NaCl, 50% ethanol, 40 m*M* sodium acetate, pH 4.2.
10. Plastic wrap.
11. Phosphorimage cassettes.
12. Phosphorimager (Molecular Dynamics).

3. Methods

3.1. In Situ *Detection of Telomerase*

The following procedure outlines the technique required for *in situ* hybridization of telomerase RNA. **Figure 2** shows the final hTR *in situ* hybridization result for an esophageal adenocarcinoma, along with a hematoxylin & eosin (H&E) stain. Because RNA probes are used, great care must be taken to main-

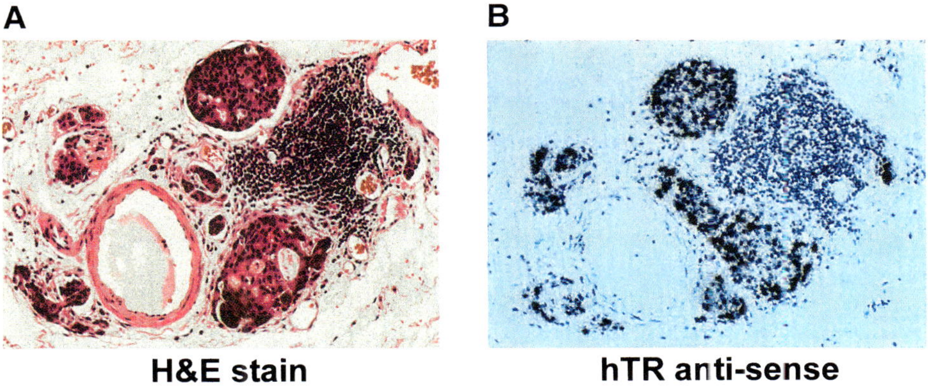

Fig. 2. *In situ* hybridization for the RNA component of human telomerase in metastatic esophageal adenocarcinoma. **(A)** An H&E stain demonstrates malignant cells adjacent to a lymphoid follicle and vascular structure, both uninvolved. **(B)** Cells are considered to be positive for telomerase RNA if they display nuclear grains in the overlying emulsion. Hybridization of a serial section with the antisense probe demonstrates an intense telomerase signal in the malignant cells whereas the endothelial cells demonstrate no detectable telomerase RNA. Note that cells of the germinal center of the lymphoid follicle are weakly positive for telomerase RNA.

tain probe integrity and avoid degradation by RNases. All solutions and dilutions should be prepared with DEPC-treated water, and all glassware should be cleaned with an appropriate RNase-free detergent. Unless otherwise indicated, all reactions are done at room temperature.

3.1.1. Pretreatment of Paraffin-Embedded Sections

1. Cut 4-µm sections from blocks and place on SuperFrost™ Plus glass slides (*see* **Note 1**).
2. Bake slides for 20 min at 80°C.
3. Deparaffinize in xylene two times for 10 min each.
4. Rehydrate in a graded ethanol series: 100% ethanol twice for 2 min each followed by 95, 85, 70, 50, and 30% ethanol for 1 min each.
5. Rinse once for 5 min with 0.85% NaCl.
6. Rinse once for 5 min with PBS.
7. Fix tissue at room temperature for 20 min with 4% paraformaldehyde.
8. Wash two times for 5 min each with PBS.
9. Permeabilize sections for 35 min at 37°C with TE buffer containing 20 µg/mL of proteinase K (*see* **Note 2**).
10. Wash once for 5 min with PBS.
11. Postfix in 4% paraformaldehyde for 5 min (reused from **step 7**).

12. Rinse in DEPC-treated water for 30 s.
13. Acetylate sections for 10 min on a rocking platform in 0.1 *M* triethanolamine containing 0.25% acetic anhydride (*see* **Note 3**).
14. Wash once for 5 min with PBS.
15. Wash once for 5 min with 0.85% NaCl.
16. Dehydrate the slides in a graded ethanol series: 30, 50, 70, 85, 95, and 100% for 1 min each.
17. Air-dry slides for 30 min. The slides may be kept in an airtight container at room temperature for up to 1 wk prior to hybridization.

3.1.2. Pretreatment of Cultured Cells

1. Grow cultured cells on sterile glass Chamber slides overnight at 37°C.
2. Wash two times for 5 min each with PBS.
3. Fix according to either of these procedures: 10 min in cold acetone and air-dried; or 10 min in cold 95% isopropanol and air-dried. Proceed directly to **step 4**.
4. Incubate for 10 min in 4% paraformaldehyde at room temperature.
5. Wash two times for 5 min each with PBS.
6. Permeabilize for 3 min with PBS containing 0.05% Triton X-100.
7. Wash two times for 5 min each with PBS.
8. Deproteinize for 10 min with 0.2 *N* HCl.
9. Wash two times for 5 min each with PBS.
10. Permeabilize sections for 5–15 min at 37°C with TE buffer containing 1–10 µg/mL of proteinase K. We regularly use 5 µg/mL for 5 min.
11. Wash two times for 5 min each in PBS containing 2 mg/mL of glycine (to inactivate the enzyme).
12. Postfix for 5 min in 4% paraformaldehyde.
13. Wash two times for 5 min each with PBS.
14. Acetylate sections for 10 min on a rocking platform in 0.1 *M* triethanolamine containing 0.25% acetic anhydride (*see* **note 3**).
15. Dehydrate the slides in a graded ethanol series: 30, 50, 70, 85, 95, and 100% for 1 min each.
16. Air-dry slides for 30 min. The slides may be kept in an airtight container at room temperature for up to 1 wk prior to hybridization.

3.1.3. Preparation of Antisense hTR DNA Template

hTR is the human telomerase template RNA sequence utilized by telomerase to add TTAGGG repeats to the 3′ ends of chromosomes ***(21)***. The 560 nucleotide cDNA sequence is cloned into the *Sac*I site of the pGEM-5Zf(+) expression vector (Boehringer Mannheim). After linearization with either *Eco*RV or *Nae*I, runoff in vitro transcription of the hTR expression plasmid with either SP6 or T7 yields the antisense (SP6) or sense (T7) RNA probe, respectively.

1. In a standard digestion at 37°C, linearize hTR expression plasmid with *Eco*RV. If desired, set up a parallel digestion with *Nae*I.

2. Purify the linearized template by standard phenol-chloroform extraction and ethanol precipitation (*see* **Note 4**).
3. Resuspend the pellet at approx 1 µg/mL in TE buffer, and quantitate by running a 200-ng equivalent on a 0.8% agarose gel with an appropriate DNA mass ladder.

3.1.4. Labeling of Antisense RNA Probe

1. Set up an in vitro transcription of the hTR template as follows 6 µL of DEPC-treated water; 1 µL of RNase inhibitor (5 U/µL); 2 µL of 10X transcription buffer; 1 µL of ATP, CTP, and GTP (all 10 m*M*); 5 µL ^{35}S-UTP; 1 µL of hTR template (1 µg/µL); and 2 µL of SP6 RNA polymerase (5 U/µL).
2. Add 1 µL of DNase (1 U/µL) for 15 min at 37°C.
3. Perform alkaline hydrolysis at 60°C by adding 50 µL of hydrolysis solution to the transcription reaction for 15 min.
4. Neutralize on ice by adding 50 µL of neutralizing solution.
5. While the tube is on ice, prepare Quick Spin columns according to the manufacturer's instructions.
6. Keeping the columns upright, carefully apply the entire RNA sample to the center of the column bed.
7. Centrifuge for 4 min at 1100*g*.
8. Save the eluate and discard the column into a radioactive waste container.
9. Add 3 µL of yeast tRNA (20 mg/mL) to the eluate and mix well.
10. Add 1/10 volume of 3 *M* sodium acetate (pH 6.0) and 2 vol of chilled 100% ethanol and precipitate for 20 min at –80°C.
11. Centrifuge for 25 min at 12,800*g*.
12. Carefully draw off the supernatant and discard.
13. Gently add 2 vol of chilled 70% ethanol.
14. Centrifuge for 20 min at 14,000*g*.
15. Draw off the supernatant and allow the pellet to air-dry.
16. Resuspend the pellet in 30 µL of 100 µ*M* DTT; count 1 µL of the final solution. Using this protocol, we usually obtain counts of approx 2 to 3×10^6 cpm/µL.

3.1.5. In Situ *Hybridization*

1. Combine probe mix and cocktail solution, vortex, and heat to 90°C for 5 min. The final hybridization solution contains probe mix and cocktail solution in a 0.14:0.86 ratio. Once the required volume of final hybridization solution is determined based on the number of slides, the amount of probe mix can be calculated. Probe mix is made of 50% yeast tRNA plus probe and DEPC-treated water for the remaining 50%. The probe mix is then added to the appropriate volume of cocktail solution. We utilize a final probe concentration of 50,000 cpm/µL and typically apply 50 µL of hybridization solution to each slide. For example, to hybridize 10 slides, 430 µL of hybridization cocktail and 70 µL of probe mix would be required. If the probe count were 2×10^6/µL, then the probe mix would be prepared with 12.5 µL of probe, 35 µL of yeast tRNA, and 22.5 µL of DEPC-treated water.

2. Quickly place hybridization solution on ice.
3. Apply 50 µL of hybridization solution over each section and cover slip. Take care not to trap air bubbles underneath the cover slip.
4. Place the slides horizontally into a clean, upright slide container (25-slide capacity).
5. Place several Kimwipes moistened with DEPC-treated water at the bottom of each box, and wrap the boxes in clear plastic wrap followed by aluminum foil.
6. Keeping the box upright, hybridize slides overnight at 50°C.

3.1.6. Washing and Detection

1. In glass staining chambers, prewarm 250 mL each of the 5X SSC solution to 50°C and the formamide wash solution to 65°C.
2. After hybridization, unwrap the box and carefully remove the cover slip from each slide.
3. Wash the slides at 50°C for 30 min in 5X SSC solution with agitation.
4. Transfer the slides to the formamide solution at 65°C for 30 min with agitation.
5. Wash two times for 10 min each at 37°C with 1X wash solution.
6. Incubate the slides for 30 min at 37°C in 250 mL of 1X wash solution containing 500 µL of RNase A.
7. Rinse once for 5 min with 1X wash solution at 37°C.
8. Wash in 2X SSC for 1 h at 37°C.
9. Wash in 0.1X SSC for 1 h at 37°C.
10. Dehydrate for 1 min each in a graded ethanol series: 30, 50, 70, 85, 95, and 100%.
11. Air-dry the slides for 30 min and proceed with emulsion.
12. Warm the emulsion in a 45°C water bath with occasional gentle swirling.
13. In a dark room, pour a small amount of emulsion in a Dip Miser or other suitable container.
14. Gently dip a blank slide in the emulsion and inspect for bubbles. If bubbles are present, allow them to clear for 10 min.
15. Dip the slides into the emulsion in a consistent fashion to minimize slide-to-slide variability (we perform two 1-s dips in rapid succession).
16. Place the slides vertically in a 50-mL conical styrofoam container and air-dry in the dark for 1 h.
17. Place the dried slides in a slide box containing desiccant wrapped in a Kimwipe, and wrap the box in two layers of foil.
18. Place the box upright at –80°C for 2–3 wk (*see* **note 5**).

3.1.7. Developing Sections

1. Prepare developer and fixer per manufacturer's directions and cool to 15°C.
2. Bring the slides to room temperature for several hours.
3. In the dark, load the slides onto a clean slide holder, while trying not to touch the emulsion.
4. Soak in full-strength developer for 3 min without agitation.
5. Rinse in distilled water for 30 s with mild agitation.

6. Fix the slides two times for 3 min each.
7. Place the slides in distilled water cooled to 15°C (*see* **Note 6**).
8. Rinse the slides twice in distilled water.
9. Using a single-edge razor blade, remove the emulsion from the back of each slide.
10. Counterstain with H&E for 2 min.
11. Rinse in running tap water for 1 min.
12. Dehydrate the slides in a graded ethanol series, clear with xylene, and cover slip.

3.2. TRAP Assay

Because the TRAP assay is PCR based, it is important to take every precaution to preserve sample integrity, prevent cross contamination, and avoid sloppiness. Separate work areas and separate pipets for each step of the assay should be used to lessen the likelihood of contamination. Gloves must be worn at all times during the assay and a surgical mask is highly recommended. Reagents should be made with DEPC-treated water, and all equipment should be cleaned with 70% ethanol prior to use (ice buckets, centrifuges, tube racks, and so on). All reagents should be used only for the TRAP assay, aliquoted in small amounts, and kept separate from general laboratory stocks. The TRAP assay is highly sensitive, which could lead to false positive results if the necessary precautions are not taken. It is absolutely required that each of the following steps be done using aerosol-resistant tips to avoid possible contamination from sample to sample.

3.2.1. Preparation of Cell Extracts from Cultured Cells and Clinical Material

3.2.1.1. Cultured Cells

1. Harvest and count cells.
2. Put an aliquot corresponding to 100,000 cells into a sterile 1.5-mL microfuge tube.
3. Pellet cells at 6000*g* for 5 min and remove the supernatant.
4. Either lyse samples immediately or store at –80°C until lysis.
5. Add 100–200 µL of ice-cold NP-40 lysis buffer and mechanically lyse the samples (by pipeting the pellet up and down a few times, avoiding bubbles). The lysis buffer is normally made with all the ingredients except for AEBSF and stored at 4°C until use. AEBSF is added fresh with each round of lysis.
6. Save a small amount of lysis buffer for use as a negative control in the TRAP reactions.
7. Incubate samples on ice for 20–30 min.
8. Centrifuge lysates at 14,000*g* for 20 min at 4°C.
9. Remove 80% of the lysate (do not disturb pellet) and flash-freeze in liquid nitrogen.
10. Store the samples at –80°C until use in the TRAP assay.

3.2.1.2. Clinical Material

1. Mechanically disperse partially thawed tissue samples on disposable Petri dishes using sterile, disposable scalpel blades.
2. Immediately transfer tissue shavings to a sterile 1.5-mL Kontes tube.
3. Add 200 μL of ice-cold CHAPS lysis (4°C) buffer to the tumor samples. Again, AEBSF is added fresh.
4. Save a small amount of lysis buffer to be used as a negative control in the TRAP reactions.
5. Homogenize samples until the tissue is well dispersed using disposable pestles (matching the Kontes tubes) and a drill, with rotation no faster than 450 rpm to preserve enzyme integrity.
6. Centrifuge lysates at 14,000*g* for 20 min at 4°C.
7. Remove 80% of the lysate (do not disturb the pellet).
8. Take an aliquot for assessment of protein concentration using the Pierce BCA assay.
9. Dilute lysates to 3 μg of protein/μL.
10. Flash-freeze the samples and store at –80°C.

3.2.2. Primer Labeling

Kinase reactions can be done at any time prior to making the TRAP master mix (*see* **Subheading 3.2.3., step 1**); the amount of primer used is 100 ng/reaction. Reactions consist of TS primer (100 ng/sample), 5X kinase buffer, DEPC water, 2.5 μCi of [γ-^{32}P]ATP/sample, and 0.25 U of T4 polynucleotide kinase/sample.

1. Incubate at 37°C for 20 min followed by heat inactivation of the kinase at 85°C for 5 min. This is generally done in a thermocycler.
2. Prior to addition to the TRAP master mix, cool the sample on ice for at least 5 min. If it is not to be used immediately, labeled primer may be stored at –20°C for up to 1 wk.

3.2.3. Telomerase Reactions Using TRAP Assay

A general schematic of the TRAP reaction is shown in **Fig. 1**.

1. Make a master mix that includes all the components necessary for TRAP, in a tube that is RNase/DNase free and able to hold the appropriate volume (*see* **Notes 7** and **8**).
2. Use 48-μL reaction volumes (to which 2 μL of sample will be added) in sterile 0.5-mL tubes. Each reaction consists of 38.6 μL of DEPC-treated water, 5 μL of 10X TRAP reaction buffer, 1 μL of 50X dNTPs, 100 ng of TS primer (generally 2-μL vol of end-labeled primer), 100 ng of RP/ACX primer, 100 ng of NT primer, 0.01 amol of TSNT internal control template, and 0.4 μL of *Taq* polymerase (2 U). Ten to 20 samples are normally done per TRAP setup, and combining all reagents into a TRAP master mix and aliquoting to each individual tube is recommended. Because of frequent pipetting error, master mix volumes should be the number of samples plus two.

3. Add 2 µL of sample (corresponding to 100–1000-cell equivalents for cultured cells or 0.1–6 µg of protein for clinical material) to each tube and write down the tube number and what the sample is.
4. Mix by flicking the tube. Do not vortex or overmix, and make certain that the entire sample remains in the bottom of the tube.
5. As a negative control, use 2 µL of lysis buffer used for making the sample lysates. In addition, use as a positive control a telomerase-positive cell line (typically 1000- and 100-cell equivalents of 293 or H1299 cells).
6. Incubate TRAP reactions at room temperature (22–25°C) for no more than 30 min.
7. Preheat the PCR machine with a heated lid to 94°C and insert the samples (i.e., a "hot start" reaction is used).
8. Proceed with the PCR at an initial hot start at 94°C for 3 min, followed by two-step PCR (94°C for 30 s, 60°C for 30 s) for 27–32 cycles. Twenty-seven or 28 cycles are sufficient for cells in culture; 30–32 cycles may be necessary for tumors. PCR takes about 75 min from start to finish.
9. Use a separate rack for storage of the samples after PCR than was used for the TRAP setup, because cross contamination of PCR products can occur.
10. Add 5 µL of TRAP loading buffer to each sample.
11. Load the samples directly onto the gel or store at 4°C or –20°C for up to 5 d without a decline in signal intensity.

3.2.4. Gel Electrophoresis and Detection

1. During the PCR, pour a 10% polyacrylamide gel (normally 20 wells) for electrophoresis of samples. Gel mixtures consist of 2.5 mL of 10X TBE, 12.5 mL of 40% acrylamide, 35 mL of deionized water, 130 µL of 10% ammonium persulfate, and 45 µL of TEMED.
2. Allow the poured gel to polymerize for at least 1 h.
3. After polymerization, remove 20-well combs from the gel and rinse the wells with deionized water to remove any unpolymerized acrylamide.
4. Submerge the gel in 0.5X TBE running buffer and flush the wells out again with running buffer and a plastic disposable transfer pipet.
5. Load 20–25 µL of each PCR sample onto the gel using aerosol-resistant gel-loading tips.
6. Run the gel at 300 V for 2 h. The bromophenol blue dye should migrate off of the gel, and the xylene cyanol should be approximately halfway. The bottom portion of the gel box contains buffer that will be highly radioactive and should be disposed of properly.
7. Remove the gel from the apparatus, remove the wells with a scalpel, and notch the top left corner (corresponding to lane 1) for orientation purposes.
8. Fix the gel for 30 min in fix solution at room temperature
9. After fixing, drain excess fix solution from the gel using paper towels.
10. Wrap the gel in plastic wrap and smooth out all the bubbles. There is no need to dry the gel unless compelled to do so.

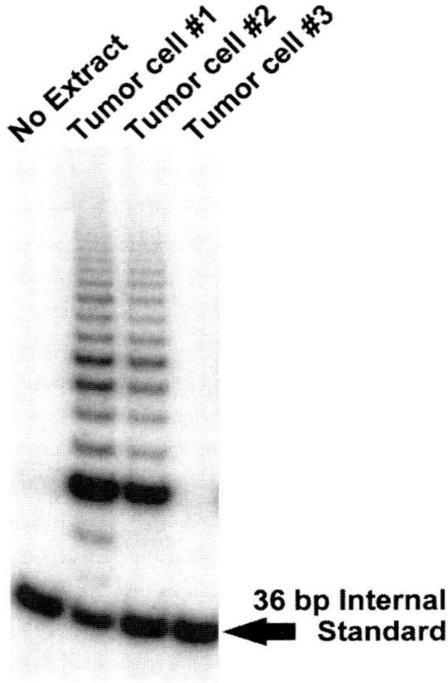

Fig. 3. Representative TRAP gel showing telomerase activity. On PCR amplification, the TRAP reactions are electrophoresed on 10% polyacrylamide gel electrophoresis. In samples that contain telomerase activity, the characteristic telomerase ladder is observed in 6-bp increments. Lane 1 serves as a negative control and contains only the lysis buffer used for sample extraction. Lanes 2–4 show varying degrees of telomerase activity, from high levels (lane 2) to lower levels (lane 3) to undetectable (lane 4). Telomerase activity is quantified by taking the ratio of the internal standard to the entire telomerase-specific ladder. Note that the difference between the amount of telomerase activity in lanes 2 and 3 is based mainly on a comparison of the amplification of the internal standard relative to the TRAP ladder (*see* **Note 9**).

11. For detection of TRAP ladders, expose the gels to a phosphorimage cassette. Exposure is generally done for at least 1 h and sometimes overnight.
12. Develop the gel per the manufacturer's protocol (Molecular Dynamics). A typical TRAP gel showing the 36 bp-internal standard and the characteristic 6-bp ladder corresponding to telomerase activity is shown in **Fig. 3** (*see* **Note 8**).
13. Quantitate telomerase activity relative to the internal standard by determining the ratio of the entire telomerase ladder to the internal standard, relative to positive control samples.

4. Notes

1. The slides can be stored at 4°C for up to 3 mo prior to pretreatment. Longer storage may result in attenuation of the hybridization signal.

2. The concentration of proteinase K varies among different tissue types. When performing the technique for the first time, we recommend varying the proteinase K concentrations (5–20 µg/mL) to determine the optimal conditions.
3. Acetic anhydride is highly unstable and should be added to the triethanolamine immediately prior to incubation.
4. The linearized template must be completely free of all phenol. As an optional step, we perform a chloroform : isoamyl (24 : 1) extraction after the phenol extraction.
5. The exact duration of this step varies considerably from 2 wk to 4 mo. We find that 3 wk is optimal for tissue sections and 2 wk is optimal for cultured cells.
6. We find that exposure of the slides to prolonged periods in water at room temperature causes the emulsion to lift off of the sections.
7. The RP/ACX, NT, and TSNT primers can be combined and stored at –20°C, in such a way that 1 µL is equivalent to 100 ng of RP/ACX primer, 100 ng of NT primer, and 0.01 amol of TSNT.
8. The TRAP assay is available as a convenient kit from Intergen (formerly Oncor) called the TRAP-eze Telomerase Detection Kit. It contains all the components for sterile detection telomerase activity in tissue samples and cultured cells using the TRAP assay.
9. For some tumor samples, PCR inhibition can occur, which is easily visible by the disappearance of the 36-bp internal standard. In cases of PCR inhibition, one of two things can be done: (1) reextraction of the tumor sample, which can result in elimination of PCR inhibitors and detectable telomerase activity; or (2) the telomerase extension, followed by phenol : chloroform extraction, ethanol precipitation, and PCR amplification of telomerase extended products. Option 1 is significantly easier than option 2, but it is also less reliable.

References

1. Shay, J. W. and Bacchetti, S. (1997) A survey of telomerase activity in human cancer. *Eur. J. Cancer* **33,** 787–791.
2. Kim, N. W., Piatyszek, M. A., Prowse, K. R., Harley, C. B., West, M. D., Ho, P. L., Coviello, G. M., Wright, W. E., Weinrich, S. L., and Shay, J. W. (1994) Specific association of human telomerase activity with immortal cells and cancer. *Science* **266,** 2011–2015.
3. Weinrich, S. L., Pruzan, R., Ma, L., et al. (1997) Reconstitution of human telomerase with the template RNA component hTR and the catalytic protein subunit hTRT. *Nat. Genet.* **17,** 498–502.
4. Olovnikov, A. M. (1971) Principle of marginotomy in template synthesis of polynucleotides. *Doklady Biochem.* **201,** 394–397.
5. Watson, J. D. (1972) Origin of concatameric T4 DNA. *Nat. New Biol.* **239,** 197–201.
6. Harley, C. B., Futcher, A. B., and Greider, C. W. (1990) Telomeres shorten with aging. *Nature* **345,** 458–460.
7. Hastie, N. D., Dempster, M., Dunlop, M. G., Thompson, A. M., Green, D. K., and Allshire, R. C. (1990) Telomere reduction in human colorectal carcinoma and with ageing. *Nature* **346,** 866–868.

8. Lindsey, J., McGill, N., Lindsey, L., Green, D., and Cooke, H. (1991) In vivo loss of telomeric repeats with age in humans. *Mutat. Res.* **256,** 45–48.
9. Shay, J. W. and Wright, W. E. (1989) Quantitation of the frequency of immortalization of normal human diploid fibroblasts by SV40 large T-antigen. *Exp. Cell Res.* **184,** 109–118.
10. Shay, J. W., Pereira-Smith, O. M., and Wright, W. E. (1991) A role for both RB and p53 in the regulation of human cellular senescence. *Exp. Cell Res.* **196,** 33–39.
11. Wright, W. E. and Shay, J. W. (1992) The two-stage mechanism controlling cellular senescence and immortalization, *Exp. Gerontol.* **27,** 383–389.
12. Ohmura, H., Tahara, H., Suzuki, M., Yoshida, M. A., Tahara, E., Shay, J. W., Barrett, J. C., and Oshimura, M. (1995) Restoration of the cellular senescence program and repression of telomerase by human chromosome 3. *Jpn. J. Cancer Res.* **86,** 899–904.
13. Yashima, K., Piatyszek, M. A., Saboorian, H. M., Virmani, A. K., Brown, D., Shay, J. W., and Gazdar, A. F. (1997) Telomerase activity and in situ telomerase RNA expression in malignant and non-malignant lymph nodes, *J. Clin. Pathol.* **50,** 110–117.
14. Soder, A. I., Hoare, S. F., Muir, S., Going, J. J., Parkinson, E. K., and Keith, W. N. (1997) Amplification, increased dosage and *in situ* expression of the telomerase RNA gene in human cancer. *Oncogene* **14,** 1013–1021.
15. Morales, C. P., Lee, E. L., and Shay, J. W. (1998) In situ hybridization for the detection of telomerase RNA in the progression from Barrett's esophagus to esophageal adenocarcinoma. *Cancer* **83,** 652–659.
16. Morales, C. P., Burdick, J. S., Saboorian, M. H., Wright, W. E., and Shay, J. W. (1998) In situ hybridization for telomerase RNA in routine cytologic brushings for the diagnosis of pancreaticobiliary malignancies. *Gastrointest. Endosc.* **48,** 402–405.
17. Ogoshi, M., Le, T., Shay, J. W., and Taylor, R. S. (1998) *In situ* hybridization analysis of the expression of human telomerase RNA in normal and pathologic conditions of the skin. *J. Invest. Dermatol.* **110,** 818–823.
18. Yashima, K., Litzky, L. A., Kaiser, L., Rogers, T., Lam, S., Wistuba, I. I., Milchgrub, S., Srivastava, S., Piatyszek, M. A., Shay, J. W., and Gazdar, A. F. (1997) Telomerase expression in respiratory epithelium during the multistage pathogenesis of lung carcinomas. *Cancer Res.* **57,** 2373–2377.
19. Piatyszek, M. A., Kim, N. W., Weinrich, S. L., Keiko, H., Hiyama, E., Wright, W. E., and Shay, J. W. (1995) Detection of telomerase activity in human cells and tumors by a telomeric repeat amplification protocol (TRAP). *Methods Cell Sci.* **17,** 1–15.
20. Holt, S. E., Norton, J. C, Wright, W. E., and Shay, J. W. (1996) Comparison of the telomeric repeat amplification protocol (TRAP) to the new TRAP-eze telomerase detection kit. *Methods Cell Sci.* **18,** 237–248.
21. Feng, J., Funk, W. D., Wang, S. S., et al. (1995) The RNA component of human telomerase. *Science* **269,** 1236–1241.

7

Detection of Microsatellite Instability

Karin D. Berg, Constance A. Griffin, and James R. Eshleman

1. Introduction

In 1993, three groups independently discovered that the lengths of microsatellites in tumors could vary from the normally constant pattern defined at birth *(1–3)* (*see* review in **ref.** ***4***). This discovery has been designated either microsatellite instability (MSI) or replication errors (RER). A recent international consensus conference convened by the National Cancer Institute defined MSI/RER as "a change in length due to either insertion or deletion of repeating units, in a microsatellite within a tumor when compared to normal tissue" *(5)*. Microsatellites are regions of repetitive DNA in which the repeating unit is small, varying in length from 1 to 6 nucleotides, and in which the number of repeating units in a microsatellite can vary from 10–60 *(6–7)*. Because microsatellite lengths generally vary from person to person, they have received widespread use in forensics, gene mapping, parentage testing, bone marrow engraftment testing, military remains testing, and so on. Microsatellite loci (markers) are generally noncoding, lying in introns and between genes. Analysis of microsatellites requires visualization of the number of repeating units that a person has at a given microsatellite locus in his or her genome (**Fig. 1**). Once a microsatellite marker is chosen for analysis, polymerase chain reaction (PCR) primers are designed in which the first anneals upstream of the microsatellite (forward primer) and the second anneals downstream of the microsatellite (reverse primer). When a person's DNA is amplified by PCR using these primers, two bands are seen on a gel if the person is a heterozygote, reflecting both paternal and maternal alleles. If the person is a homozygote, possibly because the locus is invariant in the population (e.g., BAT25 and BAT26), only a single band will be seen. By comparing to molecular weight markers (not shown in **Fig. 1**), one can extrapolate from the relative band size to the precise number of repeating units in the microsatellite.

From: *Methods in Molecular Medicine, vol. 49: Molecular Pathology Protocols*
Edited by: A. A. Killeen © Humana Press Inc., Totowa, NJ

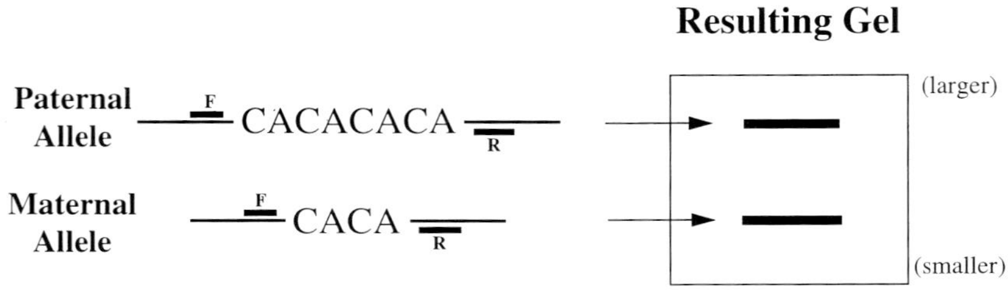

Fig. 1. A theoretical "microsatellite" locus is shown in which an individual has inherited a large paternal allele containing 4 CA repeats and a smaller maternal allele containing 2 CA repeats. Forward (F) and reverse (R) primers are designed to anneal at fixed genomic positions upstream and downstream of the microsatellite. Following amplification, the number of repeating units within the microsatellite determines the size of the PCR product and therefore the position of migration on a gel. The size of the bands on the gel can thus be precisely correlated with the number of repeating units within an individual's alleles at any microsatellite locus. Very short "microsatellites" are used in this illustration for clarity. Research Genetics (Huntsville, AL; http://www.resgen.com) currently has more than 5500 microsatellite loci listed in their on-line catalog.

During chromosome mapping experiments, microsatellite length was serendipitously discovered to have deviated from normal in the tumors of certain patients. As illustrated in **Fig. 2A** in a "normal" tumor, the alleles are the same size in both the normal and the tumor DNA samples. By contrast, a tumor with microsatellite instability shows novel alleles. Faint germline alleles are often still visible owing to residual stromal cells despite microdissection of the tumor from adjacent stromal tissue to enrich for tumor cell DNA. Stutter or shadow bands arise during PCR owing to slippage (*see* **Fig. 2B**) because *Taq* polymerase lacks proofreading function and DNA repair systems are not present. Note that the difference between the parental band and the stutter bands is exactly the number of bases of the repeating unit within the microsatellite (e.g., microsatellites with dinucleotide repeats give rise to –2 and –4 base stutter bands). On first consideration, stutter bands seem distracting and could obscure true MSI in which the shift in the tumor is small (e.g., –2 bases). However, stutter bands are probably helpful because, for a given band, they serve as a "signature" of what is contained within the PCR primers. For example, note that in **Fig. 2A**, the true instability in the tumor sample from patient #2 can be distinguished from the spurious band by the presence or absence of the signature stutter bands. Interestingly, stutter is an in vitro artifact resulting from a molecular mechanism somewhat analogous to the in vivo MSI/RER phenomenon arising from defective mismatch repair (MMR).

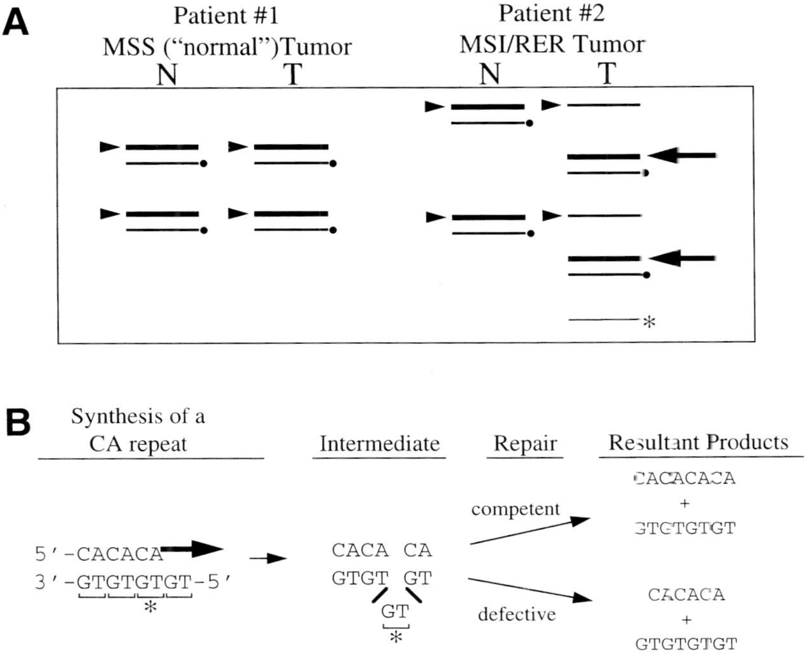

Fig. 2. **(A)** Microsatellite assay (radioactive version, see text): Paired normal (N) and tumor (T) samples are amplified from two patients at a single microsatellite locus. Patient #1 demonstrates the pattern seen in a microsatellite stable (MSS) tumor, and patient #2 shows that seen with an MSI or RER tumor. Arrowheads, germline bands; dots, stutter bands; arrows, shifted allele lengths, indicative of microsatellite instability; asterisk, nonspecific PCR product. **(B)** Template strand slippage during synthesis of a CA repeat from a 4 GT dinucleotide template repeat. The third GT is identified by an asterisk. The large arrow symbolizes the DNA polymerase during active replication in which three of the CA repeats have already been synthesized. Before the polymerase finishes synthesis, the third GT of the template strand undergoes slippage and the third CA is now annealing with the fourth GT. In the presence of competent DNA repair, this intermediate is recognized and repaired such that both strands now contain the full-length repeat. If repair is defective, one product contains a shortened length repeat.

Microsatellite instability in tumors is a relatively recently discovered phenomenon whose diagnostic utility continues to expand *(8)*. It is a functional surrogate marker for MMR defective cells *(9,10)*. MMR, first identified in yeast and bacteria, is responsible for the rapid repair of mistakes made by DNA polymerases. The principle clinical utility of the MSI/RER assay is currently for the discovery of families with hereditary nonpolyposis colorectal cancer

(HNPCC), which is owing to defects in MMR. Additionally, in colorectal cancer, the presence of MSI in a tumor probably portends a better prognosis ***(2,11)*** and may ultimately prove a predictor of tumor chemosensitivity. The following protocol to assay for MSI/RER is written primarily for use with a fluorescent primer format, but the assay can also be performed using radiolabeled PCR primers.

2. Materials

All materials used in specimen acquisition, DNA extraction, and PCR must be handled using DNA/PCR precautions. Reagents should be PCR grade. Aerosol-resistant tips should be used throughout.

2.1. Specimen Acquisition

1. Paraffin-embedded specimens:
   a. N: normal block, no histologically identifiable lesions (the block containing the margin of resection is often the best source) or a peripheral blood sample.
   b. T: tumor block, histologically verified section of tumor.
2. Clean microdissection area containing the following equipment:
   a. UV illumination source.
   b. 37°C water bath.
   c. Heating block to hold Eppendorf tubes.
   d. Sterile Eppendorf tubes.
   e. Sterile razor blades.
   f. Microfuge.
   g. Kimwipes.

2.2. DNA Extraction

1. Xylene.
2. 100% Ethanol.
3. Digestion buffer at the following final concentrations: 50 m*M* Tris-HCl (pH 8.5), 1 m*M* EDTA, 0.5% Tween-20, 200 µg/mL of proteinase K (Boehringer Mannheim). Store buffer as single-use aliquots at –20°C.

2.3. Polymerase Chain Reaction

1. Thermocycler (PE 9600 or PE 9700).
2. Reagents: AmpliTaq Gold™ Polymerase (5 U/µL; Perkin Elmer/Roche), AmpliTaq Gold Buffer containing 1.5 m*M* MgCl (Perkin Elmer/Roche), PCR-grade water, 10 m*M* dNTPs (Perkin Elmer/Roche).
3. PCR Primers (Research Genetics; *see* **Note 1** and **Table 1**). Fluorescent: forward primer 5′ labeled as indicated in **Table 1**; radioactive: forward primer 5′ end-labeled with ^{32}P or ^{33}P.

Table 1
Microsatellite Marker Characteristics[a]

Locus (Fluor) primer sequence	Genome Data Base/ Genbank numbers	Product size (bp)
BAT 25 (Tet)		
Forward:		
5'-TCGCCTCCAAGAATGTAAGT-3'	GDB:9834508/	120[d]
Reverse:	U63834	
5'-TCTGCATTTTAACTATGGCTC-3'		
BAT 26 (Hex)		
Forward:		
5'-TGACTACTTTTGACTTCAGCC-3'	GDB:9834505/	116[d]
Reverse:	U41210	
5'-AACCATTCAACATTTTTAACCC-3'[b]		
D2S123 (Hex)		
Forward:		
5'-AAACAGGATGCCTGCCTTTA-3'	GDB:187953/	197–227[e]
Reverse:	Z16551	
5'-GGACTTTCCACCTATGGGAC-3'		
D5S346 (Fam)		
Forward:		
5'-ACTCACTCTAGTGATAAATCGGG-3'	GDB:181171/	96–122[e]
Reverse:	M73547	
5'-AGCAGATAAGACAGTATTACTAGTT-3'		
D17S250[c] (Fam)		
Forward:		
5'-GGAAGAATCAAATAGACAAT-3'	GDB:177030/	151–169[e]
Reverse:	X54562	
5'-GCTGGCCATATATATATTTAAACC-3'		

[a]Sizes listed do not reflect addition of the nontemplated adenine. The primer sequences were obtained from GDB. Single genbank numbers are listed even though the microsatellites may be present in multiple entries.

[b]Note that this reverse primer has a one-base mispair from the gene sequence found in the genbank database.

[c]The locus D17S250 is also known as Mfd15.

[d]BAT25 and BAT26 (Big A-Tract) are generally invariant in size because these amplicons have not been reported to be polymorphic in humans.

[e]The base pair size ranges for the dinucleotide microsatellites do not in all cases include the full range of sizes in the population. We have noted several germline alleles that are outside of these ranges.

2.4. Detection

1. Fluorescent: ABI 310 Genetic Analyzer or comparable capillary electrophoresis apparatus, deionized formamide.
2. Radioactive: Standard DNA sequencing gel reagents and apparatus, autoradiography supplies.

3. Methods

Preventing cross contamination of cases is essential (individual disposable pipet tips for each specimen must be used at each step).

3.1. Specimen Acquisition

1. Cut five sections from blocks submitted as normal (N, no tumor) and tumor (T). Submit the first and last sections (5-µm sections) from each set for standard hematoxylin & eosin (H&E) staining. Mount the three "sandwiched" middle sections (5–10 µm thick) on standard histology slides unstained, without a cover slip (*see* **Note 2**).
2. Mark ("dot") normal (N) and tumor (T) areas of the H&E slides (this should be done by an anatomic pathologist).

3.2. Microdissection

1. Perform microdissection in a laminar flow hood, after the empty hood has undergone UV treatment for at least 20 min.
2. Label 1.5-mL Eppendorf tubes: N for normal, T for tumor, and the specimen number for each case.
3. Match the first unstained slide (level 2) grossly by tissue shape to the first (level 1) H&E-stained slide. Superimpose the unstained slide exactly over the stained, marked slide, and using a razor or scalpel blade, microdissect the relevant (dotted) areas of the H&E slide from the unstained slide. Save levels 3 and 4 for additional analyses if needed.
4. Place the section directly from the razor blade into the appropriately labeled 1.5-mL Eppendorf tube after microdissection and seal the lid. Xylene may prevent static electricity from affecting the tissue (*see* **Note 3**). Make certain that no paraffin or tissue is left on the external aspect of the Eppendorf tube; wipe the closed tube surfaces with xylene.
5. Clean all surfaces thoroughly with xylene between samples, and use fresh Kimwipes and a new razor blade for each specimen. At no time should material from one specimen (even from the same case) come in contact with another specimen. Accurate results rely on a meticulous, clean microdissection technique.
6. Centrifuge the tissue to the bottom of the Eppendorf tubes, and microfuge for 2 min at the maximum setting (e.g., 12,800*g* for the Eppendorf 5414).

3.3. DNA Extraction

1. Remove paraffin using serial xylene washes. (**Caution:** xylene solubilizes most inks. It is important to verify frequently that the specimen number is intact.) Add 1 mL of xylene to each Eppendorf tube containing microdissected tissue.

2. Mix the specimen tube contents by gently inverting each closed tube for 3 min.
3. Centrifuge in a microfuge at the maximum setting for 5 min.
4. Identify the pellet (be careful, it is usually translucent, and may be floating), and pipet off the xylene.
5. Repeat xylene wash steps (**steps 1–4**) two additional times.
6. After the third xylene wash has been removed, add 1 mL of absolute (100%) ethanol to each tube (to remove the residual xylene).
7. Mix the tube contents by gentle inversion for 3 min. The pellet should break up to some extent.
8. Centrifuge in a microfuge as in **step 3** for 5 min.
9. Remove the ethanol supernatant carefully (the pellet may still be difficult to identify).
10. Repeat the ethanol wash one additional time (**steps 6–9**).
11. Remove the last ethanol wash and cover each uncapped tube with parafilm. Poke several small holes in the parafilm (use an individual, sterile needle, and do not touch the sides).
12. Dry the pellets approx 5 min in a speed-vac (Savant). Do not overdry, because this can make DNA difficult to resuspend.
13. Depending on the size of the pellet, add 100–200 µL of thawed digestion buffer to the dried pellets. Large samples require closer to 200 µL, and smaller pellets may require 100 µL or less to ensure sufficient postdigestion DNA concentrations.
14. Vortex each tube (*see* **Note 4**) to break up the pellet and spin for 10 s. Make sure all tissue is in the buffer.
15. Incubate the specimens overnight at 37°C or for 3 h at 55°C.
16. Microfuge the tubes for 10 s (maximum setting) to collect the sample at the bottom of the tube.
17. Inactivate the proteinase K by boiling the specimen for 10 min or placing in a 95°C heat block for 10 min. Be sure to securely close the tube lids.
18. Microfuge for 1 min at maximum speed to collect the fluid at the bottom of the tube.
19. Determine the A_{260} and A_{280} absorbance using a UV spectrophotometer. The DNA concentration should ideally be between 30 and 100 µg/mL (*see* **Note 5**).
20. Samples should be stored in a non-self-defrosting –20°C freezer.

3.4. PCR Conditions

PCR conditions have been proven reliable using both the PE 9600 and the PE 9700 thermocyclers.

1. Reaction mix (10 µL total volume, but should be master mixed and aliquoted prior to sample addition): 4.7 µL of PCR-grade H_2O; 1.0 µL of 10X AmpliTaq Gold PCR buffer; 1.5 µL of forward primer (1.33 m*M*); 1.5 µL of reverse primer (20 m*M*) (*see* **Note 6**); 0.2 µL of dNTPs (10 m*M*); 0.1 µL of AmpliTaq Gold Polymerase (5 U/µL); 1.0 µL of sample, or control. For a description of primers, *see* **Table 1** and **Notes 1** and **6**.

2. Controls (for each locus):
   a. Water negative control.
   b. "Normal" cell line (transformed lymphoblasts).
   c. "Tumor" cell line from the same patient (known to be shifted at that locus).
3. Thermal-cycling conditions:
   a. Initial denaturation: 95°C for 9 min.
   b. Thirty-five cycles of denaturation at 94°C for 45 s, anneal at 55°C for 45 s, and extension at 72°C for 1 min.
   c. Final extension at 60°C for 45 min (adds nontemplated A).

3.5. Detection

3.5.1. Fluorescent

1. Aliquot to ABI 9600 PCR tubes 12.0 µL of deionized formamide, 0.75 µL of internal size standard-Tamara (red), and 1.5 µL of PCR product.
2. Denature for 3–5 min at 95°C in a heat block (PCR block works well).
3. Load ABI 310 or other capillary electrophoresis apparatus per manufacturer's directions. The instrument settings for the ABI 310 are as follows:
   a. Matrix: C.
   b. Polymer: GS POP-4.
   c. Size marker: Tamara labeled GS350 or GS500.
   d. Buffer: 1X GS buffer.
   e. Capillary temperature: 60°C.
   f. Run time: 20 min.
   g. Voltage: 15 kV.
   h. Laser: 9.9 mW.
   i. Smoothing: light.
   j. Peak amplitude threshold: 200.

3.5.2. Radioactive

1. Use standard DNA sequencing gel and autoradiography.

3.6. Interpretation

Figure 3 provides an example of the MSI/RER assay using both the radioactive and fluorescent formats. Interpretation of this assay can appear straightforward at first glance; however, one must be aware of potential pitfalls to ensure accurate and consistent interpretation of the data. First, inspect the water lanes for each primer set. There should be no banding or significant peak height data in these lanes. Next, inspect the normal sample results (**Fig. 3A** and **Fig. 3B**, top). Provided that there is no contamination, these bands or peaks represent the germline microsatellite length(s) for the patient for each of the loci (*see* **Table 1** for expected amplicon size ranges). Note that BAT25 and BAT26 are thought to be invariant in size in the population. True alleles can be identified by a dominant band or peak (**Fig. 3**) surrounded by stutter (shadow) peaks of diminishing intensity, which are generally smaller than the predominant peaks. Peaks and bands without stutter should be very carefully evaluated, because they almost invariably represent spurious amplification.

After identifying, recording, and verifying that the germline (nontumor) amplicon sizes lie in the appropriate size range for each locus, look at the tumor electropherograms and determine the predominant amplicon sizes for each locus in the tumor specimens (**Fig. 3A** and **Fig. 3B**; bottom). A direct comparison between the germline amplicon sizes and tumor amplicon sizes is now possible. For example, when one compares 1N to 1T, it is easy to appreciate that this tumor has shifted from the germline pattern at the BAT25 locus. No germline bands derived from residual stromal tissue are seen in the electropherogram of 1T shown in **Fig. 3A** or **3B**, because 1N and 1T are cell line controls and thus contain pure normal allele length or pure shifted allele length PCR products. By contrast, residual germline bands are seen in **Fig. 3A** (2N and 2T) that were amplified following microdissection of paraffin blocks. Whereas the normal patient sample (2N) shows normal length BAT25 amplicon lengths, the tumor tissue (2T) shows both shifted alleles and germline alleles, the latter likely owing to contaminating germline stromal tissue.

After identifying heterozygous and homozygous alleles identifying the germline and tumor amplicon sizes for each locus, one then counts the number of markers showing instability. One may then make the appropriate diagnosis using the guidelines from the National Cancer Institute (NCI) consensus conference (*see* **ref. 5**):

1. MSI high: two or more of five loci demonstrating instability.
2. MSI low: one of five loci demonstrating instability.
3. MSS/Non-RER: None of the markers showing instability.

The MSI high result most probably indicates a functional MMR defect in the tumor. The human MMR genes currently known to be defective in tumors are *hMSH2*, *hMLH1*, *hPMS1*, *hPMS2*, *hMLH3*, *GTBP/hMSH6*, and *hMSH3* (reviewed in **refs. *9*** and ***10***). However, this is an area of active investigation, and consequently this list may not be inclusive. The finding of MSI high can be due to a germline defect, such as exists in an HNPCC family, in combination with a second hit in the tumor or can arise owing to biallelic inactivation in the tumor in the absence of a germline defect. As a follow-up to this result, a detailed family history, immunohistochemistry of the tumor for MMR protein expression (at least hMSH2 and hMLH1 proteins), and germline DNA sequencing for MMR defects (and testing for methylation status) may all be indicated. It is probably appropriate to encourage genetic counseling when this result is obtained (if not already established). While this protocol is written using the

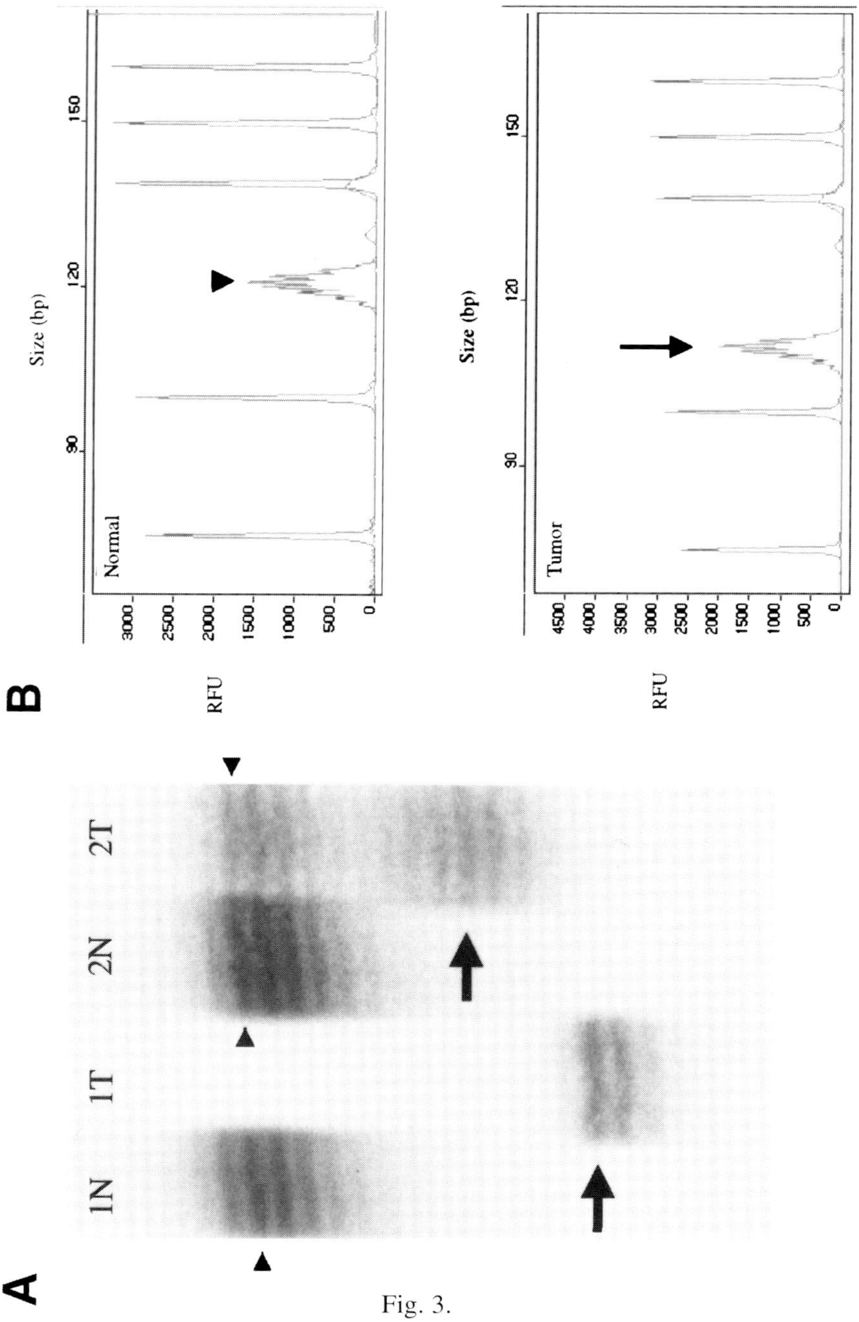

Fig. 3.

five primary loci recommended at the NCI consensus conference, MSI high also may be diagnosed with a larger number of microsatellites in which the percentage showing instability is ≥30–40% *(5)*.

The clinical implications of finding only one microsatellite shifted (MSI low) is uncertain for two reasons. First, microsatellites are inherently difficult to replicate and accordingly display a higher mutation rate than nonrepetitive regions of DNA in the presence of functional repair. Therefore, having only one marker shifted sometimes may be of no importance. Second, there are well-established "muted" phenotypes, such as *GTBP/hMSH6*, in which one would expect low-level microsatellite instability. A defect in *GTBP* produces selective mononucleotide instability in the presence of stable dinucleotides. The study of additional markers in this setting may be appropriate to assess the significance of one of five markers shifted. When more markers are analyzed, MSI low is designated when <30–40% of markers analyzed are found to be shifted *(5)*.

4. Notes

1. Primers that we currently use are those recommended by the NCI consensus conference and are synthesized by Research Genetics. The Food and Drug Administration is interested in ensuring the quality of oligonucleotide primers used in "home-brew" assays. Accordingly, one may need to purchase oligonucleotides only from vendors approved to provide these as analyte-specific reagents. Irrespective of the source of the primers, it is important to run the primers themselves on the column when they are obtained to exclude contamination resulting in extraneous bands.
2. The laboratory needs to ensure that tissue and DNA are not contaminated with any other specimen. If this occurs, novel bands representing foreign alleles could be inappropriately misinterpreted as demonstrating MSI/RER.

Fig. 3. *(see opposite page)* **(A)** Autoradiograph of BAT25 amplified from a tumor bearing a defect in the mismatch repair gene, *hMSH2*. The normal sample is derived from transformed lymphoblasts (L670) from this patient, and the tumor sample is a cell line (Vaco 670) derived from the patient's tumor. Both cell lines were generous gifts from Dr. James Willson at Case Western Reserve University. Samples 2N and 2T from the second patient consist of normal colonic epithelium (2N) and colonic adenocarcinoma (2T), prepared from paraffin blocks as per the protocol described herein. **(B)** Electropherograms of amplicons of BAT25 amplified from cell lines 1N and 1T as shown in (A). Red peaks are size standard peaks at 75, 100, 139, 150, and 160 in which the *x*-axis size is in base pairs. Peak heights are quantified as random fluorescent units (RFUs) on the *y*-axis. The green peaks at and around 120 bp (normal, arrowhead) and 116 bp (tumor shifted, arrow) represent the BAT25 amplicons. The predominant peak in 1N (arrowhead) represents the expected amplicon length and stutter (owing to slippage) is visualized as serration extending above and below the predominant peak.

3. One problem encountered during microdissection is static electricity, which can cause the microdissected tissue to fly off the razor blade. This can be avoided by applying 15 µL of xylene to the tissue on the slide prior to microdissection.
4. Vortexing solutions containing protein promotes denaturation and generally is not done. However, vortexing at this step is empirically advantageous presumably because fragmenting the tissue outweighs the protein denaturation.
5. A formal A_{260}/A_{280} reading is suggested. Because there is no precipitation step in the protocol, this reading should be inaccurate owing to the presence of amino acids, which should still contribute to absorbance. It is useful nonetheless because it is a crude measurement of the approximate amount of DNA that has been isolated. We have empirically found that a more extensive DNA preparation is not necessary.
6. We have done a substantial number of titration experiments testing various relative primer ratios. At the labeled:unlabeled primer ratio of 1:1, one gets many spurious bands, whereas at 1:40, one begins to see loss of signal. Ratios of 1:15 or 1:20 appear optimal in both regards (lack of spurious amplification and robustness of specific signal).

References

1. Aaltonen, L., Peltomaki, P., Leach, F., Sistonen, P., Pylkkanen, L., Mecklin, J., Jarvinen, H., Powell, S., Jen, J., Hamilton, S., Petersen, G., Kinzler, K., Vogelstein, B., and de la Chapelle, A. (1993) Clues to the pathogenesis of familial colorectal cancer. *Science* **260,** 812–816.
2. Thibodeau, S., Bren, G., and Schaid, D. (1993) Microsatellite instability in cancer of the proximal colon. *Science* **260,** 816–819.
3. Ionov, Y., Peinado, M., Malkhosyan, S., Shibata, D., and Perucho, M. (1993) Ubiquitous somatic mutations in simple repeated sequences reveal a new mechanism for colonic carcinogenesis. *Nature* **363,** 558–561.
4. Eshleman, J. R. and Markowitz, S. D. (1995) Microsatellite instability in inherited and sporadic neoplasms. *Curr. Opin. Oncol.* **7,** 83–89.
5. Boland, C. R., Thibodeau, S. N., Hamilton, S. R., Sidransky, D., Eshleman, J. R., Burt, R. W., Meltzer, S. J., Fodde, R., Rodriguez-Bigas, M. A., Fodde, R., Ranzani, G. N., and Srivastava, S. (1998) A National Cancer Institute workshop on microsatellite instability for cancer detection and familial predisposition: development of international criteria for the determination of microsatellite instability in colorectal cancer. *Cancer Res.* **58,** 5248–5257.
6. Litt, M. and Luty, J. A. (1989) A hypervariable microsatellite revealed by in vitro amplification of a dinucleotide repeat within the cardiac muscle actin gene. *Am. J. Hum. Genet.* **44,** 397–401.
7. Weber, J. L. and May, P. E. (1989) Abundant class of human DNA polymorphisms which can be typed using the polymerase chain reaction, *Am. J. Hum. Genet.* **44,** 388–396.
8. Rodriguez-Bigas, M., Boland, C. R., Hamilton, S. R., Henson, D. E., Jass, J. R., Khan, P. M., Lynch, H., Perucho, M., Smyrk, T., Sobin, L., and Srivastava, S.

(1997) A National Cancer Institute workshop on Hereditary Nonpolyposis Colorectal Cancer syndrome: meeting highlights and Bethesda guidelines. *JNCI* **89,** 1758–1762.
9. Eshleman, J. R. and Markowitz, S. D. (1996) Mismatch repair defects in human carcinogenesis. *Hum. Mol. Genet.* **5,** 1489–1494.
10. Toft, N. J. and Arends, M. J. (1998) DNA mismatch repair and colorectal cancer. *J. Pathol.* **185,** 123–129.
11. Sankila, R., Aaltonen, L. A., Jarvinen, H. J., and Mecklin, J. P. (1996) Better survival rates in patients with *MLH1*-associated hereditary colorectal cancer. *Gastroenterology* **110,** 682–687.

8

Polymerase Chain Reaction Clonality Assays Based on X-Linked Genes

Langxing Pan and Huaizheng Peng

1. Introduction

During embryogenesis in females, in each cell either the paternal or the maternal X chromosome is randomly inactivated through methylation *(1,2)*. This event is stably inherited by daughter progeny of each cell. Therefore, in adult women, polyclonal cell populations will comprise a random mixture of paternally and maternally derived X-inactivated cells, but monoclonal cells will contain the same inactivated X chromosome as their progenitor. The paternal and maternal X chromosomes can be distinguished by identification of polymorphisms at certain alleles, and differences in methylation of DNA sequences within these alleles can be detected by digestion of the DNA with methylation-sensitive restriction enzymes. Based on these principles, researchers have developed several X-linked clonality assays, and most are performed using Southern blot hybridization *(3–5)*.

The polymorphic and methylation sites of some X-linked genes are closely clustered within a short region, which allows clonality analysis by polymerase chain reaction (PCR) after methylation-sensitive enzyme digestion. One of the early targets is the phosphoglycerate kinase gene *(6)*. However, the usefulness of this locus as a clonal marker is limited by its low frequency of polymorphism (20–40%) *(3)*. Recently, two other genes, the human androgen receptor gene (AR gene or HUMARA) *(7)* and monoamine oxidase A gene (MAOA gene) *(8,9)* have been reported to have a very high rate of heterozygosity (AR 90%, MAOA 75%) *(7,9,10)*. In an earlier study, based on the inactivation patterns of these genes, we developed two PCR assays for detection of clonality in female patients *(11)*. We describe these assays in detail in this chapter.

From: *Methods in Molecular Medicine, vol. 49: Molecular Pathology Protocols*
Edited by: A. A. Killeen © Humana Press Inc., Totowa, NJ

2. Materials

2.1. DNA Samples

Prepare high molecular weight DNA using the standard proteinase K/phenol/chloroform method ***(12)*** or a commercial kit (Puregene; Gentra Systems, Minneapolis, MN). DNA from a male individual can serve as a control for endonuclease digestion efficiency.

2.2. Restriction Endonuclease

Use *Hpa*II, a methylation-sensitive restriction endonuclease (Boehringer Mannheim, Mannheim, Germany) for both AR and MAOA PCR analyses.

2.3. Polymerase Chain Reaction

1. 10X PCR buffer (supplied with *Taq* DNA polymerase or cat. no. M190A; Promega, Madison, WI): 100 m*M* Tris-HCl (pH 9.0), 500 m*M* KCl, 0.1% Triton X-100.
2. *Taq* DNA polymerase (5 U/μL) (cat. no. M1862A; Promega).
3. 25 m*M* each dNTP (cat. no. U1240; Promega).
4. 25 m*M* $MgCl_2$ (supplied with the *Taq* polymerase or cat. no. A351; Promega)
5. Primers: (5′ to 3′)
   a. AR sense primer (AR1): GCT GTG AAG GTT GCT GTT CCT CAT
   b. AR antisense primer (AR2): TCC AGA ATC TGT TCC AGA GCG TGC
   c. MAOA sense primer (MAOA1): ACA TTC TAA ACC TAA TAA CTC
   d. MAOA antisense primer (MAOA2): CAA TAA ATG TCC TAC ACC TT
   e. Inner MAOA antisense primer (MAOA3): GGT AGA CTC CTT TAA GAA AAG GTT AAA A

2.4. Denaturing Polyacrylamide Gel Electrophoresis

1. SequaGel™ sequencing system consisting of SequaGel™ diluent, SequaGel™ buffer, and SequaGel™ concentration (EC-833; National Diagnostics, Atlanta, GA).
2. Ammonium persulfate (A-9164; Sigma, St. Louis, MO).
3. TEMED (T-7024; Sigma).
4. 10X TBE: 0.9 *M* Tris-HCl, pH 8.3, 0.9 *M* boric acid, 0.02 *M* EDTA.
5. Loading buffer (sequencing stop buffer): 98% formamide, 10 m*M* NaOH, 20 m*M* EDTA, 0.05% bromophenol blue, and 0.05% xylene cyanol FF.

2.5. Background-Free Silver Staining

1. Acetic acid (100016; BDH).
2. Methanol (10158; BDH).
3. Formaldehyde (10113; BDH).
4. Ethanol (10107; BDH).
5. Sodium thiosulfate (72049; Fluka).
6. $AgNO_3$ (S-0139; Sigma).
7. Na_2CO_3 (10240; BDH).
8. Glass trays (30 × 30 cm or larger).

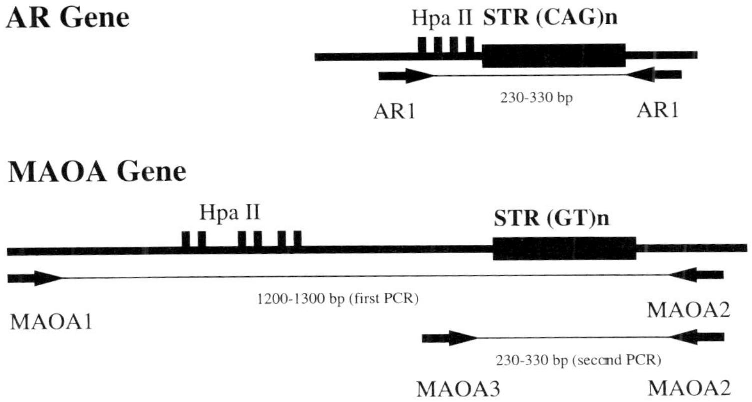

Fig. 1. AR and MAOA gene structure and PCR strategies. PCR primers are designed to flank the STR and methylation sites of the AR and MAOA genes. Amplification of this region by PCR is performed from both undigested and *Hpa*II-digested DNA samples in each case. PCR performed on undigested DNA samples amplified both methylated (inactive) and unmethylated (active) alleles of the gene and disclosed whether the sample is polymorphic. By contrast, PCR of the digested DNA samples amplified only the methylated allele of the gene because the unmethylated allele is destroyed by the restriction enzyme. Amplification of trinucleotide repeat and methylation sites of AR genes is performed in a single round of PCR. Amplification of dinucleotide repeat and methylation sites of MAOA genes is performed in two rounds of PCR. (Reproduced from **ref. *11*** with permission. © John Wiley & Sons Limited.)

9. 3MM filter paper (3030917; Whatman).
10. Cling film.
11. Cellophane membrane, optional.

2.6. Equipment

1. Thermocycler (oil free).
2. Protean II xi vertical electrophoresis cell with gel mold (200 × 240 mm) and 0.75-mm thick spacers and comb (165-1933; Bio-Rad, Hercules, CA).
3. Vacuum gel dryer, optional (Bio-Rad).

3. Methods

Figure 1 illustrates the principles of both methods. Both digested and undigested DNA samples are analyzed in parallel. To obtain accurate results, it is crucial to ensure a complete digestion of DNA samples. Because male individuals have only one X chromosome, DNA from a male can serve as a control of digestion efficiency (*see* **Subheading 3.6.**).

3.1. DNA Digestion

1. Digest 1 µg of DNA in a 20-µL vol with 10 U of *Hpa*II at 37°C overnight.
2. Dilute the digested DNA to a concentration of 20 ng/µL with water.

3.2. PCR to Amplify AR Gene (HUMARA)

1. Prepare a master mix (based on a total 25-µL vol for each reaction) containing 1X PCR buffer; 1.5 m*M* $MgCl_2$; 0.2 m*M* each of dATP, dCTP, dGTP and dTTP; 0.2 µ*M* of each primer (AR1 and AR2); and an appropriate amount of *Taq* DNA polymerase (0.2 U/25 µL of final reaction volume). Place 24 µL of the master mix into individual microtubes.
2. Add 1 µL of digested or undigested sample DNA (20 ng) to each tube and perform 30 cycles of denaturation at 95°C for 30 s, primer annealing at 54°C for 30 s, and primer extension at 72°C for 45 s. Conclude the reaction with a final extension at 72°C for 5 min.

3.3. PCR on MAOA Gene

For the MAOA gene, two rounds of PCR are performed using the same master mix used for HUMARA with different primers. In the first round, MAOA1 and MAOA2 primers are used to amplify the fragment containing both the simple tandem repeat (STR) and methylation sites in the DNA samples. In the second round of PCR, MAOA2 and MAOA3 primers are used to amplify the STR site.

1. For the first round of PCR, add 24 µL of the master mix (*see* **Subheading 3.2., step 1**) with MAOA1 and MAOA2 primers to each tube and add 1 µL (20 ng) of digested or undigested DNA sample.
2. Perform 20 PCR cycles of denaturation at 95°C for 30 s, primer annealing at 54°C for 30 s, and primer extension at 72°C for 45 s.
3. Dilute a fraction of the first-round PCR products 100-fold with water. Add 1 µL of the diluted first-round products to each tube containing 24 µL of the master mix with MAOA2 and MAOA3 primers. Run the second PCR using the same cycling conditions as for the first round for a further 30 cycles. Conclude the reaction with a final extension at 72°C for 5 min.

3.4. Polyacrylamide Gel Electrophoresis

1. For a 200 × 240 × 0.75 mm, 8% denaturing polyacrylamide gel, mix 58 mL of SequaGel diluent, 10 mL of SequaGel buffer, and 32 mL of SequaGel concentration in a beaker.
2. Add 500 µL of 10% ammonium persulfate and 50 µL of TEMED to the beaker and mix gently.
3. Quickly pour the mixture into the gel mold and allow it to set at room temperature for 1 h.
4. Assemble the electrophoresis apparatus with the gel and fill the tank with 1X TBE buffer.

5. Dilute 5 µL of each PCR product with 15 µL of loading buffer and load 10 µL of sample per track onto the gel.
6. Run the gel at 40 W constant power for 2–3 h at 40°C maintained by flowing hot tap water through the built-in water jacket of the gel apparatus (*see* **Note 1**).

3.5. Background-Free Silver Staining

1. Fix the gel in a solution containing 12% acetic acid, 50% methanol, and 0.02% formaldehyde for 2–16 h with gentle agitation.
2. Wash the gel with 50% ethanol for 20 min twice.
3. Place the gel into freshly prepared 0.02% sodium thiosulfate solution for 1 min, and rinse the gel with distilled water three times.
4. Soak the gel in silver solution containing 0.2% $AgNO_3$ and 0.03% formaldehyde for 20–30 min and then rinse twice with distilled water.
5. Soak the gel in a solution containing 6% Na_2CO_3, 0.02% formaldehyde, and 0.0005% sodium thiosulfate for 3–5 min, to develop the color.
6. Stop the reaction by placing the gel into a solution containing 50% methanol and 16% acetic acid.
7. Transfer the gel onto a piece of 3MM filter paper or cellophane membrane. Cover the gel with cling film, and dry it in a vacuum gel dryer at 80°C for 40 min.

3.6. Interpretation of Results

Undigested control male DNA should show a single band for both AR and MAOA STR sites, whereas completely digested male DNA should show no PCR products. DNA from homozygous (noninformative) females should show a single band with or without enzyme digestion. In heterozygous (informative) females, DNA from polyclonal cell populations shows two bands with equal intensity with or without enzyme digestion. Undigested DNA of monoclonal cell populations from an informative female shows two bands with equal intensity, whereas completely digested DNA shows a single band if the DNA is from a pure cell population such as a cell line, or two bands with unequal intensity if the sample contains normal or polyclonal cells (*see* **Fig. 2**).

It has been reported that similar PCR methods based on AR gene can be applied to minute amounts of paraffin-embedded tissue ***(13)***. We find that complete digestion of DNA from paraffin section is extremely difficult to achieve. However, DNA purified from microdissected fragments of frozen tissue sections can be adequately digested in the presence of both *Hpa*II and *Hha*I restriction enzymes (unpublished data) and used for the AR gene–based PCR clonality assay. Further experiments for the reliability and reproducibility in the microdissected frozen materials are needed.

A skewing phenomenon is the major disadvantage of any clonality assay based on X-linked gene ***(14,15)***, especially when DNA samples are prepared from hemopoietic cells of elderly females ***(16)***. When dealing with these materials, it is important to have DNA from samples of the patient's normal tissue as control.

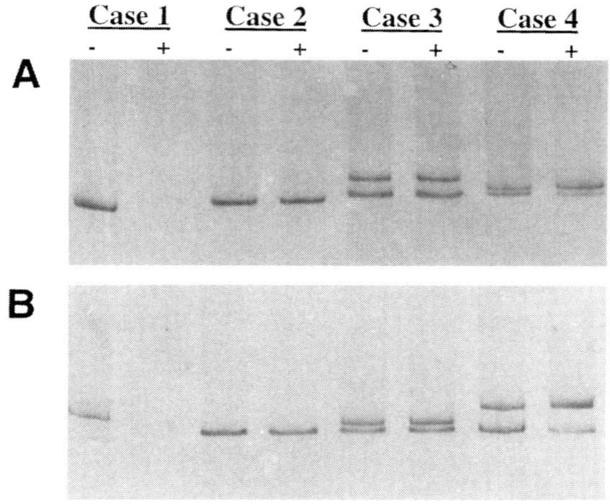

Fig. 2. Clonality detection by **(A)** MAOA-PCR and **(B)** AR-PCR. Case 1, control DNA from a male; case 2, DNA from a female, showing homozygous; case 3, tonsil DNA from a female, showing polyclonality; and case 4, breast carcinoma DNA from a female, showing monoclonality. Lanes (–) and (+) show PCR amplification before and after *Hpa*II digestion, respectively. (Reproduced from **ref.** ***11*** with permission. © John Wiley & Sons Limited.)

4. Note

1. The 8% denaturing polyacrylamide gel may be stained with ethidium bromide. Electrophoresis may be run at room temperature, but unexpected bands caused by heteroduplex DNA in the gel may occur and confuse the results.

References

1. Mandel, J. L., Manaco, A. P., Nelson, D. L., Schlessinger, D., and Willard, H. (1993) Genome analysis and the human x chromosome. *Science* **258,** 103–109.
2. Riggs, A. D. and Pfeifer, G. P. (1992) X-chromosome inactivation and cell memory. *Trends. Genet.* **8,** 169–174.
3. Vogelstein, B., Fearon, E. R., Hamilton, S. R., Preisinger, A. C., Willard, H. F., Michelson, A. M., Riggs, A. D., and Orkin, S. H. (1987) Clonal analysis using recombinant DNA probes from the X-chromosome. *Cancer Res.* **47,** 4806–4813.
4. Lucas, G. S., Padua, R. A., Masters, G. S., Oscier, D. G., and Jacobs, A. (1989) The application of X-chromosome gene probes to the diagnosis of myeloproliferative disease. *Br. J. Haematol.* **72,** 530–533.
5. Fey, M. F., Peter, H. J., Hinds, H. L., Zimmermann, A., Liechti Gallati, S., Gerber, H., Studer, H., and Tobler, A. (1992) Clonal analysis of human tumors with M27 beta, a highly informative polymorphic X chromosomal probe. *J. Clin. Invest.* **89,** 1438–1444.

6. Gilliland, D. G., Blanchard, K. L., Levy, J., Perrin, S., and Bunn, H. F. (1991) Clonality in myeloproliferative disorders: analysis by means of the polymerase chain reaction. *Proc. Natl. Acad. Sci. USA* **88,** 6848–6852.
7. Allen, R. C., Zoghbi, H. Y., Moseley, A. B., Rosenblatt, H. M., and Belmont, J. W. (1992) Methylation of HpaII and HhaI sites near the polymorphic CAG repeat in the human androgen-receptor gene correlates with X chromosome inactivation. *Am. J. Hum. Genet.* **51,** 1229–1239.
8. Hornstra, I. K. and Yang, T. P. (1992) Multiple in vivo footprints are specific to the active allele of the X-linked human hypoxanthine phosphoribosyltransferase gene 5′ region: implications for X chromosome inactivation. *Mol. Cell. Biol.* **12,** 5345–5354.
9. Hendriks, R. W., Chen, Z. Y., Hinds, H., Schuurman, R. K. B., and Craig, I. W. (1992) An X chromosome inactivation assay based on differential methylation of a CpG island coupled to a VNTR polymorphism at the 5′ end of the monoamine oxidase A gene. *Hum. Mol. Genet.* **1(3),** 187–194.
10. Willman, C. L., Busque, L., Griffith, B. B., Favar, B. E., McClain, K. L., Duncan, M. H., and Gilliland, D. G. (1994) Langerhans'-cell histocytosis (Histocytosis X)—a clonal proliferative disease. *N. Engl. J. Med.* **331,** 154–160.
11. Peng, H. Z., Du, M. Q., Diss, T. C., Isaacson, P. G., and Pan, L. X. (1997) Clonality analysis in tumours of women by PCR amplification of X-linked genes. *J. Pathol.* **181,** 223–227.
12. Sambrook, J., Fritsch, E. F., and Maniatis, T. (1989) *Molecular Cloning: A Laboratory Manual*, Cold Spring Harbor Laboratory Press, Cold Spring Harbor, NY.
13. Mashal, R. D., Lester, S. C., and Sklar, J. (1993) Clonal analysis by study of X chromosome inactivation in formalin-fixed paraffin-embedded tissue. *Cancer Res.* **53,** 4676–4679.
14. Gale, R. E. and Wainscoat, J. S. (1993) Clonal analysis using X-linked DNA polymorphisms. *Br. J. Haematol.* **85,** 2–8.
15. Gale, R. E., Wheadon, H., Boulos, P., and Linch, D. C. (1994) Tissue specificity of X-chromosome inactivation patterns. *Blood* **10,** 2899–2905.
16. Gale, R. E. and Linch, D. C. (1998) Clonality studies in acute myeloid leukaemia. *Leukaemia* **12,** 117–120.

9

Fluorescent *In Situ* Hybridization

Evaluation for Ploidy and Gene Amplification

Susan Sheldon

1. Introduction

In situ hybridization was first described in the late 1960s by Pardue and Gall *(1)*, who hybridized mouse ribosomal DNA sequences to a mouse chromosome spread. The technique came into broader use with the description of DNA probes for various viral sequences, and in the late 1980s with the publications of Lichter and Ward *(2)*, Pinkel et al. *(3)*, and others *(4–7)* on the use of fluorescence *in situ* hybridization (FISH) probes. To perform FISH, or an *in situ* hybridization technique, a DNA sequence is prepared with its thymidine tagged with a compound such as fluorescein (direct labeling), biotin, or digoxigenin to create a probe for a given sequence located on a specific chromosome. Both the probe and the fixed cellular DNA are denatured using a combination of heat and formamide, and allowed to renature together. The nonspecifically bound probe is removed, and the probe-cellular DNA complex is visualized directly, with a fluorochrome-labeled avidin or a fluorochrome-tagged anti-digoxigenin. For general reviews of the technique, *see* **refs.** ***8–10***.

This chapter supplies background information for persons using commercially prepared FISH probes. As with many commercial reagents, they do not always perform as advertised, nor are the directions always complete or correct. To illustrate the differences between using unique sequence and repeated sequence probes, I discuss two examples. The first is an enumeration of the copies of several chromosomes using an alpha satellite probe in the placenta from a patient with a possible partial molar pregnancy. Three copies of mul-

From: *Methods in Molecular Medicine, vol. 49: Molecular Pathology Protocols*
Edited by: A. A. Killeen © Humana Press Inc., Totowa, NJ

tiple chromosomes are suggestive of a triploid (69 chromosome) karyotype *(11,12)*. This example also illustrates the issues associated with working with paraffin-embedded tissue *(13,14)*. The second example involves the quantitation of the number of copies of the gene for *N-myc* in a touch imprint from a patient with neuroblastoma.

In the first example, the distinction between a complete mole vs a partial mole vs hydropic changes secondary to a fetal demise can be difficult to make on histologic grounds alone. Yet, the management of the patient is quite different depending on the final diagnosis. Often the discovery of hydropic villi is made after the entire specimen is in formalin, precluding standard cytogenetic analysis. However, the question is raised: Is this a complete mole, with 46 chromosomes, or a partial mole, with 69, or merely a hydropic placenta with a badly macerated fetus *(11)*? FISH, using several alpha satellite probes, can at least approach the question of how many chromosomes are present. In the study patient (**Fig. 1**) an alpha satellite probe for the centromere of chromosome 7 was used; on scoring 250 nuclei, most had two fluorescent signals from the probe, suggesting either a complete mole or normal tissue.

In the second example, the *N-myc* gene is normally present on chromosome 2; there are two copies per nucleus. In patients with neuroblastoma, the gene will often be amplified or present in many copies in the tumor, but not in the patient's somatic cells. The DNA sequence within the gene itself is not amplified or highly repeated, however, so the probe used is a unique sequence probe. Those patients with multiple copies of this gene have an unfavorable prognosis, regardless of the histology or stage *(15–17)*. The study patient's tumor had multiple copies of the *N-myc* gene (**Fig. 2**) in the 20 cells scored. An unfavorable prognosis is associated with this finding.

There are several different types of DNA probes:

1. Alpha satellites—These sequences are at the centromeres of each chromosome. They are specific to that chromosome, so, e.g., there is a different alpha satellite for chromosome 1 and chromosome 10. Their sequences are highly repeated, making them "sticky" and subject to nonspecific binding. A high-stringency, posthybridization wash is required to achieve specificity, i.e., so that chromosome 1 probes do not bind to those of chromosome 10. These probes are among the easiest to work with, and are readily used for chromosome enumeration, provided that one is not looking for translocations.
2. Painting probes—These contain a collection of unique sequences specific for a given chromosome. The precise identity of the genes in this mixture of probes is not usually known. Depending on the density of the given sequences, the so-called paint may cover the entire chromosome with equal intensity. These probes are useful for characterizing chromosomal translocations, but are less useful for paraffin sections.

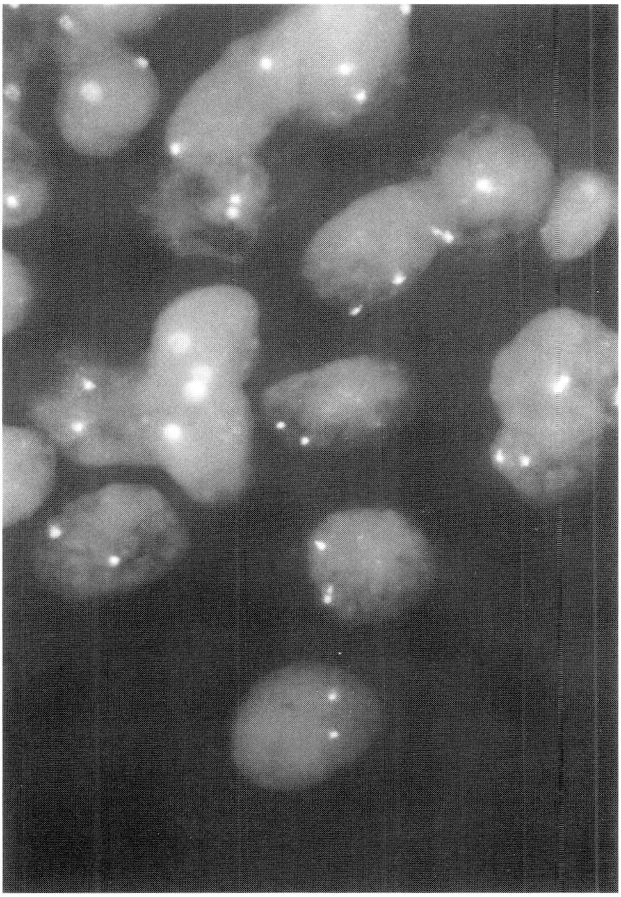

Fig. 1. Section through a formalin-fixed, paraffin-embedded section of a placenta showing hydropic changes consistent with a partial mole. Most nuclei show two brightly fluorescent signals, although not necessarily in the same focal plane.

3. Unique sequence probes—These are probes for specific genes or diseases closely linked to a known chromosomal location. They are available for a variety of microorganisms, genetic diseases (such as DiGeorge syndrome), and malignancies (such as *N-myc* in neuroblastoma). In general, probes for microdeletions associated with genetic diseases contain both a probe for the disorder of interest and a marker probe for the chromosome on which the disease gene is located. These probes require a posthybridization wash of lower stringency than that used for the alpha satellite probes.

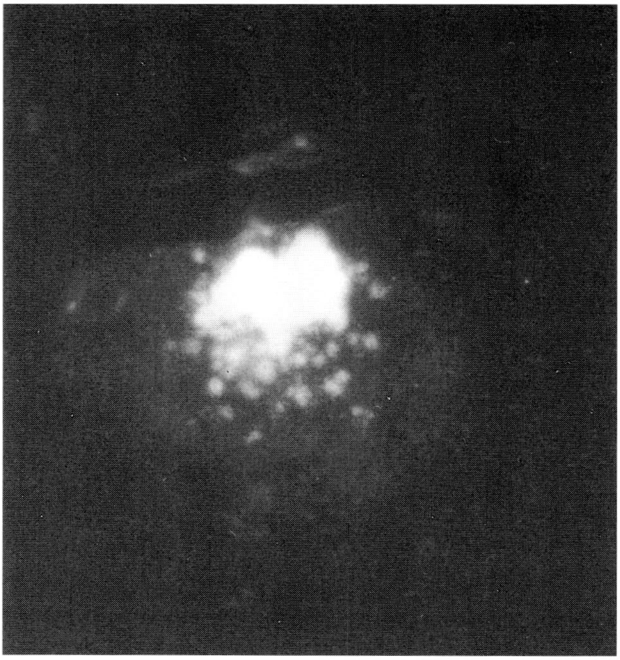

Fig. 2. Touch or imprint preparation of a neuroblastoma probed with *N-myc*. There are multiple bright signals over the nucleus, extending into the cytoplasm, suggesting that the gene is highly amplified. All cells should show two signals in the nucleus corresponding to the location of the normal gene.

Unlike Southern and polymerase chain reaction-based analyses, much of the specificity of FISH probes is derived from the posthybridization wash. The concept of "stringency" has been alluded to. This refers to the ability of DNA sequences to bind to one another when the sequence homology is not exact; for instance, sequences that are rich in adenine and thymine (A-T) and highly repeated will often hybridize to one another. To eliminate this nonspecific binding, one would use a high-stringency wash. Factors that increase the stringency and make it more difficult for inexactly matched hybrids to remain bound include increasing the temperature (from 37 to 43°C), increasing the formamide concentration (from 50 to 70%), and decreasing the salt concentration (from 0.4 to 0.25X saline sodium citrate [SSC]).

2. Materials

2.1. Tissues

For analysis of ploidy in placenta, cut routine 4-μ paraffin sections and place on positively charged slides, heat in a 60°C oven for no more than 15 min. The internal controls, both positive and negative, are blood cells present in the specimen, which should have a diploid number of signals.

For the evaluation of *N-myc* amplification, make a series of touch or imprint preparations of the neuroblastoma fresh tissue sample. One slide should be fixed and stained with Wright-Giemsa to confirm the presence of tumor, and the remaining slides are fixed as in **Subheading 3.1.2.**, then processed beginning with the denaturation step as in **Subheading 3.2.** Internal controls include the presence of two signals in the majority of cells (corresponding to the normal cellular gene) and the absence of multiple signals in stroma and nucleated blood cells.

2.2. Fixing Smears and Imprints

1. Methanol.
2. Glacial acetic acid.
3. A mixture of 3 parts methanol to 1 part acetic acid ("acid alcohol") is prepared and used within 1 h.

2.3. Dewaxing Paraffin Sections

1. Xylene.
2. Absolute ethanol, 95% ethanol, 80% ethanol, 70% ethanol.
3. Deionized water.

2.4. Thiocyanate Pretreatment of Paraffin Sections

1. 1 *M* Sodium thiocyanate solution, store protected from light.

2.5. Enzymatic Digestion of Paraffin Sections

Prepare the solutions using sterile reagents and containers; thaw at 37°C and use immediately.

1. Pepsin (4 mg/mL) in 0.2 *M* HCl (store stock at –20°C) or proteinase K (25 μg/mL) in phosphate-buffered saline (store stock at –20°C).

2.6. Denaturation

Prepare the following solutions using sterile water and containers:

1. 20X SSC: 3 *M* NaCl (175.32 g/L) and 0.3 *M* sodium citrate (88.23 g/L) in deionized water. Dissolve the two salts separately and mix. This is a stock solution. The pH will need to be adjusted to 6.8–7.0 on dilution.
2. 70% Formamide, pH 7.0, in 2X SSC (*see* **Note 1**).

2.7. Probes

The probes used are commercially available and should be used with the manufacturers' hybridization buffer. The exact ingredients of the hybridization buffers are proprietary, but they generally contain 50% formamide, 10% dextran sulfate, 0.01% sheared salmon sperm DNA in 2X SSC. The *N-myc* probe (Oncor, Gaithersburg, MD) does not require dilution. The alpha satellite or chromosome enumeration probe (Cytocell, Ltd., Oxfordshire, UK) is supplied affixed to a plastic cover slip and comes with hybridization buffer.

2.8. Hybridization

1. Hybridization chamber: These are available commercially, or you can use a plastic box with a lid or a glass baking dish covered with plastic wrap. Place one or two damp paper towels in the bottom to maintain humidity.
2. Rubber cement.
3. 37°C incubator without CO_2, 37°C oven, or hot plate.

2.9. Posthybridization Wash

1. 50% Formamide in 2X SSC, pH 7.0, or 0.4X SSC, pH 7.0.
2. Phosphate-buffered detergent (PBD): 130 m*M* NaCl, 7 m*M* dibasic sodium phosphate, 3 m*M* monobasic sodium phosphate, pH 6.8. Dissolve salts in deionized water in the order given, and then add 0.05% Triton X-100 (0.05 mL/L).

2.10. Localization of Probe

1. Antidigoxigenin antibody labeled with appropriate fluorochrome or avidin labeled with appropriate fluorochrome as supplied by the manufacturer.
2. Counterstains include 4',6-diamidino-2-phenylindole (DAPI) or propidium iodide in Antifade (Sigma, St. Louis, MO).

3. Methods

3.1. Preparing Target Tissue

When working with paraffin-embedded tissue, one must remove the paraffin (deparaffinization or dewaxing), the protein that has been crosslinked to the DNA, and the DNA crosslinks. Many manufacturers of DNA probes recommend that the sections not be baked at 60°C; this depends on the probe. It may be helpful to bake for 15 min or so to improve adhesion of the section to the slide. Slides should be positively charged, such as silanized slides, to improve adhesion.

3.1.1. Paraffin Sections

1. Dewax tissues by immersion in a series of Coplin jars at room temperature as follows: xylene, two changes for 10 min each; xylene:ethanol (50:50) 5 min; ethanol, two changes for 5 min each; air-dry at least 5 min.

2. For thiocyanate pretreatment, incubate slides for 10 min at 80°C in 1 *M* sodium thiocyanate. This can be done on a slide warmer. Flood the slide with about 2 mL of the reagent to avoid evaporation. Following incubation, rinse the slide with deionized water, two changes for 2 min each. Briefly drain the slides to remove excess water.
3. Incubate the slide at 37°C for 5–15 min in pepsin solution (this may require up to 45 min; *see* **Note 2**). The placental sample in the illustrated case was treated for 20 min.
4. Rinse with deionized water, two changes for 2 min each.
5. Dehydrate through graded alcohols (70, 80, 95, and 100%) and allow to air-dry. This is critical to avoid diluting the formamide in the denaturation step. Proceed to **Subheading 3.2.**

3.1.2. Smears and Imprints

1. Fix cells by placing the slides on a horizontal surface and covering the surface with acid alcohol for 2 min.
2. Drain excess liquid by tilting the slide.
3. Air-dry for at least 1 h.

3.2. Denaturation

Generally, both the probe and the target DNA will require denaturation, but this depends on the manufacturer's instructions. Some probes require no denaturation, and some will tolerate codenaturation, in which the probe solution is placed on the target area of the slide, a cover slip is sealed in place with rubber cement, and then the slide is heated to between 75 and 100°C for 2–10 min.

3.2.1. Denaturation Protocol

1. Place a heated solution of 70% formamide in 2X SSC, pH 7.0 (the pH is critical; *see* **Note 1**) in a Coplin jar as follows (*see* **Note 3**):
   a. For paraffin-embedded sections, denature for 8–12 min at 85°C. The section of placenta in the illustrated case (**Fig. 1**) was denatured for 10 min, although this step is not in the manufacturer's directions.
   b. For touch preparations, smears, and chromosome spreads, denature for 2 min at 72°C. The touch preparation of neuroblastoma in the illustrated case (**Fig. 2**) was denatured for 2 min.
2. Immediately place the slide in cold (–20°C) 70% ethanol to stop the denaturation. After 2 min (*see* **Note 4**), transfer to 90, 95, and 100% ethanol for 2 min each, and then allow to air-dry. Serial dehydration is crucial for paraffin sections, but immersion in 70% ethanol followed by absolute ethanol is adequate for thin smears, chromosome preparations, and so on.

3.3. Hybridization

Some probes require dilution into hybridization buffer. This buffer generally contains 70% formamide, carrier DNA, buffers, and dextran sulfate (to keep the solution in place on the slide). The last ingredient makes it difficult to pipet when cold. Bring the stock solution of probe to room temperature, briefly vortex, and centrifuge in a microfuge for 2 to 3 s to collect the contents at the bottom of the tube. If the probe is labeled with a fluorochrome, it may be useful to work in subdued light at this point (*see* **Note 5**). If the probe has passed its expiration date, altering the dilution is often useful (*see* **Note 6**).

Other probes require predenaturation and/or preannealing; the manufacturer will state this in the package insert. An aliquot is removed to a microcentrifuge tube and heated to 72°C for 5–10 min. It is then placed on ice for a few minutes (for alpha satellites, to prevent reannealing) or at 37°C for 30 min (for painting probes, to allow the repeated sequences to preanneal and prevent their nonspecific binding to all chromosomes).

The alpha satellite probe used on the section of placenta is usually denatured by a codenaturation step, as per the manufacturer's instructions. Codenaturation is a procedure by which the probe is placed on the slide, and it and the target DNA are denatured simultaneously and then allowed to hybridize. This technique must be used with probes supplied affixed to cover slips (Cytocell). **Notes 5–7** are applicable.

1. Alpha satellite probe: Place 10 µL of hybridization buffer on the section, apply the cover slip with the attached probe on the slide, and seal with rubber cement. Allow to dry for 5 min.
2. Place on a 75°C hot plate for 5 min to denature. Proceed to **step 4**.
3. *N-myc* probe: Place 10 µL of *N-myc* probe on the surface of the slide or smear and cover with a 22-mm^2 cover slip. Seal with rubber cement. This probe does not require denaturation or dilution.
4. Place the slides in the hybridization chamber, and incubate at 37°C for 30 min to overnight. For paraffin sections and new probes, it is useful to start with the longer incubation and decrease the time on subsequent trials. In these examples, the probe is incubated for 16 h.

3.4. Posthybridization Wash

1. Remove the rubber cement from the cover slip; often the cover slip comes off too. If it does not, swish the slide in a beaker of PBD to float the cover slip off.
2. Immediately place the slide in one of the following solutions (for both *N-myc* and the alpha satellite used in this example, the 50% formamide wash was used):
   a. 50% Formamide at 37°C, 15 min (paraffin sections, irrespective of the type of probe).
   b. 65% Formamide at 43°C, 15 min (alpha and beta satellite probes).
   c. 0.4X SSC at 72°C, 2 min, for directly labeled probes; this is the rapid wash technique (*see* **Note 8**).
3. Place the slides in 2X SSC at 37°C, 5 min; for the rapid SSC wash, follow with 30 s in PBD. Hybridized slides can be held in PBD at 4°C overnight prior to the next step.

3.5. Localization of Probe

1. Directly conjugated probes require only a rinse with PBD and mounting with a glass cover slip (*see* **step 5**).
2. Rinse the slides with PBD to remove the SSC. At this point, the placenta section is counterstained (*see* **step 5**).
3. Apply 15–20 µL of antidigoxigenin/fluorochrome conjugate or avidin/fluorochrome conjugate and cover with a plastic cover slip (*see* **Note 9**), and incubate at 37°C for 15–30 min. The *N-myc* probe required a fluorescein-conjugated avidin incubation for 30 min, but is now available directly conjugated.
4. Working in subdued light, remove the cover slip and rinse with PBD three times for 2 min each.
5. Apply counterstain such as propidium iodide for fluorescein-labeled probes or DAPI for probes labeled with a red fluorochrome, in "antifade." Cover with a glass cover slip (22 × 40 or 24 × 50 mm).

3.6. Visualization of Probe

A 100-W, mercury vapor light source is recommended, particularly for unique sequence probes (*see* **Note 11**). Locate the sections or cells under low power; air bubbles are in the same focal plane as the cells. The presence of label is scored under high power with either a ×100 or ×60 oil objective. For some larger probes, such as some alpha satellites a ×40 or ×50 water objective may be adequate. Score a minimum of 250–500 nuclei for interphase karyotype preparations. This is particularly necessary for tissue sections, because the entire nucleus may not be in the section. Cells to be scored for *N-myc* amplification should have at least two signals present in the nucleus, one for each gene on chromosome 2. Slides may be stored either before or after viewing (*see* **Note 11**). If results are unsatisfactory, many specimens can successfully be rehybridized (*see* **Note 12**).

4. Notes

1. Formamide becomes basic as it degrades; adjust the pH of the solution with HCl. Deionizing the formamide and freezing it in polypropylene tubes will increase the stability. Ultrapure formamide (BRL, Bethesda, MD) stored frozen will maintain its pH for years.
2. To determine whether the digestion is adequate, cover slip the wet slide and view with a fluorescent microscope using a fluorescein isothiocyanate filter. If there is green fluorescence, more digestion time is needed. If distinct nuclei are not seen, the tissue is overdigested.
3. For specimens to be denatured in formamide, it is useful to prewarm the slides on a slide warmer prior to placing them in the formamide. Denature no more than four slides at a time to maintain the temperature of the formamide, and recheck the temperature between batches of slides.

4. For most specimens, there is a trade-off between denaturation sufficient to allow the probe to bind and overdenaturation so that morphology is lost. In general, do not exceed 2 min unless the specimen is paraffin embedded. Older specimens can be denatured for 2.5–3 min.
5. For most commercial probes, subdued light is more than adequate. When working with only a few slides, and the fluorochrome is *not* directly conjugated, the relatively brief exposure to room light does not appear to cause loss of fluorescent signal.
6. Probes that are 6 mo to 1 yr or more past their stated expiration date have been used successfully by using a higher ratio of probe to diluent (twice the recommended amount of probe works well). If the probe does not require dilution, a larger volume (20 rather than 10 μL for a 22-mm^2 area) is often successful.
7. At least one vendor (Cytocell) supplies its probes bound to cover slips. These can be used quite successfully. After placing the cover slip over the hybridization solution on the target area of the slide and sealing with rubber cement, it is important to wait at least 5 min before doing the denaturation step, because the probe requires this time to dissolve off the cover slip.
8. A variety of posthybridization washes are described. For probes that are conjugated to a fluorochrome, a "quick wash" is preferable.
9. Some manufacturers of fluorochrome conjugates sell kits that include a variety of "blocking reagents" designed to reduce nonspecific binding of avidin to the tissue, buffers for washing, and polypropylene cover slips for use during incubation of the conjugate. "Plastic" cover slips, which reduce scratching of the specimen during this incubation, can be cut from Parafilm. A 22 × 50 mm surface area is preferable for this step.
10. Most commercial probes are designed for viewing with a 100- rather than 50-W mercury vapor lamp or equivalent. Signals may not be visible at 50 W. A 100-W bulb cannot be put in a 50-W lamp socket.
11. Slides can be stored in the dark in a refrigerator for 3–7 d. Some slides may be usable for several months if stored in a freezer. In either case, wipe the oil off the cover slip before storing, because it may be necessary to remount the cover slip prior to further viewing.
12. Most specimens can be rehybridized at least once. Remove the cover slip, rinse in PBD, and dehydrate. The existing probe will be removed during denaturation.

References

1. Pardue, M. and Gall, J. (1970) Chromosomal localization of mouse satellite DNA. *Science* **168,** 1356–1358.
2. Lichter, P. and Ward, D. (1990) Is non-isotopic in situ hybridization finally coming of age? *Nature* **354,** 93,94.
3. Pinkel, D., Landegent, J., Collins, C., Fuscoe, J., Seagraves, R., Lucas, J., and Gray, J. (1988) Fluorescence in situ hybridization with human chromosome specific libraries. *Proc. Natl. Acad. Sci. USA* **85,** 9138–9142.

4. Van Dilla, M., Deaven, L., Albright, K., et al. (1986). Human chromosome-specific DNA libraries: construction and availability. *Biotechnology* **4,** 537–552.
5. Trask, B. (1991) Fluorescence in situ hybridization: applications in cytogenetics and gene mapping. *Trends Genet.* **7,** 149–154.
6. Nelson, D., Ledbetter, S., Corbo, L., et al. (1989) Alu polymerase chain reaction: a method for rapid isolation of human-specific sequences from complex DNA sources. *Proc. Natl. Acad. Sci. USA* **86,** 6686–6690.
7. Ledbetter, S., Nelson, D., Warren, S., and Ledbetter, D. (1990) Rapid isolation of DNA probes within specific chromosome regions by interspersed repeated sequence polymerase chain reaction. *Genomics* **6,** 475–481.
8. Mark, H. F., Jenkins, R., and Miller, W. (1997) Current applications of molecular cytogenetic technologies. *Ann. Clin. Lab. Sci.* **27,** 47–56.
9. Wolman, S. (1995) Applications of fluorescent in situ hybridization (FISH) to genetic analysis of human tumors. *Pathol. Annu.* **30(pt. 2),** 227–243.
10. Wolfe, K. and Herrington, C. (1997) Interphase cytogenetics and pathology: a tool for diagnosis and research. *J. Pathol.* **181,** 359–361.
11. Poddighe, P., Ramaekers, F., and Hopman, A. (1992) Interphase cytogenetics of tumors. *J. Pathol.* **166,** 215–224.
12. Hopman, A., van Hooren, E., van de Kaa, C., Vooijs, P., and Ramaekers, F. (1991) Detection of numerical chromosome aberrations using in situ hybridization in paraffin sections of routinely processed bladder cancers. *Mod. Pathol.* **4,** 503–513.
13. van de Kaa, C., Nelson, K., Ramaekers, F., Vooijs, P., and Hopman, A. (1991) Interphase cytogenetics in paraffin sections of routinely processed hydatidiform moles and hydropic abortions. *J. Pathol.* **165,** 281–287.
14. Long, A., Mueller, J., Schwartz, J., Barrett, K., Schwartz, R., and Wolfe, H. (1992) High specificity in situ hybridization. *Diagn. Mol. Pathol.* **1,** 45–57.
15. Brodeur, G., Seeger, R. C., Schwab, M., et al. (1984) Amplification of N-myc in untreated human neuroblastomas correlates with advanced disease stage. *Science* **224,** 1121–1124.
16. Seeger, R., Brodeur, G., Sather, H., et al. (1985) Association of multiple copies of the N-myc oncogene with rapid progression of neuroblastomas. *New Engl. J. Med.* **313,** 1111–1116.
17. Shiloh, Y., Shipley, J., Brodeur, G., et al. (1985) Differential amplification, assembly, and relocation of multiple DNA sequences in human neuroblastomas and neuroblastoma cell lines. *Proc. Natl. Acad. Sci. USA* **82,** 3761–3765.

10

HER-2/*neu* Oncogene Amplification Determined by Fluorescence *In Situ* Hybridization

Jeffrey S. Ross, Christine E. Sheehan, and Jonathan A. Fletcher

1. Introduction

1.1. Background and Clinical Significance

The proto-oncogene HER-2/*neu* (C-*erb*B-2) has been localized to chromosome 17q and encodes a transmembrane tyrosine kinase growth factor receptor. The name for the HER-2 protein is derived from human epidermal growth factor receptor (EGFR) because it features substantial homology with the EGFR ***(1,2)***. HER-2/*neu* gene amplification has been associated with the development of breast cancer in animal models ***(1)***. The HER-2/neu protein is a component of a four-member family of closely related growth factor receptors including EGFR or HER-1 (*erb*-B1), HER-2 (*erb*-B2), HER-3 (*erb*-B3), and HER-4 (*erb*-B4) ***(3)***. In addition to its association with disease outcome in gastrointestinal, pulmonary, genitourinary, and other neoplasms, amplification of the HER-2/*neu* gene or overexpression of the HER-2/neu protein has been identified in from 10 to 34% of breast cancers ***(4–50)***. The techniques used to evaluate HER-2/*neu* status in breast cancer have included gene-based assays such as Southern and slot blotting, polymerase chain reaction methods, and, more recently, *in situ* hybridization featuring both fluorescent and nonfluorescent techniques ***(4–50)***.

Given that Southern and slot-blotting procedures are expensive, and time-consuming, and require fresh or frozen tissue, the fluorescence *in situ* hybridization (FISH) technique was implemented to measure HER-2/*neu* gene copy number on formalin-fixed, archival specimens (**Fig. 1**). In two previous studies, the FISH method was found to be more sensitive than Southern blotting for the detection of HER-2/*neu* gene amplification ***(48,51)***. The FISH technique

From: *Methods in Molecular Medicine, vol. 49: Molecular Pathology Protocols*
Edited by: A. A. Killeen © Humana Press Inc., Totowa, NJ

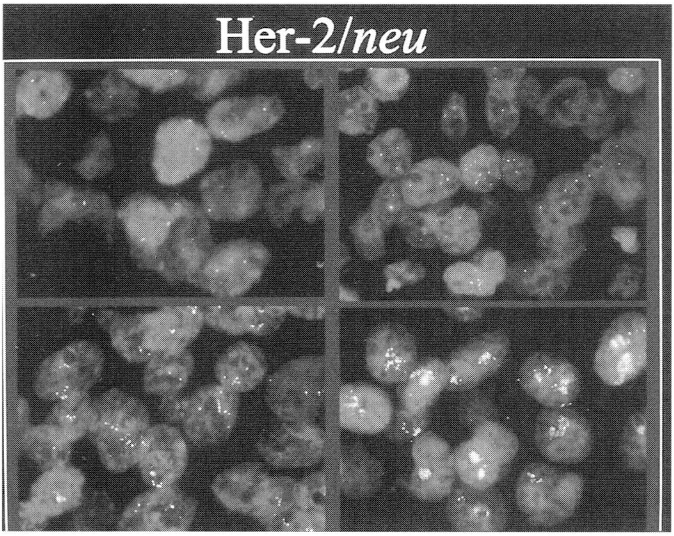

Fig. 1. Four-part photomicrograph of HER-2/*neu* gene amplification detection by FISH. (Upper left) Unamplified case with a mean signal count of 1.5 signals per nucleus; (upper right) breast cancer with a borderline result featuring a mean signal count of 4.1 signals per nucleus; (lower left) significantly amplified breast tumor with a mean signal count of 17.5 signals per nucleus. (Lower right) Another example of a significantly amplified breast cancer with a mean HER-2/*neu* signal count of 24.9 signals per nucleus.

has outperformed a number of solid matrix blotting techniques designed to detect HER-2/*neu* DNA and RNA as well as immunohistochemistry designed to detect HER-2/neu protein in formalin-fixed, paraffin-embedded tissues ***(48)***. The FISH technique has been described as a rapid, reproducible, and extremely reliable method of detecting HER-2/*neu* gene amplification ***(48)***. In addition, FISH can readily be performed on archived paraffin blocks stored for long periods and has been successfully applied to fine-needle aspiration biopsies ***(52)***. In a study using the FISH method, Xing et al. ***(43)*** reported that HER-2/*neu* gene amplification was more predictive than lymph node status and was the strongest independent predictor of outcome in breast cancer. In a recently published study, Press et al. ***(48)*** successfully utilized FISH on archived specimens to predict short- and long-term outcome in node-negative breast cancer. This study employed a two-category system of HER-2/*neu* amplification status: four or fewer signals per nucleus = unamplified and greater than four signals per nucleus = amplified. A recent study derived from a subset of the cases reported by Press et al. ***(48)*** features a three-tiered amplification scoring system with an equivocal borderline amplified group featuring greater than 3 but less than 10 signals per nucleus ***(49)***. The results of the three-tiered system are similar to those of the two-tiered system and confirm the significant association of HER-2/*neu* gene amplification with early recurrence, recurrence at any time, and disease-related death in node-negative breast cancer initially treated by surgery alone. Both the two-tiered and the three-tiered amplification scoring systems similarly found the adverse impact of HER-2/*neu* gene amplification to be independent of tumor size, grade, and estrogen receptor status ***(48,49)***. In another study using a two-tiered system, HER-2/*neu* gene amplification again predicted disease-related death independent of the original nodal status in a combined series of node-negative and node-positive patients ***(50)***.

*1.2. Comparison of Methods of Detection of HER-2/*neu *Abnormalities*

Immunohistochemistry has been the predominant method utilized to measure HER-2/neu protein abnormalities in breast cancer. However, significant issues can have an impact on immunohistochemistry, especially when performed on archival fixed paraffin-embedded tissues. Many laboratories perform the staining on referred specimens and cannot control the time and nature of tissue fixation, the method of tissue processing, and the temperature of the paraffin-embedding procedure, all of which can influence HER-2/neu protein antigen loss. Prolonged storage can also be a problem, and significant loss of tumor-marker immunostaining intensity has been identified, particularly when specimens are stored as unstained slides ***(53)***. The impact of the fixative has been considered and shown to have a significant impact on HER-2/neu immunostaining ***(54)***. Using cell-line controls, different antibodies have differing staining patterns depending on how the cells were fixed ***(54)***. Studies of the various commercially available antibodies have also demonstrated a wide variety of sensitivity and specificity for fixed paraffin-embedded tissues. In a study by Busmanis et al. ***(55)***, a panel of six antibodies showed a wide variation in staining patterns including occasional cytoplasmic immunoreactivity (a pattern considered to be nonspecific by most investigators). In a study of a large panel of antibodies, Press et al. ***(56)*** similarly reported a wide range of detection rates using a large tissue block containing multiple breast tumors. The use of nonstandardized antigen retrieval (amplification) techniques further compounds the problem and introduces the potential for false-positive staining. The lack of an agreed-upon scoring system for interpreting HER-2/neu protein immunohistochemistry is another significant issue. Recent attempts to reach consensus on the interpretation of immunohistochemical staining show promise for dealing with this issue. Note that immunohistochemistry on frozen sections has shown substantial correlation with HER-2/*neu* gene–based assays ***(48)*** and would be an ideal method of detection if it were not obviously limited by the general lack of availability of fresh or frozen material for this approach.

The enzyme-linked immunosorbent assay (ELISA) technique when performed on tumor cytosols made from fresh tissue samples avoids the potential antigen damage associated with fixation, embedding, and uncontrolled storage. In three published studies including 315 patients, ELISA-based measurements of HER-2/neu protein in tumor cytosols have uniformly correlated with disease outcome ***(39,41,43)***. However, the small size of breast cancers diagnosed in an era of enhanced screening generally precludes tumor tissue ELISA methods because insufficient tumor tissue is available to produce a cytosol. Western blotting can also detect HER-2/neu protein overexpression in both tumor cytosols and archival tissues, but is generally cumbersome and impractical for routine specimens. Southern and slot blotting were the first gene-based HER-2/*neu* detection methods used in breast cancer specimens. These methods can be significantly hampered when tumor cell DNA extracted from the primary carcinoma sample is diluted by DNA from benign breast tissue and inflammatory cells. The FISH technique allows simultaneous morphologic assessment, such that evaluation of gene amplification can be restricted to invasive carcinoma cells. This approach has been proven to be more sensitive than Southern analysis for the detection of HER-2/neu abnormalities in breast cancer ***(48)***. Of the 15 published gene-based studies of HER-2/*neu* in breast cancer, the 2 noncorrelating studies used Southern (50 patients) and slot-blotting (362 patients) methods. As already mentioned, the FISH-based assays of HER-2/*neu* gene amplification have uniformly predicted an adverse disease outcome.

In summary, both HER-2/*neu* gene amplification and protein overexpression have been associated with an adverse outcome in breast cancer with gene-based methods and protein detection on fresh or frozen samples obtaining the most consistent results. Many of the published studies have used a relatively short clinical follow-up period for a disease prone to late recurrences. Thus, abnormalities of HER-2/neu may actually identify patients at greater risk for early disease relapse, and evidence confirming the ability of the marker to predict overall relapse rates must await continuing long-term studies of tumor outcome.

The following technique for the determination of amplification of the HER-2/*neu* gene in breast cancer by FISH is based on the Oncor® INFORM™ HER-2/*neu* Gene Detection System using a unique sequence biotinylated probe (Oncor, Gaithersburg, MD) ***(26)***. Many of the materials are included in this system.

2. Materials

2.1. Buffers and Solutions

1. Pretreatment powder.
2. Protein digesting enzyme (proteinase K).
3. 20X saline sodium citrate (SSC): 3 *M* NaCl, 0.3 *M* sodium citrate.
4. 10X phosphate-buffered detergent (PBD).
5. Biotinylated HER-2/neu DNA probe.
6. Detection reagent (fluorescein-labeled avidin).
7. 4′,6-Diamidino-2-phenylindole (DAPI)/antifade counterstain.
8. Antifade.
9. Plastic cover slips.
10. Distilled deionized water.
11. Sterile deionized water.
12. Ethanol: 70, 80, 90, and 100%.
13. Xylene.
14. 6 *N* HCl.

2.2. Laboratory Supplies

1. Silanized slides.
2. Glass Coplin jars.
3. Glass cover slips.
4. Micropipettor tips.
5. Microcentrifuge tubes.
6. Microcentrifuge tube rack and float.
7. Graduated cylinders.
8. 50-mL Polypropylene tubes.

2.3. Equipment

1. Fluorescence microscope equipped with the following:
   a. 100-W Mercury arc light source.
   b. DAPI/fluorescein isothiocyanate (FITC)/Texas Red triple band-pass filter set.
   c. DAPI filter set.
   d. FITC/Texas Red dual band-pass filter set.
   e. ×10 dry, ×40 dry, and ×100 oil fluorescence objectives.
   f. Nonfluorescing immersion oil.
2. Humidified chambers.
3. Incubator at 37 ± 2°C.
4. Oven at 65 ± 5°C.
5. Water baths and ice baths.
6. Calibrated thermometers.
7. Adjustable micropipettors.
8. Vortex.
9. pH meter.
10. Balance.
11. Microcentrifuge.

2.4. Preparation of Reagent

1. 2X SSC: Add 180 mL of 20X SSC to 1620 mL of deionized water. Adjust the pH of the 2X SSC to 7.0 with 6 *N* HCI. The reagent may be prepared in advance and stored in a glass or plastic vessel at 18 to 25°C until the expiration date of the 20X SSC. Check and adjust the pH to 7.0 before use.
2. Protein-digesting enzyme stock solution (25 mg/mL): Add 4 mL of sterile distilled water to 100 mg of lyophilized protein-digesting enzyme. Aliquot 400 mL each into microcentrifuge tubes. Store this stock solution at –20°C until expiration of powder.
3. Protein-digesting enzyme working solution (0.25 mg/mL): Add 400 mL of protein-digesting enzyme stock solution to 40 mL 2X SSC. This solution must be used the same day as it is diluted and heated.
4. 1X PBD: Add 200 mL of thoroughly mixed 10X PBD to 1800 mL of distilled water. Store at 4°C until the expiration date of the stock.

3. Methods

3.1. Preparation of Specimen Slides

1. Cut 4-μm sections and apply to silanized or positively charged slides.
2. Allow to air-dry. Bake at 65 ± 5°C overnight.
3. Deparaffinize in xylene.
4. Wash in 100% ethanol two times for 2 min each.
5. Air-dry.

3.2. Pretreatment

1. Immerse a maximum of four slides in a Coplin jar containing 40 mL of prewarmed 30% pretreatment solution in a 43 ± 2°C water bath for 15 min.
2. Wash twice in 40 mL of 2X SSC at room temperature for 1 min.
3. Dehydrate in 70, 80, 90, and 100% ethanol for 2 min each.
4. Air-dry.

3.3. Protein Digestion

1. Immerse 40 mL of prewarmed protein digesting enzyme working solution in a 37°C water bath for 10 min.
2. Wash twice in 40 mL of 2X SSC at room temperature for 1 min.
3. Dehydrate in 70, 80, 90, and 100% ethanol for 2 min each.
4. Air-dry.

3.4. Denaturation and Hybridization of Probe

1. Prewarm the HER-2/*neu* probe for 5 min at 37°C.
2. Apply 10 μL of probe to each denatured tissue section and cover with a 25 × 25 mm cover slip.
3. Hybridize at 37°C in a humidified chamber for 12–16 h.

3.5. Posthybridization Wash

1. Carefully remove the cover slip.
2. Immerse in 2X SSC at 72°C for 5 min (*see* **Note 1**).
3. Transfer to 40 mL of 1X PBD at room temperature.

3.6. Detection

1. Remove the slide from the 1X PBD and drain excess fluid without drying the section.
2. Add 60 µL of detection reagent. Cover with a plastic cover slip.
3. Perform fluorescence detection and counterstaining with fluorescein-labeled avidin, antiavidin antibody, and DAPI/antifade as described in the Oncor INFORM HER-2/*neu* Gene Detection System package insert.
4. Wash three times in 40 mL of 1X PBD at room temperature for 2 min each.

3.7. Nuclear Counterstaining and Storage

1. Remove the slide from the PBD and drain excess fluid without drying the section.
2. Add 20 µL of DAPI/antifade to each slide.
3. Cover with a glass cover slip.
4. Store in the dark at –15 to –25°C for up to 5 d before scoring.

3.8. Scoring

1. Use the DAPI filter set and ×10 or ×40 objective to confirm that the tissue section contains areas of invasive breast carcinoma.
2. Use the DAPI/FITC/Texas Red triple band-pass filter set and ×100 oil immersion objective to confirm the FITC signal is present (*see* **Note 2**).
3. Record the number of signals over 20 nonoverlapping tumor cell nuclei from each of 2 noncontinguous fields.
4. Calculate the mean number of signals per tumor cell nucleus.

3.9. Reporting Results

If the mean signal count is ≤4, report as unamplified (*see* **Note 3**). If the mean signal count is >4, report as amplified.

4. Notes

1. Place a clean thermometer in the solution for accurate temperature monitoring. The temperature will drop approx 1°C for each slide placed in the solution. Therefore, adjust the initial temperature accordingly and do not remove the slides from 37°C hybridization until ready to place immediately into 2X SSC, to prevent slides from cooling down and resulting in greater temperature drop.
2. Use the DAPI filter set to select non-overlapping nuclei. Slide to dual or triple band pass to count the signals. Background signals are generally smaller and

finer ("dustlike") whereas actual signals are slightly larger and brighter, as well as on a different plane of focus. To begin signal counting, focus very slowly through the background plane until the nuclear border and signal come into focus, begin counting, and count all the signals as you focus through the nucleus. Some cells with no signal are expected in cut sections. Record more than 20 signals as 20+, but use 20 in the calculation of the mean.

3. Although the test is reported as "not amplified" if the mean signal per nucleus score is 4.0 or less and "amplified" if the mean score is greater than 4.0, it is customary to add a comment when the mean score is between 3.5 and 4.5 signals per nucleus. This comment may include a statement such as "Borderline result. Please interpret in concert with other breast cancer prognostic factors such as tumor size, tumor grade, and hormone receptor status." For lymph node–negative breast cancer, it is anticipated that approx 5–8% of the tumors will fall into the "borderline" 3.5–4.5 signals per nucleus range. Of the lymph node–negative tumors with mean signal counts outside the borderline range, approx 18–28% will be amplified and 72–82% will be unamplified.

References

1. Slamon, D. J. and Clark, G. M. (1988) Amplification of C-ERB-B2 and aggressive breast tumors? *Science* **240,** 1795–1798.
2. De Potter, C. R. (1994) The neu oncogene: more than a prognostic indicator? *Hum. Pathol.* **25,** 1264–1268.
3. Lupu, R., Cardillo, M., Harris, L., et al. (1995) Interaction between ERB-receptors and heregulin in breast cancer tumor progression and drug resistance. *Semin. Cancer Biol.* **6,** 135–145.
4. Slamon, D. J., Clark, G. M., Wong, S. G., et al. (1987) Human breast cancer: correlation of relapse and survival with amplification of the Her-2/*neu* oncogene. *Science* **235,** 177–182.
5. Berger, M. S., Locher, G. W., Saurer, S., et al. (1988) Correlation of c-*erb* B2 gene amplification and protein expression in human breast carcinoma with nodal status and nuclear grading. *Cancer Res.* **48,** 1238–1243.
6. van de Vivjer, M. J., Peterse, J. L., Mooi, W. J., et al. (1988) *Neu*-protein overexpression in breast cancer. *N. Engl. J. Med.* **319,** 1239–1245.
7. Heintz, N. H., Leslie, K. O., Rogers, L. A., and Howard, P. L. (1990) Amplification of the c-*erb* B-2 oncogene in prognosis of breast adenocarcinoma. *Arch. Pathol. Lab. Med.* **114,** 160–163.
8. Tsuda, H., Hirohashi, S., Shimosato, Y., et al. (1990) Correlation between histologic grade of malignancy and copy number of *c-erbB-2* gene in breast carcinoma: a retrospective analysis of 176 cases. *Cancer* **65,** 1794–1800.
9. Borg, A., Tandon, A. K., Sigurdsson, H., et al. (1990) HER-2/neu amplification predicts poor survival in node-positive breast cancer. *Cancer Res.* **50,** 4332–4337.
10. Paik, S., Hazan, R., Fisher, E. R., et al. (1990) Pathologic findings from the National Surgical Adjuvant Breast and Bowel Project: prognostic significance of erb B2 protein overexpression in primary breast cancer. *J. Clin. Oncol.* **8,** 103–112.

11. Battifora, H., Gaffey, M., Esteban, J., et al. (1991) Immunohistochemical assay of *neu/c-erb B-2* oncogene product in paraffin-embedded tissues in early breast cancer: retrospective follow-up study of 245 stage I and II cases. *Mod. Pathol.* **4,** 466–474.
12. Kallioniemi, O. P., Holli, K., Visakorpi, T., et al. (1991) Association of C-erb B2 protein over-expression with high rate of cell proliferation, increased risk of visceral metastasis and poor long-term survival in breast cancer. *Int. J. Cancer* **49,** 650–655.
13. Clark, G. M. and McGuire, W. L. (1991) Follow-up study of HER-2/neu amplification in primary breast cancer. *Cancer Res.* **51,** 944–948.
14. Lovekin, C., Ellis, I. O., Locker, A., et al. (1991) C-erb B2 oncoprotein expression in primary and advanced breast cancer. *Br. J. Cancer* **63,** 439–443.
15. McCann, A. H., DeDervan, T. A., O'Regan, M., et al. (1991) Prognostic significance of C-erb B2 and estrogen receptor status in human breast cancer. *Cancer Res.* **51,** 3296–3303.
16. Dykens, R., Corbett, I. P., Henry, J., et al. (1991) Long term survival in breast cancer related to overexpression of the C-erb B2 oncoprotein: an immunohistochemical study using monoclonal antibody NCL-CB11. *J. Pathol.* **163,** 105–110.
17. Rilke, F., Colnaghi, M. I., Cascinelli, N., et al. Prognostic significance of HER-2/neu expression in breast cancer and its relationship to other prognostic factors. *Int. J. Cancer* **49,** 44–49.
18. Winstanley, J., Cooke, T., Murray, G. D., et al. (1991) The long term prognostic significance of C-erb B2 in primary breast cancer. *Br. J. Cancer* **63,** 447–450.
19. O'Reilly, S. M., Barnes, D. M., Camplejohn, R. S., et al. (1991) The relationship between C-erb B2 expression, and s-phase fraction in prognosis in breast cancer. *Br. J. Cancer* **63,** 444–446.
20. Paterson, M. C., Dietrich, K. D., Danyluk, J., et al. (1991) Correlation between C-erb B2 amplification and risk of recurrent disease in node-negative breast cancer. *Cancer Res.* **51,** 556–567.
21. Toikkanen, S., Helin, H., Isola, J., et al. (1992) Prognostic significance of Her-2 oncoprotein expression in breast cancer: a 30-year follow up. *J. Clin. Oncol.* **10,** 1044–1048.
22. Molina, R., Ciocca, D. R., Candon, A. K., et al. (1992) Expression of HER-2/neu oncoprotein in breast cancer: a comparison of immunohistochemical and western blot techniques. *Anticancer Res.* **12,** 1965–1991.
23. Noguchi, M., Koyasaki, M., Ohta, N., et al. (1992) c-*erb* B-2 oncoprotein expression versus internal mammary lymph node metastases as additional prognostic factors in patients with axillary lymph node-positive breast cancer. *Cancer* **69,** 2953–2960.
24. Allred, D. C., Clark, G. M., Tandon, A. K., et al. (1992) HER-2/neu node-negative breast cancer: prognostic significance of overexpression influenced by the presence of in-situ carcinoma. *J. Clin. Oncol.* **10,** 599–605.
25. Babiak, J., Hugh, J., and Poppeme, S. (1992) Significance of c-*erb* B-2 amplification in DNA aneuploidy: analysis in 78 patients with node-negative breast cancer. *Cancer* **70,** 770–776.

26. Tiwari, R. K., Borgen, P. I., Wong, G. Y., et al. (1992) HER-2/*neu* amplification and overexpression in primary human breast cancer is associated with early metastasis. *Anticancer Res.* **12,** 419–426.
27. Gusterson, B. A., Gelber, R. D., Goldhirsch, A., et al. (1992) Prognostic importance of C-erb B2 expression in breast cancer. *J. Clin. Oncol.* **10,** 1049–1056.
28. Bianchi, S., Paglierani, M., Zampi, G., et al. (1993) Prognostic significance of C-erb B2 expression in node negative breast cancer. *Brit. J. Cancer* **67,** 625–629.
29. Press, M. F., Pike, M. C., Chazin, V. R., et al. (1993) Her-2/*neu* expression in node-negative breast cancer: direct tissue quantification by computerized image analysis and association of overexpression with increased risk of recurrent disease. *Cancer Res.* **53,** 4960–4970.
30. Seshadri, R., Firgaira, F. A., Horsfall, D. J., et al. (1993) Clinical significance of Her-2/*neu* oncogene amplification in primary breast cancer. *J. Clin. Oncol.* **11,** 1936–1942.
31. Descotes, F., Pavy, J. J., and Adessi, G. L. (1993) Human breast cancer: correlation study between Her-2/*neu* amplification and prognostic factors in an unselected population. *Anticancer Res.* **13,** 119–124.
32. Giai, M., Roagna, R., Ponzone, R., et al. (1994) Prognostic and predictive relevance of C-erb B2 and ras expression in node positive and negative breast cancer. *Anticancer Res.* **14,** 1441–1450.
33. Muss, H. B., Thor, A. D., Berry, D. A., et al. (1994) C-erb-B2 expression and response to adjuvant therapy in women with node-positive early breast cancer. *N. Engl. J. Med.* **330,** 1260–1266.
34. Tetu, B. and Brisson, J. (1994) Prognostic significance of Her-2/*neu* oncogene expression in node-positive breast cancer: the influence of the pattern of immunostaining and adjuvant therapy. *Cancer* **73,** 2359–2365.
35. Hartmann, L. C., Ingle, J. N., Wold, L. E., et al. (1994) Prognostic value of CerbB2 overexpression in axillary lymph node positive breast cancer: results from a randomized adjuvant treatment protocol. *Cancer* **74,** 2956–2963.
36. Jacquemeier, J., Penault-Llorca, P., Viens, P., et al. (1994) Breast cancer response to adjuvant chemotherapy in correlation with *erb* B2 and p53 expression. *Anticancer Res.* **14,** 2773–2778.
37. Marks, J. R., Humphrey, P. A., Wu, K., et al. (1994) Overexpression of p53 and Her-2/*neu* proteins as prognostic markers in early stage breast cancer. *Ann. Surg.* **219,** 332–341.
38. Rosen, P. P., Lesser, M. L., Arroyo, C. D., et al. (1995) Immunohistochemical detection of Her-2/*neu* expression in patients with axillary lymph node-negative breast carcinoma: a study of epidemiologic risk factors, histologic features and prognosis. *Cancer* **75,** 1320–1326.
39. Quenel, N., Wafflart, J., Bonichon, F., et al. (1995) The prognostic value of c-erbB2 in primary breast carcinomas: a study on 942 cases. *Breast Cancer Res. Treat.* **35,** 283–291.

40. Sundblad, A. S., Pellicer, E. M., and Ricci, L. (1996) Carcinoembryonic expression in stages I and II breast cancer: its relationship with clinicopathologic factors. *Hum. Pathol.* **27,** 297–300.
41. O'Malley, F. P., Saad, Z., Kerkvliet, N., et al. (1996) The predictive power of semiquantitative immunohistochemical assessment of p53 and C-*erb*B2 in lymph node-negative breast cancer. *Hum. Pathol.* **27,** 955–963.
42. Hieken, T. J., Mehta, R. R., Shilkaitis, A., et al. (1996) Her-2/neu and p53 expression in breast cancer: valid prognostic markers when assessed by direct immunoassay, but not by immunochemistry. *Proc. Annu. Meet. Am. Soc. Clin. Oncol.* **15,** A113.
43. Xing, W. R., Gilchrist, K. W., Harris, C. P., et al. (1996) FISH detection of HER-2/neu oncogene amplification in early onset breast cancer. *Breast Cancer Res. Treat.* **39,** 203–212.
44. Dittadi, R., Brazzale, A., Pappagallo, G., et al. (1997) ErbB2 assay in breast cancer: possibly improved clinical information using a quantitative method. *Anticancer Res.* **17,** 1245–1247.
45. Fernandez Acenero, M. J., Farina Gonzalez, J., and Arangoncillo Ballesteros, P. (1997) Immunohistochemical expression of p53 and c-erbB-2 in breast carcinoma: relation with epidemiologic factors, histologic features and prognosis. *Gen. Diagn. Pathol.* **142,** 289–296.
46. Eissa, S., Khalifa, A., el-Gharib, A., et al. (1997) Multivariate analysis of DNA ploidy, p53, c-erbB-2 proteins, EGFR, and steroid hormone receptors for short-term prognosis in breast cancer. *Anticancer Res.* **17,** 3091–3097.
47. Charpin, C., Garcia, S., Bouvier, C., et al. (1997) c-erbB-2 oncoprotein detected by automated quantitative immunocytochemistry in breast carcinomas correlates with patients' overall and disease-free survival. *Br. J. Cancer* **75,** 1667–1673.
48. Press, M. J., Bernstein, L., Thomas, P. A., et al. (1997) Her-2/*neu* gene amplification characterized by fluorescence in situ hybridization: poor prognosis in node-negative breast carcinomas. *J. Clin. Oncol.* **15,** 2894–2904.
49. Ross, J. S., Muraca, P. J., Jaffe, D., et al. (1998) Multivariate analysis of prognostic factors in lymph node negative breast cancer. *Mod. Pathol.* **11,** 26A.
50. Depowski, P. L., Brien, T. P., Sheehan, C. E., et al. (1998) Prognostic significance of $p34^{cdc2}$ cyclin dependent kinase and MIB1 overexpression, and HER-2/*neu* gene amplification detected by fluorescence in-situ hybridization in breast cancer. *Mod. Pathol.* **11,** 18A.
51. Pauletti, G., Godolphin, W., Press, M. F., et al. (1996) Detection and quantitation of HER-2/*neu* gene amplification in human breast cancer archival material using fluorescence *in situ* hybridization. *Oncogene* **13,** 63–72.
52. Sauter, G., Feichter, G., Torhorst, J., et al.(1996) Fluorescence in-situ hybridization for detecting ERBB-2 amplification in breast tumor fine needle aspiration biopsies. *Acta Cytol.* **40,** 164–173.
53. Jacobs, T. W., Prioleau, J. E., Stillman, I. E., et al. (1996) Loss of tumor marker-immunostaining intensity on stored paraffin slides of breast cancer. *J. Natl. Cancer Inst.* **88,** 1054–1059.

54. Penault-Llorca, F., Adelaide, J., Houvenaeghel, G., et al. (1994) Optimization of immunohistochemical detection of ERBB2 in human breast cancer: impact of fixation. *J. Pathol.* **173,** 65–75.
55. Busmanis, I., Feleppa, F., Jones, A., et al. (1994) Analysis of C-erb B2 expression using a panel of six commercially available antibodies. *Pathology* **26,** 261–267.
56. Press, M. F., Hung, G., Godolphin, W., et al. (1994) Sensitivity of Her-2/*neu* antibodies in archival tissue samples: potential source of error in immunohistochemical studies of oncogene expression. *Cancer Res.* **54,** 2771–2777.

11

A Nested Reverse Transcriptase-Polymerase Chain Reaction Assay to Detect BCR/*abl*

Linda M. Wasserman

1. Introduction

Chronic myelogenous leukemia (CML), a clonal myeloproliferative disorder in adults, and some pediatric and adult acute lymphoblastic leukemias (ALLs) are characterized by the presence of a Philadelphia chromosome, t(9;22)(q34;q11) *(1)*. In this chromosomal translocation, exons from a major breakpoint cluster region (M-bcr), located on chromosome 22q11, are joined to the c-*abl* proto-oncogene, located on chromosome 9q34. When this chromosomal translocation occurs in a hematopoietic stem cell, the resulting BCR/*abl* fusion protein has increased tyrosine kinase activity and a transforming capacity that is critical to the pathogenesis of these leukemic disorders.

The Philadelphia chromosome can be detected in 95% of adults with CML and 23–50% of adult ALL and 11% of childhood ALL *(2)*. In the M-bcr, most translocations occur within intronic sequences between the second and fourth exons. Most translocations in c-*abl* occur across a large region 5′ to c-*abl* exon II. Although breakpoints in the M-bcr and c-*abl* can be widely distributed along their respective chromosomes, mRNA processing of the fusion transcript consistently links either M-bcr exons b1–b3 or exons b1 and b2 to c-*abl* exon II, or occasionally to c-*abl* exon Ia (*see* **Fig. 1**). Because of the consistent processing of the fusion transcript, reverse transcriptase-polymerase chain reaction (RT-PCR) assays, which use mRNA as a starting material, can readily detect almost all Philadelphia chromosome translocations despite the variability in the location of chromosomal breakpoints.

Detection of the BCR/*abl* fusion transcript by RT-PCR is used clinically either to confirm a CML or ALL diagnosis or to detect and monitor the pres-

From: *Methods in Molecular Medicine, vol. 49: Molecular Pathology Protocols*
Edited by: A. A. Killeen © Humana Press Inc., Totowa, NJ

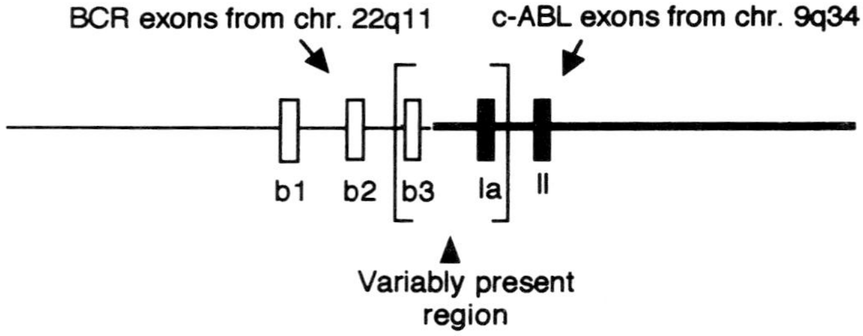

Fig. 1. The Philadelphia chromosome.

ence of minimal residual disease in leukemic patients following treatment *(3)*. The sensitivity of an RT-PCR assay, particularly if it is a nested, two-step PCR, typically enables the detection of one positive cell within a background of 10^5–10^7 normal cells. In the multiplexed, nested RT-PCR assay described herein, RNA is extracted either from peripheral blood leukocytes or from bone marrow hematopoietic cells. The RNA is first reverse transcribed and then subjected to two rounds of PCR. The final PCR product is electrophoresed through an ethidium bromide–stained agarose gel and detected by fluorescence under ultraviolet light.

The multiplexed PCR reactions described in this chapter contain primers for the BCR/*abl* translocation *(4)* as well as a set of control primers for the β-catenin gene *(5)* to confirm the quality and amplifiability of the cDNAs being tested. The positive control β-catenin primers ensure that the cDNA in each specimen is intact and that the RNA extraction and reverse transcription procedures are successful. A BCR/*abl* cDNA containing M-Bcr exons b1–b3 generates a 194-bp second-round PCR product whereas a BCR/*abl* cDNA containing only M-Bcr exons b1 and b2 generates a 119-bp second-round PCR product. Presence of the second-round β-catenin PCR amplicon is detected by the presence of a 372-bp product. **Table 1** gives the round 1 and round 2 PCR primer sequences for both BCR/*abl* and β-catenin. In the round 2 PCR, an aliquot of the PCR product from round 1 is amplified using BCR/*abl* primers that are both internal to the round 1 primers and β-catenin primers that are internal to the round 1 antisense primer.

2. Materials

2.1. Positive Control Cell Line

The K562 cell line is available from ATCC (cat. no. CCL 243) (http://www.atcc.org) and contains a BCR/*abl* translocation containing M-bcr exons b1–b3.

Table 1
BCR/*abl* and β-Catenin Primer Sequences

Sequence	Genset code no.
BCR/*abl*	
Oligo A: 5′-ggA gCT gCA gAT gCT gAC CAA C-3′	Genset HG099
Oligo B: 5′-CTg Agg CTC AAA gTC AgA Tg-3′	Genset HG101
Oligo C: 5′-gCT TCT CCC TgA CAT CCg Tg-3′	Genset HG098
Oligo D: 5′-CgA gCg gCT TCA CTC AgA CC-3′	Genset HG100
β-Catenin:	
Sense 4: 5′-TTC CAC gAC TAg TTC AgT TgC-3′	
Antisense 4: 5′-CTA CAg gCC AAT CAC AAT gC-3′	
Antisense 3: 5′-AAC AgC AgC TgC ATA TgT Cg-3′	

2.2. RNA Extraction (see Note 1*)*

1. 1.5-mL sterile plastic microcentrifuge tubes.
2. Sterilized aerosol-resistant pipet tips.
3. Purescript RNA Isolation Kit (cat. no. R-5000; Gentra Systems, Minneapolis, MN).
4. Sterile, double-deionized water treated with diethylpyrocarbonate (DEPC) and autoclaved (*see* **Note 2**).
5. Glycogen (20 mg/mL) (cat. no. 901 393; Boehringer Mannheim).
6. 100% Isopropanol, dedicated to only RNA extraction use, stored at 4°C.
7. 70% Ethanol, dedicated to only RNA extraction use, stored at 4°C.
8. Agarose DNA Grade (cat. no. BP164-100; Fisher).
9. Ethidium bromide (10 mg/mL).
10. 1X Tris-borate EDTA (TBE) prepared with DEPC-treated water.
11. 80% Glycerol/bromophenol blue loading buffer.

2.3. Reverse Transcription

1. GeneAmp RNA PCR Core Kit (cat. no. N808-0143; Perkin Elmer).
2. 200-µL Sterile microcentrifuge tubes.
3. Sterilized aerosol-resistant pipet tips.
4. RNA extracted from the K562 cell line.
5. RNA extracted from a "normal" subject, i.e., an individual with no evidence of leukemia, to use as a negative control.
6. RNA extracted from patient sample(s).

2.4. PCR Rounds 1 and 2

1. GeneAmp RNA PCR Core Kit (Perkin Elmer), which includes dNTPs, *Taq* polymerase, PCR Buffer II, and 25 m*M* $MgCl_2$).
2. 200-µL Sterile microcentrifuge tubes.

3. Sterilized aerosol-resistant pipet tips.
4. Patient and control cDNAs.
5. Sterile double-deionized water.

2.5. Gel Electrophoresis

1. NuSieve 3:1 Agarose (cat. no. 50090; FMC BioProducts).
2. 1X TBE.
3. Ethidium bromide (10 mg/mL).
4. 80% Glycerol–bromophenol blue loading buffer: 80% glycerol, 10 m*M* EDTA, 0.1% bromophenol blue.
5. DNA size standards: either pBR322/*Hae*III (cat. no. D 9655; Sigma, St. Louis, MO) or ϕ X174 DNA/*Hae*III (cat. no. D 0672; Sigma).

3. Methods

3.1. RNA Extraction (*see* Note 3)

RNA is more labile than DNA and degrades relatively quickly. Thus, RNA should be extracted from blood or bone marrow specimens as soon as possible after the specimen is received and accessioned in your laboratory. The specimen should be stored at 4°C from the time it is received in the laboratory until the RNA is extracted. The following method uses components of the Purescript RNA Isolation Kit (Gentra Systems) and includes some modifications of the original protocol found useful in our laboratory to increase RNA yield.

1. For best results, use at least 3 mL of peripheral blood or bone marrow. If the patient's specimen is <3 mL, use the entire specimen.
2. Use pipets dedicated to nucleic acid extraction, ideally dedicated to RNA extraction. Do not use these pipets when assembling the master mixes for the reverse transcription and PCR steps.
3. For each milliliter of peripheral blood or bone marrow, add 3 mL of red blood cell lysis solution in a Corning 15-mL centrifuge tube. Cap the tube and invert once to mix. Incubate at room temperature for 10 min, inverting the tube once more in the middle of the incubation.
4. Centrifuge at high speed in a bench-top centrifuge for 1 min to pellet the white cells.
5. Discard the supernatant and vortex the pellet to loosen it from the bottom of the tube.
6. Add 300 µL of cell lysis solution and pipet up and down no more than three times to lyse the white cells. Place the cell lysate in a 1.5-mL microcentrifuge tube.
7. Add 175 µL of protein precipitation solution, cap the tube, and invert it gently 10 times to mix. Place the microcentrifuge tube on ice for 5 min (*see* **Note 4**).
8. Centrifuge at 12,800*g* for 3 min.
9. Carefully remove the supernatant with a pipet and place it in a new microcentrifuge tube. Using the pipet, measure the approximate volume of the supernatant.

10. Add an equal volume of 100% isopropanol and 1 µL of glycogen (20 mg/mL). Cap the tube and invert gently 50 times.
11. Centrifuge at 12,800*g* for 5 min.
12. Carefully pour off the isopropanol and drain the tube on clean paper towels or absorbent paper.
13. Carefully pipet 300 µL of 70% ethanol into the microcentrifuge, directing the stream of fluid along the side of the tube rather than directly onto the pellet, in order to avoid dislodging it. Centrifuge at highest speed for 1 min.
14. Either carefully pour off the 70% ethanol without dislodging the pellet or remove most of it with a pipet, and allow the remainder of the ethanol to drain out of the microcentrifuge tube onto paper towels.
15. When no drops of ethanol remain on the sides of the microcentrifuge tube, rehydrate the pellet with 20–40 µL of RNA hydration solution (*see* **Note 5**).

3.2. Quantifying RNA Yield

There are two methods of quantifying RNA yield: spectrophotometric analysis of the absorption at 260 and 280 nm, and visual inspection on an agarose gel. Determining the ratio of absorption at 260:280 nm is used to calculate the concentration (micrograms/microliter) of nucleic acid in the preparation but is subject to positive interference from DNA. Electrophoresis of an aliquot of RNA in an agarose gel with ethidium bromide staining demonstrates the 18S and 28S bands of RNA, and is a visual check of the presence of high molecular weight RNA.

3.2.1. Absorption at 260 nm

Dilute 6 µL of RNA into 600 µL of DEPC-treated sterile double-deionized water. The RNA concentration in nanograms/microliter is obtained by multiplying the absorption at 260 nm by 4000. The ratio of absorptions at 260:280 nm should be ≥1.8.

3.2.2. Agarose Gel Analysis

1. Make a 1% agarose gel using 1X TBE prepared with DEPC-treated double-deionized water (ddH_2O).
2. For a small gel, add 0.4 g of agarose to 40 mL of TBE and melt in a microwave oven.
3. Add 4 µL of ethidium bromide (10 mg/mL) to the molten agarose prior to pouring the gel.
4. When the gel sets, submerge with 1X TBE and remove the comb.
5. Mix 3 µL of RNA with 3 µL of 80% glycerol/bromophenol blue loading buffer and load into the gel.
6. Run at 80 V until the dye front is two thirds of the way down the gel.
7. Photograph the gel under UV light. 18S RNA has an electrophoretic migration equivalent to a DNA molecule of 1.9 kb. 28S RNA migrates at the equivalent of a 4.7-kb DNA molecule.

3.3. Storage of RNA

RNA can be either frozen at –80°C indefinitely until needed for reverse transcription or used immediately in the reverse transcription step. If the RNA is frozen prior to reverse transcription, it should be thawed on ice.

3.4. Reverse Transcription

1. Prepare a master mix for reverse transcription according to the kit directions, calculating the total volume needed based on the number of patient and control reactions needed. Volumes of ingredients per reaction are as follows: 4 µL of 25 m*M* $MgCl_2$; 2 µL of 10X PCR Buffer II; 2 µL of each dNTP, at 10 m*M* initial concentration; 1 µL of RNAsin (20 U/µL); 1 µL of MULV reverse transcriptase (50 U/µL); and 1 µL of either random hexamers (50 µ*M*) or oligo dT (50 µ*M*).
2. Set up the reactions in a biosafety hood, if available, or in a space in your laboratory dedicated to assembling PCR ingredients. Use pipets dedicated to setting up PCR reactions.
3. Make duplicate reverse transcription reactions for each patient sample, one positive control reaction each for the BCR/*abl* exons b1–b3 translocation (i.e., K562) and the BCR/*abl* exons b1 and b2 translocation, if available, and one reaction for the negative RNA control (i.e., an RNA known not to contain a BCR/*abl* translocation).
4. Pipet 17 µL of master mix into each 200-µL microcentrifuge tube. Each tube should be and remain capped after addition of the master mix and should be opened only when pipeting in the appropriate RNA aliquot.
5. Add 3 µL of RNA to each patient sample, positive and negative control tubes, recapping each tube. Allow the tubes to sit at room temperature for 10 min to enhance binding of the random hexamers or oligo dT primer to the RNA.
6. Place the tubes in a thermocycler. Program the thermocycler for 1 cycle at 42°C for 60 min followed by 1 cycle at 90°C for 5 min to inactivate the reverse transcriptase.
7. Either use the cDNA immediately for the first PCR round or store at –20°C until needed.

3.5. PCR Round 1

1. Prepare the first round PCR master mix with dedicated PCR reagents, pipets, and consumable supplies in a location in your laboratory dedicated to preparing PCR reactions. Include duplicate tubes for each patient specimen, single tubes for the positive and negative control reactions, and a single tube for a water-alone control (*see* **Notes 6–8**). Prepare the round 1 PCR master mix according to the following reaction volumes (a total of 40.0 µL):
   a. 23.5 µL of sterile double deionized water.
   b. 3.0 µL of 25 m*M* $MgCl_2$ (1.5 m*M* final concentration).
   c. 5.0 µL of 10X PCR Buffer II (1X final concentration).
   d. 1.0 µL of 10 m*M* dATP (200 µ*M* final concentration).

   e. 1.0 μL of 10 m*M* dGTP (200 μ*M* final concentration).
   f. 1.0 μL of 10 m*M* dCTP (200 μ*M* final concentration).
   g. 1.0 μL of 10 m*M* dTTP (200 μ*M* final concentration).
   h. 1.0 μL of 10 m*M* β-catenin sense 4 primer (200 n*M* final concentration).
   i. 1.0 μL of 10 m*M* β-catenin antisense 4 primer (200 n*M* final concentration)
   j. 1.0 μL of 25 m*M* Oligo C (500 n*M* final concentration).
   k. 1.0 μL of 25 m*M* Oligo D (500 n*M* final concentration).
   l. 0.5 μL of *Taq* (5 U/μL) (2.5 U per reaction).
2. Aliquot 40 μL of master mix into each reaction tube. Cap the tubes and carry them to the area in your laboratory dedicated to the addition of DNA, cDNA, or PCR products to PCR reactions.
3. Using pipets dedicated to the addition of DNA, cDNA, or PCR reaction products and aerosol-resistant pipet tips, add 10 μL of the appropriate cDNA to each PCR tube or 10 μL of sterile double-deionized water to the water-alone control, uncapping each tube only to add the appropriate cDNA or sterile water and then recapping each tube prior to uncapping the next tube.
4. Vortex or pulse spin the tubes and place them in the thermocycler.
5. Use the following PCR cycle conditions:
   a. Step 1: 94°C for 10 min for 1 cycle.
   b. Step 2: 94°C for 1 min, 50°C for 1 min, 72°C for 1 min.
   c. Step 3: 72°C for 10 min for 1 cycle.
6. Repeat **step 5b** for 30 cycles for PCR round 1.
7. Allow the tubes to cool to room temperature. Store at 4°C until ready to assemble PCR round 2.

3.6. PCR Round 2

PCR Round 2 is the nested PCR reaction and uses an aliquot of the PCR round 1 product.

1. Prepare the PCR round 2 master mix in your laboratory's PCR setup area using dedicated reagents, pipets, and aerosol-resistant pipet tips according to the following reaction volumes (a total of 46.0 μL):
   a. 29.5 μL of Sterile double-deionized water.
   b. 3.0 μL of 25 m*M* $MgCl_2$ (1.5 m× final concentration)
   c. 5.0 μL of 10X PCR Buffer II (1X final concentration).
   d. 1.0 μL of 10 m*M* dATP (200 μ*M* final concentration).
   e. 1.0 μL of 10 m*M* dGTP (200 μ*M* final concentration).
   f. 1.0 μL of 10 m*M* dCTP (200 μ*M* final concentration).
   g. 1.0 μL of 10 m*M* dTTP (200 μ*M* final concentration).
   h. 1.0 μL of 10 μ*M* β-catenin sense 4 primer (200 n*M* final concentration).
   i. 1.0 μL of 10 μ*M* β-catenin antisense 3 primer (200 n*M* final concentration).
   j. 1.0 μL of 25 μ*M* Oligo A (500 n*M* final concentration).
   k. 1.0 μL of 25 m*M* Oligo B (500 n*M* final concentration).
   l. 0.5 μL of *Taq* (5 U/μL) (2.5 U per reaction).

2. Aliquot 46 µL into each reaction tube. Cap each tube and carry to the area in your laboratory dedicated to the addition of DNA or PCR products. Using dedicated pipets and aerosol-resistant pipet tips, add 4 µL of PCR round 1 product to each tube, recapping each tube immediately afterward.
3. Vortex or pulse spin each tube and insert in the thermocycler.
4. Use the same PCR cycling conditions as for round 1.
5. Allow the tubes to cool to room temperature and store at 4°C until ready for gel electrophoresis.

3.7. Gel Electrophoresis

1. For 100 mL of molten agarose, add 9 g of NuSieve 3:1 to 100 mL of 1X TBE and melt in a microwave oven to make a 3% gel. Add 10 µL of ethidium bromide (10 mg/mL) and pour into a gel apparatus, using a wide-tooth comb.
2. When the gel is set, add enough 1X TBE to just cover the agarose, and carefully remove the comb.
3. Mix 20 µL of each PCR round 2 product with 4 µL of 80% glycerol/bromophenol blue loading buffer and load into the gel.
4. Use either pBR322/*Hae*III (1 µg/µL) (Sigma) or ϕ X174 DNA/*Hae*III (1 µg/µL) (Sigma) as DNA size markers.

4. Notes

1. All buffers and consumable plastics needed for this assay should be kept dedicated to work with RNA. They should be kept separate from similar laboratory supplies used for work with DNA and should be labeled "FOR RNA USE ONLY."
2. All glassware used to measure reagents or to contain buffers and any sterile double-deionized water used to work with RNA should first be treated with 0.1% DEPC (cat. no. D 5758, Sigma) to inactivate RNases. One milliliter of DEPC is added to each liter of sterile ddH_2O, allowed to sit for at least 12 h at room temperature, and then autoclaved for 15 min on the liquid cycle. Glassware can be filled to the brim with sterile ddH_2O, an appropriate amount of DEPC added and allowed to sit in the vessel for 12 h at room temperature. The DEPC-H_2O is removed from the glassware prior to autoclaving. DEPC is unstable in the presence of Tris buffers and breaks down to ethanol and carbon dioxide. Thus, when preparing the 5X TBE buffer that will be used to check the quality of the RNA on an agarose gel prior to the reverse transcriptase step, prepare the buffer in DEPC-treated glassware, using DEPC-treated ddH_2O rather than adding DEPC directly to the 5X TBE.
3. If you have never extracted RNA before, it is wise to practice on specimens of peripheral blood prior to extracting a patient's sample in order to acquaint yourself with the extraction protocol you are using, to become familiar with manipu-

lating the RNA pellet following isopropanol precipitation and ethanol wash, and to become familiar with rehydrating the RNA pellet following the ethanol wash. The RNA extraction step is critical to the success of the assay because it is the starting material on which the remainder of the assay depends. Many RNA extraction kits are available and you may wish to try several to determine which kit or extraction method gives the best results in your laboratory. No matter which kit or RNA extraction protocol you use, it is wise to keep the white RNA cell pellet on ice, to complete the extraction protocol without interruption once you start it; and when precipitating the RNA, to use equal volumes of supernatant to isopropanol.

4. After completing the protein-DNA precipitation step using the Purescript reagents, the red-brown pellet, consisting of residual red cell debris, protein, and DNA, should be tight and well compacted at the bottom of the microcentrifuge tube. If the pellet is rather loose and not well compacted, adding additional protein precipitation reagent may be beneficial. When the pellet is loose and has a mucous-like appearance, it can be difficult to remove the supernatant, and the volume of supernatant recovered is often reduced. Loss of supernatant reduces the ultimate RNA yield.
5. If the RNA pellet appears small, you might wish to rehydrate it in half the recommended volume of rehydration solution as recommended in order to maximize the concentration of RNA that goes into the reverse transcription step. Because the volume of RNA in the reverse transcription step is fixed, it is advantageous to maximize the RNA concentration being reverse transcribed, in order to detect the BCR/*abl* transcript, should it be rare in your specimen.
6. Awareness of the ways in which a PCR reaction can become contaminated, as evidenced by a PCR product seen in the water-alone control reaction, is always required when amplifying DNA. However, when a PCR reaction is nested, such as in this protocol, contamination can occur much more easily and must be more vigorously anticipated and guarded against. Because an aliquot of the water-alone control reaction is reamplified in round 2, any slight, otherwise undetectable contamination occurring in the round 1 step could be detected when an aliquot is reamplified in round 2.
7. Ways to avoid contamination include the following:
   a. Assembling the PCR mixes in a laboratory area dedicated to that purpose, using dedicated pipetmen and aerosol-resistant pipet tips.
   b. Capping each tube after aliquoting the PCR master mix, keeping each tube capped except when adding each respective cDNA or PCR aliquot, and then recapping each tube prior to uncapping the next.
   c. Adding cDNA or PCR product only in a laboratory area dedicated to that purpose, using dedicated pipetmen and aerosol-resistant pipet tips.
8. Should contamination be detected in the blank lane, it is imperative that all solutions or reagents, including double-deionized water, dNTPs, primer dilutions, and *Taq*, be discarded and new dilutions prepared.

References

1. Melo, J. V. (1996) The molecular biology of chronic myeloid leukemia. *Leukemia* **10,** 751–756.
2. McClure, J. S. and Litz, C. E. (1994) Chronic myelogenous leukemia: molecular diagnostic considerations. *Hum. Pathol.* **25,** 594–597.
3. Campana, D. and Pui, C.-H. (1995) Detection of minimal residual disease in acute leukemia: methodological advances and clinical significance. *Blood* **85,** 1416–1434.
4. Genset Corp. (1991) *Human Genes. Oligonucleotide Handbook*, vol. 2, La Jolla, CA.
5. Oyama, T., Kanai, Y., Ochiai, A., Akimoto, S., Oda, T., Yanagihara, K., Nagafuchi, A., Tsukita S., Shibamoto, S., Ito, F., Takeichi, M., Matsuda, H., and Hirohashi, S. (1994) A truncated β-catenin disrupts the interaction between E-cadherin and α-catenin: a cause of loss of intercellular adhesiveness in human cancer cell lines. *Cancer Res.* **54,** 6282–6287.

12

Detection of t(15;17)(q24;q21), inv(16)/t(16;16)(p13;q22), and t(8;21)(q22;q22) Anomalies in Acute Myeloid Leukemias

David S. Viswanatha

1. Introduction

The acute myeloid leukemias (AMLs) are a relatively heterogeneous group of diseases. However, there is growing awareness that the clinical features and subclassification of morphologic leukemia types is often highly correlated with tumor genetics. Furthermore, distinct genetic subgroups of AML are associated with improved therapeutic sensitivity and a more favorable clinical outcome. These observations have prompted suggestions for a revision of the current French-American-British leukemia classification *(1)*, utilizing genetically defined principles *(2)*. Three recurrent chromosomal translocations are identified in approx 25–30% of *de novo* adult AMLs. These include the t(15;17), associated with acute promyelocytic leukemia ([APL]; AML-M3); the inv(16) and related t(16;16), associated with AML-M4Eo; and the t(8;21), associated most commonly with AML-M2. Each of these abnormalities results in the formation of a chimeric leukemia-specific fusion gene, which is transcribed and expressed as a fusion protein. The widespread genetic deregulation caused by such fusion proteins is thought to interfere with proliferative control and cell differentiation mechanisms, leading to the leukemic state. The presence of these and other fusion gene events can be specifically and sensitively detected by reverse transcriptase-polymerase chain reaction (RT-PCR) analysis.

The t(15;17) anomaly is associated with fusion of the *PML* (15q24) and RARα (17q21) genes *(3)*. The *PML* gene product is localized to specific nuclear body complexes and may function as a negative transcriptional regulator *(4–6)*. In addition, *PML* expression is required for myeloid cell differentiation induced via the retinoic acid pathway and further exhibits antiproliferative and antitumor effects *(7)*. Recent evidence also suggests a role for PML in cellular

From: *Methods in Molecular Medicine, vol. 49: Molecular Pathology Protocols*
Edited by: A. A. Killeen © Humana Press Inc., Totowa, NJ

apoptosis *(8,9)* and perhaps in immunomodulation by interactions with the major histocompatibility system *(10)*. The *RARα* gene encodes a nuclear receptor for retinoic acid; members of the retinoid receptor family are critically involved in myeloid cell maturation. As part of the chimeric PML-RARα protein, the latter moiety is important for conferring sensitivity of the leukemic blasts to all-*trans* retinoic acid ([atRA]; vitamin A), a now well-established differentiative therapy in APL *(11,12)*. At the genomic level, breakpoints in the *PML* gene occur in either introns 3 or 6, or rarely, within exon 6. Breakpoints in the *RARα* gene are distributed within intron 2. Thus, one of three types of *PML-RARα* mRNA fusion can occur and be detected in a given case of APL (**Fig. 1A**): Short (S)-form, or BCR-3 (*PML* exon 3-*RARα* exon 3, approx 45–50%); Long (L)-form, or BCR–1 (*PML* exon 6-*RARα* exon 3, approx 50–55%); and Variable (V)-form, or BCR-2 (*PML* exon 6 variable-*RARα* exon 3, approx 5–10%). The relative frequency of *PML-RARα* types differs in pediatric APL, in which V-form cases are more commonly encountered than S-form cases *(13)*.

The inv(16)/t(16;16)(p13;q22) abnormality results in the fusion of the gene encoding core binding factor-β subunit (*CBFβ*), with the *MYH11* gene *(14)*. The CBF protein complex is formed by heterodimerization of CBFβ with its heterodimeric DNA binding partner CBFα and acts transcriptionally at critical genetic loci required for myeloid and lymphoid cell differentiation (reviewed in **ref. *15***). The *MYH11* gene encodes a type II smooth muscle myosin heavy chain protein (SMMHC) and is not normally expressed in hematopoietic cells. The *CBFβ-MYH11* gene fusion and resultant CBFβ-SMMHC fusion protein is thought to disrupt CBF transcriptional function in immature myeloid cells, leading to interference with normal differentiation pathways in myelopoiesis and, subsequently, AML *(15)*. Several different chimeric mRNA types can arise from the *CBFβ-MYH11* gene fusion, owing mainly to breakpoint heterogeneity in MYH11 (**Fig. 1B**). Fortunately, for diagnostic purposes, one fusion type accounts for approx 90% of occurrences in inv(16)/t(16;16) AML and is easily detected by RT-PCR analysis.

Interestingly, the t(8;21)(q22;q22) abnormality in AML also results in a genetic fusion leading to disruption of CBF transcriptional regulation. In this translocation, the *AML1* gene encoding the CBFα subunit of CBF is fused to a putative transcription factor gene, *ETO* (also designated *MTG8*), on the der(8) chromosome (reviewed in **ref. *16***). The AML1 (CBFα) protein shares significant homology to the Drosophila pair rule gene *runt (17,18)*, and binds to DNA "core" transcriptional sites in conjunction with CBFβ. The AML1 gene is a common target in leukemias, being involved in the t(3;21) associated with myelodysplasia or therapy-induced AML *(16)*, and the t(12;21) anomaly present in approx 25% of pediatric acute lymphoblastic leukemia *(19,20)*. In the case of

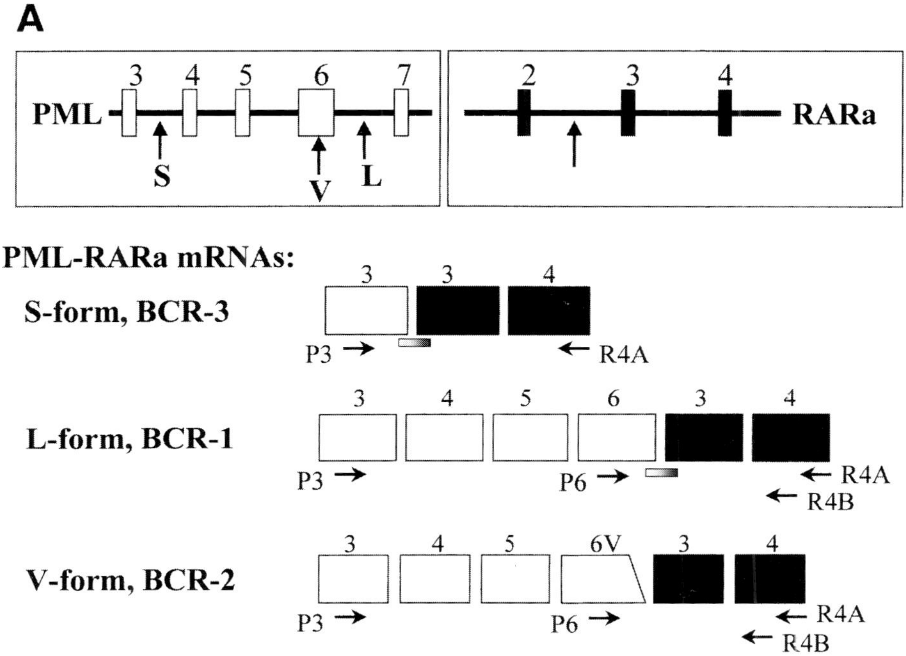

Fig. 1. (**A**) Schematic of *PML-RARα* Fusion in t(15;17) acute promyelocytic leukemia. (**Top**) Partial genomic map of *PML* (15q24) and *RARα* (17q21) genes. Vertical arrows indicate breakpoint regions. *PML* break sites can occur in intron 3, intron 6, or rarely within exon 6. By contrast, *RARα* breakpoints occur uniformly in intron 2. (**Bottom**) Potential chimeric mRNAs produced by *PML-RARα* break-fusion events: S (short)-form/BCR-3, L (long)-form/BCR-1, and V (variable)-form/BCR-2. V-form cases have a variable proportion of retained exon 6 nucleotides, usually with additional nontemplated base additions or deletions. Alternative splicing out of *PML* exon 5 or exons 5 and 6 is also seen in L- and V-form fusion transcripts. Relative locations of primers for first-round PCR (P3 and R4A) and second-round (nested) PCR (P6 and R4B) are shown. Junction-specific oligoprobes for detection of S- and L-form fusions are displayed as short bars.

t(8;21) AML, the resulting AML1(CBFα)-ETO fusion protein is similarly believed to disrupt normal processes in myelopoietic differentiation and lead to leukemia. Murine gene knock-out (for *CBFβ* and *AML1*) and knock-in (for *CBFβ-MYH11* and *AML1-ETO*) models have identified a critical role for CBF in embryonic survival and, most significantly, in definitive hematopoiesis ***(21–24)***. Although alternative splice sites have been determined in both *AML1* and *ETO* mRNAs ***(25)***, the chimeric fusion transcript is highly uniform in the vast majority of cases of t(8;21)-positive AML (**Fig. 1C**).

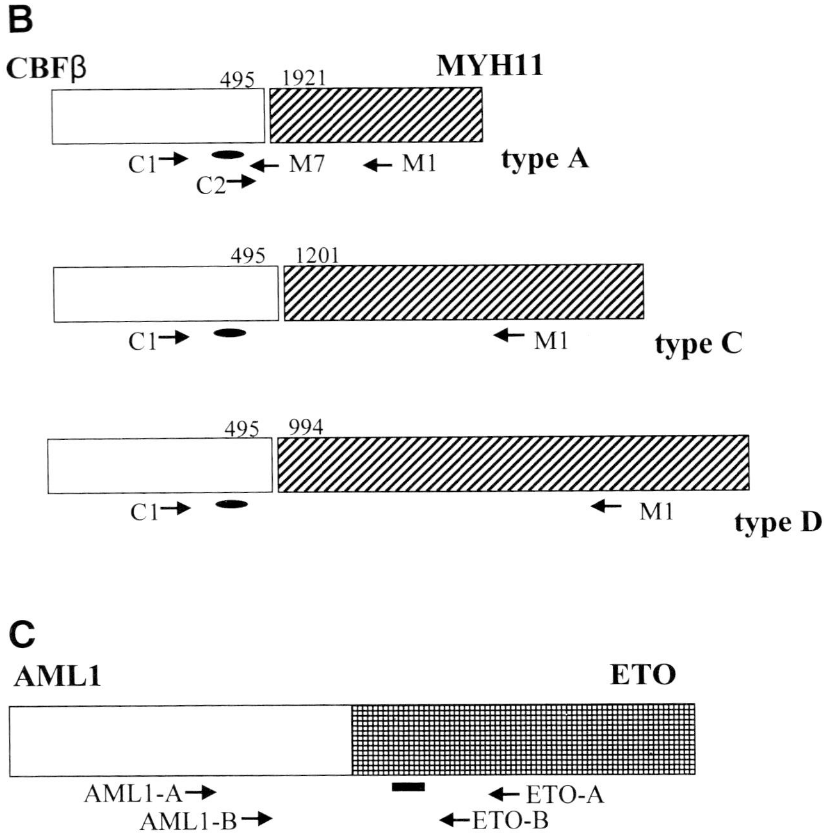

Fig. 1. *(continued)* **(B)** Schematic of major *CBFβ-MYH11* fusions in inv(16)/t(16;16) AML. The three most common *CBFβ-MYH11* fusion mRNA types are illustrated. The type A chimeric mRNA is encountered in approx 90% of cases, whereas types C and D are each detected in <5% of cases. Locations of C1 and M1 PCR primers are shown. C2 and M7 primers can be utilized in allele-specific nested PCR confirmation of the type A fusion transcript, as discussed in **Note 17**. Detection of *CBFβ-MYH11* fusion PCR products is accomplished by hybridization with an internal *CBFβ* sequence oligoprobe, indicated by the solid ovals. **(C)** Schematic of *AML1-ETO* fusion in t(8;21) AML. The diagram demonstrates the chimeric *AML1-ETO* mRNA, with relative locations of first-round PCR primers (AML1-A and ETO-A) and second-round (nested) PCR primers (AML1-B and ETO-B) indicated. Confirmation of the *AML1-ETO* fusion is accomplished by hybridization to an internal *ETO* sequence oligoprobe, indicated by the black bar.

An enhanced understanding of the genetic basis of leukemogenesis will permit more precise correlation of molecular abnormalities with clinical disease features and generate more-focused therapeutic efforts in AML. Such is the case with the *PML-RARα* fusion and the basis for the efficacy of atRA therapy in APL. Data are accumulating that these "favorable outcome" fusion gene leukemias (and perhaps others) may have a common molecular pathogenesis involving interference with histone acetylation status and, correspondingly, disruption of gene transcription processes required for cellular differentiation ***(26–30)***. This may provide yet another target for therapeutic intervention and further underscores the importance of molecular diagnosis in AML. Finally, in addition to detection of specific gene fusions for the identification of leukemic subtypes, these abnormalities also serve as sensitive markers for monitoring of minimal residual disease (MRD) in patients achieving remission status following therapy. An emerging paradigm in successful leukemia treatment is the realization that clonal disease is not fully eradicated by conventional therapies, but rather exists at submicroscopic levels (detectable by quantitative PCR methods), with the propensity to fluctuate in quantity and activity over time. Although beyond the scope of this chapter, the quantitative monitoring of MRD will likely form a cornerstone of posttherapeutic disease evaluation in the leukemias; this is briefly mentioned at the end of the chapter.

2. Materials

2.1. RNA Isolation

1. RNAqueous small-scale RNA isolation kit (Ambion, Austin, TX) (*see* **Note 1**).
2. 3 *M* Sodium acetate (pH 5.2).
3. Cold 100% (absolute) ethanol.
4. Cold 75% ethanol.
5. 1 m*M* EDTA in diethylpyrocarbonate (DEPC) distilled water (*see* **Note 2**).

2.2. Reverse Transcription Reaction/cDNA Synthesis

1. 10X RT buffer: 100 m*M* Tris-HCl (pH 8.4), 500 m*M* KCl, 50 m*M* $MgCl_2$ (*see* **Note 3**).
2. 10 m*M* stock dNTPs solution (Boehringer Mannheim, Indianapolis IN).
3. Random hexamer solution (50 pmol/μL) (Perkin-Elmer, Foster City, CA).
4. RNasin RNase inhibitor (40 U/μL) (Promega, Madison, WI).
5. 50 m*M* Dithiothreitol (DTT).
6. MMLV-RT (200 U/μL) (Gibco-BRL/Life Technologies, Gaithersburg MD).
7. DEPC distilled H_2O.

2.3. Polymerase Chain Reaction

1. 10X PCR buffer: 100 m*M* Tris-HCl (pH 8.4), 500 m*M* KCl, 15 m*M* $MgCl_2$ (*see* **Note 3**).

Table 1
DNA Sequences for Primers and Probes (all 5′–3′)

t(15;17)/*PML-RARα*
P3: ACCGATGGCTTCGACGAGTTC
R4A: AGCCCTTGCAGCCCTCACAG
P6: AATACAACGACAGCCCAGAAG
R4B: CTCACAGGCGCTGACCCCAT
L-form junction probe[a]: GGTCTCAATGGCTGCCTCCCC
S-form junction probe[a]: AATGGCTTTCCCCTGGGTGA
inv(16)/t(16;16)/*CBFB-MYH11*
C1: GCAGGCAAGGTATATTTGAAGG
M1: CTCTTCTCCTCATTCTGCTC
C2: ACACGCGAATTTGAAGATAGAG
M7: TTCTCCAGCTCATGGACCTCC
CBFB oligoprobe[a]: ATAGAGACAGGTCTCATCGG
t(8;21)/*AML1-ETO*
AML1-A: AGCCATGAAGAACCAGG
ETO-A: AGGCTGTAGGAGAATGG
AML1-B: TACCACAGAGCCATCAAA
ETO-B: GTTGTCGGTGTAAATGAA
ETO oligoprobe[a]: GTCTTCACATCCACAGGTGAGTCT
Beta2-microglobulin
B2 I sense GAAAAAGATGAGTATGCCTG
B2 II antisense: ATCTTCAAACCTCCATGATG

[a]Oligonucleotide probes are 5′-biotinylated.

2. 10 m*M* Stock dNTPs.
3. Sense and antisense primers (15–20 pmol/μL of each) (*see* **Table 1**).
4. AmpliTaq DNA polymerase (5 U/μL) (Perkin-Elmer/Roche, Foster City, CA).
5. DEPC distilled H_2O.

2.4. Gel Analysis of PCR Product and Vacuum Blot Transfer

1. Standard powdered agarose for 1.5% agarose gel (3 g) (SeaKem ME, FMC Bioproducts, ME).
2. Ethidium bromide (EtBr) solution (10 mg/mL) (Gibco-BRL/Life Technologies).
3. Stock 10X Tris-borate EDTA (TBE) buffer solution: 107.8 g of Tris-HCl, 55 g of boric acid, 7.4 g of Na_2EDTA per 1 L of sterile distilled H_2O (0.5X TBE is used for gel and 1X TBE for running buffer).
4. 10X Sample loading dye: 1 vol of 1% bromophenol blue, 1 vol of 1% xylene cyanol, 2 vol of glycerol.
5. Horizontal gel box (40 cm) with 20-well combs (BRL Horizon 20.25; Life Technologies).

6. UV light box and instant camera setup with Polaroid 667 B+W film (Polaroid, Cambridge, MA).
7. Nylon membrane (11 × 20 cm) (Biodyne PA; Pall-Biodyne, East Hills, NY) to encompass area of gel being transferred.
8. Two clean plastic tubs.
9. Dilute (0.05 *N*) HCl (500 mL).
10. 0.4 *M* NaOH (2 L).
11. Bio-Rad Model 785 vacuum transfer apparatus with vacuum regulator (Bio-Rad, Hercules, CA) (*see* **Note 4**).
12. UV crosslinking apparatus (UV Stratalinker; Stratagene, La Jolla, CA).

2.5. Nonisotopic Probe Hybridization

1. Stock 20X SSPE buffer: 210.4 g of NaCl, 27.6 g of $NaH_2PO_4{\cdot}H_2O$, 4.4 g of NaOH, and 7.4 g of Na_2EDTA per 1 L of sterile distilled H_2O; buffer usually requires gentle heat with constant stirring to solubilize completely. From this buffer prepare the following:
   a. Prehybridization solution (100 mL): 0.1X SSPE/0.5% sodium dodecyl sulfate (SDS—from 10% SDS stock solution).
   b. Blot wash solution (2 L): 2X SSPE/0.1% SDS.
   c. 50-mL Aliquots of hybridization buffer: 5X SSPE/0.1% SDS (*see* **Note 5**).
2. 5′-Biotinylated specific oligonucleotide probe (5 pmol/µL) (*see* **Table 1**).
3. Heat-sealable plastic hybridization bags.
4. Several clean plastic tubs with lids.
5. Streptavidin-horseradish peroxidase (SA-HRP) (1 mg/mL) (Vector, Burlingame, CA).
6. Enterochromaffin-like (ECL) chemiluminescence reagent solutions 1 and 2 (Amersham, Arlington Heights, IL).
7. Fluorescent marking pen.
8. Standard filter (blotting) paper.
9. Plastic wrap.
10. Radiographic film (Kodak XAR; Eastman-Kodak, Rochester, NY).

3. Methods

The PCR methods detailed herein are based on previously published protocols ***(14,31,32)***, optimized for use in my laboratory (*see* **Note 6**). General laboratory principles pertaining to the performance of PCR and analysis of PCR products should be followed (*see* **Note 7**).

3.1. Isolation of RNA

1. Obtain washed peripheral blood or bone marrow cell suspension following Ficoll density gradient separation or RBC lysis (*see* **Note 8**). Gently pellet the cells and decant all the supernatant.
2. Use the Ambion RNAqueous kit per the manufacturer's directions.

3. Following RNA elution from the column filter, collect in a 100 µL vol. Add 30 µL of 3 *M* Na acetate and 250 µL of cold absolute ethanol. Leave at –80°C for 15 min.
4. Centrifuge for 15 min at 12,000*g* and 4°C. Remove the supernatant carefully.
5. Gently wash the pellet with cold 75% ethanol. Air-dry the pellet for 5 min.
6. Resuspend the pellet in a volume of 1 m*M* EDTA to give an approximate concentration of 1 µg/µL. Calculate the concentration and yield by standard absorbance spectrophotometry.
7. Store the RNA samples at –70°C.

3.2. Detection of t(15;17)-Associated PML-RARα Fusion by RT-PCR (*see* Note 9)

3.2.1. Reverse Transcription Reaction/cDNA Synthesis

1. Thaw RNA samples on ice. Aliquot 1 µg of each RNA sample into labeled MicroAmp PCR tubes. Adjust the volume to 5 µL with sterile DEPC H_2O. Keep on ice or in a cold block.
2. Assemble RT master mix in a 1.5-mL microfuge tube, on ice, as follows: 7 µL DEPC H_2O, 2 µL of 10X RT buffer, 2 µL of 10 m*M* dNTPs, 1 µL (100 pmol) of random hexamers, 0.5 µL of RNasin, 2 µL of DTT, 0.5 µL of MMLV-RT. These amounts are per sample reaction and need to be multiplied by the number of samples (*n*) being assayed. It is advisable to make enough RT master mix for one extra reaction (i.e., *n* + 1). Gently vortex to mix.
3. Aliquot 15 µL of RT master mix to each sample tube proceeding in order from the test samples to the positive control and finally the negative control (no RNA). Mix by gentle, not vigorous, pipeting.
4. Place in a thermal cycler programmed as follows: 23°C for 10 min, 42°C for 30 min, 95°C for 5 min, then cooled to 4°C.

3.2.2. PCR for PML-RARα Fusion

1. Label a new set of MicroAmp tubes corresponding to the RT reaction set.
2. Transfer completed RT-reaction tubes to a PCR hood and aliquot 15 µL of synthesized cDNA to appropriately labeled new MicroAmp tubes proceeding in order from the test samples to the positive control and finally the negative control. This leaves 5 µL of cDNA remaining in the original tubes. Close the tube caps and keep the samples on ice or in a cold block in the hood. Use 15 µL of the cDNA product for the *PML-RARα* PCR amplification and reserve 5 µL of product for the control β_2-microglobulin amplification reaction.
3. Assemble the first-round *PML-RARα* PCR master mix in a 1.5-mL microfuge tube, on ice, as follows: 26.5 µL of DEPC H_2O, 5 µL of 10X PCR buffer, 1 µL of 10 m*M* dNTPs, 1 µL each of primers P3 (sense) and R4A (antisense), 0.5 µL of *Taq* DNA polymerase. This total of 35 µL of PCR master mix is per sample and needs to be multiplied by the number of samples being tested, plus one extra (*n* + 1). Gently vortex the tube with the lid closed.

4. Assemble the β_2-microglobulin control PCR master mix in a separate 1.5-mL microfuge tube in exactly the same manner as in **step 3**; however, use 1 µL each of primers β_2M-sense and β_2M-antisense instead. Gently vortex the tube to mix.
5. Start with the β_2-microglobulin PCR tube set and add 35 µL of β_2M master mix to each of the respective MicroAmp tubes (resulting in a total volume of 40 µL per reaction). Mix the contents of each tube gently and carefully. Similarly, add 35 µL of *PML-RARα* master mix to each of the respective MicroAmp tubes in the *PML-RARα* PCR set, and mix the contents of each tube carefully (resulting in a total volume of 50 µL per reaction). In either case, proceed in the order from the test samples to the positive control and finally the negative (no RNA) control.
6. Place all the tubes in the thermal cycler, programmed as follows: 95°C for 5 min (initial denaturation); 5 cycles of 95°C for 45 s, 62°C for 60 s, and 72°C for 30 s; 32 cycles of 95°C for 30 s, 60°C for 45 s, and 72°C for 60 s; then 72°C for 5 min (final extension) and cool to 4°C. Following the PCR reaction, remove the tubes from the thermal cycler and transfer the first-round *PML-RARα* product tubes to the PCR hood in a cold block. Put the completed β_2-microglobulin PCR tubes on ice or in a refrigerator.
7. Label one final set of fresh MicroAmp PCR tubes. Transfer 1 µL from the first-round *PML-RARα* product tubes to the corresponding new PCR tubes. Close the tube caps.
8. Assemble the second-round *PML-RARα* master mix in a 1.5-mL microfuge tube, on ice, as follows: 40.5 µL of DEPC H_2O, 5 µL of 10X PCR buffer, 1 µL of 10 m*M* dNTPs, 1 µL each of second-round primers P6 (sense) and R4B (antisense), 0.5 µL of *Taq* DNA polymerase. This total of 49 µL of PCR master mix is per sample and needs to be multiplied by the number of samples being tested, plus one extra ($n + 1$). Gently vortex the tube with the lid closed.
9. Add 49 µL of second-round *PML-RARα* master mix to each MicroAmp tube, proceeding in the order from the test samples to the positive control and finally the negative control. Mix the contents of each tube carefully (resulting in a total volume of 50 µL per reaction).
10. Place the tubes in the thermal cycler, programmed as follows: 95°C for 3 min (initial denaturation); 5 cycles of 95°C for 45 s, 62°C for 60 s, and 72°C for 30 s; 25 cycles of 95°C for 30 s, 62°C for 45 s, and 72°C for 60 s; then 72°C for 5 min (final extension) and cool to 4°C.
11. Keep the first- and second-round *PML-RARα* PCR products and β_2-microglobulin products in a refrigerator or –20°C freezer until ready for gel electrophoresis.

3.2.3. Gel Electrophoresis Analysis and Vacuum Blot Transfer of PML-RARα PCR Products

1. Prepare a 1.5% agarose gel (with 0.5X TBE) (*see* **Note 10**).
2. In a microtiter plate, add 15 µL of PCR products to 2.5 µL of 10X sample loading dye. A DNA size marker is also used, such as the 123-bp ladder (Gibco-BRL/Life Technologies). Mix briefly and load the first-round P3-R4A PCR products

in one set of lanes, followed by the second-round P6-R4B products, separating the two groups of PCR products by one or two empty lanes. Load β_2-microglobulin products in a separate set of lanes. Carry out electrophoresis at 180 V for 1.5–2 h.

3. Following electrophoresis, observe and photograph the gel under UV illumination. Proper eye protection is mandatory when viewing gels by UV light. Standard black-and-white Polaroid photographs are obtained with a photograph stand and instant film (*see* **Note 11**). Expected PCR product sizes are as follows (**Fig. 2**):
   a. t(15;17)/*PML-RAR*α: L-form (BCR-1) first round—3 bands, range 280–700 bp; second round—380 bp; V-form (BCR-2) first round—3 bands, range 280 to approx 700 bp; second round—<380 bp; S-form (BCR-3) first round only—221 bp.
   b. β_2-microglobulin: 120 bp.
4. Place the gel in a plastic tub and cover with 300–400 mL of dilute (0.05 *N*) HCl (acid-nicking step). Place on a gyrating platform on the gentle setting for 10 min. During this time, allow the precut nylon membrane to equilibrate in 300–400 mL of 0.4 *M* NaOH.
5. Decant dilute HCl and add an equal amount of 0.4 *M* NaOH over the gel.
6. Assemble the vacuum transfer apparatus according to the manufacturer's directions. Align the gel over the nylon membrane, ensuring that the wells are outside of the vacuum gasket seal. Slowly engage the vacuum to negative pressure of 4 to 5 mmHg. Pour approx 250 mL of 0.4 *M* NaOH over the gel to cover the area for transfer. Transfer the gel products to the nylon membrane for 1 h.
7. Disassemble the vacuum transfer apparatus and remove the nylon membrane. Place the membrane in a UV crosslinker and crosslink the DNA to the membrane at a 500-μJ power setting. Label the well locations at the top of the gel using a soft pencil and allow the membrane to dry.
8. Cut and separate a section containing P3-R4A PCR products from the section containing P6-R4B PCR products, label appropriately, and trim off the excess membrane. If β_2-microglobulin products have been transferred on the same membrane, cut away the area containing β_2-microglobulin product lanes and discard. The P3-R4A reaction products will be hybridized with the S-form junction probe whereas the P6-R4B products will be hybridized with the L-form junction probe (*see* **Subheading 3.2.4.**). V-form *PML-RAR*α type fusions are not amenable to junctional oligoprobe analysis; this is discussed in **Subheading 3.2.5.**

Fig. 2. *(see facing page)* t(15;17)/*PML-RAR*α PCR product analysis. (**Top**) Agarose gel electrophoresis of *PML-RAR*α PCR products. L, size marker (123-bp ladder). Lanes A–E, first-round amplification products (with P3 and R4A primers): A, NB4 positive control for L-form fusion; B, APL patient positive for L-form fusion; C, APL patient positive for V-form fusion; D, APL patient positive for S-form fusion; E, negative control (no RNA). For L- and V-form fusions, a three-band pattern is observed owing to alternative splicing out of *PML* exons 5, and 5 + 6. The full-length transcript

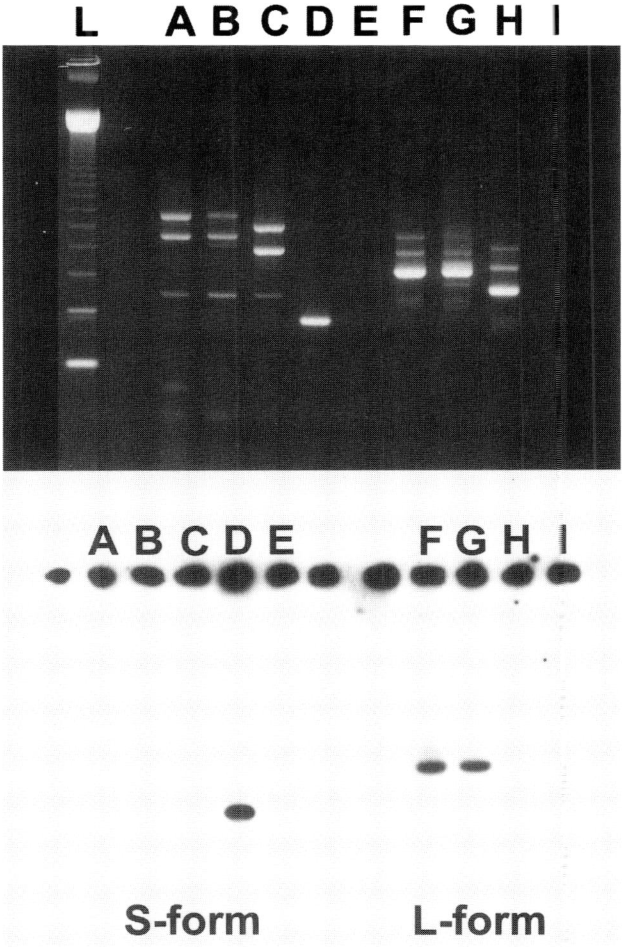

Fig. 2. *(continued)* PCR product (uppermost band) is 700 bp for L-form fusions and typically less than this for V-form fusions. The S-form fusion PCR product is 221 bp. Lanes F–I, second-round (nested) PCR of samples A, B, C, and E (with primers P6 and R4B): F, NB4 cell line; G, L-form positive APL patient; H, V-form positive APL patient; I, negative control (no RNA). L-form nested PCR products reveal a prominent band at 380 bp, whereas the V-form product is slightly smaller. (**Bottom**) Two blots of junction-specific oligoprobe hybridization to detect S- and L-form fusions. Lanes A–E correspond to the PCR products from the gel above and represent first-round amplification products. These have been hybridized with the S-form oligoprobe. Lanes F–I correspond to the PCR products from the gel above and represent second-round amplification products, hybridized with the L-form oligoprobe. Note the absence of hybridization signal for the V-form PCR product (lane H), a useful distinguishing feature when V-form PCR products are similar in size to L-form *PML-RAR*α fusions.

3.2.4. Nonisotopic (Chemiluminescent) Probe Hybridization for PML-RARα Fusions

1. Warm to 60°C in a water bath 50 mL of prehybridization solution (0.1X SSPE/ 0.5% SDS) and two 15-mL aliquots (one per separate hybridization reaction) of hybridization buffer (5X SSPE/0.1% SDS).
2. Place nylon membranes of the (first round) P3-R4A and (second round) P6-R4B PCR products in appropriately labeled, heat-sealable plastic bags and add 15 mL of prehybridization buffer to each. Displace bubbles through the open end of the bag, and then heat-seal the bag and place in a 60°C oven, on a rocking platform. Allow 30 min for prehybridization.
3. Add 5 µL of the biotinylated junction-specific oligoprobes (S-form junction and L-form junction) to respective 15-mL aliquots of warm hybridization buffer and gently mix (final probe concentrations approx 1.5–2 pmol/mL of buffer). Remove and cut the plastic bags open across the top. Drain the prehybridization buffer and carefully add the 15 mL of the hybridization buffer with the specific oligoprobe to the corresponding bags (i.e., S-form junction to the membrane with P3-R4A products and L-form junction to the membrane with P6-R4B products). Express excess air and bubbles, and then heat-seal the bags just above the nylon membrane. Check for leaks and place in a 60°C oven for 1 h. The hybridization reactions can be extended to overnight for convenience.
4. Prepare 2 L of blot wash solution (2X SSPE/0.1% SDS). Aliquot 500 mL of wash solution and heat to 60°C in a water bath. Be sure to verify the temperature of the solution. Leave the remaining wash solution covered at room temperature. Warm two clean empty plastic tubs in a 60°C oven.
5. Remove the hybridization bags, cut across to open, and drain the hybridization solution. Remove the nylon membranes and place in separate plastic tubs, and then add approx 125 mL of warm (60°C) blot wash buffer to each. Cover the tubs and place in a 60°C oven on a rocking platform for 10 min. Repeat this step once with the remaining warm blot wash solution (*see* **Note 12**).
6. Prepare SA-HRP solution in a clean plastic tub using 250 mL of room temperature blot wash solution and 10 µL of SA-HRP (final concentration of 40 ng/mL).
7. Following the second warm (60°C) wash, briefly rinse the membranes with approx 100 mL of room temperature wash solution, and transfer to the SA-HRP solution. Place on a slowly gyrating platform for 15 min.
8. Drain the SA-HRP solution, briefly rinse with 100 mL of room temperature blot wash solution and decant, and add another 400 mL of blot wash solution. Place on a gyrating platform for 5–10 min. Repeat the wash with another 400 mL of room temperature solution (*see* **Note 13**).
9. Place the wet membranes on clean dry filter paper. Quickly pipet 5 mL each of ECL chemiluminescence reagents 1 and 2 into a clean glass tray and mix by gentle agitation. Place each membrane in the tray and coat thoroughly with ECL reagents for 1 min. Remove and affix the membranes to clean precut filter paper. Mark well locations with a fluorescent pen, label blots as to probe type, and seal

the membranes over with plastic wrap. Develop chemiluminescent image on X-ray film as usual (*see* **Note 14**).

*3.2.5. Interpretation: t(15;17)/*PML-RARα *Results*

As indicated in **Subheading 1.**, the *PML-RARα* gene fusion may produce three distinct chimeric transcript types: Long (L)-form, or BCR-1 (*PML* exon 6-*RARα* exon 3); Short (S)-form, or BCR-3 (*PML* exon 3-*RARα* exon 3); Variable (V)-form, or BCR-2 (*PML* exon 6 variable-*RARα* exon 3). Overall, the L- and S-forms account for approx 90% of *PML-RARα* fusions, with the V-form being relatively rare (*see* **Note 15**). The V-form is unique in that the *PML* breakpoint occurs within exon 6 and nontemplated nucleotides are often inserted or nucleotides deleted to maintain an open reading frame in the fusion mRNA. For the first-round PCR products, the L- and V-form products give rise to three distinct bands (**Fig. 2, Top**, lanes A–E; also *see* **Note 16**). The upper two bands in V-form cases are typically smaller in size than for L-form cases, although rare V-form tumors may have similar, or longer transcript lengths. This reflects the "variable" nature of the *PML* exon 6 breakpoint in V-form cases. The S-form PCR product forms a single band of much shorter length. Second-round (nested) PCR analysis confirms the presence of the L- and V-form *PML-RARα* fusions (**Fig. 2, Top**, lanes F–I) and, in combination with L-form junction oligoprobe hybridization (**Fig. 2, Bottom**, lanes F–I), allows distinction of these fusion types when they may be of similar size. Junction-specific oligoprobe hybridization for the S-form *PML-RARα* fusion is also illustrated in **Fig. 2** (bottom panel, lane D). More important, for the RT-PCR analysis described herein, gel electrophoresis will detect all three fusion types. However, because of the variable nature of the junctional sequence in V-form cases, a specific probe for this region cannot be developed as for the L- and S-form PCR products. Hence, V-form cases are recognized on agarose gel alone. In some cases, we have resorted to direct DNA sequence analysis of suspected V-form products to confirm the fusion type.

3.3. Detection of the inv(16)/t(16;16)-Associated CBFβ-MYH11 *Fusion by RT-PCR*

3.3.1. Reverse Transcription Reaction/cDNA Synthesis (see Note 9*)*

1. Thaw RNA samples on ice. Aliquot 1 to 2 μg of each RNA sample into labeled MicroAmp PCR tubes. Adjust the volume to 5 μL with sterile DEPC H_2O. Keep on ice or in a cold block.
2. Assemble RT master mix in a 1.5-mL microfuge tube, on ice, as follows: 7 μL of DEPC H_2O, 2 μL of 10X RT buffer, 2 μL of 10 m*M* dNTPs, 1 μL of random hexamers, 0.5 μL of RNasin, 2 μL of DTT, 0.5 μL of MMLV-RT. These amounts are per sample reaction and need to be multiplied by the number of samples being assayed. It is advisable to make enough RT master mix for one extra reaction ($n + 1$). Gently vortex to mix.

3. Aliquot 15 µL of RT master mix to each sample tube proceeding in order from the test samples to the positive control and finally the negative control (no RNA). Mix by gentle, not vigorous, pipeting.
4. Place in a thermal cycler programmed as follows: 23°C for 10 min, 42°C for 60 min, 95°C for 5 min, then cooled to 4°C.

3.3.2. PCR for CBFβ-MYH11 Fusion

1. Label a new set of MicroAmp tubes corresponding to the RT reaction set.
2. Transfer completed RT-reaction tubes to a PCR hood and aliquot 15 µL of synthesized cDNA to appropriately labeled new MicroAmp tubes tube proceeding in order from the test samples to the positive control and finally the negative control (no RNA). This leaves 5 µL of cDNA remaining in the original tubes. Close the tube caps and keep the samples on ice or in a cold block in the hood. Use 15 µL of the cDNA product for the *CBFβ-MYH11* PCR amplification and reserve 5 µL of product for the control β_2-microglobulin amplification reaction.
3. Assemble the *CBFβ-MYH11* PCR master mix in a 1.5-mL microfuge tube, on ice, as follows: 26.5 µL of DEPC H_2O, 5 µL of 10X PCR buffer, 1 µL of 10 m*M* dNTPs, 1 mL each of primers C1 (sense) and M1 (antisense), 0.5 µL of *Taq* DNA polymerase. This total of 35 µL PCR master mix is per sample and needs to be multiplied by the number of samples being tested, plus one extra ($n + 1$). Gently vortex the tube with the lid closed.
4. Assemble the β_2-microglobulin control PCR master mix in a separate 1.5-mL microfuge tube in exactly the same manner as in **step 3**; however, use 1 µL each of primers β_2M-sense and β_2M-antisense instead. Gently vortex the tube to mix.
5. Start with the β_2-microglobulin PCR tube set and add 35 µL of β_2M master mix to each of the respective MicroAmp tubes (resulting in a total volume of 40 µL per reaction). Mix the contents of each tube gently and carefully. Similarly, add 35 µL of *CBFβ-MYH11* master mix to each of the respective MicroAmp tubes in the *CBFβ-MYH11* PCR set, and mix the contents of each tube carefully (resulting in a total volume of 50 µL per reaction). In either case, proceed in the order from the test samples to the positive control and finally the negative control.
6. Place all the tubes in the thermal cycler, programmed as follows: 95°C for 5 min (initial denaturation); 3 cycles of 95°C for 30 s, 59°C for 45 s, and 72°C for 90 s; 30 cycles of 95°C for 30 s, 57°C for 30 s, and 72°C for 60 s; then 72°C for 8 min (final extension) and cool to 4°C. Keep the *CBFβ-MYH11* PCR products and β_2-microglobulin products in a refrigerator or –20°C freezer until ready for gel electrophoresis.

3.3.3. Gel Electrophoresis Analysis and Vacuum Blot Transfer of CBFβ-MYH11 PCR Products

1. Prepare a 1.5% agarose gel (with 0.5X TBE) (*see* **Note 10**).
2. In a microtiter plate, add 15 µL of PCR products to 2.5 µL of 10X sample loading dye. A DNA size marker is also used, such as the 123-bp ladder (Gibco-BRL/Life Technologies). Mix briefly and load C1-M1 PCR products in one set of lanes, followed by β_2-microglobulin products, separating the two groups of PCR products by one or two empty lanes. Carry out electrophoresis at 180 V for 1.5–2 h.

3. Following electrophoresis, observe and photograph the gel under UV illumination. Proper eye protection is mandatory when viewing gels by UV light. Standard black-and-white Polaroid photographs are obtained with a photograph stand and instant film (*see* **Note 11**). Expected PCR product sizes are as follows (**Fig. 3A**):
   a. inv(16)/t(16;16) *CBFβ-MYH11*: Type A, 415 bp; Type C, 1.2 kb; Type D, 1.4 kb; other types rare. (Types A, C, and D collectively account for approx 95% of *CBFβ-MYH11* fusions [*see* **Subheading 3.3.5.**])
   b. β_2-Microglobulin: 120 bp.
4. Place the gel in a plastic tub and cover with 300–400 mL of dilute (0.05 *N*) HCl (acid-nicking step). Place on a gyrating platform on gentle setting for 10 min. During this time, allow the precut nylon membrane to equilibrate in 300–400 mL of 0.4 *M* NaOH.
5. Decant the dilute HCl and add an equal amount of 0.4 *M* NaOH over the gel.
6. Assemble the vacuum transfer apparatus according to the manufacturer's directions. Align the gel over the nylon membrane, ensuring that the wells are outside of the vacuum gasket seal. Slowly engage the vacuum to negative pressure of 4 to 5 mmHg. Pour approx 250 mL of 0.4 *M* NaOH over the gel to cover the area for transfer. Transfer the gel products to the nylon membrane for 1 h.
7. Disassemble the vacuum transfer apparatus and remove the nylon membrane. Place the membrane in a UV crosslinker and crosslink the DNA to the membrane at a 500-µJ power setting. Label the well locations at the top of the gel using a soft pencil and allow the membrane to dry.
8. Cut and separate the section containing C1-M1 PCR products, label appropriately, and then trim off the excess membrane. If β_2-microglobulin products have been transferred on the same membrane, cut away the area containing the β_2-microglobulin product lanes and discard.

3.3.4. Nonisotopic (Chemiluminescent) Probe Hybridization for CBFβ-MYH11 Fusions

1. Warm to 60°C in a water bath 50 mL of prehybridization solution (0.1X SSPE/0.5% SDS) and a 15-mL aliquot of hybridization buffer (5X SSPE/0.1% SDS).
2. Place a nylon membrane of C1-M1 PCR products in an appropriately labeled, heat-sealable plastic bag and add 15 mL of prehybridization buffer. Displace bubbles through the open end of the bag, and then heat-seal the bag and place in a 60°C oven, on a rocking platform. Allow 30 min for prehybridization.
3. Add 5 µL of the biotinylated *CBFβ* internal sequence oligoprobe (CBFβ oligoprobe) to a 15-mL aliquot of warm hybridization buffer and gently mix (final probe concentration of approx 1.5–2 pmol/mL of buffer). Remove and cut the plastic bag open across the top. Drain the prehybridization buffer and carefully add 15 mL of the hybridization buffer with the specific oligoprobe to the bag. Express excess air and bubbles, and then heat-seal the bag just above the nylon membrane. Check for leaks and place in a 60°C oven for 1 h. The hybridization reaction can be extended to overnight for convenience.

A

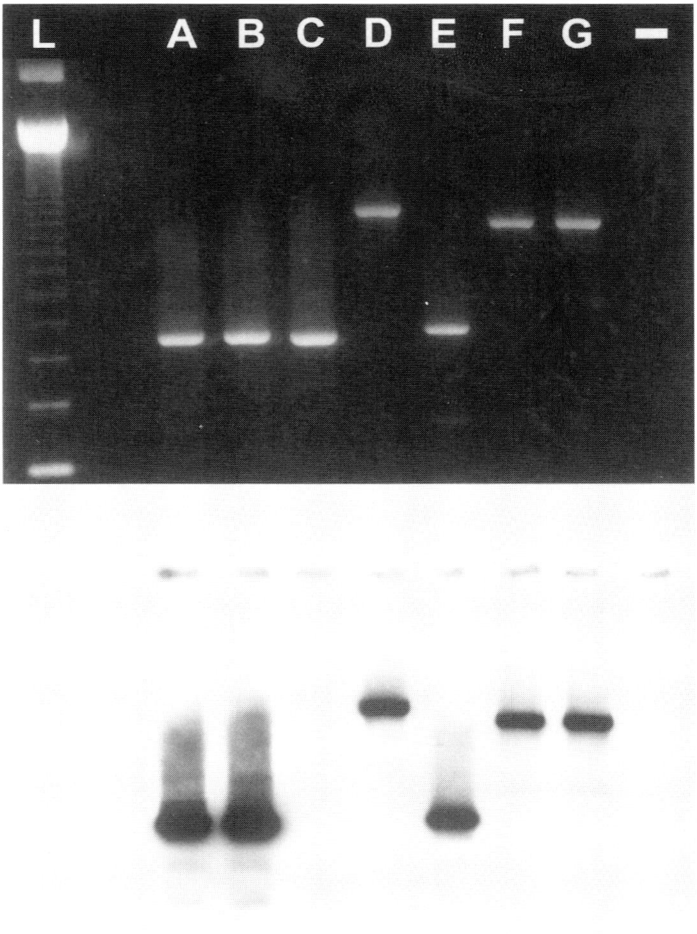

Fig. 3A. inv(16)/t(16;16)*CBFβ-MYH11* PCR product analysis. (**Top**) Agarose gel electrophoresis of C1-M1 PCR products. L, size marker (123-bp ladder). Lanes A, B, and E: type A fusion product (415 bp). Lane D: type D fusion product (1.4 kb). Lanes F and G: type C fusion product (1.2 kb). Lane marked (–) is a negative control (no RNA). Lane C is a novel *CBFβ-MYH11* fusion product that closely mimics the type A fusion in size. (**Bottom**) Internal *CBFβ* oligoprobe hybridization for detection of *CBFβ-MYH11* PCR products. Lanes are exactly as depicted at top. Novel *CBFβ-MYH11* fusion (lane C) does not hybridize with this probe and required sequencing for confirmation (*see* **Note 18**). Figures reprinted with permission of publisher, with minor modifications *(52)*.

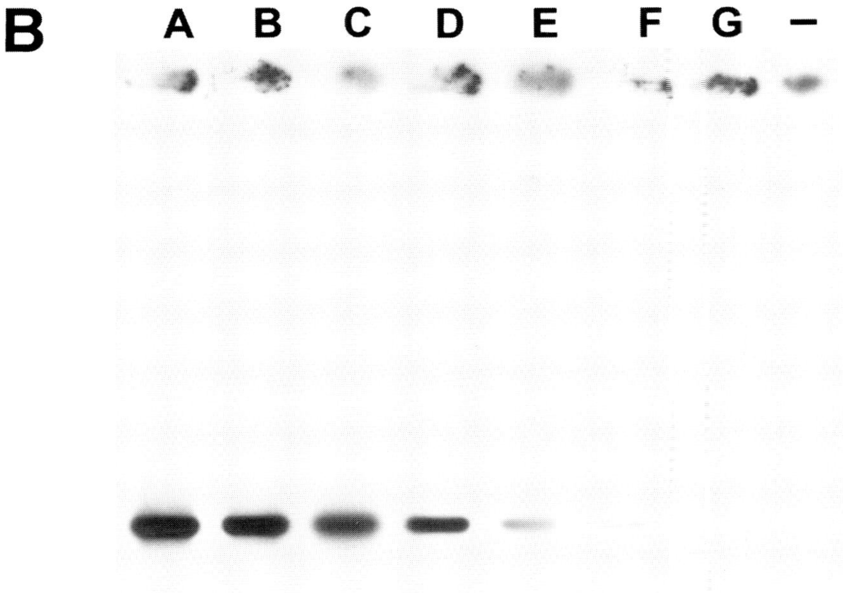

Fig. 3B. Application of type A *CBFβ-MYH11* junctional oligoprobe. Detection of type A *CBFβ-MYH11* fusion in a cell dilution experiment using a junction-specific oligonucleotide probe. Patient cells positive for type A *CBFβ-MYH11* fusion transcript were serially diluted in normal bone marrow cells and analyzed by C1-M1 RT-PCR. Lane A, undiluted patient cells; lane B, 1 : 10 dilution; lane C, 1 : 20 dilution; lane D, 1 : 100 dilution; lane E, 1 : 10^3 dilution; lane F, 1 : 10^4 dilution; lane G, pure normal bone marrow. Lane marked (–) is a negative control (no RNA). Figure reprinted with permission of publisher, with minor modifications *(52)*.

4. Prepare 2 L of blot wash solution (2X SSPE/0.1% SDS). Aliquot 500 mL of wash solution and heat to 60°C in a water bath. Be sure to verify the temperature of the solution. Leave the remaining wash solution covered at room temperature. Warm a clean empty plastic tub in the 60°C oven.
5. Remove the hybridization bag, cut across to open, and drain the hybridization solution. Remove the nylon membrane and place in a plastic tub, and then add 250 mL of warm (60°C) blot wash buffer. Cover the tub and place in a 60°C oven on a rocking platform for 10 min. Repeat this step once with the remaining warm blot wash solution (*see* **Note 12**).
6. Prepare SA-HRP solution in a clean plastic tub using 250 mL of room temperature blot wash solution and 10 µL of SA-HRP (final concentration of 40 ng/mL).
7. Following the second warm (60°C) wash, briefly rinse the membranes with approx 100 mL of room temperature wash solution, and transfer to the SA-HRP solution. Place on a slowly gyrating platform for 15 min.

8. Drain the SA-HRP solution, briefly rinse with 100 mL of room temperature blot wash solution and decant, and then add another 400 mL of blot wash solution. Place on a gyrating platform for 5–10 min. Repeat the wash with another 400 mL of room temperature solution (*see* **Note 13**).
9. Place the wet membranes on clean dry filter paper. Quickly pipet 5 mL each of ECL chemiluminescence reagents 1 and 2 into a clean glass tray and mix by gentle agitation. Place each membrane in the tray and coat thoroughly with the ECL reagents for 1 min. Remove and affix the membranes to clean precut filter paper. Mark the well locations with a fluorescent pen, label the blots as to probe type, and seal over the membranes with plastic wrap. Develop chemiluminescent image on X-ray film as usual (*see* **Note 14**).

3.3.5. Interpretation: inv(16)/t(16;16) CBFβ-MYH11 Results

The inv(16)/t(16;16)-associated *CBFβ-MYH11* fusion results in formation of a type A chimeric transcript in approx 90% of positive cases. The longer type C and type D fusion PCR products account for approx 5% of *CBFβ-MYH11* fusions overall; thus, the PCR assay and hybridization reaction described will detect nearly all the commonly encountered *CBFβ-MYH11* fusions occurring in AML. Although several other *CBFβ-MYH11* fusion types have been described ***(15)***, these are relatively rare and arise mainly owing to significant heterogeneity in *MYH11* gene break point–fusion sites. By contrast, the *CBFβ* fusion site in chimeric *CBFβ-MYH11* mRNAs is constant with very rare exceptions ***(33)***. Therefore, an internal *CBFβ* oligoprobe can be utilized to identify *CBFβ-MYH11* PCR products following Southern blot transfer (**Fig. 3A**). The type A fusion can also be specifically confirmed by using a junctional sequence oligoprobe (inv(16) junction A, 5′-3′:GCTCATGGACCTCCATTTCC) applied to blots of C1-M1 PCR products, although this may be a more useful reagent in RT-PCR assessment of minimal residual disease (**Fig. 3B**).

Confirmation of the common type A *CBFβ-MYH11* fusion product (415 bp) can also be obtained following C1-M1 primer PCR, by allele-specific nested PCR ***(34)***, usually obviating the need to perform a probe hybridization (*see* **Note 17**). However, this nested PCR method will not detect other (non–type A) *CBFβ-MYH11* types (*see* **Note 18**).

3.4. Detection of the t(8;21)-Associated AML1-ETO Fusion by RT-PCR

3.4.1. Reverse Transcription Reaction/cDNA Synthesis (*see* **Note 9**)

1. Thaw RNA samples on ice. Aliquot 1 μg of each RNA sample into labeled MicroAmp PCR tubes. Adjust the volume to 5 μL with sterile DEPC H_2O. Keep on ice or in a cold block.
2. Assemble RT master mix in a 1.5-mL microfuge tube, on ice, as follows: 7 μL of DEPC H_2O, 2 μL of 10X RT buffer, 2 μL of 10 m*M* dNTPs, 1 μL of random

hexamers, 0.5 µL of RNasin, 2 µL of DTT, 0.5 µL of MMLV-RT. These amounts are per sample reaction and need to be multiplied by the number of samples being assayed. It is advisable to make enough RT master mix for one extra reaction ($n + 1$). Gently vortex to mix.

3. Aliquot 15 µL of RT master mix to each sample tube proceeding in order from the test samples to the positive control and finally the negative control (no RNA). Mix by gentle, not vigorous, pipetting.
4. Place in a thermal cycler programmed as follows: 23°C for 10 min, 37°C for 60 min, 95°C for 5 min, then cooled to 4°C.

3.4.2. PCR for AML1-ETO Fusion

1. Label a new set of MicroAmp tubes corresponding to the RT reaction set.
2. Transfer the completed RT-reaction tubes to a PCR hood and aliquot 15 µL of synthesized cDNA to appropriately labeled new MicroAmp tubes tube proceeding in order from the test samples to the positive control and finally the negative control (no RNA). This leaves 5 µL of cDNA remaining in the original tubes. Close the tube caps and keep the samples on ice or in a cold block in a hood. Use 15 µL of cDNA product for the *AML1-ETO* PCR amplification and reserve 5 µL of product for the control β_2-microglobulin amplification reaction.
3. Assemble the first-round *AML1-ETO* PCR master mix in a 1.5-mL microfuge tube, on ice, as follows: 26.5 µL of DEPC H_2O, 5 µL of 10X PCR buffer, 1 µL of 10 m*M* dNTPs, 1 µL each of primers AML1-A (sense) and ETO-A (antisense), 0.5 µL of *Taq* DNA polymerase. This total of 35 µL of PCR master mix is per sample and needs to be multiplied by the number of samples being tested, plus one extra ($n + 1$). Gently vortex the tube with the lid closed.
4. Assemble the β_2-microglobulin control PCR master mix in a separate 1.5-mL microfuge tube in exactly the same manner as in **step 3**; however, use 1 µL each of primers β_2M-sense and β_2M-antisense instead. Gently vortex the tube to mix.
5. Start with the β_2-microglobulin PCR tube set and add 35 µL of β_2M master mix to each of the respective MicroAmp tubes (resulting in a total volume of 40 µL per reaction). Mix the contents of each tube gently and carefully. Similarly, add 35 µL of *AML1-ETO* master mix to each of the respective MicroAmp tubes in the *AML1-ETO* PCR set and mix the contents of each tube carefully (resulting in a total volume of 50 µL per reaction). In either case, proceed in the order from the test samples to the positive control and finally the negative control.
6. Place all the tubes in the thermal cycler, programmed as follows: 95°C for 3 min (initial denaturation); 30 cycles of 95°C for 30 s; 55°C for 30 s; 72°C for 60 s; then 72°C for 5 min (final extension) and cool to 4°C. Following the PCR reaction, remove the tubes from the thermal cycler and transfer the first-round *AML1-ETO* product tubes to the PCR hood in a cold block. Put the completed β_2-microglobulin PCR tubes on ice or in a refrigerator.
7. Label one final set of fresh MicroAmp PCR tubes. Transfer 2 µL from the first-round *AML1-ETO* product tubes to the corresponding new PCR tubes. Close the tube caps.

8. Assemble the second-round (nested) *AML1-ETO* master mix in a 1.5-mL microfuge tube, on ice, as follows: 39.5 µL of DEPC H_2O, 5 µL of 10X PCR buffer, 1 µL of 10 m*M* dNTPs, 1 µL each of second-round internal primers AML1-B (sense) and ETO-B (antisense), 0.5 µL of *Taq* DNA polymerase. This total of 48 µL of PCR master mix is per sample and needs to be multiplied by the number of samples being tested, plus one extra ($n + 1$). Gently vortex the tube with the lid closed.
9. Add 48 µL of second-round *AML1-ETO* master mix to each MicroAmp tube, proceeding in the order from test samples to the positive control and finally the negative control. Mix the contents of each tube carefully (resulting in a total volume of 50 µL per reaction).
10. Place the tubes in the thermal cycler, using the same program parameters as for the first-round *AML1-ETO* PCR.
11. Keep the first- and second-round *AML1-ETO* PCR products and β_2-microglobulin products in a refrigerator or –20°C freezer until ready for gel electrophoresis.

3.4.3. Gel Electrophoresis Analysis and Vacuum Blot Transfer of AML1-ETO *PCR Products*

1. Prepare a 1.5% agarose gel (with 0.5X TBE) (*see* **Note 10**).
2. In a microtiter plate, add 15 µL of PCR products to 2.5 µL of 10X sample loading dye. A DNA size marker is also used, such as the 123-bp ladder (Gibco-BRL/ Life Technologies). Mix briefly and load first-round AML1-A/ETO-A PCR products in one set of lanes, followed by second-round AML1-B/ETO-B products, separating the two groups of PCR products by one or two empty lanes. Load β_2-microglobulin products in a separate set of lanes. Carry out electrophoresis at 180 V for 1.5–2 h.
3. Following electrophoresis, observe and photograph the gel under UV illumination. Proper eye protection is mandatory when viewing gels by UV light. Standard black-and-white Polaroid photographs are rendered with a photograph stand and instant film (*see* **Note 11**). Expected PCR product sizes are as follows (**Fig. 4**):
   a. t(8;21)/*AML1-ETO*: first round, 338 bp (May not be observed after first-round amplification [*see* **Subheading 3.4.5.**]); second round, 185 bp.
   b. β_2-microglobulin: 120 bp.
4. Place the gel in a plastic tub and cover with 300–400 mL of dilute (0.05 *N*) HCl (acid-nicking step). Place on a gyratory platform on gentle setting for 10 min. During this time, allow the precut nylon membrane to equilibrate in 300–400 mL of 0.4 *M* NaOH.
5. Decant the dilute HCl and add an equal amount of 0.4 *M* NaOH over the gel.
6. Assemble the vacuum transfer apparatus according to the manufacturer's directions. Align the gel over the nylon membrane, ensuring that wells are outside of the vacuum gasket seal. Slowly engage the vacuum to negative pressure of 4 to 5 mmHg. Pour approx 250 mL of 0.4 *M* NaOH over the gel to cover the area for transfer. Transfer the gel products to the nylon membrane for 1 h.

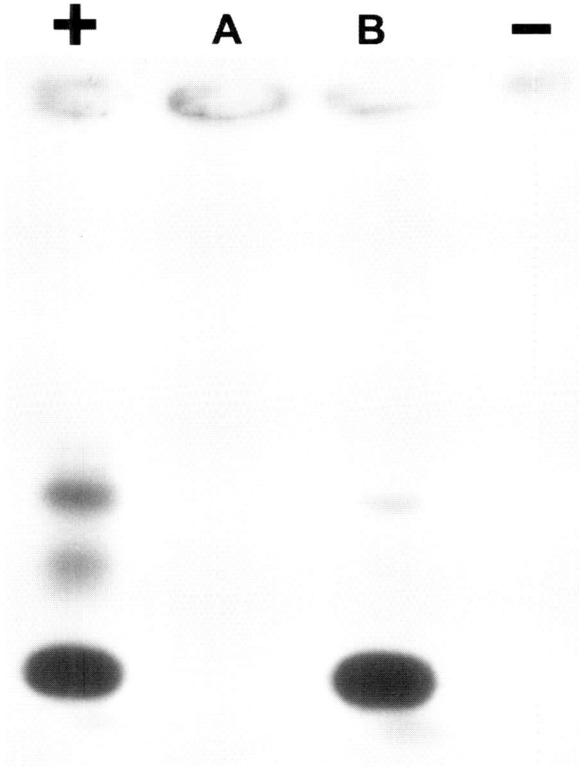

Fig. 4. t(8;21)/*AML1-ETO* PCR product analysis. Gel blot illustrating detection of *AML1-ETO* fusion PCR products with internal *ETO* sequence oligoprobe. Figure shows hybridized blot of second-round amplification products (with AML1-B and ETO-B primers). Lane marked (+) is the positive control (Kasumi-1 cell line). Lanes A and B are patient samples, with B demonstrating the presence of the *AML1-ETO* fusion. Lane marked (–) is a negative control (no RNA).

7. Disassemble the vacuum transfer apparatus and remove the nylon membrane. Place the membrane in a UV crosslinker and crosslink the DNA to the membrane at a 500-μJ power setting. Label the well locations at the top of the gel using a soft pencil and allow the membrane to dry.
8. Cut and separate the sections containing first-round AML1-A/ETO-A and second-round AML1-B/ETO-B PCR products, label appropriately, and then trim off the excess membrane from each. If β_2-microglobulin products have been transferred on the same membrane, cut away the area containing β_2-microglobulin product lanes and discard.

3.4.4. Nonisotopic (Chemiluminescent) Probe Hybridization for AML1-ETO Fusion

1. Warm to 60°C in a water bath 50 mL of prehybridization solution (0.1X SSPE/ 0.5% SDS) and a 15-mL aliquot of hybridization buffer (5X SSPE/0.1% SDS).
2. Place nylon membranes of first- and second-round *AML1-ETO* PCR products back-to-back in an appropriately labeled, heat-sealable plastic bag and add 15 mL of prehybridization buffer. Displace bubbles through the open end of the bag, and heat-seal the bag, and place in a 60°C oven, on a rocking platform. Allow 30 min for prehybridization.
3. Add 5 µL of the biotinylated *ETO* internal sequence oligoprobe (ETO oligoprobe) to a 15-mL aliquot of warm hybridization buffer and gently mix (final probe concentration of approx 1.5–2 pmol/mL of buffer). Remove and cut the plastic bag open across the top. Drain the prehybridization buffer and carefully add 15 mL of the hybridization buffer with the specific oligoprobe to the bag. Express excess air and bubbles, and then heat-seal the bag just above the nylon membranes. Check for leaks and place in a 60°C oven for 1 h. The hybridization reaction can be extended to overnight for convenience.
4. Prepare 2 L of blot wash solution (2X SSPE/0.1% SDS). Aliquot 500 mL of wash solution and heat to 60°C in a water bath. Be sure to verify the temperature of the solution. Leave the remaining wash solution covered at room temperature. Warm a clean empty plastic tub in a 60°C oven.
5. Remove the hybridization bag, cut across to open, and drain the hybridization solution. Remove the nylon membranes, place both in a plastic tub, and add 250 mL of warm (60°C) blot wash buffer. Cover and place in a 60°C oven on a rocking platform for 10 min. Repeat this step once with the remaining warm blot wash solution (*see* **Note 12**).
6. Prepare SA-HRP solution in a clean plastic tub using 250 mL of room temperature blot wash solution and 10 µL of SA-HRP (final concentration of 40 ng/mL).
7. Following the second warm (60°C) wash, briefly rinse the membranes with approx 100 mL of room temperature wash solution and transfer to the SA-HRP solution. Place on a slowly gyrating platform for 15 min.
8. Drain the SA-HRP solution, briefly rinse with 100 mL of room temperature blot wash solution, and decant. Then add another 400 mL of blot wash solution. Place on a gyrating platform for 5–10 min. Repeat the wash with another 400 mL of room temperature solution (*see* **Note 13**).
9. Place the wet membranes on clean dry filter paper. Quickly pipet 5 mL each of ECL chemiluminescence reagents 1 and 2 into a clean glass tray and mix by gentle agitation. Place each membrane in the tray and coat thoroughly with ECL reagents for 1 min. Remove and affix the membranes to clean precut filter paper. Mark the well locations with a fluorescent pen, label the blots as to probe type, and seal over the membranes with plastic wrap. Develop chemiluminescent image on X-ray film as usual (*see* **Note 14**).

3.4.5. Interpretation: t(8;21)/AML1-ETO Results

In contrast to the t(15;17)/*PML-RAR*α and inv(16) or t(16;16)/ *CBF*β-*MYH11* chimeric fusions, the *AML1-ETO* abnormality is characterized by a constant and predictable fusion type (**Fig. 4**). In a minority of cases, detection of a slightly larger transcript has been described in addition to the usual *AML1-ETO* transcript, owing to an additional 68 bp of *ETO* sequence *(25)*. However, significant heterogeneity in *AML1-ETO* breakpoint-fusion sites is not a feature of this genetic abnormality. Nested PCR is performed in this assay to detect the presence of the *AML1-ETO* mRNA, because first-round PCR alone may not achieve sufficient sensitivity. Some protocols have been described that appear to obtain good results with a single round of PCR *(35)*.

3.5. Conclusion

The results of gel electrophoresis and blot hybridization analyses are used to determine whether the specific PCR assay is positive (i.e., whether the presence of the translocation fusion mRNA in question has been detected). The clarity and strength of specific oligoprobe hybridization, as well as the molecular size of the PCR product, are considered to establish a result as positive. The absence of appropriately sized PCR products and lack of specific probe hybridization denote negative results. Concomitant demonstration of intact and amplifiable control RNA (cDNA) is always required in order to exclude a sample or technical failure, particularly in the case of a negative PCR analysis. In the latter case, amplification of a segment of β_2-microglobulin RNA (cDNA) is commonly utilized.

Although an in-depth discussion is beyond the scope of this chapter, the choice of RT-PCR control(s) is important. I have illustrated β_2-microglobulin herein, because it is relatively well expressed in hematopoietic cells and has proven to be informative in most cases. However, more substantial guidelines are emerging regarding this issue *(36)*. In particular, care should be taken to exclude amplification of genomic DNA (e.g., genes with short intron segments spanning the area amplified), control gene products should be relatively unique and lack pseudogenes, and the expression level of the chosen control gene should not be greater than that of the target gene. Notably, high-purity isolation and proper storage (at least –80°C) of high-quality RNA from viable, fresh, or well-preserved cells is essential; sensitivity of the RT-PCR assay can be significantly compromised in poorly preserved material. Although this may be somewhat less critical in examples with abundant target mRNA and short amplicon length (e.g., *BCR-ABL* fusion in chronic myeloid leukemia), detection of other labile or low-abundance fusion mRNAs may be adversely affected (e.g., *PML-RAR*α fusion in acute promyelocytic leukemia).

Finally, brief mention is made here regarding the sensitivity of RT-PCR assays of leukemic fusion genes, in the context of monitoring MRD. In my experience, the sensitivity of the inv(16)/*CBFβ-MYH11* and t(8;21)/*AML1-ETO* RT-PCR assays is typically 1 in 10^4–10^5 cells. Further enhancements can be gained by the use of radiolabeled PCR primers or probes, although the clinical utility of this goal is uncertain. Although the reported data are not yet clear concerning the presence of MRD and risk of relapse in inv(16)/*CBFβ-MYH11* leukemia ***(37)***, low-level t(8;21)/*AML1-ETO* fusion transcript is commonly detected in patients with persistent long-term clinical remissions ***(38–40)***. By contrast, RT-PCR for the t(15;17)/*PML-RARα* has a sensitivity of one or two orders of magnitude less than for the other described RT-PCR assays. This likely reflects a combination of factors, of which mRNA instability and relatively low transcript abundance are important. However, this relatively lower level of sensitivity in detection of *PML-RARα* MRD is of substantial clinical prognostic significance and can be utilized for prediction of impending disease relapse ***(41,42)***. An emerging paradigm for the management of acute leukemic patients is the realization that despite attainment of clinical remission, residual disease persists and can be detected by sensitive molecular methods. The development of novel technologies such as the fluorescence-based automated quantitative real-time PCR (e.g., ABI 7700 TaqMan system [Applied Biosystems, Foster City, CA] and LightCycler system [Roche Diagnostics, Indianapolis, IN]) now permits extremely accurate and reproducible measurements of specific molecular disease markers over a dynamic range of 10^5–10^6. Application of this technology in our laboratory has revealed dramatic fluctuations in the level of residual *PML-RARα* positive clonal leukemic cells over time in patients treated for acute promyelocytic leukemia, with increasing levels of fusion transcript heralding impending overt relapse. Similar data are also emerging for other leukemia-associated fusion translocations ***(43–45)***. Thus, it appears that both the quantitative ("threshold") level of residual leukemia and the temporal behavior of the clonal population are determinants of disease activity and potential for relapse. Automated quantitative PCR monitoring of patients will likely play an increasing role in this context.

4. Notes

1. RNA quality and recovery are vital to the success of RT-PCR reactions, particularly if sensitive MRD studies are also being performed. The integrity of RNA is also especially important for transcripts such as the t(15;17)-associated *PML-RARα* fusion, which are relatively labile and in low abundance. We have had excellent results with proprietary complete RNA isolation kits, such as those from Ambion or Qiagen (Santa Clarita, CA) and have opted to utilize these in favor of standard guanidinium-based isolation methods. Despite an increase in cost over

more traditional methods, the consistency in RNA quality and yield is better suited to meet the stringent quality assurance issues required in a clinical laboratory and to provide RNA sufficient for routine monitoring of MRD.

2. All stock solutions utilized in reverse transcription and PCR reactions are prepared with DEPC-treated double-distilled water and are stored or manipulated in similarly treated, autoclaved, and dedicated glassware.
3. Stock solution tubes of 10X RT buffer, 10X PCR buffer, and 10 m*M* dNTPs are made in quantity and labeled with a specific lot number. New reagent tubes are tested prior to use in actual assays. The stock buffer and dNTP tubes are kept at –20°C.
4. The Bio-Rad model 785 vacuum transfer system (Bio-Rad) is used in my laboratory with reliable and excellent results. The setup parameters described in **Subheading 3.** refer to this system and will vary slightly for different types of apparatus.
5. Hybridization buffer can be made in quantity and aliquots stored at –20°C, then removed, and warmed in a 60°C water bath when performing hybridization.
6. For positive controls, these sources can be obtained with appropriate permission as required: the NB4 cell line for the t(15;17)/*PML-RARα* L-form (BCR-1) fusion ***(46)***; the UF-1 cell line for the t(15;17)/*PML-RARα* S-form (BCR-3) fusion ***(47)***; the Kasumi-1 cell line for the t(8;21)/*AML1-ETO* fusion ***(48)***; and a cytogenetically confirmed anonymous patient sample for the inv(16)/t(16;16)/*CBFβ-MYH11* anomaly (type A fusion). Finally, in addition to positive control reactions, negative controls (blanks) containing everything except nucleic acid template should be routinely utilized to monitor for contamination.
7. Because PCR techniques are generally quite robust and capable of detecting small amounts of initial nucleic acid target, control of potential contamination during every step of the assay is paramount. My laboratory utilizes separate areas for sample preparation (RNA and DNA isolation), PCR set-up and gel analysis/hybridization. Analyzed PCR products (post-PCR) should *never* be returned to or circulated through PCR setup, and nucleic acid isolation areas. Nucleic acid isolation and PCR stock and working solutions are kept separate from all other laboratory reagents. Positive displacement micropipets (e.g., Rainin Microman, Rainin, Emeryville, CA) and sterile, RNase-free, barrier-type, disposable pipet tips are used throughout. Separate dedicated pipets are utilized in the nucleic acid isolation and PCR areas.
8. The red blood cell lysis method is less favored owing to the presence of residual heme, which can inhibit PCR efficiency.
9. The reverse transcription and PCR steps are performed in thin-walled 100-µL MicroAmp tubes (Perkin-Elmer), for use in a Perkin-Elmer model 9600 or 9700 thermal cycler, or equivalent instrument. Mineral oil overlay is avoided with this approach. Other instruments may require different PCR sample tubes and possibly addition of an oil layer before PCR.
10. For ease of analysis, I add 15 µL of 10 mg/mL of EtBr directly to the warm, prepoured gel.

11. If β_2-microglobulin PCR products are on a separate gel, or are clearly separated from the fusion gene PCR products (e.g., on the other half of a double-comb gel), these are not transferred to the nylon membrane. If they are on the same part of the gel, the β_2-microglobulin PCR products are transferred along with the fusion gene PCR products; the section of membrane containing β_2-microglobulin PCR products is then separated and discarded prior to probe hybridization.
12. Following the specific probe hybridization and warm blot wash steps, several blots can be combined and processed together in the SA-HRP and subsequent room temperature wash steps.
13. During the SA-HRP and room temperature wash steps, the plastic tubs can be kept loosely covered to prevent possible precipitation of the SSPE/SDS solution. Precipitation can occasionally occur in laboratories with lower ambient temperature.
14. Typical exposure times are between 5 and 15 min; however, strong signals are often present on film within 1–3 min. The chemiluminescent output decays rapidly after a few hours.
15. The type of *PML-RARα* fusion in APL does not appear to be associated with clinical outcome. Some previous studies have suggested a more aggressive course for S-form (BCR-3) positive tumors ***(49,50)***. However, the results of a large Intergroup Cooperative trial ***(51)*** did not confirm a significant independent association of this fusion type. Thus, specific chimeric *PML-RARα* mRNA types do not appear to have prognostic value in APL. However, identification of the transcript type in individual patients is important to serve as a marker in MRD studies. We have also encountered rare situations in which different *PML-RARα* transcript types may coexist at diagnosis (e.g., both L- and S-forms), or change from one type to another over time in follow-up samples (personal observations).
16. The three-band pattern observed in first-round L- and V-form *PML-RARα* amplification products arises from alternative splicing. The largest (uppermost) PCR fragment represents the full-length fusion of *PML* exon 6 to *RARα* exon 3. The two lower molecular weight bands occur owing to alternative splicing out of *PML* exon 5 and exons 5 and 6, respectively. The upper two bands of V-form (BCR-2) cases typically are of smaller size compared to the L-form fusion product, owing to the variable break point–fusion events situated within *PML* exon 6; however, rare V-form cases may demonstrate larger or similarly sized PCR bands. For any of these V-form cases, no hybridization signal is expected with the L-form fusion junction oligoprobe.
17. Nested allele-specific PCR ***(34)*** to confirm the presence of the type A *CBFβ-MYH11* fusion mRNA is usually performed in our laboratory. Following first-round PCR, transfer 5 μL from each of the C1-M1 product tubes to a new set of labeled MicroAmp PCR tubes. Assemble the second-round *CBFβ-MYH11* master mix in a 1.5-mL microfuge tube, on ice, as follows: 36.5 μL of DEPC H_2O, 5 μL of 10X PCR buffer, 1 μL of 10 m*M* dNTPs, 1 μL each of second-round primers C2 (sense) and M7 (allele-specific antisense), 0.5 μL of *Taq* DNA polymerase (*see* **Fig. 1B** for location of nested primers). This total of 45 μL of PCR master mix is per sample and needs to be multiplied by the number of samples being tested, plus one extra (n + 1). Add 45 μL of second-round *CBFβ-MYH11*

master mix to each MicroAmp tube and mix the contents of each tube carefully (resulting in a total volume of 50 µL per reaction). Place the tubes in the thermal cycler, programmed as follows: 95°C for 3 min (initial denaturation); 25 cycles of 95°C for 30 s, 57°C for 30 s, and 72°C for 60 s; then 72°C for 5 min (final extension) and cool to 4°C. The C2-M7 PCR products are 65 bp in size on standard gel electrophoresis. This method will specifically confirm the presence of the type A *CBFβ-MYH11* transcript and extends the sensitivity of detection of MRD for this particular fusion by one or two orders of magnitude over first-round (C1-M1) PCR alone in cell dilution experiments (personal observations).

18. As a cautionary note, a rare *CBFβ-MYH11* fusion PCR product with a size almost indistinguishable from the type A product has been identified ***(52)***, resulting from novel fusion sites in both *CBFβ* and *MYH11* genes. This PCR product did not amplify with the allele-specific PCR (**Note 17**) and did not hybridize with the internal *CBFβ* or the inv(16) junction A oligoprobes. Thus, although the use of probe hybridization is generally recommended, DNA sequencing of the PCR product is reserved for rare cases with unusual break points in the *CBFβ* gene.

References

1. Bennett, J. M., Catovsky, D., Daniel, M. T., Flandrin, G., Galton, D. A., Gralnick, H. R., and Sultan, C. (1985) Proposed revised criteria for the classification of acute myeloid leukemia: a report of the French-American-British Cooperative Group. *Ann. Intern. Med.* **103,** 620–625.
2. Head, D. R. (1996) Revised classification of acute myeloid leukemia. *Leukemia* **10,** 1826–1831.
3. Grignani, F., Fagioli, M., Alcalay, M., Longo, L., Pandolfi, P. F., Bonti, E., Biondi, A., LoCoco, F., Grignani, F., and Pelicci, P. G. (1994) Acute promyelocytic leukemia: from genetics to treatment. *Blood* **83,** 10–25.
4. Dyck, J. A., Maul, G. G., Miller, W. H. Jr., Chen, J. D., Kakizuka, A., and Evans, R. M. (1994) A novel macromolecular structure is a target of the promyelocyte-retinoic acid receptor oncoprotein. *Cell* **76,** 333–343.
5. Weism K., Rambaud, S., Lavau, C., Jansen, J., Carvalho, T., Carmo-Fonseca, M., Lamond, A., and Dejean, A. (1994) Retinoic acid regulates aberrant nuclear localization of PML-RARα in acute promyelocytic leukemia cells *Cell* **76,** 345–356.
6. Lamond, A. I. and Earnshaw, W. C. (1998) Structure and function in the nucleus. *Science* **280,** 547–553.
7. Wang, Z. G., Delva, L., Gaboli, M., Rivi, R., Giorgio, M., Cordon-Cardo, C., Grosveld, F., and Pandolfi, P. P. (1998) Role of PML in cell growth and the retinoic acid pathway. *Science* **279,** 1547–1551.
8. Quignon, F., De Bels, F., Koken, M., Feunteun, J., Ameisen, J C., and de The, H. (1998) PML induces a novel caspase-independent death process. *Nat. Genet.* **20,** 259–265.
9. Wang, Z. G., Ruggero, D., Ronchetti, S., Zhong, S., Gaboli, M., Rivi, R., and Pandolfi, P. P. (1998) PML is essential for mulitple apoptotic pathways. *Nat. Genet.* **20,** 266–272.

10. Zheng, P., Guo, Y., Niu, Q., Levy, D. E., Dyck, J. A., Lu, S., Sheiman, L. A., and Liu, Y. (1998) Proto-oncogene *PML* controls genes devoted to MHC class I antigen presentation. *Nature* **396,** 373–376.
11. Degos, L., Dombret, H., Chomienne, C., Daniel, M. T., Micléa, J. M., Chasting, C., Castaigne, S., and Fenaux, P. (1995) All-*trans*-retinoic acid as a differentiating agent in the treatment of acute promyelocytic leukemia. *Blood* **85,** 2643–2653.
12. Tallman, M. S., Andersen, J. W., Sciffer, C. A., Appelbaum, F. R., Feusner, J. H., Ogden, A., Shepherd, L., Willman, C., Bloomfield, C. D., Rowe, J. M., and Wiernik, P. H. (1997) All-*trans*-retinoic acid in acute promyelocytic leukemia. *N. Engl. J. Med.* **337,** 1021–1028.
13. Kane, J. R., Head, D. R., Balazs, L., Hulshof, M. G., Motroni, T. A., Raimondi, S. C., Carroll, A. J., Behm, F. G., Krance, R. A., Shurtleff, S. A., and Downing, J. R. (1996) Molecular analysis of the PML/RAR alpha chimeric gene in pediatric acute promyelocytic leukemia. *Leukemia* **10,** 1296–1302.
14. Liu, P., Tarlé, S. A., Hajra, A., Claxton, D. F., Marlton, P., Freedman, M., Siciliano, M. J., and Collins, F. S. (1993) Fusion between transcription factor CBFβ and a myosin heavy chain in acute myeloid leukemia. *Science* **261,** 1041–1044.
15. Liu, P. P., Hajra, A., Wijmenga, C., and Collins, F. S. (1995) Molecular pathogenesis of the chromosome 16 inversion in the M4Eo subtype of acute myeloid leukemia. *Blood* **85,** 2289–2302.
16. Nucifora, G. and Rowley, J. D. (1995) *AML1* and the 8;21 and 3;21 translocations in acute and chronic myeloid leukemia. *Blood* **86,** 1–14.
17. Daga, A., Tighe, J. E., and Calabi, F. (1992) Leukemia/*Drosophila* homology. *Nature* **356,** 484.
18. Erickson, P., Gao, J., Chang, K. S., Look, T., Whisenant, E., Raimondi, S., Lasher, R., Trujillo, J., Rowley, J. D., and Drabkin, H. (1992) Identification of breakpoints in t(8;21) AML and isolation of a fusion transcript with similarity to *Drosophila* segmentation gene *runt*. *Blood* **80,** 1825.
19. Shurtleff, S. A., Buijs, A., Behm, F. G., Rubnitz, J. E., Raimondi, S. C., Hancock, M. L., Chan, CG. F., Pui, C. H., Grosveld, G., and Downing, J. R. (1995) TEL/AML1 fusion resulting from a cryptic t(12;21) is the most common genetic lesion in pediatric ALL and defines a subgroup of patients with excellent prognosis. *Leukemia* **9,** 1985–1989.
20. Borkhardt, A., Cazzaniga, G., Viehmann, S., Valsecchi, M. G., Ludwig, W. D., Burci, L., Mangioni, S., Schrappe, M., Riehm, H., Lampert, F., Basso, G., Masera, G., Harbott, J., and Biondi, A. (1997) Incidence and clinical relevance of TEL/AML1 fusion genes in children with acute lymphoblastic leukemia enrolled in the German and Italian multicenter therapy trials. *Blood* **90,** 571–577.
21. Wang, Q., Stacy, T., Miller, J. D., Lewis, A. F., Gu, T. L., Huang, X., Bushweller, J. H., Bories, J. C., Alt, F. W., Ryan, G., Liu, P. P., Wynshaw-Boris, A., Binder, M., Marín-Padilla, M., Sharpe, A. H., and Speck, N. A. (1996) The CBFβ subunit is essential for CBFα2 (AML1) function in vivo. *Cell* **87,** 697–708.

22. Wang, Q., Stacy, T., Binder, M., Marín-Padilla, M., Sharpe, A. H., and Speck, N. A. (1996) Disruption of the *Cbfa2* gene causes necrosis and hemorrhaging in the central nervous system and blocks definitive hematopoiesis. *Proc. Natl. Acad. Sci. USA* **93,** 3444–3449.
23. Castilla, L. H., Wijmenga, C., Wang, Q., Stacy, T., Speck, N. A., Eckhaus, M., Marín-Padilla, M., Collins, F. S., Wynshaw-Boris, A., and Liu, P. P. (1996) Failure of embryonic hematopoiesis and lethal hemorrhages in mouse embryos heterozygous for a knocked-in leukemia gene CBFB-MYH11. *Cell* **87,** 687–696.
24. Okuda, T., Cai, Z., Yang, S., Lenny, N., Lyu, C. J., van Deursen, J. M., Harada, H., and Downing, J. R. (1998) Expression of a knocked-in AML1-ETO leukemia gene inhibits the establishment of normal differentiative hematopoiesis and directly generates dysplastic hematopoietic progenitors. *Blood* **91,** 3134–3143.
25. Van de Locht, L. T., Smetsers, T. F., Wittebol, S., Raymakers, R. A., and Mensink, E. J. (1994) Molecular diversity in AML1/ETO fusion transcripts in patients with t(8;21) positive acute myeloid leukaemia. *Leukemia* **8,** 1780–1784.
26. Lin, R. J., Nagy, L., Inoue, S., Shao, W., Miller, W. H. Jr., and Evans, R. M. (1998) Role of the histone deacetylase complex in acute promyelocytic leukaemia. *Nature* **391,** 811–814.
27. Grignani, F., De Matteis, S., Nervi, C., Tomassoni, L., Gelmetti, V., Cioce, M., Fanelli, M., Ruthardt, M., Ferrara, F. F., Zamir, I., Seiser, C., Grignani, F., Lazar, M. A., Minucci, S., and Pelicci, P. G. (1998) Fusion proteins of the retinoic acid receptor-α recruit histone deacetylase in promyelocytic leukaemia. *Nature* **391,** 815–818.
28. Guidez, F., Ivins, S., Zhu, J., Söderström, M., Waxman, S., and Zelent, A. (1998) Reduced retinoic acid-sensitivities of nuclear receptor corepressor binding to PML- and PLZ-RARα underlie molecular pathogenesis and treatment of acute promyelocytic leukemia. *Blood* **91,** 2634–2642.
29. Wang, J., Hoshino, T., Redner, R. L., Kajigaya, S., and Liu, J. M. (1998) ETO, fusion partner in t(8;21) acute myeloid leukemia, represses transcription by interaction with the human N-COR/mSIN3/HDAC1 complex. *Proc. Natl. Acad. Sci. USA* **95,** 10,860–10,865.
30. Lutterbach, B., Westendorf, J. J., Linggi, B., and Hiebert, S. W. (1998) AML-1, a target of multiple chromosomal translocations in acute leukemia, interacts with mSIN3 to repress transcription from the *p21WAF1/CIP1* promoter. *Blood* **92(Suppl.),** 508a.
31. Gallagher, R. E., Li, Y. P., Rao, S., Paietta, E., Andersen, J., Etkind, P., Bennett, J. M., Tallman, M. S., and Wiernik, P. H. (1995) Characterization of acute promyelocytic leukemia cases with PML-RARα break/fusion sites in PML exon 6: identification of a subgroup with decreased in vitro responsiveness to all-*trans* retinoic acid. *Blood* **86,** 1540–1547.
32. Downing, J. R., Head, D. R., Curcio-Brint, A. M., Hulshof, M. G., Motroni, T. A., Raimondi, S. C., Carroll, A. J., Drabkin, H. A., Willman, C., Theil, K. S., Civin, C. I., and Erickson, P. (1993) An *AML1/ETO* fusion transcript is consistently detected by RNA-based polymerase chain reaction in acute myelogenous leukemia containing the (8;21)(q22;q22) translocation. *Blood* **81,** 2860–2865.

33. Shurtleff, S. A., Meyers, S., Hiebert, S. W., Raimondi, S. C., Head, D. R., Willman, C. L., Wolman, S., Slovak, M. L., Carroll, A. J., Behm, F., Hulshof, M. G., Motroni, T. A., Okuda, T., Liu, P., Collins, F. S, and Downing, J. R. (1995) Heterogeneity in CBFβ/MYH11 fusion messages encoded by the inv(16)(p13q22) and the t(16;16)(p13;q22) in acute myelogenous leukemia. *Blood* **85,** 3695–3703.
34. Hébert, J., Cayuela, J. M., Daniel, M. T., Berger, R., and Sigaux, F. (1994) Detection of minimal residual disease in acute myelomonocytic leukemia with abnormal marrow eosinophils by nested polymerase chain reaction with allele specific amplification. *Blood* **84,** 2291–2296.
35. Barragan, E., Bonanad, S., Lopez, J. A., Bolufer, P., and Sanz, M. A. (1998) Comparison of two reverse transcription-polymerase chain reaction methods for detection of AML1/ETO rearrangement in the M2 subtype of acute myeloid leukaemia. *Clin. Chem. Lab. Med.* **36,** 137–142.
36. Watzinger, F. and Lion, T. (1998) Multiplex PCR for quality control of template RNA/cDNA in RT-PCR assays. *Leukemia* **12,** 1930–1936.
37. Marcucci, G., Caligiuri, M. A., and Bloomfield, C. D. (1997) Defining the "absence" of the CBFβ/MYH11 fusion transcript in patients with acute myeloid leukemia and inversion of chromosome 16 to predict long-term complete remission: a call for definitions. *Blood* **90,** 5022–5025 (letter).
38. Kusec, R., Laczika, K., Knöbl, P., Friedl, J., Greinix, H., Kahls, P., Linkesh, W., Schwarzinger, I., Mitterbauer, G., Purtscher, B., Hass, O. A., Lechner, K., and Jaeger, U. (1994) AML1/ETO fusion mRNA can be detected in remission blood samples of all patients with t(8;21) acute myeloid leukemia after chemotherapy or autologous bone marrow transplantation. *Leukemia* **8,** 735–739.
39. Jurlander, J., Caligiuri, M. A., Ruutu, T., Baer, M. R., Strout, M. P., Oberkircher, A. R., Hoffmann, L., Ball, E. D., Frei-Lahr, D. A., Christiansen, N. P., Block, A. W., Knuutila, S., Herzig, G. P., and Bloomfield, C. D. (1996) Persistence of the AML1/ETO fusion transcript in patients treated with allogeneic bone marrow transplantation for t(8;21) leukemia. *Blood* **88,** 2183–2191.
40. Tobal, K. and Liu Yin, J. A. (1996) Monitoring of minimal residual disease by quantitative reverse transcriptase-polymerase chain reaction for AML1-MTG8 transcripts in AML-M2 with t(8;21). *Blood* **88,** 3704–3709.
41. Diverio, D., Rossi, V., Avvisati, G., De Santis, S., Pistilli, A., Pane, F., Saglio, G., Martinelli, G., Petti, M. C., Santoro, A., Pelicci, P. G., Mandelli, F., Biondi, A., and Lo Coco, F. (1998) Early detection of relapse by prospective reverse transcriptase-polymerase chain reaction analysis of the PML/RARα fusion gene in patients with acute promyelocytic leukemia enrolled in the GIMEMA-AIEOP multicenter "AIDA" trial. *Blood* **92,** 784–789.
42. Diverio, D., Pandolfi, P. P., Rossi, V., Biondi, A., Pelicci, P. G., and Lo Coco, F. (1994) Monitoring of treatment outcome in acute promyelocytic leukemia by RT-PCR. *Leukemia* **8(Suppl. 2),** S63–S65.
43. Marcucci, G., Livak, K. J., Bi, W., Strout, M. P., Bloomfield, C. D., and Caligiuri, M. A. (1998) Detection of minimal residual disease in patients with AML1/ETO-

associated acute myeloid leukemia using a novel quantitative reverse transcription polymerase chain reaction assay. *Leukemia* **12**, 1482–1489.

44. Zhao, S., Xu, H., Xie, Z., Chang, S., Konopleva, M., Kavka, K., Calvert, L., Guo, J. Q., Arlinghaus, R., Siciliano, M., and Andreef, M. (1998) Preliminary comparison of real-time QPCR with cytogenetic karyotype, hypermetaphase FISH and western blot analysis in CML patients in clinical remission. *Blood* **92(Suppl.),** 72a.
45. Mensink, E., van de Locht, A., Schattenberg, A., Linders, E., Schaap, N., Geurts van Kessel, A., De Witte, T. (1998) Quantitation of minimal residual disease in Philadelphia chromosome positive chronic myeloid leukaemia patients using real-time quantitative RT-PCR. *Br. J. Haematol.* **102,** 768–774.
46. Lanotte, M., Martin-Thouvenin, V., Najman, S., Balerini, P., Valensi, F., and Berger, R. (1991) NB4, a maturation inducible cell line with t(15;17) marker isolated from a human acute promyelocytic leukemia (M3). *Blood* **77,** 1080–1086.
47. Kizaki, M., Matsushita, H., Takayama, N., Muto, A., Ueno, H., Awaya, N., Kawai, Y., Asou, H., Kamada, N., and Ikeda, Y. (1996) Establishment and characterization of a novel acute promyelocytic leukemia cell line (UF-1) with retinoic acid-resistant features. *Blood* **88,** 1824–1833.
48. Asou, H., Tashiro, S., Hamamoto, K., Otsuji, A., Kita, K., and Kamada, N. (1991) Establishment of a human acute myeloid leukemia cell line (Kasumi-1) with t(8;21) chromosome translocation. *Blood* **77,** 2031–2036.
49. Huang, W., Sun, G. L., Li, X. S., Cao, Q., Lu, Y., Jang, G. S., Zhang, F. Q., Chai, J. R., Wang, Z. Y., Waxman, S., Chen, Z., and Chen, S. J. (1993) Acute promyelocytic leukemia: clinical relevance of two major PML-RARα isoforms and detection of minimal residual disease by retro-transcriptase/polymerase chain reaction to predict relapse. *Blood* **82,** 1264.
50. Vahdat, L., Maslak, P., Miller, H. W., Eardley, A., Heller, G., Scheinberg, D. A., and Warrell, R. P. Jr. (1994) Early mortality and the retinoic acid syndrome in acute promyelocytic leukemia: impact of leukocytosis, low-dose chemotherapy, PMN/RAR-α isoform, and CD13 expression in patients treated with all-*trans* retinoic acid. *Blood* **84,** 3843–3849.
51. Gallagher, R. E., Willman, C. L., Slack, J. L., Andersen, J. W., Li, Y. P., Viswanatha, D., Bloomfield, C. D., Appelbaum, F. R., Schiffer, C. A., Tallman, M. S., and Wiernik, P. H. (1997) Association of PML-RARα fusion mRNA type with pretreatment hematologic characteristics but not treatment outcome in acute promyelocytic leukemia: an intergroup molecular study. *Blood* **90,** 1656–1663.
52. Viswanatha, D. S., Chen, I. M., Liu, P. P., Slovak, M. L., Rankin, C., Head, D. R., and Willman, C. L. (1998) Characterization and use of an antibody detecting the CBFβ-SMMHC fusion protein in inv(16)/t(16;16)-associated acute myeloid leukemias. *Blood* **91,** 1882–1890.

13

Detection of t(14;18)(q32;q21)-Associated *BCL-2/J_H* Gene Fusion in Non-Hodgkin Lymphoma

David S. Viswanatha

1. Introduction

The identification and study of nonrandom recurrent chromosomal translocations has substantially increased our understanding of the non-Hodgkin lymphomas. Cytogenetic and molecular genetic data now form an integral part of current lymphoma classifications ***(1)*** and provide important information for diagnosis, tumor biology, and in some cases prognosis. The t(14;18)(q32;q21) abnormality is the most common translocation detected in B-lineage lymphoma and results in juxtaposition of the *BCL-2* gene (18q21) and the J_H locus of the immunoglobulin (Ig) heavy chain gene (14q32) ***(2–5)***. More specifically, in the North American population, alterations of the *BCL-2* gene are detected in approx 75 to 85% of low-grade follicular lymphomas, 20–30% of aggressive large B-cell lymphomas, and rarely in other B-cell tumors (e.g., chronic lymphocytic leukemia (CLL), acute lymphoblastic leukemia) ***(2,6–9)***. As a consequence of the *BCL-2/J_H* fusion, deregulated overexpression of the antiapoptotic bcl-2 protein occurs owing to constitutive transcriptional activation of the *BCL-2* gene by the Ig heavy chain gene enhancer. The unbridled expression of bcl-2 protein in lymphoid tumors confers resistance to programmed cell death ***(10,11)*** and is implicated in primary therapeutic failure and a less favorable prognosis ***(12–14)***. Although karyotypic detection of lymphoma-associated translocations such as the t(14;18) has proved to be useful in disease diagnosis and subcategorization, molecular genetic approaches including polymerase chain reaction (PCR) and fluorescence *in situ* hybridization (FISH) have gained substantial popularity owing to their rapidity, relatively low cost, and increased sensitivity ***(6,15–22)***.

From: *Methods in Molecular Medicine, vol. 49: Molecular Pathology Protocols*
Edited by: A. A. Killeen © Humana Press Inc., Totowa, NJ

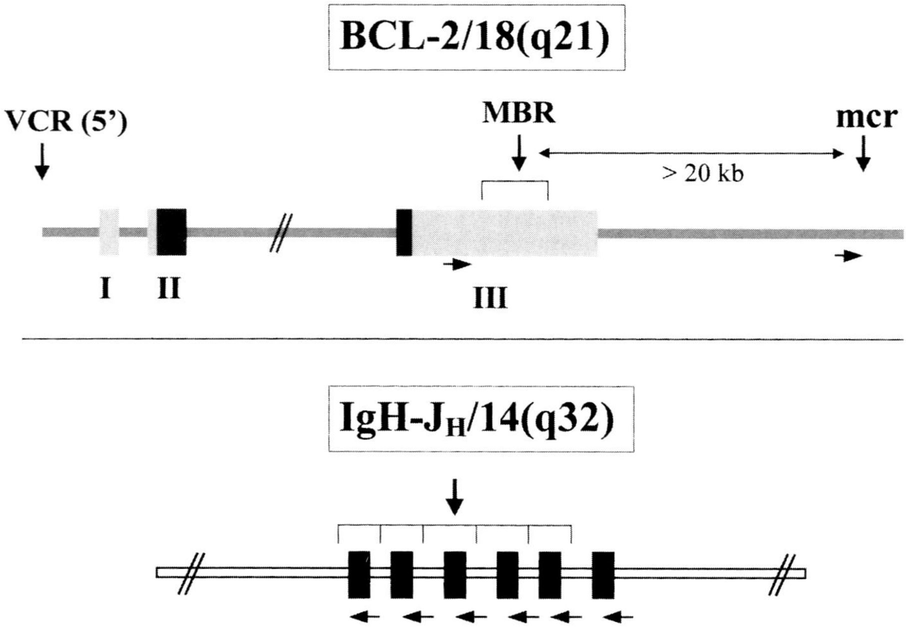

Fig. 1. Schematic diagrams of *BCL-2* and immunoglobulin J_H gene regions. (**Top**) *BCL-2* gene. Exons are rectangular boxes (I–III). Gray shading indicates noncoding exon regions. Relative locations of principal breakpoint regions are indicated by vertical arrows: VCR, variant cluster region; MBR, major breakpoint region; mcr, minor cluster region. The MBR is situated in the 3 noncoding area of *BCL-2* exon 3 and encompasses a tightly clustered segment of approx 150 bp. Positions of MBR and mcr locus primers for PCR are indicated by short horizontal arrows. Oligonucleotide probes for MBR and mcr rearrangement detection are situated internal to the respective primers (not shown). (**Bottom**) Immunoglobulin heavy chain gene J_H locus. The six J_H exons are shown as rectangular boxes. Breakpoints can be distributed in any of the J_H intron areas. Consensus J_H primer for PCR is illustrated by short horizontal arrows (one primer, complementary to conserved J_H sequence).

The partial genomic structures of the *BCL-2* and Ig heavy chain genes are illustrated schematically in **Fig. 1**. In the case of the Ig heavy chain gene locus, the vast majority of breakpoints arising from the t(14;18) are distributed within the joining region (J_H) introns. The largest proportion (60%) of break-fusion sites in the *BCL-2* gene occurs in a tightly clustered area in the 3′ noncoding segment of exon 3, known as the major breakpoint region (MBR) ***(3)***, whereas a small number (15–20%) involves a second clustered region called the minor cluster region (mcr) ***(23,24)***. Rarely, a 5′ region of *BCL-2* called the variant cluster region (*VCR*) is rearranged in B-cell CLL; typically, the VCR locus is involved in translocations with the Ig light chain genes ***(25,26)***. As a result of the relatively tight clustering of genomic breakpoints in the MBR and mcr loci of the *BCL-2* gene, PCR techniques can be employed to detect the majority of t(14;18)-associated *BCL-2/*J_H fusions. This strategy, depicted in **Fig. 1**, can be accomplished using MBR and mcr oligonucleotide primers placed upstream of the clustered regions, in combination with a consensus J_H primer.

The identification of BCL-2 gene rearrangements in lymphoid proliferations is quite useful in several clinical contexts including the diagnosis and subclassification of non-Hodgkin lymphoma. Demonstration of clonality represents an important means of confirming the diagnosis of lymphoma in cases in which morphologic and phenotypic methods have been inconclusive. Clonal Ig gene rearrangements are often not detected by standard PCR techniques in follicular center cell lymphomas ***(27)***. However, the *BCL-2/*J_H abnormality is readily detected by PCR, providing an alternative clonal marker for distinguishing follicular lymphoma from an atypical or florid but benign follicular hyperplasia. As a corollary, PCR analysis for the *BCL-2/*J_H fusion can be used to differentiate subtypes of non-Hodgkin lymphoma with similar morphologic features, such as follicular lymphoma versus lymphomas of mantle or marginal zone type. As knowledge of lymphoma biology continues to broaden, the recognition of specific entities based on molecular genetic criteria will likely form an integral aspect of "tumor-directed" therapies. Finally, sensitive PCR detection of the *BCL-2/*J_H fusion can serve as a patient-specific marker for monitoring of minimal residual disease (MRD) in individuals undergoing intensive chemotherapy or bone marrow transplantation for follicular lymphoma; this aspect is discussed briefly in **Subheading 3.6.**

2. Materials

2.1. Isolation of DNA

2.1.1. Isolation of DNA from Cell Pellets and Fresh or Frozen Tissues

1. DNA isolation kit (Puregene; Gentra Systems, Minneapolis MN) (*see* **Note 1**).
2. Proteinase K solution (20 µg/µL) (Puregene; Gentra Systems).
3. RNase A solution (4 µg/µL) (Puregene; Gentra Systems).
4. Isopropanol, reagent grade (EM Science, Gibbstown, NJ).
5. Cold 70% ethanol.

2.1.2. Isolation of DNA from Fixed, Paraffin-Embedded Tissues

1. Xylene (Fisher, Fair Lawn, NJ).
2. Absolute ethanol (Midwest Grain Products, Pekin, IL).
3. QIAamp DNA Mini kit (Qiagen, Santa Clarita, CA) (*see* **Note 1**).
4. Proteinase K solution (approx 18 µg/µL) (Qiagen).

Table 1
Primer and Probe Sequences for *BCL-2/J_H* PCR Analysis

Primer or Probe	Sequence (5′ → 3′)[a]
MBR	CCAAGTCATGTGCATTTCCACGTC
mcr	ACAGCGTGGTTAGGGTTAGGTCGTA
J_H	ACCTGAGGAGACGGTGACC
β-Globin I	GGTTGGCCAATCTACTCCCAGG
β-Globin II	GCTCACTCAGTGTGGCAAAG
MBR probe	*TAGAGAGTTGCTTTACGTGGCCTG
mcr probe	*AGTGCCTGGCATAGAGCAAG

[a]An asterisk denotes 5′-biotin label for use in chemiluminescent probe hybridization and detection.

2.2. PCR for BCL-2/J_H Fusion

1. 10 m*M* stock dNTPs (Perkin-Elmer, Foster City, CA) (*see* **Note 2**).
2. 10X PCR buffer (Perkin-Elmer): 100 m*M* Tris-HCl (pH 8.4), 500 m*M* KCl, 15 m*M* $MgCl_2$.
3. Sense and antisense primers (15–20 pmol/μL of each) (*see* **Table 1**).
4. AmpliTaq DNA polymerase (5 U/μL) (Perkin-Elmer/Roche, Foster City, CA).
5. Diethylpyrocarbonate (DEPC) distilled H_2O.

2.3. Gel Analysis of PCR Product and Vacuum Blot Transfer

1. Standard powdered agarose for 1.5% agarose gel (3g) (SeaKem ME, FMC Bioproducts, ME).
2. Ethidium bromide (EtBr) solution (10 mg/mL) (Gibco-BRL/Life Technologies, Gaithersburg, MD).
3. Stock 10X Tris-borate EDTA (TBE) buffer solution: 107.8 g of Tris-HCl, 55 g of boric acid, 7.4 g of Na_2EDTA per 1 L of sterile distilled H_2O (0.5X TBE is used for gel and 1X TBE for running buffer).
4. 10X Sample loading dye: 1 vol of 1% bromophenol blue, 1 vol of 1% xylene cyanol, 2 vol of glycerol.
5. Horizontal gel box (40 cm) with 20-well combs (BRL Horizon 20.25; Gibco-BRL/Life Technologies).
6. UV light box and instant camera setup with Polaroid 667 B+W film (Polaroid, Cambridge, MA).
7. Biodyne B nylon membrane (11 × 20 cm) (Pall-Biodyne, East Hills, NY) to encompass area of gel being transferred.
8. Two clean plastic tubs.
9. Dilute (0.05 *N*) HCl (500 mL).
10. 0.4 *M* NaOH (1 L).

11. Bio-Rad Model 785 vacuum transfer apparatus with vacuum regulator (Bio-Rad, Hercules, CA) (*see* **Note 3**).
12. UV crosslinking apparatus (UV Stratalinker; Stratagene, La Jolla, CA).

2.4. Nonisotopic Probe Hybridization

1. Stock 20X SSPE buffer: 210.4 g of NaCl, 27.6 g of $NaH_2PO_4 \cdot H_2O$, 4.4 g of NaOH, 7.4 g of Na_2EDTA per 1 L of sterile distilled H_2O; the buffer usually requires gentle heat with constant stirring to completely solubilize. From this prepare the following:
   a. Prehybridization solution (100 mL): 0.1X SSPE/0.5% sodium dodecyl sulfate (SDS) (from 10% SDS stock solution).
   b. Blot wash solution (2 L): 2X SSPE/0.1% SDS.
   c. 50-mL Aliquots of hybridization buffer: 5X SSPE/0.1% SDS (*see* **Note 4**).
2. 5′-Biotinylated oligonucleotide probes (10–15 pmol/µL) (*see* **Table 1**).
3. Heat-sealable plastic hybridization bags.
4. Several clean plastic tubs with lids.
5. Streptavidin-horseradish peroxidase (SA-HRP) (1mg/mL) (Vector, Burlingame, CA).
6. ECL chemiluminescence detection reagent solutions 1 and 2 (Amersham Pharmacia Biotech, Piscataway, NJ).
7. Fluorescent marking pen.
8. Standard filter (blotting) paper.
9. Plastic wrap.
10. Radiographic film (Kodak XAR; Eastman-Kodak, Rochester, NY).

3. Methods

The PCR method detailed is based on a previously described protocol ***(6)***, optimized for use in my laboratory. General laboratory principles pertaining to the performance of PCR and analysis of PCR products should be followed (*see* **Note 5**).

3.1. Isolation of DNA

3.1.1. Isolation of DNA from Cell Pellets and Fresh or Frozen Tissues

1. Obtain a cell pellet (of blood or bone marrow) or minced tissue sample in a 15-mL conical centrifuge tube.
2. Follow manufacturer's general guidelines for the Puregene kit, for cell pellets ($10–20 \times 10^6$ cells) or tissue samples (10–20 mg) (*see* **Note 6**).
3. Resuspend the DNA pellet in a volume of DNA hydration buffer (e.g., 1X TE or equivalent) to give an approximate concentration of 1 µg/µL. Hydration may be accomplished overnight at ambient temperature for large sample isolates. Calculate the concentration and yield by standard 260-nm UV absorbance spectrophotometry.
4. Store the DNA samples at –20°C.

3.1.2. Isolation of DNA from Fixed, Paraffin-Embedded Tissues

1. Obtain three to four 10-µm thick sections of paraffin-embedded tissue. Generally, only two of these are required for isolation and the remaining material can be kept for reisolation if the initial yield or PCR is inadequate. Place the tissue sections in a 1.5-mL microfuge tube (*see* **Note 7**).
2. Add 1 mL of xylene to the tube and vortex vigorously to mix well. Centrifuge in a tabletop microcentrifuge on the highest setting for 5 min (*see* **Note 8**). Carefully draw off the xylene and discard in an appropriate organic waste container.
3. Add 1 mL of absolute ethanol, vortex, and centrifuge on highest setting for 5 min. Draw off and discard the ethanol into an appropriate waste container. Repeat this step once more.
4. Follow the manufacturer's directions for the Qiagen QiaAmp DNA Mini kit, for fixed, paraffin-embedded tissues.
5. Calculate the concentration and yield by standard 260-nm UV absorbance spectrophotometry.
6. Store the DNA samples at –20°C.

3.2. PCR for MBR and mcr Region BCL-2/J_H Rearrangements

1. Label three sets of MicroAmp tubes for the samples being tested (*see* **Note 9**), positive controls (*see* **Note 10**), and negative control (blank—no DNA). One set of tubes is for the MBR-J_H PCR, one for the mcr-J_H PCR, and one for the control amplification of the β-globin gene. Similarly, label three 1.5-mL microfuge tubes for each of the PCR master mix solutions.
2. Thaw the DNA tubes and keep on ice. Aliquot 1 µg of DNA into respective MicroAmp tubes, proceeding in order of the sample tubes and then the positive control. Do not add DNA template to the negative control (blank) tubes. Adjust the volume of each tube to 5 µL with sterile DEPC H_2O. Keep on ice or in a cold block.
3. Assemble the PCR master mixes in the corresponding 1.5-mL microfuge tubes, on ice, as follows:
   a. For MBR-J_H: 36.5 µL of DEPC H_2O, 5 µL of 10X PCR buffer, 1 µL of 10 m*M* dNTPs, 1 µL each of primers MBR (sense) and J_H (antisense), 0.5 µL of *Taq* DNA polymerase.
   b. For mcr-J_H: 36.5 µL of DEPC H_2O, 5 µL of 10X PCR buffer, 1 µL of 10 m*M* dNTPs, 1 µL each of primers mcr (sense) and J_H (antisense), 0.5 µL of *Taq* DNA polymerase.
   c. For β-globin: 36.5 µL of DEPC H_2O, 5 µL of 10X PCR buffer, 1 µL of 10 m*M* dNTPs, 1 µL each of primers βI (sense) and βII (antisense), 0.5 µL of *Taq* DNA polymerase. (Note that this total 45-µL vol of each specific PCR master mix is per sample and needs to be multiplied by the number of samples being tested, plus one extra (n + 1). Gently vortex the tubes with lids closed to mix the contents.)
4. Begin with the β-globin PCR tube set and add 45 µL of master mix to each of the respective MicroAmp tubes (resulting in a total volume of 50 µL/tube). Mix the contents of each tube gently and carefully. Proceed similarly, adding 45 µL of

MBR-J_H and mcr-J_H master mixes to each of the MicroAmp tubes in the respective PCR sets, mixing the contents of tubes carefully (resulting in a total volume of 50 µL/tube). In each PCR reaction set, proceed in the order from the test samples to the positive control and finally the negative control.

5. Place all the tubes in a thermal cycler, programmed as follows: 95°C for 5 min (initial denaturation); 2 cycles of 95°C for 30 s, 61°C for 15 s, and 72°C for 30 s; then 30 cycles of 95°C for 15 s, 58°C for 15 s, and 72°C for 30 s; then 72°C for 5 min (final extension) and cool to 4°C. Following the PCR reaction, remove the tubes from the thermal cycler and store the PCR products in a refrigerator or –20°C freezer until ready for gel electrophoresis.

3.3. Gel Electrophoresis Analysis and Vacuum Blot Transfer of BCL-2/J_H PCR Products

1. Prepare a 1.5% agarose gel (with 0.5X TBE) (*see* **Note 11**).
2. In a microtiter plate, add 15 µL of PCR products to 2.5 µL of 10X sample loading dye. A DNA size marker is also used, such as the 100-bp ladder (Gibco-BRL/Life Technologies). Mix briefly and load the MBR-J_H PCR products in one set of lanes, followed by mcr-J_H products, separating the two groups of PCR products by two empty lanes. Load β-globin products in a separate set of lanes. Carry out electrophoresis at 180 V for 1.5–2 h.
3. Following electrophoresis, observe and photograph the gel under UV illumination. Proper eye protection is required when viewing gels by UV light. Standard black-and-white Polaroid photographs are obtained using a photograph stand (*see* **Note 12**).
4. Place the gel in a plastic tub and cover with 300–400 mL of dilute (0.05 *M*) HCl (acid-nicking step). Place on a gyratory platform on gentle setting for 10 min. During this time, allow the precut nylon membrane to equilibrate in 300–400 mL of 0.4 *M* NaOH.
5. Decant the dilute HCl and add an equal amount of 0.4 *M* NaOH over the gel.
6. Assemble the vacuum transfer apparatus according to the manufacturer's directions. Align the gel over the nylon membrane, ensuring that the wells are outside of the vacuum gasket seal. Slowly engage the vacuum to negative pressure of 4 to 5 mmHg. Pour approx 250 mL of 0.4 *M* NaOH over the gel to cover the area for transfer. Transfer the gel products to the nylon membrane for 1 h.
7. Disassemble the vacuum transfer apparatus and remove the nylon membrane. Place the membrane in a UV crosslinker and crosslink the DNA to the membrane at a 500-µJ power setting. Label the well locations at the top of the gel using a soft pencil and allow the membrane to dry.
8. Cut and separate sections containing MBR-J_H and mcr-J_H PCR products, label each appropriately, and trim off the excess membrane. If β-globin products have been transferred on the same membrane, cut away the area containing β-globin product lanes and discard. The MBR-J_H reaction products will be hybridized with the internal sequence MBR oligoprobe whereas the mcr-J_H products will be hybridized with the internal sequence mcr oligoprobe.

3.4. Nonisotopic (Chemiluminescent) Probe Hybridization for BCL-2/J_H Fusion

1. Warm to 60°C in a water bath 50 mL of prehybridization solution (0.1X SSPE/0.5% SDS) and two 15-mL aliquots (one per separate hybridization reaction) of hybridization buffer (5X SSPE/0.1% SDS).
2. Place nylon membranes of MBR-J_H and mcr-J_H PCR products in appropriately labeled, heat-sealable plastic bags and add 15 mL of prehybridization buffer to each. Displace bubbles through the open end of the bag, heat-seal the bag, and place in a 60°C oven, on a rocking platform. Allow 30 min for prehybridization.
3. Add 5 µL of the biotinylated oligoprobes (MBR and mcr) to respective 15-mL aliquots of warm hybridization buffer and gently mix (final concentration of approx 1 to 2 pmol/mL of buffer). Remove and cut open the plastic bags across the top. Drain the prehybridization buffer and carefully add 15 mL of the hybridization buffer with the specific oligoprobe to the corresponding bags. Express excess air and bubbles and heat-seal the bags just above the nylon membrane. Check for leaks and place in a 60°C oven for 1 h. The hybridization reactions can be extended to overnight for convenience.
4. Prepare 2 L of blot wash solution (2X SSPE/0.1% SDS). Aliquot 500 mL of wash solution and heat to 60°C in a water bath. Be sure to verify the temperature of the solution. Leave the remaining wash solution covered at room temperature. Warm two clean empty plastic tubs in a 60°C oven.
5. Remove the hybridization bags, cut across to open, and drain the hybridization solution. Remove the nylon membranes and place in separate plastic tubs. Then add approx 125 mL of warm (60°C) blot wash buffer to each. Cover the tubs and place in 60°C oven on a rocking platform for 10 min. Repeat this step once with the remaining warm blot wash solution (*see* **Note 13**).
6. Prepare SA-HRP solution in a clean plastic tub using 250 mL of room temperature blot wash solution and 10 µL of SA-HRP (final concentration of 40 ng/mL).
7. Following the second warm (60°C) wash, briefly rinse the membranes with approx 100 mL of room temperature wash solution and transfer to the SA-HRP solution. Place on a slowly gyrating platform for 15 min.
8. Drain the SA-HRP solution, briefly rinse with 100 mL of room temperature blot wash solution, and decant. Then add another 400 mL of blot wash solution. Place on a gyrating platform for 5–10 min. Repeat the wash with another 400 mL of room temperature solution (*see* **Note 14**).
9. Place the wet membranes on clean dry filter paper. Quickly pipet 5 mL each of ECL chemiluminescence reagents 1 and 2 into a clean glass tray and mix by gentle agitation. Place each membrane in the tray and coat thoroughly with ECL reagents for 1 min. Remove and affix the membranes to clean precut filter paper. Mark the well locations with a fluorescent pen, label the blots as to probe type, and seal over the membranes with plastic wrap. Develop chemiluminescent image on X-ray film as usual (*see* **Note 15**).

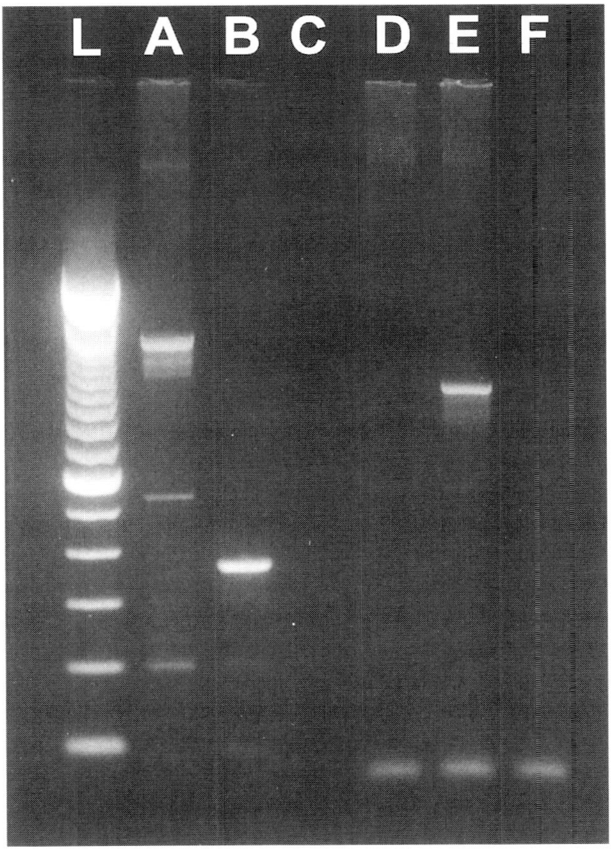

Fig. 2. Agarose gel electrophoresis of *BCL-2/J$_H$* PCR (MBR and mcr). Lanes A–C and MBR/J$_H$ PCR products: A, patient sample; B, positive control; C, negative control (no DNA). Note the difference in PCR amplicon fragment length between patient and positive control, illustrating the range of size that can be generated by the *BCL-2/J$_H$* fusion. Lanes D–F are mcr/J$_H$ PCR products: D, patient sample; E, positive control; F, negative control (no DNA). Lane L is a 100-bp molecular weight marker.

3.5. Interpretation: t(14;18)/BCL-2/J$_H$ Results

Both agarose gel and chemiluminscent blot results are examined to determine the presence or absence of a *BCL-2/J$_H$* fusion. A prominent ethidium-stained gel band with corresponding positivity on the blot denotes a positive result (**Figs. 2** and **3**). Conversely, the lack of gel and hybridization signals is

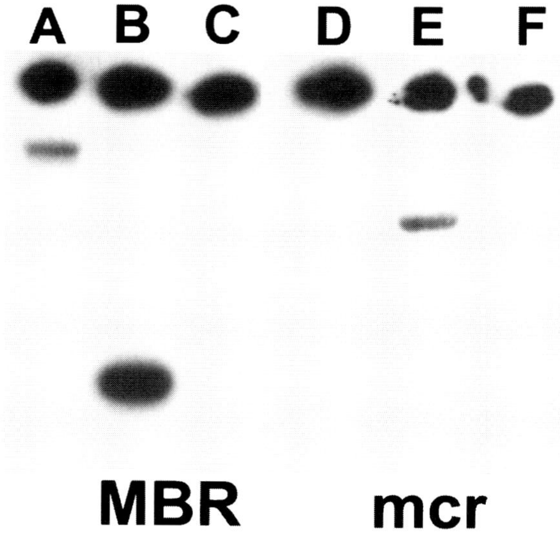

Fig. 3. Chemiluminescent oligoprobe hybridization to detect MBR/J_H and mcr/J_H fusions. *BCL-2/J_H* PCR products hybridized with biotinylated internal MBR or mcr oligoprobes. Lane (sample) designations are the same as for **Fig. 2**.

consistent with the absence of the *BCL-2/J_H* rearrangement. In any case, demonstration of a positive β-globin amplification is also required to exclude the possibility of poor-quality DNA or PCR failure, prior to concluding that a PCR test is negative. Occasionally one or more low-intensity bands may be observed on agarose gels with diagnostic specimens; in my experience, these low-intensity (low-quantity) PCR products are nearly always artifactual in nature and do not hybridize with the oligoprobes.

PCR product fragments will be of unique size in individual cases (**Figs. 2** and **3**), owing to the variability of breakpoint sites in the MBR or mcr loci, as well as the possibility of fusion to any of six J_H Ig heavy chain gene segments. This feature can help to distinguish between true *BCL-2/J_H* rearrangements and false-positive bands resulting from contamination, in assays with multiple samples. For the MBR locus, PCR product sizes may range between 300 and >1000 bp *(6)*. The typical size range for most MBR BCL-2/J_H amplicons is approx 400–500 bp. PCR analysis of the mcr locus as presented herein can be expected to identify amplified fragments in the 400-bp size range, although, again, larger products up to 1000 bp can be encountered ***(6,23)***.

3.6. Conclusion

With the use of the single-round PCR technique described, one can expect to identify slightly more than two thirds of all *BCL-2/J*$_H$ gene fusions arising from the t(14;18)(q32;q21) in non-Hodgkin lymphoma ***(6)***. PCR therefore represents a powerful tool to detect this abnormality in a rapid and cost-effective manner. The majority of fusions involving the MBR locus will be detected by this PCR method; however, mcr locus fusions have a lower overall detection rate (approx 50%). The latter situation arises in part because of a looser and less well-defined clustering of break-fusion sites in the mcr such that breakpoints upstream or far downstream of the mcr primer will not be detected. Notably, large amplicon PCR targets created by both MBR and mcr locus *BCL-2/J*$_H$ fusions may be inconsistently detected owing to PCR inefficiency and may require nested PCR techniques. The presence of large PCR amplicons is also of considerable significance when using archival (fixed) tissues, because DNA extracted from paraffin-embedded sources is frequently compromised owing to crosslinking and degradation of high molecular weight strands. As a result, the detection rate of *BCL-2/J*$_H$ for both MBR and mcr locus fusions is usually lower in paraffin tissue specimens compared to fresh or frozen tissue samples.

Other investigators have recently described the application of long distance PCR (LD-PCR) to identify and further characterize the molecular anatomy of *BCL-2/J*$_H$ fusions ***(28)***. LD-PCR and sequencing analyses have revealed extended breakpoint sites occurring in the far 3′ MBR region and also 5′ of the mcr locus, largely accounting for the remainder of *BCL-2/J*$_H$ fusions not identified by standard PCR techniques ***(28)***. To achieve a more comprehensive detection rate for *BCL-2* gene rearrangements, Southern blot hybridization or FISH methods have been described ***(6,16,21,22,29)***. However, these approaches can be laborious and require the availability of genomic or cloned probes. Nonetheless, Southern blot hybridization or FISH remain important modalities for the detection of rare *BCL-2* rearrangements, such as those involving the VCR.

Brief mention is made here regarding the distinction of detection rate versus sensitivity of this PCR assay. Detection rate refers to the number of truly positive *BCL-2* gene–rearranged cases that can be identified by the assay (against an established standard method). PCR sensitivity is defined in a dilutional sense: that is, how capable is the assay of identifying low levels of the specific gene fusion in question? Although *BCL-2/J*$_H$ PCR is used in my laboratory primarily to assist in the diagnosis and classification of lymphoid tumors, the sensitivity of this assay can be optimized for detection of *BCL-2/J*$_H$ fusions at a level of 1 in 10^4–10^5 cells. The high sensitivity of PCR and unique *BCL-2/J*$_H$ amplicon size (and sequence) for a given patient sample creates a clonal "fingerprint" for assessment of MRD during or following therapy for lymphoma.

This concept has been applied to patients with follicular lymphoma undergoing intensive chemotherapy with or without autologous bone marrow transplantation, in which the detection of residual *BCL-2/*J_H fusion DNA can serve as a prognostic marker of posttherapeutic outcome. In general, the molecular clearance of residual *BCL-2/*J_H DNA, or its absence in preinfusion peripheral blood or bone marrow progenitor cell autografts, has been correlated with significantly prolonged disease-free and relapse-free survival ***(30–34)***. Finally, the advent of highly sensitive and automated real-time fluorescent PCR techniques promises to revolutionize the measurement of MRD in these clinical settings, by greatly increasing the accuracy and reproducibility of detection ***(35,36)***. However, as a cautionary note, *BCL-2/*J_H fusion events have been reported at very low levels in normal individuals or in patients without lymphoproliferative disease ***(37–42)***, implying that errant *BCL-2/*J_H rearrangements may occur in lymphoid cells in the absence of frank neoplasia. Although standard PCR methods have not been shown to detect false-positive *BCL-2/*J_H fusions in histologically benign tissues ***(43)***, the finding of rare event positivity is of potential concern in more sensitive MRD analyses, unless sequencing and design of patient tumor-specific primers or probes is employed ***(44)***.

In conclusion, PCR evaluation of the *BCL-2/*J_H fusion abnormality can be a valuable adjunct to the diagnosis and assessment of MRD of B-cell lymphoproliferative disorders. As with any ancillary investigation, the results of *BCL-2/*J_H PCR analyses should be correlated with clinical, histologic, and laboratory data to be of the greatest use in diagnostic medicine.

4. Notes

1. The use of proprietary DNA isolation kits has been adopted in my laboratory, both for fresh or frozen tissue and paraffin-embedded tissue extractions. Many "homemade" reagents are used for DNA isolation, some of which may be as effective, or less costly. However, the consistent reagent quality of the former products has been an added benefit to quality control issues in my clinical molecular diagnostic setting.
2. All stock solutions utilized in PCR reactions are prepared with DEPC-treated double-distilled water and stored or manipulated in similarly treated, autoclaved, and dedicated glassware. Stock solution tubes of 10 m*M* dNTPs are made in quantity and labeled with a specific lot number. New reagent tubes are tested prior to use in actual assays. The dNTPs, buffer, primers, and enzyme tubes are stored at –20°C.
3. The Bio-Rad model 785 vacuum transfer system (Bio-Rad) is used in my laboratory with reliable and excellent results. The setup parameters described in **Subheading 3.** refer to this system and will vary slightly for different types of apparatus.

4. Hybridization buffer can be made in quantity and aliquots stored at –20°C, then removed, and warmed in a 60°C water bath when performing hybridization.
5. Because PCR techniques are generally very robust and capable of detecting small amounts of initial nucleic acid target, control of potential contamination during every step of the assay is paramount. My laboratory utilizes separate areas for sample preparation (RNA and DNA isolation), PCR setup, and gel analysis/hybridization. Analyzed PCR products (post-PCR) should *never* be returned to or circulated through PCR setup and nucleic acid isolation areas. Nucleic acid isolation and PCR stock and working solutions are kept separate from all other laboratory reagents. Positive displacement micropipets (e.g , Rainin Microman; Rainin, Emeryville, CA) and sterile, RNase-free, barrier-type, disposable pipet tips are used throughout. Separate dedicated pipets are utilized in the nucleic acid isolation and PCR areas.
6. For cell pellets (e.g., from blood, bone marrow, or body fluid samples), cells can be obtained by the density gradient method (Ficoll Hypaque; Pharmacia) or red cell lysis. The latter can result in the presence of residual heme, which may inhibit PCR efficiency. Cell pellets are easily lysed and DNA can generally be extracted without a proteinase K digestion. For tissue samples, the specimen is quickly diced as finely as possible using a sterile disposable blade, and then placed in lysis buffer with proteinase K. Larger tissue volumes or fibrotic specimens may require prolonged (i.e., overnight) digestion at 37 or 55°C.
7. Procurement of paraffin tissue sections must be done with considerable attention to detail. The microtome area must be extremely clean, and preferably a new disposable blade should be used between samples. Tissue curls can be carefully placed in a 1.5-mL microfuge tube; however, tissue "flaking" is common and may increase the risk of contamination. Generally, unknown samples are cut first, then positive control(s), then negative control. As an alternative, unstained paraffin sections can be provided on glass slides and either scraped into the sample tubes or carefully dissolved in xylene before transfer to the tube. The issue of section thickness is controversial; although some anecdotal reports suggest that thicker sections increase the concentration of PCR inhibitors, I have had good results from sections between 5 and 20 μm thick. If adequate DNA has been obtained and PCR inhibition is suspected, 1:10 and 1:50 dilutions of the DNA extract can be made for PCR, to dilute out the effect of a potential inhibitor.
8. Xylene is a biohazardous organic chemical and must be used cautiously, preferably in a ventilated hood area. Following dissolution of the paraffin and centrifugation, the xylene must be removed slowly, because the tissue pellet tends to be poorly compacted and may be disrupted, leading to lower tissue (and thus DNA) yield.
9. PCR steps are performed in thin-walled 100-μL MicroAmp tubes (Perkin-Elmer) for use in a Perkin-Elmer model 9600 or 9700 thermal cycler, or equivalent instrument. Mineral oil overlay is avoided with this approach. Other instruments may require different PCR sample tubes and possibly the addition of an oil layer before PCR.

10. For the *BCL-2* MBR positive control, DNA from an anonymous patient lymphoma with a documented t(14;18) and MBR-J_H fusion was used. Several cell lines containing *BCL-2*/J_H MBR rearrangements have been reported, including the DOHH-2 and SU-DHL-4 lines. For the *BCL-2* mcr positive control, the DHL-16 cell line was used (kindly provided by Dr. J. Gribben, Dana Farber Cancer Institute).
11. For ease of analysis, I add 15 µL of 10 mg/mL EtBr directly to the warm, prepoured gel.
12. If β-globin PCR products are on a separate gel, or are clearly separated from the *BCL-2*/J_H fusion gene PCR products (e.g., on the other half of a double-comb gel), these are not transferred to the nylon membrane. If they are on the same part of the gel, the β-globin PCR products are transferred along with the fusion gene PCR products. The section of membrane containing β-globin PCR products is then separated and discarded prior to probe hybridization.
13. Following the specific probe hybridization and warm blot wash steps, several blots can be combined and processed together in the SA-HRP and subsequent room temperature wash steps.
14. During the SA-HRP and room temperature wash steps, the plastic tubs can be kept loosely covered to prevent possible precipitation of the SSPE/SDS solution. Precipitation occasionally can occur in laboratories with lower ambient temperature.
15. Typical exposure times are between 5 and 15 min; however, strong signals are often present on film within 1–3 min. The chemiluminescent output decays rapidly after a few hours.

References

1. Harris, N. L., Jaffe, E. S., Stein, H., et al. (1994) A revised European-American classification of lymphoid neoplasms: a proposal from the International Lymphoma Study Group. *Blood* **84,** 1361–1392.
2. Weiss, L. M., Warnke, R. A., Sklar, J., and Cleary, M. L. (1987) Molecular analysis of the t(14;18) chromosomal translocation in malignant lymphomas. *N. Engl. J. Med.* **317,** 1185.
3. Cleary, M. L. and Sklar, J. (1985) Nucleotide sequence of t(14;18) chromosomal translocation breakpoint in follicular lymphoma and demonstration of a breakpoint cluster region near a transcriptionally active locus on chromosome 18. *Proc. Natl. Acad. Sci. USA* **82,** 7439.
4. Bakhshi, A., Jensen, J. P., Goldman, P., Wright, J. J., McBride, O. W., Epstein, A. L., and Korsmeyer, S. J. (1985) Cloning the chromosomal breakpoint of t(14;18) human lymphomas: clustering around J_H on chromosome 14 and near a transcriptional unit on 18. *Cell* **41,** 899.
5. Tsujimoto, Y., Cossman, J., Jaffe, E., and Croce, C. M. (1985) Involvement of the bcl-2 gene in human follicular lymphomas. *Science* **228,** 1440.
6. Horsman, D. E., Gascoyne, R. D., Coupland, R. W., Coldman, A. J., and Adomat, S. A. (1995) Comparison of cytogenetic analysis, Southern analysis, and polymerase chain reaction for the detection of t(14;18) in follicular lymphoma. *Am. J. Clin. Pathol.* **103,** 472–478.

7. Yabumoto, K., Akasaka, T., Muramatsu, M., Kadowaki, N., Hayashi, T., Ohno, H., Fukuhara, S., and Okuma, M. (1996) Rearrangement of the 5′ cluster region of the bcl-2 gene in lymphoid neoplasm: a summary of nine cases. *Leukemia* **10,** 970–977.
8. Adachi, M., Cossman, J., Longo, D., Croce, C. M., and Tsujimoto, Y. (1989) Varian translocation of the bcl-2 gene to immunoglobulin light chain gene in chronic lymphocytic leukemia. *Proc. Natl. Acad. Sci. USA* **86,** 2771.
9. Kouides, P. A., Phatak, P. D., Wang, N., and Bennett, J. M. (1994) B-cell acute lymphoblastic leukemia with L1 morphology and coexistence of t(1;19) and t(14;18) chromosome translocations. *Cancer Genet. Cytogenet.* **78,** 23–27.
10. Yang, E. and Korsmeyer, S. J. (1996) Molecular thanatopsis: a discourse on the BCL2 family and cell death. *Blood* **88,** 386–401.
11. Hockenberry, D., Nunez, G., Milliman, C., Schreiber, R. D., and Korsmeyer, S. J. (1990) Bcl-2 is an inner mitochondrial membrane protein that blocks programmed cell death. *Nature* **348,** 334.
12. Gascoyne, R. D., Adomat, S. A., Krajewski, S., Krajewska, M., Horsman, D. E., Tolcher, A. W., O'Reilly, S. E., Hoskins, P., Coldman, A. J., Reed, J. C., and Connors, J. M.(1997) Prognostic significance of Bcl-2 protein expression and Bcl-2 gene rearrangement in diffuse aggressive non-Hodgkin's lymphoma. *Blood* **90(1),** 44–51.
13. Hill, M. E., MacLennan, K. A., Cunningham, D. C., et al. (1996) Prognostic significance of BCL-2 expression and bcl-2 major breakpoint region rearrangement in diffuse large cell non-Hodgkin's lymphoma: a British National Lymphoma Investigation Study. *Blood* **88(3),** 1046–1051.
14. Hermine, O., Haioun, C., Lepage, E., et al. (1996) Prognostic significance of bcl-2 protein expression in aggressive non-Hodgkin's lymphoma. Groupe d'Etude des Lymphomes de l'Adulte (GELA). *Blood* **87(1),** 265–272.
15. Liu, J., Johnson, R. M., and Traweek, S. T. (1993) Rearrangement of the BCL-2 gene in follicular lymphoma: detection by PCR in both fresh and fixed tissue samples. *Diagn. Mol. Pathol.* **2,** 241–247.
16. Ladanyi, M. and Wang, S. (1992) Detection of rearrangements of the BCL2 major breakpoint region in follicular lymphomas: correlation of polymerase chain reaction results with southern blot analysis. *Diagn. Mol. Pathol.* **1,** 31–35.
17. Shibata, D., Hu, E., Weiss, L. M., Brynes, R. K., and Nathwani, B. N. (1990) Detection of specific t(14;18) chromosomal translocations in fixed tissues. *Hum. Pathol.* **21,** 199–203.
18. Pezella, F., Gatter, K. C., and Mason, D. Y. (1989) Detection of 14;18 chromosomal translocation in paraffin-embedded lymphoma tissue. *Lancet* **1,** 779,780.
19. Crescenzi, M., Seto, M., Herzig, G. P., et al. (1988) Thermostable DNA polymerase chain amplification of t(14;18) chromosome breakpoints and detection of minimal residual disease. *Proc. Natl. Acad. Sci. USA* **85,** 4869–4873.
20. Lee, M., Chang, K., Cabanillas, F., et al. (1987) Detection of minimal residual cells carrying the t(14;18) by DNA sequence amplification. *Science* **230,** 1350–1354.

21. Poetsch, M., Weber-Matthieson, K., Plendl, J. J., Grote, W., and Schlegelberger, B. (1996) Detection of the t(14;18) chromosomal translocation by interphase cytogenetics with yeast-artificial-chromosome probes in follicular lymphoma and nonneoplastic lymphoproliferation. *J. Clin. Oncol.* **14,** 963–969.
22. Taniwaki, M., Silverman, G. A., Nishida, K., Horike, S., Misawa, S., Shimazaki, C., Miura, I., Nagai, M., Abe, M., Fukuhara, S., and Kashima, K. (1995) Translocations and amplification of the BCL2 gene are detected in interphase nuclei of non-Hodgkin's lymphoma by in situ hybridization with yeast artificial chromosome clones. *Blood* **86,** 1481–1486.
23. Ngan, B., Nourse J., and Cleary, M. L. (1989) Detection of chromosomal translocation t(14;18) within the minor cluster region of bcl-2 by polymerase chain reaction and direct genomic sequencing of the enzymatically amplified DNA in follicular lymphomas. *Blood* **73,** 1759–1762.
24. Cleary, M. L., Galili, N., and Sklar, J. (1986) Detection of a second t(14;18) breakpoint cluster region in follicular lymphomas. *J. Exp. Med.* **164,** 315.
25. Dyer, M. J. S., Zani, V. J, Lu, W. Z., et al. (1994) BCL2 Translocations in leukemias of mature B cells. *Blood* **83,** 3682–3688.
26. Adachi, M., Tefferi, A., Greipp, P. R., Kipps, T. J., and Tsujimoto, Y. (1990) Preferential linkage of BCL-2 to immunoglobulin light chain gene in chronic lymphocytic leukemia. *J. Exp. Med.* **171,** 559.
27. Segal, G. H., Jorgensen, T., Scott, M., and Braylan, R. C. (1994) Optimal primer selection for clonality assessment by polymerase chain reaction analysis: II. Follicular lymphomas. *Hum. Pathol.* **25,** 1276–1282.
28. Akasaka, T., Akasaka, H., Yonetani, N., Ohno, H., Yamabe, H., Fukuhara, S., and Okuma, M. (1998) Refinement of the BCL2/immunoglobulin heavy chain fusion gene in t(14;18)(q32;q21) by polymerase chain reaction amplification for long targets. *Genes Chromosomes Cancer* **21,** 17–29.
29. Pezzella, F., Ralfkiaer, E., Gatter, K. C., and Mason, D. Y. (1990) The 14;18 translocation in European cases of follicular lymphoma: comparison of Southern blotting and the polymerase chain reaction. *Br. J. Haematol.* **76,** 58.
30. Lopez-Guillermo, A., Cabanillas, F., McLaughlin, P., et al. (1998) The clinical significance of molecular response in indolent follicular lymphomas. *Blood* **91,** 2955–2960.
31. Corradini, P., Astolfi, M., Cherasco, C., Ladetto, M., Voena, C., Caracciolo, D., Pileri, A., and Tarella, C. (1997) Molecular monitoring of minimal residual disease in follicular and mantle cell non-Hodgkin's lymphomas treated with high-dose chemotherapy and peripheral blood progenitor cell autografting. *Blood* **89,** 724–731.
32. Freedman, A. S., Gribben, J. G., Neuberg, D., et al. (1996) High-dose therapy and autologous bone marrow transplantation in patients with follicular lymphoma during first remission. *Blood* **88,** 2780–2786.
33. Gribben, J. G., Neuberg, D., Freedman, A. S., et al. (1993) Detection by polymerase chain reaction of residual cells with the bcl-2 translocation is associated with increased risk of relapse after autologous bone marrow transplantion for B-cell lymphoma. *Blood* **81,** 3449–3457.

34. Gribben, J. G., Saprito, L., Barber, M., Blake, K. W., Edwards, R. M., Griffin, J. D., Freedman, A. S., and Nadler, L. M. (1992) Bone marrows of non-Hodgkin's lymphoma patients with a bcl-2 translocation can be purged of polymerase chain reaction-detectable lymphoma cells using monoclonal antibodies and immunomagnetic bead depletion. *Blood* **80,** 1083–1089.
35. Luthra, R., McBride, J. A., Cabanillas, F., and Sarris, A. (1998) Novel 5′ exonuclease-based real-time PCR assay for the detection of t(14,18)(q32;q21) in patients with follicular lymphoma. *Am. J. Pathol.* **153,** 63–68.
36. Heid, C. A., Stevens, J., Kivak, K. J., and Williams, P. M. (1996) Real time quantitative PCR. *Genome Res.* **6,** 986–994.
37. Rauzy, O., Galoin, S., Chale, J. J., Adoue, D., Albarede, J. L , Delsol, G., and al Saati, T. (1998) Detection of t(14;18) carrying cells in bone marrow and peripheral blood from patients affected by non-lymphoid diseases. *Mol. Pathol.* **51,** 333–338.
38. Dolken, G., Illerhaus, G., Hirt, C., and Mertelsmann, R. (1996) BCL-2/J_H rearrangements in circulating B cells of healthy blood donors and patients with nonmalignant diseases. *J. Clin. Oncol.* **14,** 1333–1344.
39. Limpens, J., Stad, R., Vos, C., de Vlaam, C., de Jong, D., van Ommen, G. B., Schuuring, E., and Kluin, P. M. (1995) Lymphoma-associated translocation t(14;18) in blood B cells of normal individuals. *Blood* **85,** 2528–2536.
40. Corbally, N., Grogan, L., Keane, M. M., Devaney, D. M., Dervan, P. A., and Carney, D. N. (1994) Bcl-2 rearrangement in Hodgkin's disease and reactive lymph nodes. *Am. J. Clin. Pathol.* **101,** 756–760.
41. Aster, J. C., Kobayashi, Y., Shiota, M., Mori, S., and Sklar, J. (1992) Detection of the t(14;18) at similar frequencies in hyperplastic lymphoid tissues from American and Japanese patients. *Am. J. Pathol.* **141,** 291–299.
42. Limpens, J., de Jong, D., van Krieken, J. H., Price, C. G., Young, B. D., van Ommen, G. J., and Kluin, P. M. (1991) Bcl-2/J_H rearrangements in benign lymphoid tissues with follicular hyperplasia. *Oncogene* **6,** 2271–2276.
43. Segal, G. H., Scott, M., Jorgensen, T., and Braylan, R. C. (1994) Standard polymerase chain reaction analysis does not detect t(14;18) in reactive lymphoid hyperplasia. *Arch. Pathol. Lab. Med.* **118,** 791–794.
44. Berinstein, N. L, Reis, M. D., Ngan, B. Y., Sawka, C. A., Jamal, H. H., and Kuzniar, B. (1993) Detection of occult lymphoma in the peripheral blood and bone marrow of patients with untreated early-stage and advanced-stage follicular lymphoma. *J. Clin. Oncol.* **11,** 1344–1352.

14

Detection of Breast Cancer Cells Using Immunomagnetic Beads and Reverse Transcriptase Polymerase Chain Reaction

Scott Luke and Karen L. Kaul

1. Introduction

Molecular methods permit the detection of cells too few in number to be detected by light microscopy, immunohistochemistry, or flow cytometry *(1–5)*. Numerous investigators are therefore developing sensitive and specific reverse transcriptase polymerase chain reaction (RT-PCR) assays for tumor cell detection. The detection of small numbers of tumor cells in blood, lymph node, and stem cell harvests may have a significant impact on our understanding of the spread of breast cancer, and eventually may impact the management of breast cancer patients as well.

These assays are based on the detection of an amplified product from an mRNA target uniquely expressed in a particular cell type. In the case of carcinoma, however, tumor-specific targets are not available. RT-PCR assays therefore demonstrate the presence of cells of a particular type such as epithelial cells, rather than tumor cells *per se*. It is important to keep in mind that normal cells may also be detectable by RT-PCR assays, as can cells showing nonspecific expression of the mRNA of interest. Assay specificity must be rigorously investigated.

Several markers for breast epithelial cells have been reported, including cytokeratins, gross cystic disease fluid protein, and mammaglobin *(2,6–10)*. However, lack of specificity has been a commonly encountered problem *(11)*. The use of immunomagnetic beads for positive selection of epithelial cells permits the elimination of false-positive signal from background expression of the

From: *Methods in Molecular Medicine, vol. 49: Molecular Pathology Protocols*
Edited by: A. A. Killeen © Humana Press Inc., Totowa, NJ

chosen marker. Additionally, enhancements in sensitivity owing to enrichment of tumor cells in the fraction used for RNA isolation have been observed ***(12,13)***. The beads used in this method are magnetic, polystyrene beads coated with mouse monoclonal antibody (Ber-EP4) directed against human epithelial antigen. The bound antiepithelial beads will target two membrane glycoproteins found in both normal and neoplastic epithelial cells ***(14)***.

This chapter outlines two RT-PCR assays that have been used successfully for the detection of breast cancer cells in a variety of sample types. The first target is cytokeratin-19 (CK-19), a widely expressed gene in cells of epithelial origin. CK-19, a member of the family of cytokeratins, is a component of the mammalian cell cytoskeleton ***(2,6,7)***. Detection of CK-19 expression is therefore potentially useful for the study of many carcinomas. By contrast, mammaglobin, a member of the uteroglobin gene family, appears to be specifically expressed in mammary epithelium and present in the majority of breast carcinomas ***(10)***. The clinical utility of these assays is currently being investigated.

The general format of these assays for the detection of breast cancer cells via RT-PCR includes the immunoselection and enrichment of epithelial cells, followed by RNA preparation. cDNA is then generated via a reverse transcription protocol and amplified by PCR using primers specific for the chosen target. The amplified products are first assessed on an agarose gel counterstained with ethidium bromide (EtBr), followed by probe hybridization to increase both the specificity and sensitivity of the assay. Additionally, when studying human samples, an internal control such as β_2-microglobulin (β_2M) must be RT-PCR amplified to demonstrate the intactness and ability to amplify isolated mRNA.

To ensure that amplification products truly reflect the presence of epithelial cell RNA, primers must be carefully chosen to avoid complementarity to processed pseudogenes that may be present, and primers must be located across exon-intron boundaries. Failure on either of these requirements may result in production of amplicons from traces of genomic DNA that are indistinguishable from the desired mRNA of the tumor cells.

2. Materials

2.1. Positive Control Cells

As a positive control for the CK-19 RT-PCR, the T47D cell line can be used (*see* **Fig. 1**). T47D is an epithelial breast cancer cell line available from the American Type Culture Collection (ATCC). Another epithelial breast cancer cell line, BT-474 (also available from ATCC), is used as a positive control for

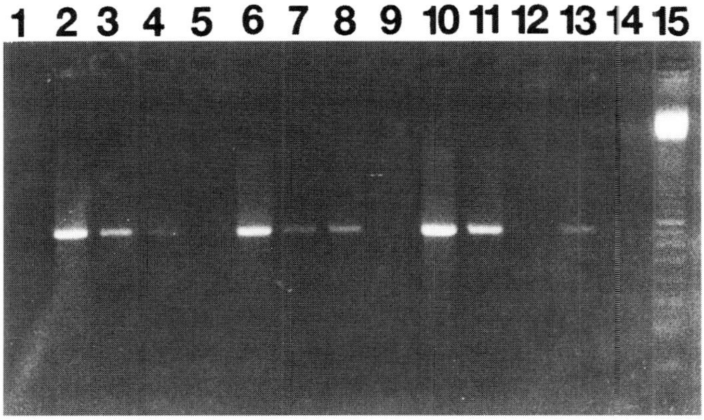

Fig. 1. CK-19 RT-PCR of immunoselected blood using Dynabeads. A 1.5% agarose gel stained with EtBr showing the sensitivity of the CK-19 RT-PCR assay. Lanes 1, 5, and 9 are mRNA prepared from blood of healthy volunteers (all negative by RT-PCR). Lanes 2–4, 6–8, and 10–12 correspond to the addition of 1000, 100, and 10 T47D cells to the volunteer blood, respectively. Lane 13 is a positive T47D control (751 bp). Lane 14 is an mRNA blank and lane 15 is a 100-bp ladder.

the mammaglobin assay. Normal blood serves as a control for the presence of the ubiquitous β_2M mRNA target. Immunoselected normal blood is used as the negative control in the CK-19 and mammaglobin assays.

2.2. Preparation of Sample

Care must be taken to avoid mRNA degradation from RNases. Gloves should be worn at all times and changed often to avoid the introduction of RNases. Diethylpyrocarbonate (DEPC)-treated water should be used in all reagents. DEPC-treated water is made in-house (*see* **Note 1**). Samples should be processed as quickly as possible (within 2 h of collection) to minimize loss of mRNA from the presence of RNases owing to cellular destruction.

1. Patient blood, 5–10 mL collected in EDTA-treated Vacutainer tubes.
2. RNase-free microcentrifuge tubes and pipet tips.
3. Wash buffer consisting of 1X phosphate-buffered saline, pH 7.4, 0.1% bovine serum albumin, and 1 m*M* EDTA.
4. Dynabeads® Epithelial Enrich immunobeads (Dynal). The beads are 4.5 µm in diameter.
5. Dynal MPC® magnetic separator (Dynal).

2.3. Isolation of RNA

Gloves should be worn and changed often to reduce the risk of contamination with RNases present in the oils of the skin and to minimize the risk of carryover between samples.

1. Trizol reagent (Life Technologies).
2. Chloroform (*see* **Note 2**).
3. RNase-free tubes and plasticware.
4. DEPC-treated deionized H_2O.
5. Glycogen (Boehringer Mannheim).
6. Isopropanol.
7. 75% Ethanol diluted with DEPC-treated water.

2.4. Reverse Transcription

Master mix for the RT reaction should be made in large batches to minimize run-to-run variability. Reagents may be susceptible to degradation via repeated freezing and thawing, and all reagents should be aliquoted appropriately to minimize this occurrence. Reverse transcription and amplification mixes utilize dUTP in place of dTTP so that amplicons can be degraded by uracil *N*-glycosylase if desired to ablate contamination by amplicon carryover.

1. 25 m*M* $MgCl_2$ (Perkin-Elmer), 10X PCR Buffer II (Perkin-Elmer), and DEPC-treated water.
2. Stock dNTP mixtures consisting of 10 m*M* for A, G, and C nucleotides (Gene Amp RNA PCR kit; Perkin-Elmer); 20 m*M* stock of dUTP (Perkin-Elmer).
3. MuLV reverse transcriptase (25 U/µL), RNase Inhibitor (10 U/µL), and 25 µM oligo $d(T)_{16}$ (Perkin-Elmer).

2.5. Polymerase Chain Reaction

1. 25 m*M* $MgCl_2$, 10X PCR Buffer II, DEPC-treated water.
2. AmpliTaq DNA polymerase (5 U/µL) (Perkin-Elmer).
3. 40 µM Stocks of each primer target.

CK-19 ***(15)*** gives a 751-bp product:
  Sense primer CK-19: GAC TAC AGC CAC TAC TAC ACG ACC
  Antisense primer CK-19: AGC CGC GAC TTG ATG TCC ATG AGC C (*see* **Note 3**).
Mammaglobin ***(10)*** gives a 430-bp product:
  Sense primer mammaglobin: CAG CGG CTT CCT TGA TCC TTG
  Antisense primer mammaglobin: CAT AAG AAA GAG AAG GTG TGG
β_2M (16) gives a 158-bp product:
  Sense primer β_2M: CTT GTC TTT CAG CAA GGA CTG G
  Antisense primer β_2M: CCT CCA TGA TGC TGC TTA CAT GTC

2.6. Agarose Gel Electrophoresis

1. 1.5% Agarose in 1X TAE buffer. A 50X stock solution consists of the following in a 1L of solution: 242.2 g of Trizma base (Sigma), 57.1 mL of glacial acetic acid, 100 mL of 0.5 *M* EDTA (pH 8.0).
2. 10X Loading dye: 0.25% bromophenol blue, 0.25% xylene cyanol, 15% Ficoll (Type 400); store at room temperature.
3. Staining box containing 1X TAE and 0.7 μg/mL of EtBr.

2.7. Solution Hybridization

1. 5% Acrylamide gel (acrylamide/*bis*-acrylamide 19:1, 40% stock solution (Sigma).
2. Loading dye: 0.25% bromophenol blue, 0.25% xylene cyanol, 15% Ficoll (Type 400); store at room temperature.
3. Adenosine 5′-[γ-^{32}P] triphosphate (9.25 MBq), triethylammonium salt (250 μCi) (Pharmacia).
4. T4 Polynucleotide kinase, cloned, pure (1000 U) (Pharmacia).
5. 10X One-Phor-All Buffer *PLUS* 10X solution (Pharmacia).
6. NAP-5 columns (Pharmacia).
7. 1X TE buffer consisting of 10 m*M* Tris-Cl (pH 7.4) and 1 m*M* EDTA (pH 8.0).
8. 1X TBE buffer: A 5X stock solution consisting of the following in a 1-L solution: 54 g of Trizma base, 27.5 g of boric acid, 20 mL of 0.5 *M* EDTA (pH 8.0).
9. DNA probe for CK-19 (100 μ*M*; sense strand): GCG GGA CAA GAT TCT TGG TG or mammaglobin (100 μ*M*; sense strand): CTT TCT GCA AGA CCT TTG GCT CAC. No probe is necessary for the β_2M product.
10. Beta counter (Bioscan/QC 2000).

3. Methods

3.1. Preparation of Sample (*see* Note 4)

1. Collect 5–10 mL of patient blood in EDTA-treated Vacutainer collection tubes.
2. Chill the blood at 4°C for 20 min.
3. Transfer the blood to a 15-mL conical polypropylene tube (Becton Dickinson).
4. Add 25 × 10^6 washed Dynabeads Epithelial Enrich immunobeads (Dynal) to each sample and rock gently at 4°C for 30 min to allow for immunomagnetic capture of any present epithelial cells.
5. Following the incubation, place the conical tube containing the blood into a Dynal Magnetic Particle Concentrator (Dynal MPC; Dynal) and rock gently for 5 min allowing the immunomagnetic beads to migrate to the side of the tube abutting the magnets.
6. Using a vacuum aspirator and a clean, sterile pipet, slowly aspirate the blood being careful to avoid the aspiration of any attached beads.
7. Remove the magnet and wash the beads by resuspending in 10 mL of cold buffer.
8. Replace the slide-out magnet and rock for 2 to 3 min allowing the beads to migrate to the magnet.
9. Aspirate the supernatant.
10. Repeat **steps 7–9** two more times.

3.2. Isolation of RNA

RNA is isolated using the Trizol (Life Technologies) kit according to the manufacturer's protocol. Aerosol-resistant pipet tips are always used along with pipettors dedicated to RNA preparation. RNA is isolated on a laboratory bench kept separate from other activities.

1. Following the last wash and aspiration, add a volume of 0.8 mL of Trizol reagent to lyse the captured cells adherent to the beads. Incubate the cells in the Trizol for at least 3 min to allow complete detachment of nucleoprotein complexes. Transfer the volume to a clean 1.5-mL tube (*see* **Note 5**).
2. Add 160 µL of chloroform to each Trizol-containing tube and briefly vortex.
3. Spin the tubes in a refrigerated centrifuge at 4°C for 15 min at 12,000*g*.
4. An upper aqueous layer, an interphase, and a lower organic layer will be evident following the centrifugation. Using a clean plastic transfer pipet (Scientific Products), gently aspirate the upper aqueous layer containing the RNA into a clean 1.5-mL microcentrifuge tube.
5. Add 1 µL of glycogen (20 mg/mL) (Boehringer Mannheim) to the RNA-containing solution and mix thoroughly.
6. Add 400 µL of 100% isopropanol and invert the tube several times. Let the solution sit at room temperature for 10 min to allow the RNA to precipitate.
7. Centrifuge the sample for 10 min at 4°C and 12,000*g*.
8. A glycogen pellet (which will contain the desired RNA) will be visible at the bottom of the tube. Discard the isopropanol supernatant and add 1 mL of 75% ethanol in DEPC water to the pellet. Dislodge the pellet and invert the tube several times to wash.
9. Spin for 5 min at 4°C and 7500*g*.
10. Discard the supernatant and place the tube with its top open in a 55°C water bath for 5 min to allow evaporation of excess ethanol. Do not overdry the pellet because this will make it difficult to resolubilize the RNA.
11. Add 7.5 µL of DEPC-treated water and place in a 55°C water bath for 10 min (*see* **Note 6**).
12. Spin the tubes down and place on ice in preparation for cDNA synthesis and subsequent PCR.

3.3. Reverse Transcription

It must be stressed that when working with RNA, gloves must be worn and changed often. Mixes to be used for cDNA synthesis and PCR reactions are prepared in a UV-equipped hood separate from the sample preparation and the amplification areas.

1. Add 1 µL of RNA sample (*see* **Note 7**) to 9 µL of the RT mix. Each RT reaction vial contains the following with final concentrations listed: 5 m*M* $MgCl_2$; 1X

PCR Buffer II; 1 mM each of dATP, dCTP, and dGTP and 2 mM dUTP; 2.5 U/µL of MuLV-RT; 1.0 U/µL of RNase Inhibitor; 2.5 µM oligo d$(T)_{16}$; and DEPC-treated water to achieve a final volume of 10 µL.
2. The RT cycle parameters (GeneAmp 2400 thermalcycler; Perkin-Elmer) are as follows: 10 min at 24°C, 15 min at 42°C, and 5 min at 99°C.
3. Store the cDNA at 4°C and proceed with the PCR reaction. If the PCR portion of the assay is not to be carried out immediately (within the same day), store the cDNA at –20°C until ready to proceed.

3.4. PCR Amplification

PCR amplification is performed in a total volume of 50 µL, which includes the 10 µL from the RT reaction.

1. The PCR mix (40 µL/sample) contains the following with final concentrations listed: 1X PCR Buffer II, 1.25 U of AmpliTaq DNA polymerase, 0.20 µM of each primer, 2.0 mM $MgCl_2$, and DEPC-treated water.
2. Add 40 µL of the PCR mix to each vial containing 10 µL of the cDNA solution from the RT reaction.
3. The cycling parameters for CK-19 are as follows: cycle 1, 5 min at 94°C; cycles 2–36, 30 s at 94°C, 30 s at 68.5°C, and 30 s at 72°C; cycle 37, 7-min final extension period at 72°C. The cycling parameters for β_2M are as follows: cycle 1, 105 s at 95°C; cycles 2–36, 15 s at 95°C and 30 s at 60°C; cycle 37, 7-min final extension period at 72°C. The cycling parameters for mammaglobin are as follows: cycle 1, 4 min at 94°C and 2 min at 80°C (*see* **Note 8**); cycles 2–36, 30 s at 94°C, 20 s at 57°C, and 30 s at 72°C; cycle 37, 7-min final extension period at 4°C. After amplification store the RT-PCR solution at 4°C.

3.5. Agarose Gel Electrophoresis

Tubes containing amplified products are opened and analyzed by electrophoresis in a room separate from the sample reagent preparation area to avoid amplicon contamination. Aerosol-resistant tips are used.

1. Mix 10 µL of each RT-PCR reaction thoroughly with 1 µL of loading dye and load the wells.
2. Load one well with a 100-bp ladder (Pharmacia) mixed with dye. This will be used as a reference for amplicon size.
3. Run the gel for 30 min to 1 h at 110 V, depending on the size of the desired amplicon. CK-19 has a 751-bp product, mammaglobin displays a 430-bp product, and β_2M has a 158-bp product.
4. Stain the gel in 1X TAE containing EtBr (0.7 µg/mL) for 20 min at room temperature.
5. Visualize the presence or absence of bands in control and sample lanes with a UV transilluminator.

3.6. Labeling Probe for Solution Hybridization

In our assays, the antisense strand of the amplified product is hybridized with a radioactively labeled probe (^{32}P). The solution hybridization is employed to increase both the sensitivity and specificity of the CK-19 and mammaglobin assays. Because of the ubiquitous nature of β_2M, a solution hybridization is unwarranted for this primer set.

1. To label the probe, add the following to a 1.5-mL tube: 17 µL of H_2O, 2.0 µL of the DNA probe, 2.5 µL of 10X One-Phor-All buffer, 1.5 µL of γ-^{32}P ATP, and 2.0 µL of T4 polynucleotide kinase.
2. Incubate the tube in a 37°C water bath for 30 min.
3. Following the 30-min incubation, add 5 µL of 0.25 *M* EDTA (pH 7.0) to stop the reaction.
4. Add 470 µL of 1X TE buffer to the labeled probe.
5. Prepare the NAP-5 column during the 30-min incubation (*see* **Note 9**).
6. Remove the top and bottom caps of the NAP-5 column and discard the liquid.
7. Wash the column with 10 mL of 1X TE buffer.
8. Following the 30-min incubation, add the 500-µL sample to the column, let the liquid run through, and discard.
9. Add 500 µL of 1X TE buffer, allow the liquid to run through, and discard.
10. Add 750 µL of 1X TE buffer and collect this portion in a 1.5-µL tube.
11. On a beta counter obtain a radioactive count on the labeled probe.

3.6.1. Solution Hybridization

1. Put 10 µL of the amplified product into a 1.5-µL tube.
2. Add 10 µL of the radioactive probe to the amplified product.
3. Incubate the probe/amplicon mixture for 10 min at 95°C.
4. Following the 95°C incubation, allow the mixture to cool at room temperature. It is during this step that the radioactive probe will hybridize to the antisense region of interest.
5. Add 5 µL of loading buffer to each sample and mix well.
6. Load the 5% acrylamide gel and run for 1.5 h at 110 V in 1X TBE buffer (the acrylamide gels are made with 1X TBE buffer).
7. Enclose the gel in plastic wrap and develop an autoradiogram. An overnight film should be sufficient for analysis.

4. Notes

1. DEPC is used to purge reagents of RNase activity for use in RNA recovery procedures. DEPC is added to stock solutions at a final concentration of 0.1% and allowed to incubate overnight. DEPC must be completely destroyed by autoclaving the solution, where it degrades into carbon dioxide and ethanol. The degrada-

tion of DEPC is absolutely necessary because even trace amounts will result in modification of adenine residues. Note also that DEPC cannot be added to any solution containing Tris or mercaptans. DEPC-treated water that has been autoclaved should be used to make solutions containing Tris or mercaptans and then autoclaved again.

2. Aged chloroform can degenerate, producing a variety of undesirable byproducts, including phosgene. Chloroform should be stabilized, ideally with alcohol, to minimize this process. Chloroform should also be stored properly in a dark glass bottle and used within a few months of opening.
3. We generally prefer amplicon sizes smaller than 300 bp, or even smaller than 200 bp if fixed tissues are to be analyzed. To avoid amplification of the CK-19 pseudogene, a published primer set amplifying a much larger amplicon was used. The CK-19 primers span five introns and were carefully chosen to possess bases that differ from the known processed pseudogene ***(4,6,15)***. A high annealing temperature is used to increase the stringency of the assay, ensuring specific binding of the primers to the desired sequence.
4. The protocol described here has been optimized for detection of breast cancer cells in peripheral whole blood samples but can also be used for other sample types. Fresh lymph nodes can be disaggregated to produce a single cell suspension suitable for immunoselection. Dimethylsulfoxide-preserved stem cell harvests can also be washed and immunoselected (unpublished observations). For samples in which immunoselection cannot be performed (fixed or frozen lymph nodes, some stem cell harvests) targets such as mammaglobin may be preferential to cytokeratin for detection of breast cancer cells because of the absence of low-level background expression.
5. There are several convenient points at which to stop during this procedure, permitting storage of the reactants.
6. RNA solutions are stored at –70°C. RNA is susceptible to degradation via freeze-thaw; therefore, we recommend that the RNA be aliquoted in single reaction quantities. However, RNA can also be stored in 100% formamide with RT formamide concentrations not to exceed 7% (http://www.nwfsc.noaa.gov/protocols/rnasoluble.html).
7. The RNA collected from patient blood is not quantified spectrophotometrically because so few cells are gathered from the immunobead selection technique. We nonetheless hydrate our RNA with 7.5 µL because that volume affords good sensitivity.
8. The mammaglobin assay goes through a "hot start." The DNA polymerase is not added to the PCR mixture until the solution is at 80°C in cycle 1. Adding the DNA polymerase at 80°C will minimize the amplification of nonspecific targets that may occur if the DNA polymerase is added at room temperature.
9. Pharmacia NAP-5 columns are prepared disposable columns containing Sephadex® G-25 medium of DNA grade for rapid and convenient desalting and buffer exchange of oligonucleotides ≥10 mers.

References

1. Brown, D. C., Purushotham, A. D., Birnie, G. D., and George, W. D. (1995) Detection of intraoperative tumor cell dissemination in patients with breast cancer by use of reverse transcription and polymerase chain reaction. *Surgery* **117,** 96–101.
2. Burchill, S. A., Bradbury, M. F., Pittman, K., Southgate, J., Smith, B., and Selby, P. (1995) Detection of epithelial cancer cells in peripheral blood by reverse transcriptase polymerase chain reaction. *Br. J. Cancer* **71,** 278–281.
3. Choy, A. and McCulloch, P. (1996) Induction of tumour cell shedding into effluent venous blood breast cancer surgery. *Br. J. Cancer* **73,** 79–82.
4. Datta, Y. H., Adams, P. T., Drobyski, W. R., Ethier, S. P., Terry, V. H., and Roth, M. S. (1994) Sensitive detection of occult breast cancer by the reverse-transcriptase polymerase chain reaction. *J. Clin. Oncol.* **12(3),** 475–482.
5. Gross, H. J., Verwer, B., Houck, D., Hoffman, R. A., and Recktenwald, D. (1995) Model study detecting breast cancer cells in peripheral blood mononuclear cells at frequencies as low as 10^7. *Proc. Natl. Acad. Sci. USA* **92,** 537–541.
6. Savtchenko, E. S., Schiff, T. A., Jiang, C. K., Freedburg, I. M., and Blumenburg, M. (1988) Embryonic expression of the human 40-kD keratin: evidence from a processed pseudogene sequence. *Am. J. Hum. Genet.* **43,** 630–637.
7. Traweek, S. T., Liu, J., and Battifora, H. (1993) Keratin gene expression in non-epithelial tissues. *Am. J. Pathol.* **142,** 1111–1118.
8. Mazoujian, G., Bodian, C., Haagensen, D. E., and Haagensen, C. D. (1989) Expression of GCDFP-15 in breast carcinomas. *Cancer* **63,** 2156–2161.
9. Mazoujian, G., Pinkus, G. S., Davis, S., and Haagensen, D. E. (1983) Immunohistochemistry of a gross cystic disease fluid protein (GCDFP-15) of the breast. *Am. J. Pathol.* **110(2),** 105–112.
10. Watson, M. A. and Fleming, T. P. (1996) Mammaglobin, a mammary-specific member of the uteroglobin gene family, is overexpressed in human breast cancer. *Cancer Res.* **56,** 860–865.
11. Luke, S. and Kaul, K. (1998) Detection of breast cancer cells in blood using immunomagnetic bead selection and reverse transcription-polymerase chain reaction. *Mol. Diagn.* **3(3),** 149–155.
12. Gomm, J. J., Browne, P. J., Coope, R. C., Liu, Q. Y., Bulawela, L., and Coombes, R. C. (1995) Isolation of pure populations of epithelial and myoepithelial cells from the normal human mammary gland using immunomagnetic separation with Dynabeads. *Analyt. Biochem.* **226,** 91–99.
13. Yaremko, M. L., Kelemen, P. R., Kutza, C., Barker, D., and Westbrook, C. A. (1996) Immunomagnetic separation can enrich fixed solid tumors for epithelial cells. *Am. J. Pathol.* **148,** 95–104.

14. Latza, U., et al. (1990) Ber-EP4; new monoclonal Ab which distinguishes epithelia from mesothelia. *J. Clin. Pathol.* **43,** 213–219.
15. Eaton, M. C., Hardingham, J. E., Kotasek, D., and Dobrovic, D. (1997) Immunobead RT-PCR: a sensitive method for detection of circulating tumor cells. *Biotechniques* **21,** 100–105.
16. Krafft, A. E., Duncan, B. W., Bijwaard, K. E., Taubenberger, J. K., and Lichy, J. H. (1997) Optimization of the isolation and amplification of RNA from formalin-embedded tissue: the Armed Forces Institute of Pathology experience and literature review. *Mol. Diagn.* **2(3),** 217–230.

15

Molecular Detection of Circulating Prostate Cancer Cells

Karen L. Kaul

1. Introduction

Molecular methods have proven extremely useful for the detection of occult tumor cells and can yield valuable clinical information as well as a better understanding of the mechanisms of metastasis and relapse of cancer *(1)*. In the case of many hematopoietic malignancies, the presence of a unique molecular marker such as a chromosomal translocation has made this task relatively straightforward. Carcinomas generally lack such markers, however. Certain oncogene mutations have been targeted, but the lack of consistent and specific markers has remained problematic.

An alternative approach has been increasingly utilized in the past decade *(2–4)*. Reverse transcriptase polymerase chain reaction (RT-PCR) assays have been designed to amplify the mRNA of a gene specifically expressed in the cells of interest. Generally, such markers are not truly tumor specific, but are expressed in both benign and malignant cells of the same origin. The mRNA of prostate-specific antigen (PSA), e.g., is one such marker that has been successfully used to detect prostate epithelial cells. The finding of such cells in the circulation, lymph nodes, or bone marrow of a patient with prostate cancer most likely reflects the spread of disease, although benign prostate epithelium will also generate a positive RT-PCR result. Several clinical studies have been performed to investigate the potential utility of RT-PCR assays in the management of patients with prostate cancer *(4–26)*. At this time, however, the role of RT-PCR has not been clearly established. Further long-term follow-up studies are needed and are under way. This chapter details one successful method for the detection of prostate epithelial cells in blood and lymph node samples.

From: *Methods in Molecular Medicine, vol. 49: Molecular Pathology Protocols*
Edited by: A. A. Killeen © Humana Press Inc., Totowa, NJ

A number of issues must be considered in the design of an RT-PCR assay for the detection of occult tumor cells. The choice of a target is perhaps the most critical. The target gene expression must be generally limited to the cells of interest, with minimal or no expression in other cells within the sample, such as leukocytes. As mentioned, target expression is generally seen in both benign and malignant cells, and thus the potential for positivity owing to the presence of benign cells must always be considered. Low-level expression of the gene by other cells in the sample can also be problematic. Once a suitable target is chosen, primer design becomes the next consideration. Primers ideally should bridge one or more intron/exon boundaries so that the amplicons generated from mRNA in the RT-PCR process can be differentiated by size from those originating from any genomic DNA that might be contaminating the RNA sample. Additionally, primers must be chosen such that amplification of genomic pseudogenes is avoided. During assay validation, it is worth investigating these possibilities.

Assay validation takes place in two phases. Analytic validation utilizes known negative and positive samples, often cultured cells, to demonstrate that positive results truly correlate with the presence of tumor cells in the sample of interest, and to further investigate the number of cells detectable. Clinical validation encompasses analysis of a sufficient number of patient samples to demonstrate that the assay detects real tumor cells in actual samples without false-positive signals in this heterogeneous sample group. This phase leads into the actual RT-PCR study, in which long-term patient follow-up may be needed to determine the clinical significance of a positive result.

2. Materials

As a positive control, the PSA-producing prostate cancer cell line LNCaP, obtained from the American Type Culture Collection (Rockville, MD) is utilized. Cultured LNCaP cells are trypsinized and mixed in known numbers into samples of prostate cell–free whole blood and used as a positive/sensitivity control for the assay. Whole blood from normal volunteers, both male and female, serves as negative control samples.

2.1. Collection and Preparation of Samples

Samples must be processed as quickly as possible to minimize loss of mRNA; a maximum of 2 h is recommended.

1. Patient blood, 5–10 mL collected in EDTA-anticoagulant (Vacutainer; Becton-Dickenson) tubes (*see* **Note 1**).
2. RNase-free microcentrifuge tubes and pipet tips.

3. Polymorphprep (Robbins Scientific) or Ficoll-Hypaque gradient density media (*see* **Note 2**).
4. Wash buffer consisting of 1X phosphate-buffered saline (PBS), pH 7.4, 0.1% bovine serum albumin, and 1m*M* EDTA.

2.2. Isolation of RNA

Care must be taken to avoid mRNA degradation. Diethylpyrocarbonate (DEPC)-treated water (*see* **Note 3**) should be used in all reagents. Gloves should be worn and changed often to lessen the risk of contamination with RNases and to minimize the risk of carryover between samples.

1. Trizol reagent (Life Technologies).
2. Chloroform (*see* **Note 4**).
3. RNase-free tubes and plasticware.
4. DEPC-treated deionized H_2O.
5. Glycogen, Rnase free.
6. Isopropanol.
7. 75% Ethanol diluted with DEPC-treated water.

2.3. Reverse Transcription

Master mix for the RT reaction should be made in large batches to minimize run-to-run variability. Reagents are susceptible to degradation via repeated freezing and thawing, and all reagents should be aliquoted appropriately to minimize this exposure. The DEPC-treated water is made inhouse (*see* **Note 3**).

1. 25 m*M* $MgCl_2$, 10X PCR Buffer II (Perkin-Elmer), DEPC-treated water.
2. Stock dNTP mixtures of 10 m*M* for A, G, and C nucleotides (GeneAmp RNA PCR kit; Perkin-Elmer); 20 m*M* stock of dUTP (Pharmacia).
3. 25 U/µL of Moloney murine leukemia virus (MuLV) RT, 10 U/µL of RNase inhibitor, and 25 µ*M* of oligo $d(T)_{16}$ (all in the GeneAMP RNA PCR kit; Perkin-Elmer).

2.4. Polymerase Chain Reaction

1. 10X PCR Buffer II (Perkin-Elmer).
2. 25 m*M* $MgCl_2$.
3. DEPC-treated water.
4. AmpliTaq DNA polymerase (2.5 U) (Perkin-Elmer).
5. 40 µ*M* Stocks of each primer target (PSA, prostate-specific membrane antigen [PSMA] [*see* **Note 5**], or β_2-microglobulin).

The following primer pair, derived from Katz, et al. ***(5)*** generates a 710-bp amplicon (*see* **Note 6**):

Sense primer PSA710: CAC AGA CAC CCC ATC CTA TC
Antisense primer PSA710: GAT GAC TCC AGC CAC GAC CT

The following primer pair, derived from the PSA sequence (Genbank accession no. #X14810) generates a 144-bp amplicon:

Sense primer PSA 144: AGG CTG GGG CAG CAT TGA ACC AGA GGA
Antisense primer PSA144: GTC CAG CGT CCA GCA CAC AGC ATG AAC T

The following primers target the PSMA gene (Genbank accession no. M99487) and yield a 165-bp amplicon:

Sense primer PSMA: AAA AGT CCT TCC CCA GAG TTC AGT
Antisense primer PSMA: ACT GTG ATA CAG TGG ATA GCC GCT

The primers for β_2-microglobulin, used to amplify mRNA as a control for RNA integrity, are taken from Krafft et al. ***(27)*** and amplify a 158-bp fragment:

Sense primer β_2M: CTT GTC TTT CAG CAA GGA CTG G
Antisense primer β_2M: CCT CCA TGA TGC TGC TTA CAT GTC

2.5. Agarose Gel Electrophoresis

1. Tris-acetate EDTA (TAE) buffer: 40 m*M* Tris acetate, pH 7.4, 1 m*M* EDTA.
2. 1.5% Agarose gel in 1X TAE buffer.
3. 10X sample-loading buffer: 0.25% bromophenol blue, 0.25% xylene cyanol, 25% Ficoll.
4. Staining box containing 1X TAE and 0.7 µg/mL of ethidium bromide (EtBr).

2.6. Probe Labeling and Hybridization

1. Oligoprobes (stock solution of 100 µ*M*):
   a. PSA 710: Use a cocktail of *Pr1*: 5′ CAA GTT CAC CCT CAG AAG GTG ACC AAG TTC AT 3′; *Pr2*: 5′ AGG CTG GGG CAG CAT TGA ACC AGA GGA GT3′; *Pr3*: 5′ TTC AGT GTG TGG ACC TCC ATG TTA TTT CCA ATG ACT TGT GT 3′.
   b. PSA 144 probe: TTC AGT GTG TGG ACC TCC ATG TTA TTT CCA ATG ACG TGT GT.
   c. PSMA 165 probe: GAG GTG TTC TTC CAA CGA CTT GGA ATT GCT.
2. $\gamma\,^{32}$P ATP (50 µCi), 3000 Ci/mmol (Amersham, Arlington Heights, IL).
3. T4 polynucleotide kinase (20 U) (Pharmacia).
4. One-Phor-All buffer (Pharmacia).
5. 0.25 *M* EDTA (pH 7.0).
6. NAP-5 Column (Pharmacia).
7. Beta counter (Bioscan QC 2000 or equivalent).
8. Boiling water bath.

2.7. Acrylamide Gel Electrophoresis

1. Vertical minigel apparatus and power supply.
2. Acrylamide/*bis*-acrylamide 19:1, 40% stock solution (Sigma, St. Louis, MO).
3. Ammonium persulfate, 10% solution, prepared fresh in distilled water.
4. TEMED (Sigma).
5. TBE buffer: 10 m*M* Tris-borate, pH 8.0, 2 m*M* EDTA.
6. 10X Sample-loading buffer: 0.25% bromophenol blue, 0.25% xylene cyanol, 25% Ficoll.

2.8. Autoradiography

1. X-ray film (Kodak, Rochester, NY).
2. Photographic developing tanks or equipment.

3. Methods

3.1. Collection and Preparation of Samples

Peripheral blood must be collected in a lavender top (EDTA) tube with a minimum volume of 5 mL. Tubes must be delivered to the laboratory immediately or within 2 h. Specimens that are clotted, drawn with incorrect anticoagulant, or frozen cannot be accepted for testing.

1. Prepare the leukocyte fraction, which includes circulating tumor cells, using Polymorphprep according to the manufacturer's suggested protocol. Ficoll-Hypaque may also be used.
2. Wash the cells with cold PBS buffer and place on ice.

3.2. Isolation of RNA

RNA is isolated using the Trizol (Life Technologies) kit according to the manufacturer's protocol. Aerosol-resistant pipet tips are always used along with pipettors dedicated to RNA preparation. RNA is isolated on a laboratory bench kept separate from other activities.

1. Following the wash, add a volume of 0.8 mL of Trizol reagent to lyse the cells. Pipet up and down several times to ensure cell lysis. Transfer to a 1.5-mL microcentrifuge tube, and incubate for 3 min at RT. If necessary, samples can be stored at –20°C at this point.
2. Add 160 µL of chloroform to each Trizol-containing tube and briefly vortex.
3. Spin the tubes in a refrigerated centrifuge at 4°C for 15 min at 12,000*g*.
4. An upper aqueous layer, an interphase, and a lower organic layer will be evident following centrifugation. Using a clean plastic transfer pipet (Scientific Products), gently aspirate the upper RNA-containing aqueous layer into a clean 1.5-mL microcentrifuge tube.
5. Add 1 µL of glycogen (20 mg/mL) (Boehringer Mannheim) to the RNA-containing solution and mix thoroughly.

6. Add 400 µL of 100% isopropanol and invert the tube several times. Let the solution sit at room temperature for 10 min to allow the RNA to precipitate. If desired, samples may be stored in alcohol at –80°C and will remain stable.
7. Centrifuge the sample for 10 min at 4°C and 12,000*g*.
8. A glycogen pellet will be visible at the bottom of the tube. Discard the isopropanol supernatant and add at least 1 mL of 75% ethanol in DEPC-treated water to the pellet; vortex to wash (*see* **Note 7**).
9. Spin for 5 min at 4°C and 7500*g*.
10. Discard the supernatant and place the tube with its top open in a 55°C water bath for 5 min to allow evaporation of excess ethanol.
11. Add 7.5 µL of DEPC-treated water and place in a 55°C water bath for 10 min.
12. Spin the tubes down and place on ice in preparation for cDNA synthesis and subsequent PCR.

3.3. Reverse Transcription

When working with RNA, gloves must be worn and changed often. Mixes to be used for cDNA synthesis and PCR reactions are prepared in a hood separate from the sample preparation and amplification areas.

1. Aliquot 2.5 m*M* oligo $d(T)_{16}$ and the desired DEPC-treated water volume to all tubes. Add RNA to a final volume of 4 µL.
2. Anneal the primers at 65°C for 5 min. Place on ice.
3. Add 16 µL of RT master mix: 5 m*M* $MgCl_2$, 1X PCR Buffer II, 1 m*M* each dNTP, 1 U of RNase inhibitor, 2.5 U of MuLV RT.
4. Incubate for 15 min at 42°C, 5 min at 99°C, and then 5 min at 5°C.

3.4. PCR Amplification

PCR amplification is performed in a total volume of 50 µL, including 10 µL from the RT reaction.

1. Aliquot 40 µL of appropriate PCR Master Mix (containing β_2-microglobulin, PSA, or PSMA primers) to the correct sets of tubes. PCR Master mix contains 2 m*M* $MgCl_2$, 1X PCR Buffer II, 2.5 U of *Taq* polymerase, 0.2 µ*M* of each primer, and DEPC water. Keep the mixture on ice until completion of RT.
2. Add 10 µL of RT reaction.
3. Perform PCR amplification in a Perkin-Elmer 9600 or 2400 thermalcycler.
   a. For PSA 710, cycle according to Katz et al. ***(5)***: 1 cycle of 4 min at 95°C; 15 cycles of 1 min at 95°C, 1 min at 60°C and 30 s at 72°C; 11 cycles of 1 min at 95°C, 1 min at 60°C, and 1 min at 72°C; 7 cycles of 1 min at 95°C, 1 min at 60°C, and 2 min at 72°C; 1 cycle of 15 min at 72°C; indefinite hold/storage at 4°C.
   b. For all other amplifications cycle as follows: 1 cycle of 4 min at 95°C; 35 cycles of 15 s at 95°C, 30 s at 60°C, and 30 s at 72°C; 1 cycle of 5 min at 72°C; indefinite hold/storage at 4°C.

3.5. Agarose Gel Electrophoresis

Tubes containing amplified products are opened and analyzed by electrophoresis in a room separate from where the samples were prepared, and separate from where the mixes for the RT and PCR reactions were made. Aerosol-resistant tips are used.

1. Mix 10 µL of each RT-PCR reaction thoroughly with 1 µL of loading dye, and load the wells.
2. Load one well with a 100-bp ladder (Pharmacia Biotech) mixed with dye. This will be used as a reference for amplicon size.
3. Run the gel for about 1 h at 110 V.
4. Stain the gel in 1X TAE containing EtBr (0.7 µg/mL) for 20 min at RT.
5. Visualize the absence or presence of bands in the control and sample lanes under UV light. A 158-bp product should be visible in all specimens amplified using β_2-microglobulin primers.
6. Further analyze negative or inconclusive specimens by probe hybridization.

3.6. Probe Labeling and Hybridization

1. End label oligoprobe: Mix 1 µL of oligoprobe stock with 2.5 µL of buffer, 2 µL of polynucleotide kinase, and 5 µL of radioactive ATP. Add sterile deionized water to 25 µL. Incubate at 37°C for 30 min. Stop the reaction by adding 5 µL of 0.25 *M* EDTA (pH 7.0).
2. Separate labeled probe from unincorporated radioactive ATP using the NAP column according to the manufacturers' directions.
3. Mix 10 µL of amplicons and 10 µL of labeled probe.
4. Incubate at 95°C for 10 min, then at room temperature for 20 min.
5. Add 5 µL of loading dye.

3.7. Acrylamide Gel Electrophoresis

1. Prepare 5% acrylamide gel using acrylamide/*bis*-acrylamide 19:1, 40% stock solution.
2. Electrophorese at 75–150 V until bromophenol blue dye reaches the end of the gel.

3.8. Autoradiography

1. Wrap the gel in plastic and place next to a sheet of film in an autoradiography cassette.
2. Expose for 4–16 h at –70°C, or as desired.
3. Develop the film using conventional methods.

4. Notes

1. CPT tubes (Vacutainer; Becton Dickenson) contain a polymeric gel that separates mononuclear cells from neutrophils and red blood cells after a short centrifugation step. Our preliminary studies indicated that these could be used as alternative collection tubes and may be particularly useful in the collection of samples from other institutions or after hours, where complete gradient separation is not possible.
2. Ficoll-Hypaque can be used in place of Polymorphprep with no apparent alteration in recovery of tumor cells from whole blood samples.
3. DEPC-treated water is prepared by adding DEPC to a final concentration of 0.1% in distilled water. After an overnight incubation, autoclave to destroy the DEPC.
4. Aged chloroform can degenerate, producing a variety of undesirable byproducts, including phosgene. Chloroform should stabilized, ideally with alcohol, to minimize this process. Chloroform should also be stored properly in a dark glass bottle, and used within a few months of opening,
5. Although PSMA has been used for the detection of prostate epithelial cells, several laboratories have reported background expression of this marker in leukocytes and nonprostate cell lines, yielding nonspecific results and making PSMA of questionable value in the detection of prostate cancer cells ***(28–30)***.
6. Although our clinical studies have generally utilized the primers developed by Katz et al. ***(5)***, which amplify a 710-bp portion of the PSA gene, we generally prefer amplicon sizes smaller than 300 bp, or even smaller than 200 bp if fixed tissues are to be analyzed.
7. RNA is most stable when stored under ethanol at –80°C. Alternatively, RNA can be reconstituted in formamide and can be used directly in reaction mixtures provided that the final concentration of formamide is less than 8–10%.
8. The sensitivity of the assay should be carefully determined. In our hands, detection of a single LNCaP cell in 5 mL of blood is possible; tenfold dilution or more of this mRNA with that of unspiked blood can be done without losing the positive signal, as shown in **Fig. 1**, because several hundred copies of PSA mRNA are estimated to be present in each LNCaP cell ***(6)***. Actual tumor cells may vary in the copy number of the target message.

References

1. Glaves, D. (1986) Detection of circulating metastatic cells, in *Cancer Metastasis: Experimental and Clinical Strategies* (Welch, D. R., Bhuyan, B. K., and Liotta, L. A., eds.), Alan R. Liss, New York, pp. 151–165.
2. Moreno, J. G., Croce, C. M., Fisher, R., et al. (1992) Detection of hematogenous micrometastasis in patients with prostate cancer. *Cancer Res.* **52,** 6110–6112.
3. Ghossein, R. A. and Rosai, J. (1996) Polymerase chain reaction in the detection of micrometastases and circulating tumor cells. *Cancer* **78,** 10–16.
4. Raj, G. V., Moreno, J. G., and Gomella, L. G. (1998) Utilization of polymerase chain reaction technology in the detection of solid tumors. *Cancer* **82,** 1419–1442.

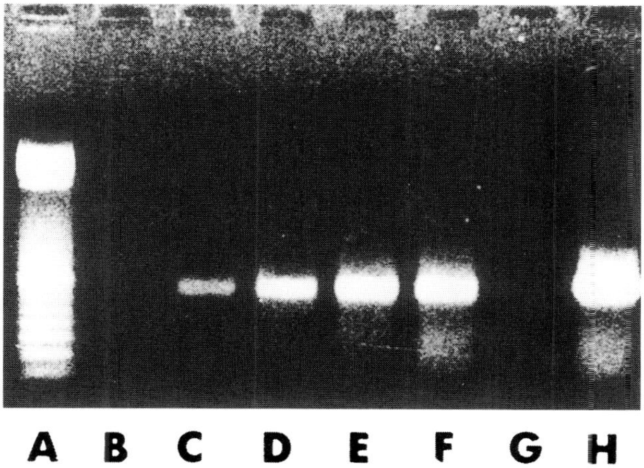

Fig. 1. Agarose gel stained with EtBr showing PSA RT-PCR assay sensitivity for the detection of LNCaP cells mixed with normal whole blood. Lane A, 100-bp molecular weight marker; lanes B–F, dilutions of LNCaP mRNA increasing from 0.01 to 100 cell equivalents/2.5 mL of whole female blood; lane G, RNA blank; lane H, LNCaP mRNA (*see* **Note 8**). (Reprinted from **ref. *6*** with permission from Lippincott Williams & Wilkins.)

5. Katz, A. E., Olsson, C. A., Raffo, A. J., et al. (1994) Molecular staging of prostate cancer with the use of an enhanced reverse transcriptase-PCR assay. *Urology* **43,** 765–775.
6. Oefelein, M. G., Kaul, K., Herz, B., Blum, M. D., Holland, J. M., Keeler, T. C., Cook, W. A., and Ignatoff, J. M. (1996) Molecular Detection of prostate epithelial cells from the surgical field and peripheral circulation during radical prostatectomy. *J. Urol.* **155,** 238–242.
7. Oefelein, M. G., Ignatoff, J. M., Clemens, Q., Watkin, W., and Kaul, K. L. (1999) Clinical and molecular followup after radical retropubic prostatectomy. *J. Urol.* **162,** 307–310.
8. Ignatoff, J. M., Oefelein, M. G., Watkin, W., et al. (1997) Prostate specific antigen-reverse transcriptase-polymerase chain reaction assay in preoperative staging of prostate cancer. *J. Urol.* **158,** 1870–1875.
9. Israeli, R. S., Miller, W. H., Su, S. L., et al. (1994) Sensitive nested reverse transcriptase polymerase chain reaction detection of circulating prostate tumor cells: comparison of prostate specific membrane antigen and prostate specific antigen based assays. *Cancer Res.* **54,** 6306–6310.
10. Seiden, M. V., Kantoff, P. W., Krithivas, K., et al. (1994) Detection of circulating tumor cells in men with localized prostate cancer. *J. Clin. Oncol* **12,** 2634–2639.

11. Jaakkola, S., Vornanen, T., Leinonen, J., et al. (1995) Detection of prostatic cells in peripheral blood: correlation with serum concentrations of prostate specific antigen. *Clin. Chem.* **41,** 182–186.
12. Loric, S., Dumas, F., Eschwege, P., et al. (1995) Enhanced detection of hematogenous circulating prostatic cells in patients with prostate adenocarcinoma by using nested reverse transcription polymerase chain reaction assay based on prostate-specific membrane antigen. *Clin. Chem.* **41,** 1698–1704.
13. Sokoloff, M. H., Tso, C. L., Kaboo, R., et al. (1996) Quantitative polymerase chain reaction does not improve preoperative cancer staging: a clinico-pathological molecular analysis of 121 patients. *J. Urol.* **156,** 1560–1566.
14. Ghossein, R. A., Rosai, J., Scher, H. I., et al. (1997) Prognostic significance of detection of prostate-specific antigen transcripts in the peripheral blood of patients with metastatic androgen-independent prostatic carcinoma. *Urology* **50,** 100–105.
15. Kawakami, M., Okaneya, T., Furihata, K., et al. (1997) Detection of prostate cancer cells circulating in peripheral blood by reverse transcription-PCR for hKLK2. *Cancer Res.* **57,** 4167–4170.
16. Corey, E., Arfman, E. W., Oswin, M. M., et al. (1997) Detection of circulating prostate cells by reverse transcriptase-polymerase chain reaction of human glandular kallikrein (hK2) and prostate-specific antigen (PSA) messages. *Urology* **50,** 184–188.
17. Corey, E., Arfman, E. W., Liu, A. Y., et al. (1997) Improved protocol for reverse transcriptase polymerase chain reaction protocol with exogenous internal competitive control for prostate specific antigen mRNA in blood and bone marrow. *Clin. Chem.* **43,** 443–452.
18. Gomella, L. G., Raj, G. V., and Moreno, J. G. (1997) Reverse transcriptase polymerase chain reaction for prostate specific antigen in the management of prostate cancer. *J. Urol.* **158,** 326–337.
19. Noguchi, M., Miyajima, J., Itoh, K., et al. (1997) Detection of circulating tumor cells in patients with prostate cancer using prostate specific membrane-derived primers in the polymerase chain reaction. *Int. J. Urol.* **4,** 374–379.
20. Wood, D. P. and Banerjee, M. (1997) Presence of circulating prostate cells in the bone marrow of patients undergoing radical prostatectomy is predictive of disease-free survival. *J. Clin. Oncol.* **15,** 3451.
21. Thiounn, N., Saporta, F., Flam, T. A., et al. (1997) Positive prostate-specific antigen circulating cells detected by reverse transcriptase-polymerase chain reaction does not imply the presence of prostatic micrometastases. *Urology* **50,** 245–250.
22. Ellis, W. J., Vessella, R. L., Corey, E., et al. (1998) The value of a reverse-transcriptase polymerase chain reaction assay in preoperative staging and follow-up of patients with prostate cancer. *J. Urol.* **159,** 1134–1138.
23. Vessela, R. L., Lange, P. H., Blumenstein, B. A., et al. (1998) Multicenter RT-PCR PSA clinical trial for preoperative staging of prostate cancer. *J. Urol.* **159,** 292A.

24. Van Nguyen, C., Song, W., Scardino, P. T., et al. (1998) RT-PCR for PSA and hK2: implications for staging and patient management in men undergoing radical prostatectomy. *J. Urol.* **159,** 292A.
25. Nejat, R. J., Katz, A. E., Benson, M. C., et al. (1998) Enhanced RT-PCR for PSA combined with serum PSA predicts pathologic stage and outcome in 300 radical prostatectomy patients. *J. Urol.* **159,** 291A.
26. Grasso, Y. Z., Gupta, M. K., Levin, H. S., et al. (1998) Combined nested RT-PCR assay for prostate-specific antigen and prostate-specific membrane antigen and prostate-specific membrane antigen in prostate cancer patients: correlation with pathological stage. *Cancer Res.* **58,** 1456–1459.
27. Krafft, A. E., Duncan, B. W., Bijwaard, K. E., Taubenberger, J. K., and Lichy, J. H. (1997) Optimization of the isolation and amplification of RNA from formalin-fixed, paraffin-embedded tissue: the Armed Forces Institute of Pathology experience and literature review. *Mol. Diagn.* **2,** 217.
28. Kaul, K. L., Hanna, W. L., Luke, S., Oda, J., and King, S. T. (1997) Molecular assays for detecting micrometastases in patient blood. *Clin. Chem.* **43,** S92.
29. Lintula, S. and Stenman, U. (1997) Expression of prostate-specific membrane antigen in peripheral blood leukocytes. *J. Urol.* **157,** 1969.
30. Gala, J.-L., Heusterspreute, M., Loric, S., Hanon, F., Tombal. B., Van Cangh, P., De Nayer, P., and Phillipe, M. (1998) Expression of prostate-specific antigen and prostate-specific membrane antigen transcripts in blood cells: implications for the detection of prostate cells and standardization. *Clin. Chem.* **44,** 472–481.

16

Methods to Detect Clonal Gene Rearrangements in Lymphomas and Leukemias

Naheed Mitha and Ronald C. McGlennen

1. Introduction

The process of lymphocyte differentiation involves structural alterations of specific genes including those for the immunoglobulin (*Ig*) and T-cell receptor (*TCR*) antigen genes. This process occurs very early in the differentiation of B- and T-lymphocytes and involves an ordered program for splicing and rearranging segments of these genes, depending on cell lineage and level of differentiation. Specific DNA cutting and splicing enzymes result in the removal of a number of constant, joining, and variable segments of the *Ig* and *TCR* genes. Rearrangement of the VDJ and C segments occurs randomly during the process of B- and T-cell development; hence, the resultant gene rearrangement varies from cell to cell. This results in a unique rearrangement of these genes that encode for a specific Ig or TCR protein. A clonal population of lymphocytes, however, will have a specific molecular structure of rearrangements. Identification of this clonal population is central to the diagnosis of lymphomas and lymphocytic leukemias, because virtually all forms of lymphoid malignancies contain rearrangements of one or more antigen receptor genes. Furthermore, as a clonal expansion, an individual neoplasm will contain the identical rearranged gene throughout the population, serving as a unique clonal marker *(1)*. However, it is important to be aware that lymphocyte clonality is not equivalent to malignancy *(2)*. Benign and reactive conditions may show monoclonal rearrangements. Correlation with histology and immunophenotypic studies is important in order to establish a definitive diagnosis of malignancy. Similarly, the absence of clonal gene rearrangement may be seen in cases that

From: *Methods in Molecular Medicine, vol. 49: Molecular Pathology Protocols*
Edited by: A. A. Killeen © Humana Press Inc., Totowa, NJ

appear malignant by histologic and immunophenotypic criteria. In these instances, it is important to be aware of technical limitations of the assays and sampling errors, which may result in a false-negative result.

Detection of either *Ig* or *TCR* gene rearrangements involves examination of DNA from lymphoid cells that may be obtained from blood, bone marrow, or tissue specimens. The polymerase chain reaction (PCR) and Southern blot analysis are methods currently used for detecting *Ig* and *TCR* gene rearrangements. In the PCR, DNA is amplified with a series of consensus primer pairs that bind to sequences of variable, diversity, and joining regions of these genes. In our laboratory, five consensus primers are used for the TCR-β chain gene rearrangements. These include one V_β, two D_β, and two J_β primers. The primers are combined into four sets as described in **Subheading 3.** Both $V_\beta J_\beta$ primer sets will detect only complete VDJ rearrangements and the $D_\beta J_\beta$ primer sets will primarily detect partial DJ and a few complete rearrangements ***(3)***.The PCR assay for the IgH chain gene employs V_H primers that anneal to frameworks I, II, or III ***(4)***. In our laboratory, the J_H primer binds to the framework III region and J_H2 to the framework II region. The detection rate with these primers varies according to the type of lymphoma ***(4)***. Framework I primers are typically not employed because they require several distinct primers to identify the rearrangement ***(4)***. The products are then analyzed by polyacrylamide gel electrophoresis (PAGE). If a significant population of cells contains a unique rearrangement of these genes, it appears as a well-defined band within a molecular size range specific for each set of primers on the electrophoretic gel. Southern blot analysis utilizes restriction endonucleases that cut genomic DNA into specific fragments in or around the *Ig* or *TCR* genes. These digested fragments are then separated by gel electrophoresis. The separated DNA is next transferred to a nylon membrane, denatured, and detected by hybridization to a radioactive probe. A clonal population of cells containing a unique rearrangement of *Ig* or *TCR* genes is indicated by the presence of a unique nongermline band on the autoradiogram.

Both techniques have advantages and disadvantages. Southern blot analysis of the IgH chain using only one probe and a limited number of restriction enzymes is highly specific. The sensitivity of Southern blot in detecting a clonal population ranges from 1 to 5% of specimen cells ***(5)***. Although PCR is more sensitive in detecting overall clonality (ability to detect 1 neoplastic cell admixed with 100,000 normal cells), it has a significant risk of contamination and a higher false-negative rate. In practice, the sensitivity of detecting IgH chain gene rearrangement by PCR lies between 0.1 and 10%, depending on the type of background cells, number of PCR cycles, and resolution of the gel ***(6,7)***. Southern blot is more expensive and has a longer turnaround time. By contrast, PCR is less expensive, has a shorter turnaround time, does not require the use of radioactivity, requires less DNA/RNA, and can be performed on DNA extracted from fixed specimens. High-quality genomic DNA necessary for Southern analysis cannot be obtained from paraffin-embedded tissues owing to the degradation that occurs during the fixation process.

2. Materials

2.1. Polymerase Chain Reaction

2.1.1. Specimens

The following specimen types may be used for PCR-based analysis of *Ig* and *TCR* gene rearrangements.

1. Blood: 10–15 mL collected in acid citrate dextrose (ACD) or EDTA. Only the mononuclear cells are required for this test. Therefore, the blood is first separated by a Ficoll-Hypaque separation procedure and the mononuclear fraction is extracted and analyzed.
2. Bone marrow: 5 mL (2 mL minimum if the white count is normal) collected in a syringe containing ACD or EDTA.
3. Tissue: 5-mm^3 tissue delivered to the laboratory within 1 h of collection or frozen in liquid nitrogen or on dry ice. Paraffin-embedded tissue can also be used (*see* **Note 1**).
4. Other: DNA extracted from any nucleated cells.

2.1.2. Equipment and Supplies

1. Perkin-Elmer thermocycler 480 (Perkin-Elmer Cetus, Norwalk, CT).
2. AmpliTaq DNA Polymerase (Perkin-Elmer). 10X Buffer and 25 m*M* $MgCl_2$ are supplied with the AmpliTaq.
3. Bulk dNTPs, 100 m*M* each of dATP, dCTP, dGTP, dTTP (Perkin-Elmer).
4. Three J_H primers have been described. J_H-A is the most common primer and is homologous with all the J_H regions *(8)*. As mentioned in **Subheading 1.**, five consensus primers combined into four sets have been described for T-cell β chain gene rearrangements. They produce bands ranging between 55 and 100 bp. Primers are as follows:
   a. $T_β$-V (19mer): 5′-TGT-A(CT)C-TCT-GTG-CCA-GCA-G-3′.
   b. $T_β$-D_1 (23mer): 5′-CAA-AGC-TGT-AAC-ATT-GTG-GGG-AC-3′.
   c. $T_β$-D_2 (23mer): 5′-TCA-TGG-TGT-AAC-ATT-GTG-GGG-AC-3′.
   d. $T_β$-J_1 (17mer): 5′-ACA-GTG-AGC-C(GT)G-GT(CT)-CC-3′.
   e. $T_β$-J_2 (20mer): 5′-AGC-AC(GCT)-GTG-AGC-C(GT)G-GTG-CC-3′.
   f. J_H1-S (25mer): 5′-CTG-TCG-ACA-CGG-CCG-TGT-ATT-ACT-G-3′.
   g. J_H-A (22mer): 5′-AAC-TGC-AGA-GGA-GAC-GGT-GAC-C-3′.
   h. J_H2-S (20mer): 5′-TGG-(AG)TC-CG(CA)-CAG-(GC)C(TC)-(TC)CN-GG-3′.
   i. MBR (20mer): 5′-TTA-GAG-AGT-TGC-TTT-ACG-TG-3′.
   j. Vg11 (20mer): 5′-TCT-GG(AG)-GTC-TAT-TAC-TGT-GC-3′.
   k. Jg11 (19mer): 5′-CAA-GTG-TTG-TTC-CAC-TGC-C-3′.
   l. bcl-1(s) (19mer): 5′-GAA-GGA-CTT-GTG-GGT-TGC-T-3′.

Table 1
Reaction Cocktail for Gene Rearrangements by PCR

Component	Volume/sample (does not include pipeting error) (μL)	Volume for 10 samples (includes 10% pipeting error) (μL)
dNTPs	8.0	88
$MgCl_2$	6.0	66
10X Buffer	5.0	55
Sterile H_2O	17.15	188.65
Taq I polymerase	0.1	1.1
Total volume	36.25	398.75

m. CF20i-5′(s) (21mer): 5′-GGT-CAG-GAT-TGA-AAG-TGT-GCA-3′.
n. CF20i-3′(A) (21mer): 5′-CTA-TGA-GAA-AAC-TGC-ACT-GGA-3′.

5. Mini-Electrophoresis System (Schleicher & Schuell, Keene, NH) or Xcell Mini-Cell Electrophoresis System (Novex, San Diego, CA).
6. FB105 Power supply (Fisher Scientific, Pittsburgh, PA).
7. 6% TBE Precast polyacrylamide gels (cat. no. EC6265; Novex) (*see* **Note 2**).
8. Ethidium bromide (EtBr) (cat. no 161-0430; Bio-Rad, Hercules, CA).
9. Molecular weight ladder: D-15 DNA Marker (cat. no. LC5825; Novex).
10. Polaroid type 667 film.
11. MilliQ Water double-distilled H_2O (ddH_2O).
12. Stock dNTPs (1.25 mmol/L): To prepare a 1.25 mmol/L solution, 400 μL (1.6 mL total) of each dNTP is mixed with 30.4 mL of sterile water (32.0 mL total volume). The dNTP solution should be aliquoted (1 mL) and stored frozen at –20°C until needed.
13. Stock primers (100 pmol/μL).
14. Working primers (3.0 pmol/μL): 30 microliters of each stock (100 pmol/μL) gene rearrangement primer and 12.5 each of CF20 5′ and CF20 3′ are added and diluted to 1000 μL with sterile water. These are then stored frozen at –20°C. The CF20 5′ and CF20 3′ are primers that amplify a region approx 460–500 bp in exon 20 of the cystic fibrosis gene; this amplification product serves as an internal control. Primer mixtures are prepared to make the following nine sets. Each mixture also contains the two CF20 primers: (T_β-V) + (T_β-J_I); (T_β-V) + (T_β-J_2); (T_β-D_1) + (T_β-J_2); (T_β-D_2) + (T_β-J_2); V_g11 + J_g11; (J_H-S) + (J_H-A); MBR + J_H-A; J_H2 + J_HA; bcl-1 + J_H-A.
15. Working PCR mix: A working mix is prepared for the total number of reactions. It is advisable to prepare a slight excess of master mix to allow for pipeting error. Typically allowing for a 10% error is adequate (*see* **Table 1**).

16. 18.5X TBE: To a 6-L Erlenmeyer flask, add 216 g of Tris base, 110 g of boric acid, and 80 mL of 0.5 *M* EDTA, pH 8.0. Add about 2 to 3 L of MilliQ water and mix until dissolved. Add MilliQ water to 4 L. Aliquot 500 mL/bottle and store at room temperature.
17. 1X TBE: Dilute 500 mL of 5X TBE to 2.5 L with MilliQ water. Store at room temperature.
18. PCR control: A "no template" control reaction in which water is substituted for a DNA specimen is included with each PCR setup; this is a check for the presence of amplified DNA contamination. It is recommended to rotate primer pairs according to the test required.
19. Gene rearrangement analysis controls: Controls may be obtained from investigators or from suppliers of cell lines, e.g., American Type Culture Collection:
    a. Ig Genes: J_H1, FJO (EBV-transformed lymphoblastoid cell line); mbr, RLBCL2 cell line; J_H2, 95-80 (positive patient sample); bcl-1, 1094 cell line.
    b. TCRB: (VJ_1), adult T-cell leukemia lymphoma.
    c. PCR amplification control: Exon 20 of the CFTR gene is used as an internal control for PCR amplification.

2.2. Southern Blot Analysis

2.2.1. Specimen

Refer to **Subheading 2.1.1.**

2.2.2. Equipment and Supplies

1. UV crosslinker (Stratalinker; Stratagene, La Jolla, CA).
2. Hybridization oven (Robbins Scientific, Sunnyvale, CA).
3. Horizontal Electrophoresis System (Bio-Rad).
4. Seal-a-meal bags.
5. Molecular weight ladder: Lambda phage DNA digested with *Bst*EII.
6. X-Ray film (cat. no. 04-441-95; Fisher, Itasca, IL).
7. Whatman 3MM chromatography paper.
8. Nick Translation System (cat. no. 18160-010); Gibco-BRL Life Technologies, Gaithersburg, MD).
9. Oligolabeling Kit (cat. no. 27-9250-01; Pharmacia Biotech). The kit contains the following components:
    a. Reagent mix: Buffered aqueous solution containing dATP, dGTP, dTTP, and random hexadeoxyribonucleotides.
    b. FPLCpure™ Klenow fragment: Buffered glycerol solution (5–10 U/µL).
    c. Control DNA: Aqueous solution or λDNA-*Hin*dIII restriction fragments.
    d. Carrier DNA: Aqueous solution of calf thymus or salmon sperm DNA at 1 mg/mL.
10. Restriction endonucleases: Purchased from Gibco-BRL Life Technologies. (*See* **Table 2**.)

Table 2
Restriction Enzymes Used in Southern Blot Analysis

Restriction enzyme	Stock concentration (U/μL)	Cat. no.
*Bam*HI	50	15201-049
*Eco*RI	50	15202-039
*Bgl*II	50	15213-036
*Hin*dIII	50	15207-038

11. Recombinant plasmid probes: The plasmids given in **Table 3** were obtained in our laboratory from investigators. However, Dako (Carpinteria, CA) offers several probes including IGHJ6 (Ig heavy chain) IGKJ5; IGKC and IHKDE (kappa light chain); TCRBC and TCRBJ2 (TCRβ locus); and TCRDJI, TCRDC4, TCRDRE (TCRδ locus). It is beneficial to run several enzyme probe combinations to maximize detection of clonal rearrangements (**Fig. 1**).
12. Blotting Solution II (0.5 *M* NaOH, 1.5 *M* NaCl): Dilute 120 g of NaOH and 528 g of NaCl to 6 L with MilliQ water (or 360 g of NaOH and 1584 g of NaCl to 18 L).
13. Blotting Solution III (3 *M* NaCl, 1 *M* Tris, pH 7.5): Dilute 1046.4 g of NaCl and 726.6 g of Tris to about 5 L with MilliQ water. Adjust the pH to 7.5 with concentrated HCl. Start with about 200 mL of acid and then measure the pH as more acid is added. This requires about 350 mL of acid.
14. EtBr (1 mg/mL): Dilute 1 tablet (11 mg) of EtBr with 11 mL of sterile MilliQ water. Make in a sterile screw-capped tube. Let it dissolve for about 4 min. Wrap in foil and store at room temperature.
15. Prehybridization solution (total volume of 150 mL): MilliQ water (77 mL); 20X SSPE (45 mL); 50X Denhardt's solution (15 mL); 25% sodium dodecyl sulfate (SDS) (3 mL); salmon sperm DNA, denatured by boiling for 5 min (10 mL).
16. Hybridization solution (total volume of 10.0 mL): 20X SSPE (3.0 mL), formamide (5.0 mL), 50% dextran sulfate (1.66 mL), 25% SDS (0.2 mL).
17. Salmon sperm DNA: In a 1-L Erlenmeyer flask add 5 g of DNA sodium salt type III from salmon testes and dissolve in 500 mL of ddH_2O. Shake until evenly dispersed. Dispense into a wide-mouthed bottle and autoclave to sterilize. Store refrigerated at 4°C.
18. 6X Loading buffer: 0.25% bromophenol blue, 0.25% xylene cyanol, 15% Ficoll. Dilute 0.25 g of bromophenol blue, 0.25 g of xylene cyanol, and 15.0 g of Ficoll to 100 mL with sterile water. Store in a 100-mL bottle at room temperature.
19. Equilibration buffer, TE, pH 7.5 (for Pharmacia nick translation columns): Dilute 5.0 mL of 1 *M* Tris-HCl, pH 7.5, and 1.0 mL of 0.5 *M* EDTA, pH 8.0, to 500 mL with MilliQ water and autoclave.
20. 10% SDS: In a 2-L Erlenmeyer flask add 100 g of SDS. Slowly add 1.0 L of ddH_2O. Heat to 68°C to assist in dissolution.

Table 3
Common Probes Used in Gene Rearrangement Analysis: Plasmid Sources

Plasmid	Insert size	Bacterial vector	Antibiotic selection	Cloning site	Bacterial strain
J_H	5.6	pUC-19	Amp	*Bam*HI-*Hin*dIII	DH5a
C-κ	2.5	pBR322	Amp	*Eco*RI	HB101
C-λ	0.7	pUC-9	Amp	*Eco*RI-*Hin*dIII	HB101
TCR-γ J1-2	0.7	pUC-18	Amp	*Eco*RI-*Hin*dIII	HB101
TCR-δ V2	0.576	pUC-18	Amp	*Eco*RI-*Hin*dIII	HB101
TCR-β	0.96	pUC-18	Amp	*Pst*I	HB101
EBV	2.3	pBR322	Amp	*Eco*RI-*Bam*HI	HB101

21. 25% SDS: In a 2-L Erlenmeyer flask add 250 g of SDS. Slowly add 1.0 L of ddH_2O. Heat to 68°C to assist in dissolution.
22. 25X saline sodium citrate (SSC): In a 4-L Erlenmeyer flask add 238.6 g of NaCl (3.75 *M)* and 220.8 g of sodium citrate (0.375 *M*). Dissolve the solid with ddH_2O to 2 L. Autoclave for sterility.
23. 18X SSC + 1 *M* ammonium acetate: In a 4-L Erlenmeyer flask add 473.4 g of NaCl (2.7 *M*) and 238.2 g of sodium citrate (0.27 *M*). Add 600 mL of 5 *M* NH_4Ac and ddH_2O to a final volume of 3 L.
24. 0.1X SSC + 0.1% SDS: In a 6-L Erlenmeyer flask add 24 mL of 25X SSC, 60 mL of 10% SDS, and 5.916 L of ddH_2O.
25. 0.2X SSC + 0.1% SDS: In a 20-L carboy add 160 mL of 25X SSC, 200 mL of 10% SDS, and 19.64 L of ddH_2O.
26. 2X SSC + 0.1% SDS: In a 10-L vessel add 800 mL of 25X SSC, 100 mL of 10% SDS, and 9.1 L of ddH_2O.
27. 20X SSPE: In a 4-L Erlenmeyer flask add 701.2 g of NaCl (3.0 *M*), 110.4 g of $NaHPO_4 \cdot H_2O$, and 29.6 g of disodium EDTA. Add approx 3.2 L of ddH_2O until the solute dissolves. Adjust the pH to 7.4 with 10 *N* NaOH. Add ddH_2O to 4 L. Sterilize by autoclaving.
28. 10X TAE: In a 6-L Erlenmeyer flask add 290.4 mL Tris base and 120 mL of 0.5 *M* EDTA (pH 8.0). Add approx 5.0 L ddH_2O and 68.52 mL of glacial acetic acid. Adjust to a final volume of 6 L with ddH_2O.
29. 1X TE (pH 7.0): In a 4-L Erlenmeyer flask add 40 mL of 1 mol/L Tris (pH 7.5) and 8 mL of 0.5 mol/L EDTA (pH 8.0). Adjust to pH 7.0 and then add ddH_2O to a final volume of 4 L. Autoclave to sterilize.
30. 1X TE (pH 8.0): In a 4-L Erlenmeyer flask add 40 mL of 1 mol/L Tris (pH 8.0) and 8 mL of 0.5 mol/L EDTA (pH 8.0). Adjust to pH 8.0 and then add ddH_2O to a final volume of 4 L. Autoclave to sterilize.
31. MilliQ water (ddH_2O).
32. Negative (germline) control: Patient samples that have previously been demonstrated to be negative for gene rearrangements are used in our laboratory.

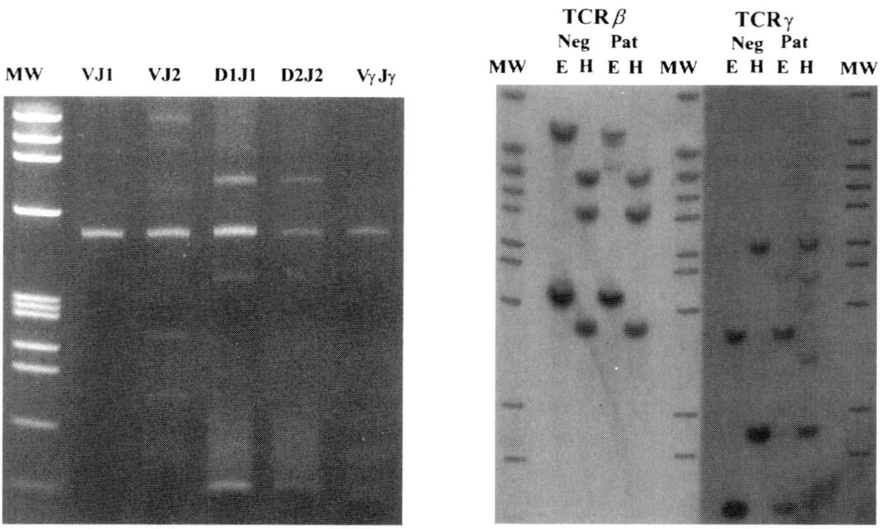

Fig. 1. PCR gel and Southern blot analysis demonstrating TCRβ chain gene rearrangement. In this case Southern blot is used to verify the rearrangement detected by PCR analysis. Abbreviations: MW = molecular weight marker; Neg = negative control sample; Pat = patient sample; E = *Eco*Ri enzyme digests; H = *Hin*dIII enzyme digests.

3. Methods

3.1. DNA Isolation

The Puregene™ DNA isolation Kit (Gentra Systems, Minneapolis, MN) allows rapid isolation of high-quality genomic DNA from whole blood, cultured cells, and tissue (*see* Chapter 34). It is based on published salting-out procedures, thus eliminating the use of toxic organic solvents. Other methods that yield intact DNA can be used (*see* Chapters 1 and 2).

3.2. Polymerase Chain Reaction

This protocol is designed for use with 0.5-mL PCR tubes. Adjustments may be required if 0.2-mL tubes are used.

1. Dilute the genomic DNA to 0.067 mg/mL.
2. Add 36.25 µL of working PCR mix to each tube and add 7.5 µL of patient sample or control to the respective tubes.
3. Vortex the tubes, spin briefly in a microcentrifuge, and add 1 drop of mineral oil to each tube before placing the tubes in a thermocycler.
4. Perform "hot start" PCR by setting the temperature of the thermocycler to 80°C. Place the tubes in the thermocycler in order according to the primer pairs to be

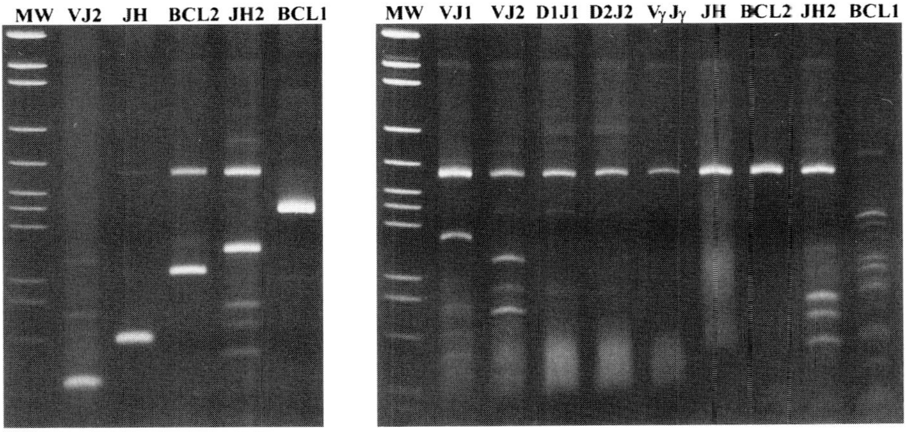

Fig. 2. PCR gels demonstrating TCR and Ig heavy-chain positive and negative controls. Note the nonspecific banding patterns seen with V_J1, V_J2, J_H2 and BCL-1. MW = molecular weight marker.

added. **Note:** Nonspecific primer annealing can be minimized by putting in tubes for two primer sets at a time, adding primers, and then putting in more tubes.

5. Add 6.25 µL of primer pairs to their respective tubes.
6. Start the program for gene rearrangement PCR using the following thermocycler parameters: 4 min at 94°C (initial denaturation step); 40 cycles of 1 min at 94°C (denature), 55 s at 60°C (anneal), 1 min at 73°C (extension) The 40 cycles are followed by a final 5-min extension at 72°C. Samples may be stored indefinitely at 4°C.

3.2.1. Gel Electrophoresis of PCR Products

1. Load 0.5 µL of the molecular weight marker in lane 1 along with 3 µL of 6X loading dye and 10 µL of H_2O. Then use 3 µL of 6X loading dye and 15 µL of PCR product (patient samples and controls) for the other lanes.
2. The recommended gel setup is as follows: lane 1: molecular weight ladder; lanes 2–10: VJ_1, VJ_2, D_1J_2, D_2J_2, Vg11Jg11, J_H1, mbr, J_H2, no template control. Run for 55 min at 100 V. The bottom dye will be about halfway between the bottom two lines on the PAGE cassette.
3. Stain with EtBr and photograph the gel using Polaroid type 667 film using f-stop 11 at 1 s.

3.2.2. Interpretation of PCR Results

Results are reported as positive or negative (**Fig. 2**). A smear pattern indicates polyclonality. A positive result is based on the presence of a sharp band with well-defined edges and a width not more than 1 mm, in the ranges for the

Table 4
Size Range for Interpretation of a Monoclonal Band and the Expected Nonspecific Bands

Primer	Expected size range (bp)	Nonspecific bands
J_H1	100–150	50, 65, 100
D1J2	55–100	65, 85, 120, 175, 185
Vg11Jg11	70–110	50, 75
MBR	222	—
J_H2	220–250	—
VJ1	55–100	—
VJ2	55–100	—
D2J2	55–100	—

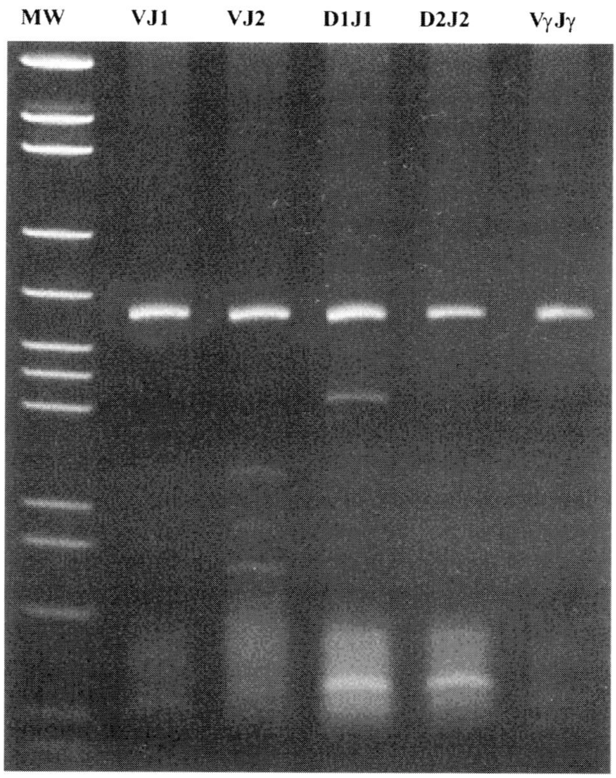

Fig. 3. PCR gels demonstrating clonal TCRβ chain gene rearrangements within a polyclonal smear. The smear most likely represents background-reactive, polyclonal T-lymphocytes in this case of a T-cell lymphoma.

primer pairs given in **Table 4** (*see* **Notes 3–5**). A clonal band may be masked in a polyclonal smear, as is sometimes seen in T-cell lymphomas (*see* **Fig. 3**).

A monoclonal population may also have two sharp bands, as is seen in some cases of chronic lymphocytic leukemia. These are usually a consequence of rearrangement of both alleles of that particular gene. Cases with more than two bands or a broad-based smear of bands are interpreted as oligoclonal and polyclonal, respectively. True clonal bands may also vary with a certain size range depending on the specific primers used. Empty lanes without smears, bands, primer/dimer artifact, or amplification of CF exon 20 should be regarded as failed PCR rather than negative, and repeated if possible.

Distinctive nonspecific primer–dependent banding patterns are seen and positive controls should be routinely performed. The primers used for the *TCR*-β chain gene rearrangement produce nonspecific bands at 65, 85, 120, 175, and 185 bp. In addition, an internal control should be used in each reaction tube to verify amplification of the individual samples. Tissues with a scant lymphoid inflammatory infiltrate may yield pseudoclonal bands owing to amplifications of normal rearrangements present in just a few lymphocytes. These polyclonal bands are usually smaller and less intense than the clonally rearranged ones and often occur in pairs.

False-negative results in true clonal populations, by PCR, are primarily owing to an inability of the selected primers to anneal effectively to selected exons of the recombined IgH chain gene. Other reasons include low DNA quality, amplification of nonclonal DNA, suboptimal conditions, chromosomal translocations, presence of deletions/mutations in the IgH chain genes, and presence of rearranged DNA below the sensitivity level of the assay ***(9,10)***. One specific protocol modification is to decrease the annealing temperature, which may increase the detection rate. Increasing the number of PCR cycles may also increase detection.

PCR has the highest false-negative rate in cases of follicular lymphomas. The PCR-based assay for the detection of t(14;18) detects a rearrangement in 50–60% of follicular lymphomas, 60% of cases with a cytogenetically proven t(14;18), and approx 70% of cases detectable by Southern blot ***(11–15)***. Both Southern blot and PCR can fail to detect a rearrangement if the breakpoint occurs outside the restriction enzyme or primer recognition site ***(16)***. Our laboratory has identified at least three *bcl*2 rearrangements of differing molecular weights by PCR (**Fig. 4**). Crossreactivity with EBV DNA may lead to false-positive results, and confirmation of these cases by Southern blot or slot blot hybridization is required ***(17)***.

"Cross-lineage" rearrangements are not uncommon ***(18–20)*** (**Fig. 5**). IgH chain gene rearrangements have been detected in some T-cell neoplasms. Approximately 25% of precursor B-cell acute lymphoblastic leukemias (ALLs) contain rearrangements of the IgH chain genes, and as many as 40% may have rearranged T-gamma genes ***(21)***. More than 50% of tdt positive acute myeloid

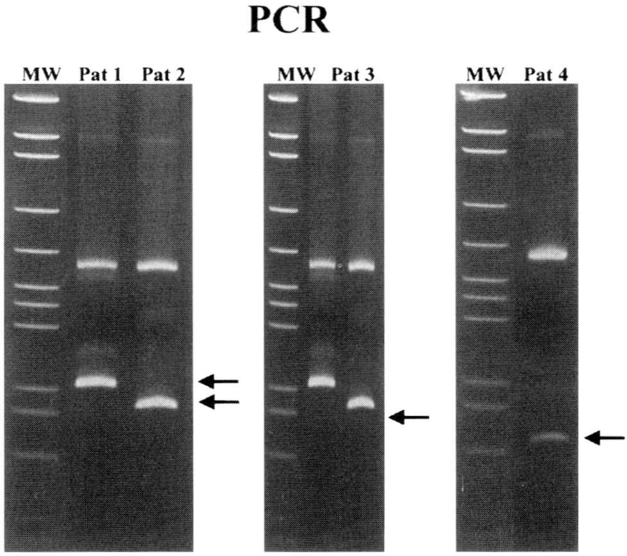

Fig. 4. Three PCR gels demonstrating four *bcl*2 rearrangements of differing molecular weight. The slot blot was performed in three of these patients and confirms the presence of an Ig heavy-chain–*bcl*2 gene fusion. Abbreviations: MW = molecular weight marker; Pat = patient sample.

leukemias show rearrangements of both IgH and TCR-β and TCR-γ chain genes *(8)*. Because of this phenomena of "lineage infidelity," both Ig and TCR assays should be routinely performed, and the results should be evaluated with morphology and immunophenotypic data. However, rearrangements of both IgH and light chain genes is a valid marker of B-cell lineage, because coexpression of these has not clearly been identified in T-lineage cells ***(22,23)***.

3.3. Southern Blot Analysis

3.3.1. DNA Isolation

Refer to **Subheading 3.1.**

3.3.2. Evaluation of Genomic DNA

Both quantitative and qualitative evaluation is done to ascertain evidence of degradation. Quantitation of DNA is performed by measuring the absorbance at 260 nm, and evidence of degradation is sought by electrophoresis of a small aliquot in an agarose gel with EtBr staining. These protocols are described in Chapter 2.

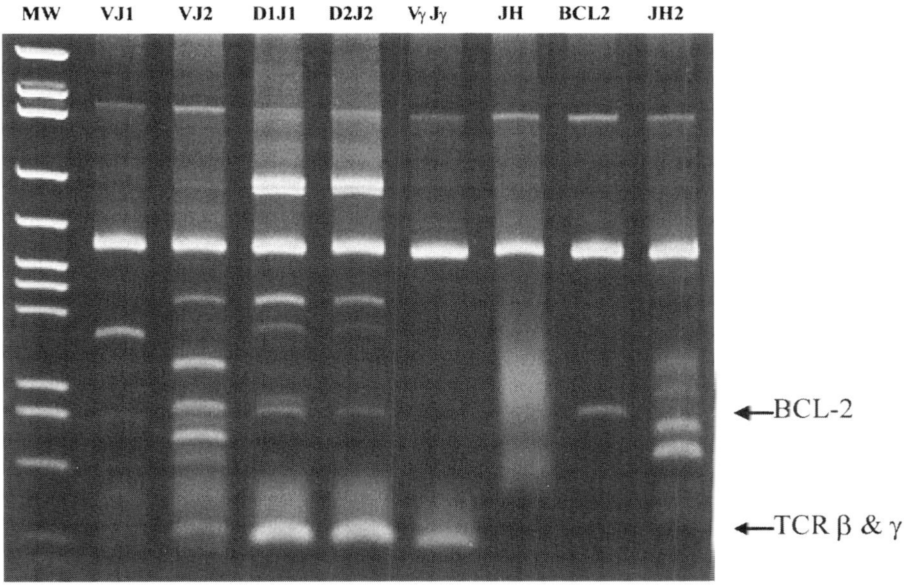

Fig. 5. PCR gels demonstrating a "cross-lineage" rearrangement. The patient had a history of follicular small cleaved lymphoma diagnosed on a lymph node biopsy. Molecular testing of the staging bone marrow biopsy (shown above) demonstrated a *bcl2* gene rearrangement as well as TCR-β and TCR-γ chain gene rearrangements. MW = molecular weight marker.

Table 5
Recommended Probe/Enzyme Combinations

Probe	Enzymes	Expected germline band sizes, kb *(3,4)*
C_T-β	*Eco*RI	11 and 4.2
	*Hin*dIII	7.2, 6.2, and 3.7
J_T-γ	*Eco*RI	3.4 and 1.5
	*Hin*dIII	5.4 and 2.2
C-κ	*Bam*HI	12
	*Hin*dIII	5.4
J_H	*Bgl*II	4
	*Hin*dIII	11 and 3.5[a]
EBV	*Bam*	None present

[a]The 3.5-kb band represents a crosshybridizing band *(4)*.

3.3.3. Restriction Digestion

Make *Bam*HI, *Eco*RI, *Bgl*II, and *Hin*dIII restriction endonuclease digests using 20 µg of genomic DNA under the appropriate digestion conditions recommended by the manufacturer. **Table 5** lists the recommended probe/enzyme combinations.

3.3.4. Submerged Gel Electrophoresis

1. Prepare 0.8% agarose gels using TAE buffer as recommended by the manufacturer. Add EtBr (final concentration of 0.1 µg/mL) to the agarose prior to pouring the gel.
2. Loading of subgels: In the first and last lanes, load 0.5 µg of molecular weight ladder prepared by adding the ladder DNA, 6 µL of 6X loading buffer, and water to a total volume of 36 µL. Leave the adjacent lanes to the ladder blank to prevent spillover into patient or control lanes. In the remaining lanes, load the control samples and patient digests. Load 10 µg of DNA diluted in 1X loading buffer.

3.3.5. Southern Transfer

This method is based on **ref.** ***24***.

1. Photograph the gel at 60–62 cm, f-stop 5.6, for 2 s to check the digest quality and amount of DNA per lane.
2. Depurinate the DNA in 500 mL of 0.1 *N* HCl for 30 min on a shaker platform. Follow depurination with rinsing with tap water.
3. Denature the DNA in 500 mL of Blotting Solution II with shaking for 15 min.
4. Neutralize the DNA in 500 mL of Blotting Solution III with shaking for 30 min.
5. Transfer the DNA to Zetabind membrane as described by the manufacturer. The layers in the Southern transfer setup are as follows:
   a. Layer 1: Two sheets of 3MM Whatman paper to serve as wicks, prewet in transfer solution.
   b. Layer 2: Denatured/neutralized gel, bottom side (DNA side) up.
   c. Layer 3: Nylon membrane (Zetabind).
   d. Layer 4: Two 3MM Whatman paper wicks.
   e. Layer 5: One dry 3MM Whatman paper wick.
   f. Layer 6: Stack of dry paper towels, 3–4 in.
   g. Layer 7: Evenly distributed weight, e.g., glass plate with two 500-mL reagent bottles on top or a glass pan.
6. Transfer overnight. Transfer can be accomplished in 4 h by removing soaked paper towels every 30 min and replacing with dry ones. Do not allow the nylon membrane to dry out.
7. Perform UV crosslinking of the membrane in a crosslinking apparatus as described by the manufacturer.
8. Prehybridize the membrane in 150 mL of prehybridization solution at 55°C for 30 min to overnight.

3.3.6. Radiolabeling of Probe

1. Perform nick translation with the Gibco-BRL nick translation system and α^{32}P-dCTP as described by the manufacturer. Oligolabel smaller probes and inserts as described by the manufacturer.
2. Isolate radiolabeled probe with the Pharmacia nick column as described by the manufacturer.
3. To quantitate the radiolabeled DNA, determine the volume in microliters of probe that is required for 2×10^7 cpm; also calculate the specific activity (disintegrations per minute/micrograms).

3.3.7. Hybridization

1. Into each hybridization bottle, add 10 mL of hybridization solution and the membranes.
2. For every 10 mL of hybridization solution, add boiled probe/salmon sperm mix (the mixture is prepared by boiling the volume of radiolabeled probe required for 2×10^7 cpm/filter with 100 μL salmon sperm DNA). **Note:** Do not drip the concentrated probe onto the filter because background hot spots may occur.
3. Hybridize at 42°C for 18 h overnight.
4. Posthybridization washes are as follows:
   a. Wash 1: 500 mL of 2X SSC + 0.1% SDS (made fresh) at room temperature with shaking for 15 min.
   b. Washes 2 and 3 (stringency washes): 500 mL of 0.1X SSC + 0.1% SDS, at 60°C except for *PFLI* (*bcl2*), which is washed at 55°C. Perform each wash with shaking for 30 min.

3.3.8. Autoradiography

Autoradiography is performed by placing the membrane in a plastic bag (e.g., Seal-a-Meal) and then in an X-ray cassette with film at –70°C for 3 d. **Note:** Do not let the membranes dry out.

3.3.9. Interpretation of Southern Blot Results

The presence of germline bands is interpreted only as a negative result. Any rearrangement of the Ig or TCR genes will appear as a band with variable intensity and a size different from the germline band. The intensity of the rearranged band is proportional to the percentage of clonal cells in the sample being tested. Generally, a positive result will be seen with both enzymes and is usually also positive by PCR. Two rearranged bands in a single lane hybridized with one gene probe may be a result of two coexisting clones within the same tissue or of rearrangements of both alleles for that specific gene ***(25)***. A marked difference in intensity of the two bands implies different dosages of

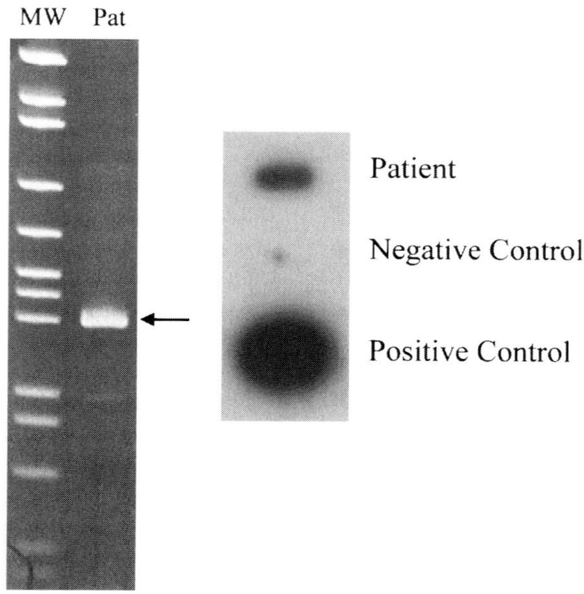

Fig. 6. PCR gel and slot blot in a patient with mantle cell lymphoma, demonstrating the classic *bcl*1 gene (t [11;14]) rearrangement. Abbreviations: MW = molecular weight marker; Pat = patient sample.

each rearranged gene and is likely to represent more than one clone. The following guidelines are useful for interpretation of Southern blots:

1. False-negative results with Southern blotting usually occur because the clonal population is below the sensitivity level of Southern analysis or because of tissue-sampling error. False-positive results may also arise from either a partial digestion or gene polymorphisms. A common example of partial digestion is *Eco*RI-digested DNA hybridized with a TCRβ probe. One usually sees an 8.5-kb band in addition to the usual 11- and 4-kb germline bands, which is owing to a relatively resistant *Eco*RI site ***(3,21)***. Additionally, certain rearrangements may produce very large restriction fragments, and hence the DNA may transfer poorly, causing these rearrangements to be missed. The use of multiple enzyme-probe combinations helps overcome this problem.
2. Several "benign" clonal lymphoproliferative conditions exist and include immunodeficiency settings associated with Wiscott-Aldrich syndrome and autoimmune deficiency syndrome, angioimmunoblastic lymphadenopathy, posttransplant immunosuppression, congenital immunodeficiency, and benign monoclonal gammopathy. It is important to be aware of these conditions to avoid erroneous diagnoses of malignancy.

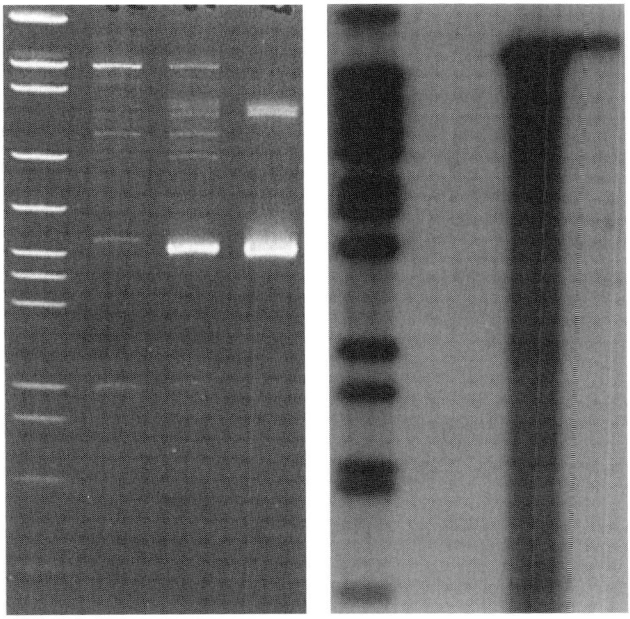

Fig. 7. Status post autologous bone marrow transplant for Hodgkin disease of a 39-yr-old female. The patient now presents with a lung mass suspicious for lymphoma. The PCR gel demonstrates the presence of EBV DNA, and the Southern blot confirms the clonal nature of the EBV DNA. The molecular findings in conjunction with morphology are suggestive of a posttransplant lymphoproliferative disorder. Abbreviations: MW = molecular weight marker; Pat = patient sample.

3. Restriction fragment length polymorphisms (RFLPs) and partially digested DNA may produce nongermline bands that are not owing to rearranged antigen receptor genes. Thus, laboratories must be aware of RFLPs generated by routinely used restriction enzymes and DNA probes. It is recommended that two enzymes be used in combination with each probe. If results from the two digests are not consistent, a third digest should be performed. This will eliminate misinterpretation of uncommon RFLPs or partial digests as a clonal rearrangement.
4. Comigration occurs when both the germline band and the rearranged band migrate to the same point in the gel. Comigration of rearranged bands with germline bands can be a major problem when using the restriction enzyme *Hin*dIII in combination with the constant region probe for the TCRβ chain. Restriction enzymes that produce large germline fragments are more likely to comigrate with nongermline bands. DNA should be digested with a second enzyme to resolve comigrations.

4. Notes

1. The quality of DNA affects the PCR-based assays. PCR detection of clonality in formalin-fixed DNA is 15% less sensitive at detecting IgH gene clonality than in unfixed DNA ***(26,27)***. Tissues obtained in mercurial-based fixations may also be difficult to amplify.
2. Polyacrylamide gels, 6–8% final concentration, provide the best resolution and clearest banding patterns.
3. The use of multiple primers improves overall clonality detection rates in the non-Hodgkin lymphomas. The use of both β and γ chain assays detects rearrangements in 90% of T-cell lymphomas. The sensitivity varies depending on the background cell population.
4. Specific PCR and data protocols for TCR gene rearrangements are not as well documented as those for B-cell gene rearrangements. However, several studies suggest that virtually all T-cell chronic lymphocytic and prolymphocytic leukemias should have clonal TCRβ and TCRγ rearrangements ***(19,28)***. T-cell ALL and lymphoblastic lymphomas show TCRβ and TCRγ rearrangement in more than 90% of cases ***(29–35)***. A corresponding IgH rearrangement is seen in 15–20% of these cases ***(36)***. Seventy to 80% of cases of mycosis fungoides/ Sezary syndrome demonstrate clonality with TCRs. In this case, clonal TCR-γ chain rearrangements are seen more frequently than TCRβ chain rearrangements ***(24,25,37)***. Peripheral T-cell lymphomas almost always have clonal TCR-γ rearrangement and often have a TRC-β rearrangement.
5. Other assays for which PCR is frequently used in our laboratory include the PCR-based assay for the detection of the t(11;14) translocation and Epstein-Barr virus (EBV) DNA, as illustrated in **Figs. 6** and **7**.

References

1. Arnold, A., Cossman, J., Bakhshi, A., et al. (1983) Immunoglobulin gene rearrangements as unique clonal markers in human lymphoid neoplasms. *N. Engl. J. Med.* **309,** 1593–1599.
2. Collins, R. D. (1997) Is clonality equivalent to malignancy: specifically is immunoglobulin gene rearrangement diagnostic of malignant lymphoma. *Hum. Pathol.* **28(7),** 757–759.
3. Coad, J. E., Olson, D. J., Lander, T. A., et al. (1997) Molecular assessment of clonality in lymphoproliferative disorders: II. T-cell receptor gene rearrangements. *Mol. Diagn.* **2,** 69–81.
4. Coad, J. E., Olson, D. J., Lander, T. A., et al. (1996) Molecular assessment of clonality in lymphoproliferative disorders: I. Immunoglobulin gene rearrangements. *Mol. Diagn.* **1,** 335–355.
5. Lehman, C. M., Sarago, C., Nasim, S., et al. (1995) Comparison of PCR with Southern hybridization for routine detection of immunoglobulin heavy chain gene rearrangements. *Am. J. Clin. Pathol.* **103,** 171–176.

6. Aubin, J., Davi, F., Nguyen-Salomon, F., et al. (1995) Description of a novel FR1 IgH PCR strategy and its comparison with three other strategies for the detection of clonality in B cell malignancy. *Leukemia* **9,** 471–479.
7. Potter, M. N., Steward, C. G., Maitland, N. J., et al. (1992) Detection of clonality in childhood B lineage acute lymphoblastic leukemia by polymerase chain reaction. *Leukemia* **9,** 289–294.
8. Segal, G. H., Wittwer, C. T., Fishleder, A. J., et al. (1992) Identification of monoclonal B cell populations by rapid cycle polymerase chain reaction: a practical screening method for the detection of immunoglobulin gene rearrangements. *Am. J. Pathol.* **141,** 1291–1297.
9. Cleary, M. L., Meeker, T. C., Levy, S., et al. (1986) Clustering of extensive somatic mutations in the variable regions of an immunoglobulin heavy chain gene from a B-cell lymphoma. *Cell* **44,** 97–106.
10. Deane, M., McCarthy, K. P., Wiedemann, L. M., et al. (1991) An improved method for detection of B-lymphoid clonality by polymerase chain reaction. *Leukemia* **5,** 726–730.
11. Kneba, M., Eick, S., Herbst, H., et al. (1991) Frequency and structure of t(14;18) major breakpoint lesions in Non-Hodgkin's lymphoma types according to the Keil classification: analysis by direct DNA sequencing. *Cancer Res.* **51,** 3243–3250.
12. Ladanyi, M. and Wang, S. (1992) Detection of rearrangements of the bcl-2 major breakpoint region in follicular lymphomas: correlation of polymerase chain reaction results with Southern blot analysis. *Diagn. Mol. Pathol.* **1,** 31–35.
13. Horsman, D. E., Gascoyne, R. D., Coupland, R. W., et al. (1995) Comparison of cytogenetic analysis, Southern blot analysis, and polymerase chain reaction for the detection of t(14;18) follicular lymphoma. *Am. J. Clin. Pathol.* **103,** 472–478.
14. Ngan, B. Y., Nourse, J., and Cleary, M. L. (1989) Detection of chromosomal translocation t(14;18) within the minor cluster region of bcl-2 by polymerase chain reaction and direct genomic sequencing of the enzymatically amplified DNA in follicular lymphomas. *Blood* **73,** 1759–1762.
15. Segal, G. H., Scott, M., Jorgensen, T., et al. (1994) Primers frequently used for detecting the t(14;18) major breakpoint also amplify Epstein-Barr virus. *Diagn. Mol. Pathol.* **3,** 15–21.
16. Klein, A., Zemer, R., Manor, Y., et al. (1997) Lymphoma with multi gene rearrangement on the level of immunoglobulin heavy chain, light chains and T-cell receptor β chain. *Am. J. Hematol.* **56,** 219–223.
17. Hanawa, H., Abo, J., Inokuchi, K., et al. (1995) Dual rearrangement of immunoglobulin and T-cell receptor genes in a case of splenic lymphoma with villous lymphocytes. *Leukemia Lymphoma* **18,** 357–360.
18. Hu, E., Weiss, L., Warnke, R., et al. (1989) Non-Hodgkins lymphoma containing both B and T cell clones. *Blood* **70,** 287–292.
19. Cossman, J., Uppenkamp, M., Sundeen, J., et al. (1988) Molecular genetics and the diagnosis of lymphoma. *Arch. Pathol. Lab. Med.* **112,** 117–127.

20. Cheng, G., Minden, M. D., Toyonaga, B., et al. (1986) T cell receptor and immunoglobulin gene rearrangements in acute myeloblastic leukemia. *J. Exp. Med.* **163,** 414.
21. Dick, F. R., Goeken, J. A., Kemp, J. D., et al. (1990) Kappa immunoglobulin light chain gene rearrangement in a T lineage chronic lymphocytic leukemia. *Am. J. Clin. Pathol.* **95,** 702.
22. Ebrahim, S. A., Ladanyi, M., Desai, S. B., Offit, K., Jhanwar, S. C., Filippa, D. A., Lieberman, P. H., and Chaganti, R. S. (1990) Immunohistochemical, molecular, and cytogenetic analysis of a consecutive series of 20 peripheral T-cell lymphomas and lymphomas of uncertain lineage, including 12 Ki-1 positive lymphomas. *Genes Chromosomes Cancer* **2,** 27–35.
23. Lust, J. A. (1996) Molecular genetics and lymphoproliferative disorders. *J. Clin. Lab. Anal.* **10,** 359–367.
24. Ralfkiaer, E., O'Conner, N. T. J., Crick, J., et al. (1987) Genotypic analysis of cutaneous T cell lymphomas. *J. Invest. Dermatol.* **88,** 762–765.
25. Bachelez, H., Bioul, L., Flageul, B., et al. (1995) Detection of clonal T cell receptor gamma gene rearrangements with the use of the polymerase chain reaction in cutaneous lesions of mycosis fungoides and Sezary syndrome. *Arch. Dermatol.* **131,** 1027–1031.
26. Achille, A., Scarpa, A., Montresor, M., et al. (1995) Routine application of polymerase chain reaction in the diagnosis of monoclonality of B-cell lymphoid proliferations. *Diagn. Mol. Pathol.* **4,** 14–24.
27. Chen, Y.-T., Whitney, K. D., and Chen, Y. (1994) Clonality analysis of B cell lymphoma in fresh frozen and paraffin embedded tissues: the effects of variable polymerase chain reaction parameters. *Mod. Pathol.* **7,** 429–434.
28. Knowles, D. M. (1989) Immunophenotypic and antigen receptor gene rearrangement analysis in T cell neoplasia. *Am. J. Pathol.* **134,** 761–785.
29. Gill, J. I. and Gulley, M. L. (1994) Immunoglobulin and T cell receptor gene rearrangement. *Hematol. Oncol. Clin.* **8,** 751–770.
30. Perl, A., DiVincenzo, J., Ryan, D., et al. (1990) Rearrangement of the T cell receptor alpha, beta, and gamma chain genes in chronic lymphocytic leukemia. *Leukemia Res.* **14,** 131–137.
31. Davey, M. P., Bongiovanni, K. F., Kaulfersch, W., et al. (1986) Immunoglobulin and T cell receptor gene rearrangement and expression in human lymphoid leukemia cells at different stages of maturation. *Proc. Natl. Acad. Sci. USA* **83,** 8759–8763.
32. Van Dongen, J. J. M. and Wolvers-Tettero, I. L. M. (1991) Analysis of immunoglobulin and T cell receptor genes. Part 11: possibilities and limitations in the diagnosis and management of lymphoproliferative diseases and related disorders. *Clin. Chem. Acta.* **198,** 93–174.
33. De Villartay, J. P., Pullman, A. B., Andrade, R., et al. (1989) Gamma/delta lineage relationship within a consecutive series of human precursor T cell neoplasms. *Blood* **74,** 2508–2518.

34. Korsmeyer, S. J., Arnold, A., Bakhshi, A., et al. (1983) Immunoglobulin gene rearrangement and cell surface antigen expression in acute lymphocytic leukemias of T cell and B cell precursor origins. *J. Clin. Invest.* **71,** 301–313.
35. Falini, B., Flenghi, L., Fagioli, M., et al. (1989) T lymphoblastic lymphomas expressing the non-disulfide-linked form of the T cell receptor. *Blood* **74,** 2501–2507.
36. Kitchingman, G. R., Rovigatti, U., Mauer, A. M., et al. (1985) Rearrangement of immunoglobulin heavy chain genes in T-cell acute lymphoblastic leukemia. *Blood* **65,** 725–729.
37. Mielke, V., Staib, G., Boehncke, W. H., et al. (1994) Clonal disease in early cutaneous T cell lymphoma. *Dermatol. Clin.* **12,** 351–360.

17

Monitoring of Bone Marrow Transplant Engraftment

Kristine P. Woronzoff-Dashkoff and Ronald C. McGlennen

1. Introduction

1.1. Background of Engraftment Testing

Bone marrow transplantation is used as a primary treatment for many diseases, including leukemia, lymphoma, and inborn errors of metabolism. The procedure involves ablation of the recipient's bone marrow by chemotherapy and/or radiation therapy, followed by transplantation of harvested bone marrow. In autologous bone marrow transplantation (BMT), the patient's own marrow is harvested and treated to remove malignant cells before it is replaced into the patient. In allogeneic BMT, bone marrow is obtained from a donor who is a close antigenic match to the patient. In either case, the goal of BMT is full, permanent replacement of the recipient's original bone marrow by donor hematopoietic elements.

Patients who have had bone marrow transplants are carefully monitored for evidence of disease remission or relapse. In addition, particularly in the early posttransplant period, it is critical to establish the extent of engraftment of the transplanted marrow. In patients who have received autologous bone marrow transplants, a morphologic estimation of bone marrow cellularity is usually adequate for determining engraftment status. In patients who have received allogeneic bone marrow transplants, however, bone marrow cellularity may not reflect true engraftment, because morphologic examination alone cannot determine whether cells are of donor or recipient origin.

Accurate identification of cell origin is achieved by examining cellular DNA at either the chromosomal or at the molecular level. Cytogenetic evaluation affords examination of the full complement of chromosomes; therefore, in addition to monitoring engraftment status, this method may detect additional

From: *Methods in Molecular Medicine, vol. 49: Molecular Pathology Protocols*
Edited by: A. A. Killeen © Humana Press Inc., Totowa, NJ

abnormalities of clinical importance, such as new or persistent chromosomal aberrations that portend a certain prognostic significance. In this case, morphologic features unique to the donor's or recipient's chromosomes, including differences in sex chromosomes, are followed serially in the posttransplant period. However, the sensitivity of this method is relatively low. Furthermore, regenerating marrow specimens, which are often very hypocellular, may not contain enough dividing cells for accurate cytogenetic analysis.

Molecular evaluation of engraftment involves the evaluation of anonymous DNA markers, a technique long used in forensic DNA testing. This testing is based on the fact that the human genome contains small sequences of repetitive DNA, or markers, located mainly at the ends and centers of chromosomes. These markers are highly polymorphic; that is, they may vary considerably in size among individuals. If a bone marrow transplant recipient carries a marker that is sized differently than the corresponding donor marker, this marker may be used in the posttransplant period to determine whether the cells repopulating the recipient's bone marrow are of donor or recipient origin. Although this type of testing does not allow examination of the entire chromosomal complement, its high sensitivity makes it uniquely suitable for routine laboratory evaluation of engraftment status.

In the past, the first-line method of monitoring bone marrow transplant engraftment involved examination of restriction fragment length polymorphisms (RFLPs) by Southern transfer analysis. In this technique, donor and recipient markers with different enzymatic restriction sites, and thus different molecular weights, are analyzed by Southern transfer blotting (**Fig. 1**). The results obtained are usually relatively unambiguous, with few artifacts, allowing simple interpretation. However, the amount of DNA required for this method of testing is relatively large, the procedure is time-consuming, and the method is inherently less sensitive than polymerase chain reaction (PCR)-based methods. Southern transfer analysis for RFLPs is still used occasionally, particul-arly when PCR analysis fails to detect informative alleles (*see* **Subheading 3.3.**).

Currently, the engraftment analysis method used by many laboratories is PCR amplification of genomic DNA. This method affords several advantages over RFLP testing, including increased sensitivity, smaller sample requirements, simpler test setup, shorter turnaround time, elimination of restriction enzymes and radioisotopes, and substantial cost savings ***(1,2)***. As in RFLP analysis, the targeted DNA regions are highly polymorphic, repetitive DNA sequences. These sequences may be classified according to the number of nucleotides in each repeated segment, and the length of the entire array of repeats. Intermediately sized units (often 0.1–20 kb long) of tandem repeat sequences are termed *minisatellites*. Under this category fall the variable number tandem repeat regions (VNTRs), in which each repeat sequence is between

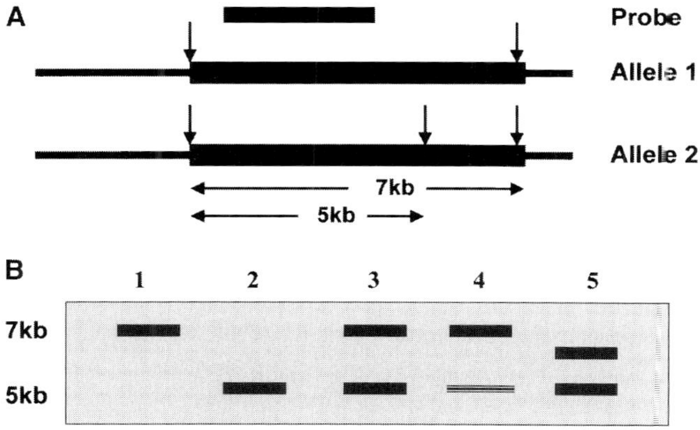

Fig. 1. **(A)** Diagram of an RFLP. Digestion of allele 1 with a restriction endonuclease produces a single 7-kb fragment, whereas digestion of allele 2 with the same restriction endonuclease produces two fragments, measuring 5 and 2 kb. **(B)** Diagram of the corresponding possibilities on Southern blotting. Lane 1: Donor (homozygous for allele 1); lane 2: recipient, pretransplant (homozygous for allele 2); lane 3: recipient, posttransplant, with 50% engraftment of donor marrow; equal amounts of donor-specific and recipient-specific allele are present; lane 4: recipient, posttransplant, with 75% engraftment of donor marrow; relatively more donor-specific allele than recipient-specific allele is present; lane 5: recipient, posttransplant, with equal amounts of recipient-specific allele and previously unidentified allele. Such results may be spurious (e.g., due to specimen mixup) or attributable to third-party engraftment (e.g., the patient has received a recent blood transfusion or another bone marrow transplant from a different donor).

5 and 64 nucleotides in length. VNTRs are used in both RFLP and PCR analysis (**Fig. 2**). Small units (<0.01 kb long) of tandem repeat sequences are termed *microsatellites*. Certain types of microsatellites, called short tandem repeat regions (STRs), contain very small repeat sequences of 1–4 nucleotides in length. STRs are evaluated using PCR, for which assay components are now available in kit format (**Fig. 3**).

1.2. Laboratory Approach to Engraftment Testing

For analysis of bone marrow transplant engraftment, a simple scheme of laboratory testing is suggested (**Fig. 4**). Prior to BMT, donor and recipient DNA is tested, with the goal of finding an informative marker suitable for following in the posttransplant period. An informative marker is defined as one for which at least one unique allele is present in the donor/recipient pair. The ideal marker would show as many independently segregating alleles as possible, i.e., two

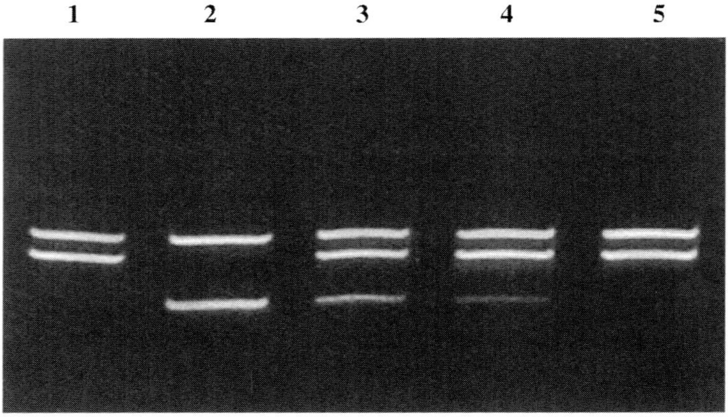

Fig. 2. Polyacrylamide gel: PCR analysis of bone marrow engraftment using ColIIA1 marker. Lane 1, Donor blood; lane 2, recipient blood, pretransplant; lane 3, control mixture (75% D, 25% R); lane 4, control mixture (90% D, 10% R); lane 5, recipient marrow, posttransplant (100% engraftment).

unique alleles in the donor and two unique alleles in the recipient (abbreviated D2R2). However, because only a limited number of differently sized alleles have been described for each marker, it is likely that the donor and recipient will have at least one allele size in common. At the minimum, at least one unique—preferably donor-specific—allele must be found in the donor/recipient pair.

In our laboratory, pretransplant specimens from donor and recipient are first analyzed by PCR for VNTR markers. In the past, analysis of PCR products was performed manually. The products were electrophoresed on a polyacrylamide gel, which was stained and photographed for visual analysis (**Fig. 2**). Currently, our laboratory uses the ABI373 GeneScan DNA sequencing system (*see* **Subheading 2.2.**) for automated quantification of allele size. Briefly, fluorescently tagged primers are used to amplify genomic DNA from the specimen. The PCR products are electrophoresed on a polyacrylamide gel, which is then analyzed by the ABI instrument using laser-based technology. The sizes of the donor and recipient alleles are determined by comparing the PCR products with internal standards, and a histogram is produced (**Fig. 3**). Most specimens show one or more unique alleles using this method, and therefore no further pretransplant testing is necessary.

VNTR analysis is used routinely in our laboratory because of our extensive experience with these markers; in addition, many of our patients' initial pretransplant screening assays were performed using VNTR markers. Laboratories new to bone marrow transplant engraftment analysis may elect to use

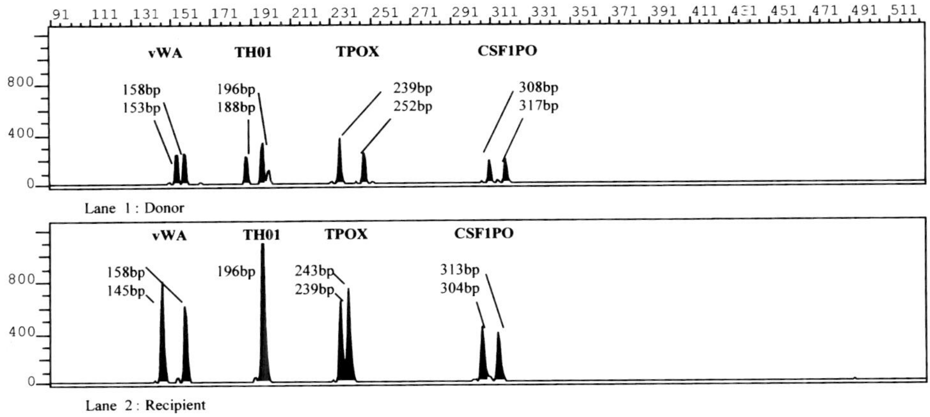

Fig. 3. Histogram of donor and recipient pretransplant alleles showing polymorphisms in 4 STRs: vWA (D1R1), TH01 (D1R0), TPOX (D1R1), and CSF1PO.

STR markers. If VNTR testing is not informative, the next line of testing in our laboratory is PCR for STRs. In the unlikely event that no STR marker is informative, Southern transfer analysis is used to identify RFLPs.

The second major segment of engraftment testing occurs following BMT (**Fig. 4**). DNA from the recipient's blood and bone marrow is amplified by PCR, and the allele sizes in each previously selected marker are deter-mined. These allele sizes are compared to those in the recipient's pretransplant marrow and the donor's marrow. The percentage of donor engraftment is determined semiquantitatively by comparing the quantity of donor-specific allele to the total quantity of donor-plus recipient-specific alleles detected (*see* **Subheading 3.3.2.**). The quantity of allele may be measured by visual estimation of band density, fluorescent quantification, or other methods.

Whichever type of assay is chosen for monitoring of engraftment status, it must be carefully optimized for each marker. The reaction must be robust, particularly since the quantity of DNA available in the posttransplant period may be very small. Hence, sensitivity controls that employ patient-derived mixes of donor and recipient cells extracted for DNA mixed in prescribed ratios (5%, 10%) ensure that interassay comparison are meaningful and precise. In addition, accurate, reliable quantification of the percentage of donor and recipient allele is necessary. In our experience, clinicians place more importance on the trend of engraftment in a patient, rather than precise numerical quantification of engraftment at any one particular time. Thus, we report results as a specific range of percentage of engraftment, rather than as fixed numerical values.

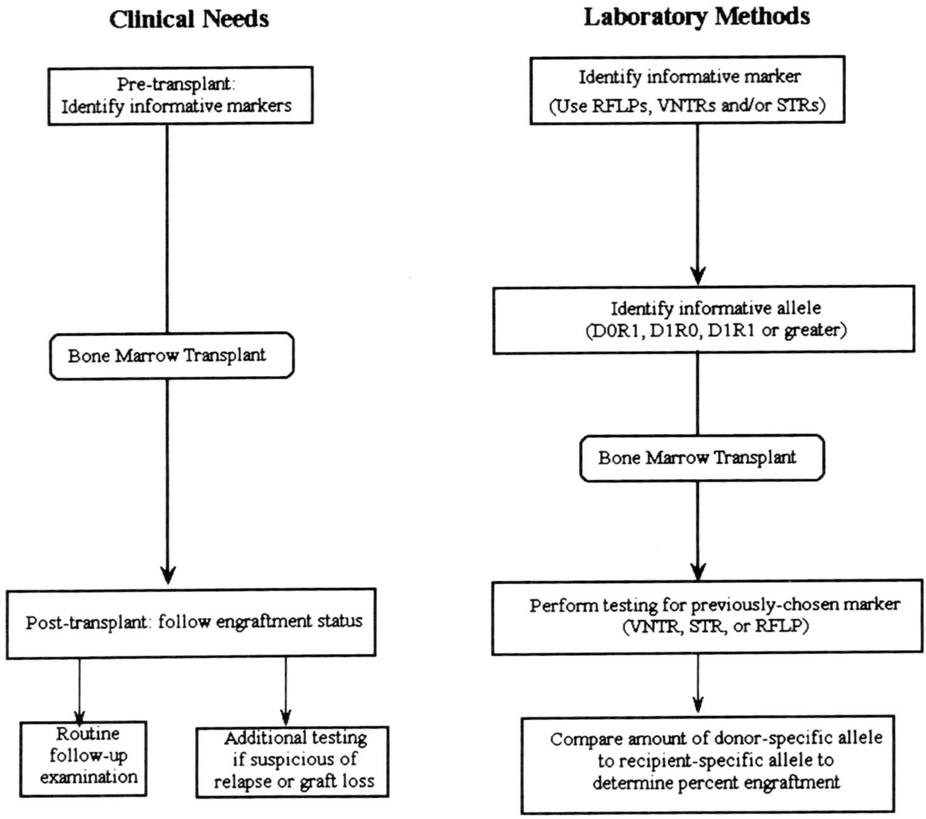

Fig. 4. Flow chart showing clinical engraftment assessment and accompanying laboratory testing.

2. Materials

Markers examined in our assay include the following VNTRs and STRs:

1. Apolipoprotein B (ApoB): This autosomal codominant VNTR lies on the short arm of chromosome 2 and is located in the 3′ flanking region of the 42-kb ApoB gene. Twelve alleles have been identified, ranging in size from 460–600 bp. The ApoB VNTR has a heterozygosity of 75% *(3)*.
2. Collagen Type II alpha 1 (ColIIA1): This autosomal codominant VNTR is located at 12q14.3, in the 3′ flanking region of the 32-kb Type II Collagen gene. Several alleles have been identified, ranging in size from 600–700 bp. The COLIIA1 VNTR has a heterozygosity of 81% *(4,5)*.

3. D1S80: This autosomal codominant VNTR is located on chromosome 1. Sixteen alleles have been identified, ranging in size from 300–700 bp. The D1S80 VNTR has a heterozygosity of 80.8% ***(6)***.
4. pYNZ22: This autosomal codominant VNTR is located at 17p23. More than 10 alleles have been identified, ranging in size from 170 –870 bp. The pYNZ22 VNTR has a heterozygosity of 86% (***[7]***; Bruce Balzar, personal communication).
5. CF-17b: This is a dinucleotide intronic STR found in the CFTR gene at chromosome 7q31. Thirty-three alleles have been identified, ranging in size from 167– 414 bp ***(8)***.
6. CSF1PO: This STR is found within the human c-*fms* proto-oncogene for CSF-1 receptor gene (*HUMCSF1PO*) located at 5q33.3-34. Ten alleles have been identified, ranging in size from 295–327 bp.
7. TPOX: This STR is found within the human thyroid peroxidase gene (*HUMTPOX*) located at 2p25-1-pter. Eight alleles have been identified, ranging in size from 224–252 bp.
8. TH01: This STR is found within the human tyrosine hydroxylase gene (*HUMTH01*) located at 11p15.5. Eight alleles have been identified, ranging in size from 179–203 bp.
9. vWA (formerly vWF): This STR is found within the human von Willebrand factor gene (*HUMVWFA31*) located at 12p12-pter. Ten alleles have been identified, ranging in size from 139–167 bp.

2.1. Specimen Collection and Processing

Prior to BMT, patient and donor blood specimens are collected. The DNA from these specimens is amplified by PCR for identification of polymorphism. These pre-BMT results are later correlated with results from post-BMT specimen testing.

2.1.1. Blood Specimens

1. Volume: For pre-BMT specimens, collect 30 mL of blood. For post-BMT specimens, the volume of blood necessary is dependent on the white blood cell (WBC) count. For WBC (10^9/L) of >1.0, 0.5, 0.25, and 0.1 the blood volume is 10, 20, 30, and 50 mL, respectively.
2. Preservative: Acid citrate dextrose (ACD) is preferred, but EDTA is acceptable.

2.1.2. Bone Marrow Specimens

1. Volume: For pre-BMT, bone marrow is not required (blood is recommended for this procedure). For post-BMT, 5 mL is required (or as little as 2 mL, if marrow is not markedly hypocellular).
2. Preservative: Collect in a syringe to which ACD has been added (EDTA is acceptable).

2.1.3. Tissue Specimens

A minimum volume of 5 mm^3 must be delivered to the laboratory within 1 h of collection or quick frozen in liquid nitrogen or dry ice. Specimens from outside the hospital should be transported frozen on dry ice.

2.2. Equipment and Supplies

1. Perkin-Elmer Thermocycler 480 (Perkin-Elmer, Norwalk, CT).
2. ABI373 DNA sequencing system (Applied Biosystems, Foster City, CA).
3. The following supplies from Applied Biosystems:
   a. GENESCAN™ 672 Software (cat. no. 672-10).
   b. Genotyper™ Software (cat. no. 401614).
   c. 6-cm S Notched Glass Plate (cat. no. 401623).
   d. 6-cm S Plain Plate (cat. no. 401624).
   e. 6-cm S Gel Spacer, Pair (cat. no. 401625).
   f. GENESCAN 24-tooth comb (cat. no. 401444).
   g. GENESCAN 36-tooth comb (cat. no. 401497).
   h. PRISM™ GENESCAN-500 Tamra Size Standard (cat. no. 401733).
   i. PRISM GENESCAN-2500 Tamra Size Standard (cat. no. 401545).
4. Acrylamide/*bis* powder (19:1) (cat. no. 161-0120; Bio-Rad, Hercules, CA).
5. Formamide, molecular biology grade (cat. no. BP227-100; Fisher, Fair Lawn, NJ).
6. TEMED (cat. no. 161-0800; Bio-Rad).
7. Ammonium persulfate (cat. no. 161-0700; Bio-Rad).
8. Urea, ultrapure (cat. no. 15505-035, Life Technologies, Rockville, MD).
9. AG 501X8 resin (cat. no. 143-6424; Bio-Rad).
10. Sterilization filter unit (0.45-µm, 115 mL) (cat. no. 245-0045; Nalge, Rochester, NY).
11. Scotch™ electrical tape) (cat. no. 1739-7; 3M, St. Paul, MN).
12. Tris crystallized free base (cat. no. BP152-5; Fisher).
13. Boric acid (cat. no. A73-500; Fisher).
14. EDTA disodium salt (cat. no. BP 120-1; Fisher).
15. Blue dextran powder (cat. no. D-5751; Sigma, St. Louis, MO).
16. Spectrophotometer (Beckman, Palo Alto, CA, or other supplier).
17. *Taq* DNA polymerase in storage Buffer A, 5 µ/µL (cat. no. M1865; Promega, Madison, WI).
18. Bulk dNTPs (40 µ*M*) 100 m*M*/L each of dATP, dCTP, dGTP, dTTP (cat. no. U1240; Promega).
19. Primers for VNTR and STR sequences: Primers for the ApoB, ColIIA1, D1S80, pYNZ22, and CF-17b markers are custom synthesized and fluorescently labeled by Microchemical Facility Laboratory, UMHC Institute of Human Genetics, Minneapolis, MN. The sequences are as follows:
   a. ApoB3′(A) (20mer): 5′-CCT-TCT-CAC-TTG-GCA-AAT-AC-3′.
   b. ApoB5′(S) (20mer): 5′-ATG-GAA-ACG-GAG-AAA-TTA-TG-3′.

Table 1
PCR Cocktail for BMT Engraftment Testing

Component	1 rxn[a] (mL)	500 rxn (mL)	2000 rxn (mL)
Peg	0.0425	21.25	85.0
dATP	0.004	2.0	8.0
dCTP	0.004	2.0	8.0
dGTP	0.004	2.0	8.0
dTTP	0.004	2.0	8.0
10X Buffer	0.010	5.0	20.0
Total volume	0.0685	34.25	137.0

[a]rxn = reaction.

c. COL2A3′(A) (20mer): 5′-GTC-ATG-AAC-TAG-CTC-TGG-TG-3′.
d. COL2A5′(S) (20 mer): 5′-CCA-GGT-TAA-GGT-TGA-CAG-CT-3′.
e. D1S80w (28mer): 5′-GAA-ACT-GGC-CTC-CAA-ACA-CTG-CCC-GCC-G-3′.
f. D1S80c (29 mer): 5′-GTC-TTG-TTG-GAG-ATG-CAC-GTG-CCC-CTT-GC-3′.
g. pYNZ223′(A) (22mer): 5′-GCC-CCA-TGT-ATC-TTG-TCC-AGT-G-3′.
h. pYNZ225′(S) (22mer): 5′-GGT-CGA-AGA-GTG-AAG-TGC-ACA-G-3′.
i. CF-17b3′(A) (20mer): 5′-GCT-GCA-TTC-TAT-AGG-TTA-TC-3′.
j. CF-17b5′(S) (20mer): 5′-AAA-CTT-ACC-GAC-AAG-AGG-AA-3′.

Primers for the CSF1PO, TPOX, TH01, and vWA STRs are obtained from Promega.

2.3. Reagents

1. MilliQ Water (double-distilled H_2O): MilliQ is the trade name of the water system purchased from Millipore. This deionized water is treated with activated carbon and deionization cartridges, and filtered to remove microorganisms larger than 0.22 µm. It meets CAP Class II Water Requirements when stored in polyethylene carboys. If microbial-free water is needed, a bottle of this water is autoclaved and is referred to as sterile water.
2. PCR master mix: A preparation for either 500 or 2000 reactions is made by combining the reagents given in **Table 1**.
3. Stock primers (100 pmol/µL): Use the following formula to calculate the amount of filtered, sterilized water to add to the primers (store at –20°C):

$$\text{Yield } (\mu g)/\text{mol wt } (\mu g/\mu mol) \times (10^6) \text{ pmol}/\mu mol \times \mu L/100 \text{ pmol} = \text{volume needed for resuspension}$$

4. Working primers (2.5 pmol/µL): Add 25 µL of each stock primer and dilute to 1000 µL with sterile water. Store at –20°C.

5. Working PCR mix: Prepare a mix for the total number of reactions plus one based on the amount of DNA template to be used. For 4 µL of DNA template, prepare the mix as follows: 40.25 µL of PCR master mix, 3.0 µL of $MgCl_2$ (25 m*M*), 2.5 µL of SIA primer, and 0.25 µL of *Taq* polymerase (for a total volume of 46.0 µL).
6. PCR control: A sample containing water in place of specimen is included with each thermocycler run. This controls for the presence of contaminating DNA in the reaction reagents.
7. Sensitivity controls: Two cell lines are mixed at a ratio of 95:5 and 10:90. These product mixes, which determine the sensitivity of the assay, are run as controls on every gel that includes an engraftment analysis. The sensitivity for a particular specimen is that of the lowest percentage of detectable control, usually 5 or 10%.

3. Methods

3.1. Isolation of DNA

Isolate DNA from the specimen following standard laboratory protocol (*see* **Note 1**).

3.2. Dilution of Genomic DNA

3.2.1. Calculating Amount of DNA to Dilute

3.2.1.1. Pretransplant Recipient and Donor Samples

Because pretreatment recipient and donor samples will be used in every patient analysis, a dilution of a large quantity of DNA is made (typically 30 µg). However, if the amount of sample is limited, avoid diluting all of it. If the donor and recipient are not polymorphic by PCR testing, DNA will be needed for Southern analysis. To determine the volume of DNA needed for 30 µg, take the inverse of the concentration in micrograms/milliliter and multiply by 30,000:

$$1/(\mu g/mL) \times 30\ \mu g \times 1000\ \mu L/mL = \mu L \text{ for } 30\ \mu g$$

To determine the amount of H_2O to add, dilute 30 µg of DNA into a total volume of 450 µL to achieve the proper concentration. Then subtract the volume needed for 30 µg from 450.

3.2.1.2. Posttransplant Recipient samples

Because posttransplant recipient samples will be analyzed only once or twice, a small dilution is made (typically 7.5 µg). If pretransplant analysis revealed at least one donor-specific and one recipient-specific allele, Southern transfer analysis will not be required, and the entire posttransplant sample may be diluted. If this is not the case, avoid diluting the entire sample. To determine the amount of DNA needed for 7.5 µg, take the inverse of the concentration in micrograms/microliter and multiply by 7500:

$$1/(\mu g/mL) \times 7.5\ \mu g \times 1000\ \mu L/mL = \mu L \text{ for } 7.5\ \mu g$$

To determine the amount of H_2O to add, dilute 7.5 µg of DNA into a total volume of 112.5 µL to achieve the proper concentration. Then subtract the volume needed for 7.5 µg from 112.5.

3.2.2. Making Dilutions for PCR

1. Use 1.5-mL microcentrifuge tubes labeled with the sample number.
2. Make dilutions using designated pipettors and sterile water reserved for PCR use.
3. Dilute the samples.
4. Vortex the dilutions after making them. Revortex prior to beginning PCR.

3.3. Setting Up Samples According to Type of Analysis

3.3.1. Pretransplant Polymorphism Determination

Pretransplant donor and recipient samples are screened for polymorphisms in the VNTRs and STRs listed previously in order to find an informative marker. A marker is considered informative when at least one allele with a unique number of repeats is found in the donor or recipient. These unique alleles have different molecular weights and are thus separable on gel electrophoresis.

Three VNTRs, ApoB, ColIIA1, and D1S80, are evaluated first; most recipient–donor pairs will be polymorphic at one or more of these VNTRs. If no polymorphism is identified, one additional VNTR (pYNZ22) and an STR (CF-17b) are examined. If these markers prove uninformative, additional STRs (CSF1PO, POX, TH01, and vWA) are examined. If these markers are also uninformative, Southern transfer analysis for RFLPs may be necessary for polymorphism determination and engraftment analysis.

3.3.2. Posttransplant Engraftment Analysis

Patient samples are analyzed using the markers determined to be informative in the pretransplant polymorphism screen (*see* **Subheading 2.**).

1. Add reagents and specimens to tubes; place the tubes in a thermocycler.
2. Into a 0.6-µL microcentrifuge tube, add 85 µL of the working PCR mix (*see* **Subheading 3.2.**), and then add 15µL of DNA template. Vortex the tubes, spin briefly in a microcentrifuge, and place the tubes in a thermal cycler. Run the thermal cycler according to predetermined PCR parameters (*see* **Note 2**).

3. Perform electrophoresis according to the ABI373 GeneScan Electrophoresis Procedure using 1–2 µL of PCR product.
4. Analyze the GeneScan collection file according to the ABI373 GeneScan Analysis Procedure.

3.4. Formats for Reporting Results

3.4.1. Pretransplant Results

The allele sizes of the donor and the recipient for the informative marker are recorded in the laboratory. Test results are reported to clinicians as "polymorphism found" or "polymorphism not found."

3.4.2. Posttransplant Results

The allele sizes of the recipient and the percentage of engraftment are recorded in the laboratory. The results are reported to clinicians as ranges, from the following choices: 0%, 1–10%, 11–25%, 26–50%, 51–75%, 76–99%, 90–94%, 95–99%, and 100%.

3.5. Interpretation of Results

3.5.1. Pretransplant Assays

A useful pretransplant assay will identify at least one unique allele in a donor/recipient pair. Although some donors will possess two alleles that are completely different from the recipient's two alleles, this is not often the case. Because engraftment testing by PCR is so sensitive, the presence of even one unique allele in either the donor or recipient is sufficient for distinguishing between the donor and the recipient.

The unique allele must, of course, be different enough in size to be distinguished from its partner allele. The necessary size difference depends on the system used to analyze the PCR products. In our computerized analysis system, alleles must be at least 4 bp different in size to be resolved by the computer. If one is analyzing the PCR products manually, one should choose a marker that shows at least one unique band in either the donor or recipient that is easily and distinctly distinguishable from its partner band.

3.5.2. Posttransplant Assays

In the monitoring of bone marrow transplant engraftment, it is essential to obtain current clinical information about the patient. The date of the bone marrow transplant should be noted, along with any current clinical information, such as whether the specimen is sent for routine follow-up examination, or whether there is a suspicion of disease relapse or graft loss. Morphologic interpretation of the specimen, if available, is also quite helpful, particularly when molecular results are not in concordance with clinical information.

One morphologic setting in which molecular testing may be particularly useful is that of a markedly hypocellular marrow. In this situation, cells are too few in number to accurately assess morphologically or cytogenetically. Because PCR requires so little DNA to provide an informative result, engraftment testing in the molecular laboratory often provides valid, critical information to the clinician at this vulnerable stage of the posttransplant period. Following transplant, testing is limited to those unique alleles identified on pretransplant testing. In most cases, examination of a single marker provides informative results. If at least one unique allele in each donor and recipient (abbreviated D1R1) is present, the assay will provide informative results. However, finding one unique allele in the donor and no unique recipient alleles (D1R0) may also be informative, particularly in the setting of minimal (<25%) engraftment. Likewise, finding no unique donor alleles but one unique recipient allele (D0R1) is informative in the setting of near-total (>75%) engraftment. In the latter two scenarios, correlation of molecular engraftment studies with bone marrow morphology is particularly crucial.

3.5.3. Semiquantitative Analysis of Data

Based on the amount of donor-specific allele (D) and recipient-specific allele (R) present, the computer calculates the percentage of bone marrow transplant engraftment. This number is reported as a range to allow for gel-to-gel variation (*see* **Subheading 3.5.2.**). The formulas for determining the percentage of engraftment are different depending on whether the results show one donor-specific allele and one recipient-specific allele (D1R1), one recipient-specific allele and no donor-specific alleles (D0R1), or one donor-specific allele and no recipient-specific alleles (D1R0). For D1R1, the formula is D/R + D; for D0R1, the formula is 1 – (2R1/R1 + R2); and for D2R0, the formula is 2D2/(D1 + D2).

4. Notes

1. On occasion, posttransplant specimens may be sent for engraftment studies on patients who have not had pretransplant polymorphism screening. In this situation, tissues such as buccal scrapings or skin biopsies may be used for obtaining DNA. However, special care must be taken when obtaining skin biopsies in order to avoid excessive blood contamination, which could lead to amplification of post-BMT donor leukocyte DNA. Another possible source of pretransplant recipient DNA is cell lysate samples from the HLA-typing laboratory. These specimens are used as is, without DNA extraction. Usually, only a very small volume of this type of specimen is available; the sample is diluted only enough to allow performance of the three most commonly polymorphic VNTRs: ApoB, ColIIA1, and D1S80.

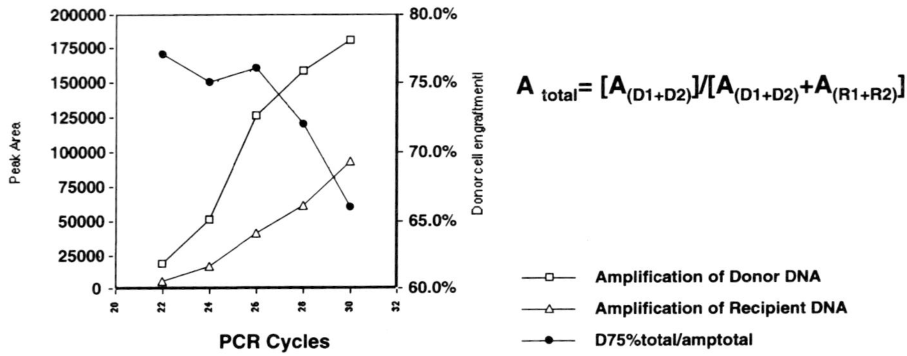

Fig. 5. Amplification kinetics of a mixture of 75% donor and 25% recipient template DNA, plotted as a function of cycle number. (Reprinted from **ref. *9*** with permission from W. B. Saunders Company.)

2. Because individual thermal cyclers may have very different characteristics, each laboratory must optimize its own PCR parameters for each marker. In a semiquantitative assay, it is particularly important to optimize not only the temperatures and segment lengths but also the cycle number. As shown in **Fig. 5**, performing only a few cycles under or over the optimum number may result in misrepresentation of the quantity of template. The following is a sample PCR protocol for the ApoB marker: 94°C for 4 min; 19 cycles of 94°C for 1 min and 58°C for 6 min; 58°C for 4 min; followed by a 4°C soak.

References

1. Sreenan, J. J., Pettay, J. D., Tbakhi, A., et al. (1997) The use of amplified variable number of tandem repeats (VNTR) in the detection of chimerism following bone marrow transplantation: a comparison with restriction fragment length polymorphism (RFLP) by Southern blotting. *Am. J. Clin. Pathol.* **107,** 292–298.
2. Martinelli, G., Trabetti, E., Farabegoli, P., et al. (1997) Early detection of bone marrow engraftment by amplification of hypervariable DNA regions. *Hematologica* **82,** 156–160.
3. Boerwinkle, E., Xiang, W., Fourest, E., et al. (1989) Rapid typing of tandem repeated hypervariable loci by the polymerase chain: application to the apolipoprotein B 3′ hypervariable region. *Proc. Natl. Acad. Sci. USA* **86,** 212–216.
4. Seino, S. W. and Bell, G. I. (1990) Human Collagen Type II Alpha I (Col2AI) Gene: variable number of tandem repeat polymorphism detected by gene amplification. *Nucleic Acid Res. **18,** 3102.*
5. Stoker, N. G., Cheah, K. E., Griffin, J. R., et al. (1985) A highly polymorphic region 3′ to the human type II collagen gene. *Nucleic Acid Res.* 13, **4613–4622.**

6. Budowle, B., Chakraborty, R., Giursti, A. M., et al. (1991) Analysis of the variable number of tandem repeat locus D1S80 by the polymerase chain reaction followed by high resolution polyacrylamide gel electrophoresis *Am. J. Hum. Genetics* **48,** 137–144.
7. Horn, T., Richards, B. R., and Klinger, K. W. (1989) Amplification of a highly polymorphic variable number of tandem repeat segment by the polymerase chain reaction. *Nucleic Acid Res.* **17,** 2140.
8. Zielinski, J., Markiewicz, D., Rininsland, F., et al. (1991) A cluster of highly polymorphic dinucleotide repeats in intron 17b of the cystic fibrosis transmembrane conductance regulator (CFTR) gene. *Am. J. Hum. Genet.* **49,** 1256–1262.
9. Crotty, P. L., Staggs, R. A., Porter, P. T., et al. (1994) Quantitative analysis in molecular diagnostics. *Hum. Pathol.* **25,** 572–579.

18

Direct Molecular Diagnosis of Multiple Endocrine Neoplasia Type 1

Elizabeth M. Petty, Michael Glynn, and Allen E. Bale

1. Introduction

1.1. Epidemiology and Clinical Phenotype

Multiple endocrine neoplasia type 1 (MEN1) is an autosomal dominant syndrome characterized by the predisposition to develop both peptic ulcer disease and a wide variety of endocrine tumors usually in adolescence and adulthood. Specifically, hyperplasia and/or tumors (most often adenomas) of the parathyroid, pancreatic islet cells, anterior pituitary, and adrenal cortical glands are classically described in affected individuals who have MEN1 *(1,2)*. MEN1 is a highly penetrant disorder whose onset is generally during adult life with the occurrence of at least one, but most often more than one, of the aforementioned tumors. The age-related penetrance of this disorder based on analysis in 63 unrelated kindreds is 7, 52, 87, 98, 99, and 100% by 10, 20, 30, 40, 50, and 60 yr, respectively *(3)*. The disorder is estimated to occur in approx 1 in 30,000 to 1 in 50,000 individuals. Most cases are associated with a positive family history of the disorder, but new germline mutations have been identified in a small percentage of individuals having a negative family history of the disorder but classic features of MEN1 *(3–7)*.

Although the tumors most commonly described in MEN1 are not malignant, they are often associated with medical conditions that require therapeutic intervention. Symptoms in this disorder are therefore related to the biology of the tumors occurring in any one affected individual. Symptoms are most often related to hypersecretion of various hormones secondary to these tumors. Glucose intolerance, hypoglycemia, hypergastrinemia with severe peptic ulcer dis-

From: *Methods in Molecular Medicine, vol. 49: Molecular Pathology Protocols*
Edited by: A. A. Killeen © Humana Press Inc., Totowa, NJ

ease, galactorrhea, and full-blown Cushing syndrome are some of the symptoms that can result from the many different tumors, including pancreatic islet cell adenomas, gastrinomas, parathyroid adenomas, prolactinomas, glucagonomas, insulinomas, and vasointestinal peptide–producing tumors that occur in this condition ***(1,2)***. Epigastric pain with intractable peptic ulcers and/or ulcerative gastritis (known as Zollinger Ellison syndrome) along with the steatorrhea and diarrhea are especially problematic for individuals who have gastrointestinal (GI) and pancreatic manifestations of the disease ***(8)***.

Occasionally tumors will undergo malignant transformation, especially those that are located in the pancreas, thymus, or bronchi ***(1,2)***. Thus, malignant tumors in the GI tract and the thymic-bronchic tract have been reported, including bronchial carcinoids or carcinomas, thymic carcinoids, and duodenal carcinoids. Cutaneous lesions, ovarian tumors, adrenocortical carcinomas, and primary nervous tissue tumors including malignant schwannomas have also been observed. In fact, angiofibromas, similar to those seen in tuberous sclerosis, are present in many affected individuals. Thus, the effect of germline mutations in the *MEN1* gene is pleiotropic and there is both inter- and intrafamilial variability in the phenotypic expression of the highly penetrant disorder.

Because MEN1 is a medical condition in which regular clinical screening studies of at-risk individuals have proven useful in helping to reduce morbidity and mortality related to the disease, owing to early symptom management and medical or surgical intervention to minimize development of symptoms, DNA or molecular diagnosis of MEN1 has demonstrated clear clinical utility in families in which the MEN1 disease phenotype segregates. At-risk individuals can be evaluated for development of parathyroid, pituitary, and pancreatic islet cell abnormalities by monitoring calcium, parathyroid hormone, prolactin, and gastrin levels. Radiographic studies are useful to screen for pulmonary carcinoids.

1.2. MEN1 *Tumor Suppressor Gene and Menin Protein*

Studies of both linkage analysis and loss of heterozygosity pinpointed the location of the *MEN1* gene to chromosome 11q13 ***(9–15)***. Studies of early loss of heterozygosity suggested that the gene would be a tumor suppressor based on the two-hit model according to Knudson ***(16)***. In 1997, the *MEN1* gene was cloned ***(17)***. The gene contains 10 exons spanning approx 9 kb of genomic DNA. Exon 1 and the last 832 bp at the 3′ end of exon 10 remained untranslated. Therefore, there are nine coding exons that contribute to the 2.9-kb MEN1 transcript that is ubiquitously expressed in most human tissues. An additional 4-kb transcript was identified in the pancreas and the thymus.

The *MEN1* gene is ubiquitously transcribed and encodes a 610 amino acid (67 kDa) protein called menin ***(17)***. Recently, clues to the possible function of menin were reported ***(18,19)***. Menin is a nuclear protein that interacts with

JunD. JunD may have transactivating and transrepressor activity through the AP-1 transcription factor depending on the specific Fos partner or promoter, but the actual role of menin and the tissue specificity of tumor involvement in individuals with germline *MEN1* mutations is not yet understood.

No one predisposing mutation has been identified in the coding region of the *MEN1* to account for the majority of the disease in patients studied to date. However, founder mutations have been described in some populations stemming from geographic isolates ***(20–23)***. Germline mutations have been reported scattered throughout the coding region of the gene and include nonsense, missense, and frameshift mutations. Mutations often predict premature truncation of the protein owing to the nonsense or frameshift mutations. Missense mutations account for approx 30% of the cases ***(3–7,24,25)***. To date, there are no well-defined genotype/phenotype correlations or prognostic predictions that can be made based solely on mutational analysis that are useful in the clinical management of individuals. In general, it appears that germline mutations can be identified in approx 90% of classic MEN1 families and slightly more than 80% of patients who themselves have isolated MEN1 with no known family history ***(3–7,25)***. *MEN1* mutations have also been identified in a wide range of related endocrine disorders and sporadic endocrine tumors ***(5,7,26–35)*** (*see* **Note 1**).

1.3. Considerations for DNA Diagnostic Testing of MEN1

Because the vast majority of *MEN1* mutations reported to date are scattered throughout the coding region of the gene, screening the nucleotide sequence of each coding exon and adjacent intron/exon boundaries is a relatively robust method for identifying mutations in the *MEN1* gene (*see* **Note 2**). This type of exon-by-exon mutation screening has the potential drawback, however, of missing large deletions or rearrangements involving one allele. The MEN1 phenotype in its classic form does not display significant genetic heterogeneity, making linkage analysis a useful diagnostic tool in large families in whom multiple blood samples are available for analysis. In fact, in families in whom a *MEN1* mutation cannot be found by direct analysis, further studies to analyze *MEN1* linkage in these kindreds may be quite useful in helping to make a diagnosis. Presumably in families in whom *MEN1* mutations cannot be identified in the coding regions, mutations may lie in promoter or other regions important to the expression of the gene that have not been fully characterized in these patients or there may be a large deletion or rearrangement involving several exons.

A variety of well-described methods to screen for point mutations have been widely published in the primary scientific literature as well as in molecular genetics or molecular biology protocol manuals ***(36–52)***. These different strategies, often involving modifications of single-strand conformation polymorphism (SSCP) analysis, have varying degrees of sensitivity, depending on the specific techniques employed. Given that there are only nine relatively small coding exons in the *MEN1* gene, direct sequence analysis proves to be the most robust, cost-effective, and sensitive strategy to screen for unknown mutations. Thus, polymerase chain reaction (PCR)-based manual or automated sequence analysis provides the most useful means for the diagnosis of MEN1 in our laboratories. Although there is no particular hot spot of mutations in *MEN1*, early studies suggested that a slightly higher percentage of mutations have been found in exons 2 and 10, potentially making these exons ideal starting places for sequence-based mutation analysis. Exons 2 and 10 are the largest of the MEN1 coding exons, which may help account for the relatively high number of mutations in these regions. Given that there is no one exon where the majority of mutations are located, full sequencing through all coding exons in a molecular diagnostic laboratory is recommended.

2. Materials

2.1. Reagents for DNA Sample Preparation

1. Reagents from peripheral blood using either standard laboratory protocols or commercial DNA extraction/purification kits that reliably yield PCR quality DNA, e.g., Puregene (Gentra Systems, Minneapolis, MN).

2.2. PCR Reagents

1. *Taq* polymerase (5 U/μL) (Perkin-Elmer).
2. 10X PCR Buffer II (Perkin-Elmer).
3. Klen*Taq1* (Ab peptides) (25 U/μL) and buffer.
4. Cloned *Pfu* Polymerase (2.5 U/μL) (Stratagene).
5. LA 16 (15 parts Klen*Taq* and 1 part *Pfu* polymerase).
6. Double-distilled H_2O (ddH_2O).
7. dNTPs (2 m*M*).
8. Spermidine (50 m*M*).
9. $MgCl_2$ (25 m*M*).
10. Dimethyl sulfoxide (DMSO).
11. 5 *M* Betaine.
12. PCR primers (10 μ*M*) (*see* **Table 1** for sequences) (*see* **Note 3**).
13. For direct mutation analysis: men1x2 (F and R), men1x3 (F and R), men1x4 (F and R), men1x5 + 6 (F and R), men1x7 (F and R), men1x8 (F and R), men1x9 (F and R), men1x10 (F and R).

2.3. Reagents for Agarose Gel Electrophoresis

1. Molecular biology grade agarose.
2. Ethidium bromide (10 mg/mL) stock.
3. 5X TBE buffer stock: 54g of Tris base, 27.59g of boric acid, 0.5 *M* Na_2 EDTA, 20 mL in 1 L of ddH_2O (pH 8.0).

Table 1
***MEN1* Primer Pairs for Mutation Analysis**

Exon	Primer name	Primer sequence 5′ to 3′	Product size (bp)	Annealing temperature (°C)	Number of cycles	PCR conditions[a]
2	men1 2F	GGT GGA ACC TTA GCG GAC	592	55	30	Betaine
	men1 2R	GGT TTT GAA GAA GTG GGT C				
3	men1 3F	CCC ATG TTA AAG CAC AGA G	299	60	30	Standard
	men1 3R	ACA GTA TGA AGG GGA CAA G				
4	men1 4F	TGT CAT TCC CTG AAG CAG	252	60	30	Standard
	men1 4R	CCC ACA GCA AGT CAA GTC				
5 and 6	men1 5 and 6F	AAG GAC CCG TTC TCC TCC C	320	60	30	Standard
	men1 5 and 6R	CCT GCC TCA GCC ACT GTT AG				
7	men1 7F	GCA TTT GTG CCA GCA GGG	268	60	30	Standard
	men1 7R	GGG TGG TTG GAA ACT GAT GGA G				
8	men1 8F	GCT ACC CCC GAT GGT GAG AC	261	55	30	Betaine
	men1 8R	ATG GCC CTG TGG AAG GGA G				
9	men1 9F	CTG CTA AGG GGT GAG TAA GAG AC	260	50	30	Betaine
	men1 9R	ACC ACC TGT AGT GCC CAG AC				
10	men1 10FB	TGC CGA TGG GAC TGA GAC	714	55 or 60	30	Betaine
	men1 10RB	CTA GGG TTT GGG TAG AGG TG				

[a]Standard and Betaine conditions are described in **Subheading 3.1.** The Betaine conditions enhance amplification of GC-rich sequences.

2.4. Sequencing Reagents

Sequencing reagents will vary because they will be specific to the laboratory's available sequencing equipment. Several different commercial kits are available for manual sequencing of PCR products. In our hands, incorporating PCR cycle sequencing with ^{33}P-radiolabeled ddNTPs provides quick, strong, optimally readable manual sequencing results as visualized after overnight autoradiography compared to methods using end-labeled primers with T_4 kinase, but lacks the advantage of being able to use one radiolabeled primer mix for a number of sample reactions over a few weeks. We routinely use the Thermosequenase kit (US 79750; Amersham Life Science Reagents), which we have found provides reproducible high-quality sequence. A 6% polyacrylamide sequencing gel (a commercial preparation mix for long-range sequencing polyacrylamide gel mix) has proven optimal for manual sequencing. For automated sequencing protocols, obtain reagents and methods for optimal analysis recommended by the manufacturer of the equipment (*see* **Note 4**).

2.5. Equipment

1. Thermocycler.
2. Agarose gel electrophoresis equipment (power supply and gel boxes).
3. Manual sequencing gel-running apparatus.
4. Sequencing gel-running apparatus.
5. Glass plates, spacers, combs.
6. Power supply to support electrophoresis.
7. Gel dryer.
8. Pipets with accurate pipetting between 1 and 200 μL.
9. Centrifuge.
10. Or automated sequencer with associated gel and analysis components.

3. Methods

Because the equipment and technical expertise available within different molecular diagnostic and research laboratories vary considerably, detailed methods for DNA extraction and sequencing are not provided here. Several different reliable protocols have been previously published in manuals on molecular genetic techniques as well as in other chapters in the *Methods in Molecular Medicine* series ***(53,54)***. Several different highly reliable commercial kits are available for both DNA extraction and sequencing.

After PCR-quality DNA has been prepared from the biological samples of interest, which are generally leukocytes (although any nucleated specimen containing nondegraded DNA such as cultured amniocytes, chorionic villus samples, buccal cells, fibroblasts, or fresh or archival tumor tissue may be used as appropriate), PCR amplification of coding exons and flanking sequences using the primers and conditions discussed next can be conducted.

The methods outlined will specifically focus on providing detailed information about useful primer pairs and optimal PCR conditions to provide appropriate template for *MEN1* analysis and general discussion of the analysis of point mutations in the *MEN1* gene by direct sequencing.

3.1. PCR of MEN1 *Coding Regions and Splice Sites*

A 50-µL (this volume may be decreased by adjusting all components appropriately, but a 50-µL sample provides an optimal amount of specimen for complete analysis and reanalysis if necessary) PCR is set up for each pair of primers using one of the two following conditions, as noted in **Table 1**. LA 16, a 15:1 mix of Klen*Taq1*:*Pfu* polymerase, may be mixed ahead of time and stored at –20°C.

1. Standard conditions:
   a. Template DNA (0.1–1 µg): 1 µL.
   b. H_2O: 34.5 µL.
   c. 10X buffer: 5 µL.
   d. dNTP (2 m*M*): 5 µL.
   e. Spermidine (50 m*M*): 0.25 µL.
   f. Primer 1(10 µ*M*): 1 µL.
   g. Primer 2 (10 µ*M*): 1 µL.
   h. *Taq* polymerase (5 U/µL): 0.25 µL.
   i. $MgCl_2$ (25 m*M*): 3 µL.
2. Betaine conditions (to enhance amplification of GC-rich templates:
   a. Template DNA (0.1–1 µg): 1 µL.
   b. H_2O: 14.3 µL.
   c. 10X Klen*Taq* buffer: 5 µL.
   d. dNTP (2 m*M*): 5 µL.
   e. DMSO: 2.5 µL.
   f. Primer 1 (10 µ*M*): 1 µL.
   g. Primer 2 (10 µ*M*): 1 µL.
   h. LA 16: 0.2 µL.
   i. 5 *M* Betaine: 20 µL.

3.2. General PCR Cycling Conditions

Annealing temperatures and cycling conditions may vary depending on the specific thermocycler used. The following conditions were optimized using an Ericomp dual-block, water-cooled thermocycler.

1. Initial denaturation step: 97°C for 2 min.
2. Cycling steps: 1: 96°C at 30 s; 2: For annealing temperatures of exon flanking primers, *see* **Table 1**. 30 s; 3: 72°C at 40 s (total cycles: 30).
3. Final extension: 72°C for 5 min.

3.3. Initial Analysis of PCR Products

Prior to direct mutation analysis by sequencing, analyze 5 µL of each PCR product in a 4% agarose gel to ensure that all PCR reactions generated specific products (a single band) of the appropriate size and concentration. If a nonspecific PCR product is obtained, adjustment of the PCR conditions to increase specificity will be necessary. Often, the simplest way to increase the specificity is to increase the annealing temperature by a few degrees or by employing a "touchdown" method of annealing. Adjustments in the PCR reaction components, such as the buffer salt or magnesium concentration, can be employed to enhance specificity if desired. Approximation of the size and concentration of the PCR products can be easily done by comparing the migration distance of the band and the band intensity of the PCR product to a well-quantified, appropriately loaded, commercially available size standard marker designed to produce bands in the 100- to 1000-bp size range. Ideally, the PCR reaction should yield approx 10–30 ng/µL of a specific amplified product.

3.4. Sequence Analysis

The PCR sample generally must be purified prior to sequencing. This can be done through commercially available spin columns designed for purifying PCR products (Qiagen or Promega) or simply by treating 5 µL of the PCR product with 1 µL of exonuclease I (10 U/µL) and 2 µL of shrimp alkaline phosphatase (1 U/µL) for 15 min at 37°C. Stop the enzyme activity by incubating the sample at 80°C for 15 min. Use approx 10–20 ng per each 100 bp of product for sequencing. Follow the specific protocol for manual or automated sequencing in your laboratory. We routinely use the forward primer fused in the initial PCR reaction for sequencing.

3.5. Analysis of Results

Sequence chromatographs and or sequencing gel autoradiographs should be read very carefully to look for any base changes. Always read the sequence against a normal control sequence for comparison of peak height in chromatographs. For optimal analysis of manual sequencing autoradiographs, it is often helpful to run multiple samples against a normal control in which samples are grouped by the ddNTP. For instance, all "A" samples should be run next to one another, all "G" samples next to one another, and so on so that mutations are easy to identify visually. Any missense mutations should be checked against a database or published literature describing previously identified polymorphisms and mutations ***(3–7,24,25)***.

If an individual who has features of MEN1 is found to have a previously undescribed missense mutation that is not a known polymorphism, other family members, including parents, should be evaluated to determine whether it is seen in affected or unaffected individuals. If the missense mutation is not seen in unaffected parents of an affected individual, it is quite likely that it may be a new disease-causing mutation. Any mutations that have been reported previously as being associated with the disease are presumed to be disease-causing mutations. Mutations that alter splice sites or cause frameshifts and nonsense mutations are presumed to be disease causing mutations. Missense mutations that affect conserved amino acid residues or make a significant change in the polarity of the residue may be associated with disease in an affected individual especially if they are not found in unaffected parents. Missense mutations that cannot be identified as clear polymorphisms based on segregation with unaffected individuals in the pedigree or polymorphism database comparisons, or that cannot be presumed to be disease causing based on the aforementioned criteria, are not diagnostic. Once a mutation is found, confirm the mutation by restriction endonuclease digestion (if the mutation changes a restriction site) or reverse sequencing using the reverse primer. If a restriction site confirms the mutation, a simple restriction digest can be used for direct mutation DNA analysis in other family members (*see* **Note 5**).

3.6. Linkage-Based Diagnosis

When multiple family members are available and the clinical affection status can be clearly documented, linkage analysis may still be useful especially in cases in which no mutation is found by sequencing analysis. Flanking and intragenic primer sequences are readily available through the Genome Database. We routinely use primers from the following loci: *PYGM*, *DS11S913*, *D11S970*, *D11S971*, and *D11S987*. Although methods for diagnostic linkage studies are beyond the scope of this chapter, incorporating 0.2 μL of ^{32}P α-dCTP in the PCR reaction and running samples on a 5% polyacrylamide gel allow for clear visualization of genotypes after autoradiography. The methods for interpretation of linkage analysis are also beyond the scope of this chapter, but note that this type of testing is dependent on many variables that must be considered in the computer analysis of linkage, including the penetrance of the disorder for the ages of the individuals in the analysis and the prior probability that this family's disease is caused by a mutation in the *MEN1* gene. Inherent potential problems in linkage analysis include problems or errors in typing owing to nonpaternity, formation of new alleles, misclassification or diagnosis of affected individuals who may have a sporadic phenocopy of the disease, and misclassification of currently nonexpressing gene carriers as unaffected. Despite these problems, linkage remains quite useful for individuals in large kindreds with MEN1 in whom no specific mutation can be identified.

3.7. Benefits and Pitfalls of Diagnosis

The medical benefit of testing for MEN1 molecular genetic susceptibility for individuals at 50% risk in early diagnosis and treatment is sometimes accompanied by the fear that this information may be misused by providing a basis for discrimination against individuals who carry a predisposing mutation. However, given the availability of screening programs, medical management based on genetic predisposition, specific genetic counseling, provision of accurate recurrence risks, patient education, and referral to appropriate support resources for patients and their at-risk relatives, there are clear benefits for identifying individuals at highest risk for MEN1. There are no clear guidelines regarding at what age *MEN1* mutation testing is optimal. Because most young children do not develop symptoms of MEN1, it could be argued that testing could wait until an individual is old enough to make an informed, educated choice about having the test. Most medical screening programs for signs and symptoms of MEN1 do not begin until late adolescence or early adulthood. However, because some tumors can occur earlier, there may be benefits in testing children, but there are not yet well-defined guidelines for MEN1 screening in young pediatric populations.

3.8. Importance of Genetic Counseling

It is critically important to remember that genetic testing encompasses more than a simple laboratory analysis. It needs to include pretesting counseling and education; provision of informed consent; accurate interpretation of the test results and their implications; follow-up conveyance of test results; and posttesting education, management, and support. This is especially true when DNA-based testing is used to determine more accurately a healthy individual's genetic risk as in predictive testing of an asymptomatic individual who, by virtue of his or her family history, is at risk of having inherited MEN1 and seeks to learn whether or not he or she has indeed inherited a *MEN1* mutation.

4. Notes

1. Of the 166 mutations in *MEN1* entered in the Human Gene Mutation Database at the Institute of Medical Genetics in Cardiff, Wales (http://www.uwcm.ac.uk/uwcm/mg/hgmd0.html), 43% are single-base substitutions, either nonsense or missense. Small deletions, generally of 1–5 bp, occur in 34%, and small insertions (up to 15 bp) occur in 13%. Nucleotide substitutions that affect splicing occur in 6%. Large deletions, insertions, or duplications have been reported in <1% of cases reported to date, but this may be because the type of mutational analysis used is biased against finding large deletions and rearrangements. Thus, at present it seems that the vast majority of mutations are substitutions of a single nucleotide or small deletions or insertions of one or more base pairs. These muta-

tions have been found throughout the coding exons of the gene, and there is no one hot spot that accounts for the majority of mutations in nonfounder populations. To date, exon 2, the first coding exon and the second largest of the coding exons (exon 10 is the largest), has the highest number of mutations reported, but only 13% of the reported mutations fall in this exon, further highlighting the fact that mutations are scattered throughout the sequence.

2. A variety of strategies to find base pair substitutions and minute insertions and deletions to identify *MEN1* mutations has been described in the literature. Standard mutational analyses including SSCP analyses and heteroduplex analysis, bi-dideoxy fingerprinting, and direct manual and automated sequencing have been employed in our research laboratories with good results. These methods are well described in protocol manuals as well as in the primary scientific literature describing *MEN1* mutations ***(4,5,17,36–52)***. A combination of SSCP/heteroduplex analysis identifies approx 80–85% of *MEN1* mutations. Given the advances in technology and the increased sensitivity of direct sequencing, the use of direct sequencing, whether manual or automated, has been favored in our laboratories for both analysis of research and diagnostic samples. Thus, we propose here that direct sequencing of coding regions of the gene and intron/exon boundaries is the analysis of choice for relatively small genes such as *MEN1* in which mutations are scattered throughout the coding region. However, if rapid high-throughput sequencing is not available in the laboratory, a modified SSCP method can be used with the primers cited in **Table 1** and analyzed using autoradiography if 0.2 µL ^{32}P α-dCTP is added to the PCR reaction. Advances in microarray and microchip hybridization technology for analyzing sequences may become an optimal way for screening sequences at a much more rapid pace than current automated methods.
3. Several other primer pairs have been reported for use in *MEN1* mutation analysis ***(6,17,29)***. The primers reported here were specifically designed at the Yale University DNA Diagnostic Laboratory to allow running PCR reactions in two general PCR buffers with the majority of samples having the same annealing temperature. However, we have also used the other reported primers with success, including those listed through the National Institutes of Health Internet database (http://www.nhgri.nih.gov/DIR/LGT/MEN1/table1.html).
4. Because sequencing one strand of a PCR product is usually sufficient to detect mutations, we do not routinely use bidirectional sequencing because it has not been proven to be cost-effective in most cases. Our diagnostic sequencing is done using an ABI-373XL automated sequencer with which we routinely are able to read through the 700 bp of exon 10 and flanking splice sites. When using manual sequencing, bidirectional sequencing using both the forward and reverse primers of the two largest exons, exons 2 and 10, is necessary. By running samples on 5% long-range sequencing polyacrylamide gels at 55 W in which the sample runs for both 1.5 and 4.0 h by doing a second loading on the same gel, we are routinely able to read approx 400 bp of DNA, spanning each exon completely.
5. A useful Web site is Online Mendelian Inheritance in Man (OMIM) (http://www3.ncbi.nlm.nih.gov/omim/searchomim.html), a regularly updated database

of inherited disorders with information on clinical presentation, molecular basis, cytogenetics, mapping, and population genetics. OMIM also has direct links to the National Library of Medicine's MEDLINE database, DNA sequence databases, and the Genome Database. As stated in **Note 1**, the Human Gene Mutation Database at the Institute of Medical Genetics in Cardiff is a useful catalog of known mutations in *MEN1*. Published reports of known mutations and polymorphisms are also available *(3–7,24,25)*. The *GeneTests*™, a searchable database (http://www.genetests.org/), provides contact and test information regarding clinical and research laboratories worldwide that are doing molecular testing for MEN1. It is a password-protected (passwords are issued free of charge to health care professionals who register) database in which laboratories offering either clinical or research-based testing for any genetic disease, including MEN1, can list their services and contact information, making their services readily available to health care professionals. Contact and discussion with other diagnostic laboratories doing *MEN1* molecular testing may help provide additional useful new information for those individuals setting up *MEN1* testing in their own molecular genetic laboratories. Currently, five laboratories worldwide (including the Yale University DNA Diagnostic Laboratory) are listed as offering clinical testing, and three additional laboratories are listed as providing research-based testing.

References

1. Miller, J. A. and Norton, J. A. (1997) Multiple endocrine neoplasia. *Cancer Treat. Res.* **90,** 213–225.
2. Thakker, R. V. (1998) Multiple endocrine neoplasia—syndromes of the twentieth century. *J. Clin. Endocrinol. Metab.* **83,** 2617–2620.
3. Bassett, J. H., Forbes, S. A., Pannett, A. A., et al. (1998) Characterization of mutations in patients with multiple endocrine neoplasia type 1. *Am. J. Hum. Genet.* **62,** 232–244.
4. Agarwal, S. K., Kester, M. B., Debelenko, L. V., et al. (1997) Germline mutations of the MEN1 gene in familial multiple endocrine neoplasia type 1 and related states. *Hum. Mol. Genet.* **6,** 1169–1175.
5. Giraud, S., Zhang, C. X., Serova-Sinilnikova, O., et al. (1998) Germ-line mutation analysis in patients with multiple endocrine neoplasia type 1 and related disorders. *Am. J. Hum. Genet.* **63,** 455–467.
6. Sato, M., Matsubara, S., Miyauchi, A., Ohye, H., Imachi, H., Murao, K., and Takahara, J. (1998) Identification of five novel germline mutations of the MEN1 gene in Japanese multiple endocrine neoplasia type 1 (MEN1) families. *J. Med. Genet.* **35,** 915–919.
7. Teh, B. T., Kytola, S., Farnebo, F., et al. (1998) Mutation analysis of the MEN1 gene in multiple endocrine neoplasia type 1, familial acromegaly and familial isolated hyperparathyroidism. *J. Clin. Endocrinol. Metab.* **83,** 2621–2626.

8. Yu, F., Venzon, D. J., Serrano, J., Goebel, S. U., Doppman, J. L., Gibril, F., and Jensen, R.T. (1999) Prospective study of the clinical course, prognostic factors, causes of death, and survival in patients with long-standing Zollinger-Ellison syndrome. *J. Clin. Oncol.* **17,** 615–630.
9. Bystrom, C., Larsson, C., Blomberg, C., Sandelin, K., Falkmer, U., Skogseid, B., Oberg, K., Werner, S., and Nordenskjold, M. (1990) Localization of the MEN1 gene to a small region within chromosome 11q13 by deletion mapping in tumors. *Proc. Natl. Acad. Sci. USA* **87,** 1968–1972.
10. Bale, S. J., Bale, A. E., Stewart, K., Dachowski, L., McBride, O. W., Glaser, T., Green, J. E. III, Mulvihill, J. J., Brandi, M. L., and Sakaguchi, K. (1989) Linkage analysis of multiple endocrine neoplasia type 1 with INT2 and other markers on chromosome 11. *Genomics* **4,** 320–322 (published erratum appears in *Genomics* 1989;**5[1],** 166).
11. Courseaux, A., Grosgeorge, J., Gaudray, P., et al. (1996) Definition of the minimal MEN1 candidate area based on a 5-Mb integrated map of proximal 11q13. The European Consortium on Men1 (GENEM 1; Groupe d'Etude des Neoplasies Endocriniennes Multiples de type 1). *Genomics* **37,** 354–365.
12. Guru, S. C., Agarwal, S. K., Manickam, P., et al. (1997) A transcript map for the 2.8-Mb region containing the multiple endocrine neoplasia type 1 locus. *Genome Res.* **7,** 725–735.
13. Larsson, C., Skogseid, B., Oberg, K., Nakamura, Y., and Nordenskjold, M. (1988) Multiple endocrine neoplasia type 1 gene maps to chromosome 11 and is lost in insulinoma. *Nature* **332,** 85–87.
14. Lemmens, I., Merregaert, J., Van de Ven, W. J., et al. (1997) Construction of a 1.2-Mb sequence-ready contig of chromosome 11q13 encompassing the multiple endocrine neoplasia type 1 (MEN1) gene. The European Consortium on MEN1. *Genomics* **44,** 94–100.
15. Nakamura, Y., Larsson, C., Julier, C., Bystrom, C., Skogseid, B., Wells, S., Oberg, K., Carlson, M., Taggart, T., and O'Connell, P. (1989) Localization of the genetic defect in multiple endocrine neoplasia type 1 within a small region of chromosome 11. *Am. J. Hum. Genet.* **44,** 751–755.
16. Knudson, A. G. (1971) Mutation and cancer: statistical study of retinoblastoma. *Proc. Natl. Acad. Sci. USA* **68,** 820–823.
17. Chandrasekharappa, S. C., Guru, S. C., Manickam, P., et al. (1997) Positional cloning of the gene for multiple endocrine neoplasia-type 1. *Science* **276,** 404–407.
18. Guru, S. C., Goldsmith, P. K., Burns, A. L., Marx, S. J., Spiegel, A. M., Collins, F. S., and Chandrasekharappa, S. C. (1998) Menin, the product of the MEN1 gene, is a nuclear protein. *Proc. Natl. Acad. Sci. USA* **95,** 1630–1634.
19. Agarwal, S. K., Guru, S. C., Heppner, C., et al. (1999) Menin interacts with the AP1 transcription factor JunD and represses JunD-activated transcription. *Cell* **96,** 143–152.

20. Bear, J. C., Briones-Urbina, R., Fahey, J. F., and Farid, N. R. (1985) Variant multiple endocrine neoplasia I (MEN IBurin): further studies and non-linkage to HLA. *Hum. Hered.* **35,** 15–20.
21. Farid, N. R., Buehler, S., Russell, N. A., Maroun, F. B., Allerdice, P., and Smyth, H. S. (1980) Prolactinomas in familial multiple endocrine neoplasia syndrome type I: relationship to HLA and carcinoid tumors. *Amer. J. Med.* **69,** 874–880.
22. Petty, E. M., Green, J. S., Marx, S. J., Taggart, R. T., Farid, N., and Bale, A. E. (1994) Mapping the gene for hereditary hyperparathyroidism and prolactinoma (MEN1Burin) to chromosome 11q: evidence for a founder effect in patients from Newfoundland. *Am. J. Hum. Genet.* **54,** 1060–1066.
23. Olufemi, S. E., Green, J. S., Manickam, P., et al. (1998) Common ancestral mutation in the MEN1 gene is likely responsible for the prolactinoma variant of MEN1 (MEN1Burin) in four kindreds from Newfoundland. *Hum. Mutat.* **11,** 264–269.
24. Krawczak, M. and Cooper, D. N. (1997) The Human Gene Mutation Database. *Trends Genet.* **13,** 121–122.
25. Lemmens, I., Van de Ven, W. J., Kas, K., et al. (1997) Identification of the multiple endocrine neoplasia type 1 (MEN1) gene. The European Consortium on MEN1. *Hum. Mol. Genet.* **6,** 1177–1183.
26. Carling, T., Correa, P., Hessman, O., Hedberg, J., Skogseid, B., Lindberg, D., Rastad, J., Westin, G., and Akerstrom, G. (1998) Parathyroid MEN1 gene mutations in relation to clinical characteristics of nonfamilial primary hyperparathyroidism. *J. Clin. Endocrinol. Metab.* **83,** 2960–2963.
27. Debelenko, L. V., Brambilla, E., Agarwal, S. K., et al. (1997) Identification of MEN1 gene mutations in sporadic carcinoid tumors of the lung. *Hum. Mol. Genet.* **6,** 2285–2290.
28. Farnebo, F., Teh, B. T., Kytola, S., Svensson, A., Phelan, C., Sandelin, K., Thompson, N. W., Hoog, A., Weber, G., Farnebo, L.O., and Larsson, C. (1998) Alterations of the MEN1 gene in sporadic parathyroid tumors. *J. Clin. Endocrinol. Metab.* **83,** 2627–2630.
29. Görtz, B., Roth, J., Speel, E. J. M., Krähenmann, A., DeKrijger, R. R., Matias-Guiu, X., Muletta-Feurer, S., Rütmann, K., Saremaslani, P., Heitz, P. U., and Komminoth, P. (1999) *MEN1* gene mutation analysis of sporadic adrenocortical lesions. *Int. J. Cancer* **80,** 373–379.
30. Shou, W., Seol, J. H., Shevchenko, A., Baskerville, C., Moazed, D., Chen, Z. W. S., Jang, J., Shevchenko, A., Charbonneau, H., and Deshaies, R. J. (1999) Exit from mitosis is triggered by Tem1-dependent release of the protein phosphatase Cdc14 from nucleolar RENT complex. *Cell* **97,** 233–244.
31. Prezant, T. R., Levine, J., and Melmed, S. (1998) Molecular characterization of the men1 tumor suppressor gene in sporadic pituitary tumors. *J. Clin. Endocrinol. Metab.* **83,** 1388–1391.
32. Sawicki, M. P., Wan, Y. J., Johnson, C. L., Berenson, J., Gatti, R., and Passaro, E. Jr. (1992) Loss of heterozygosity on chromosome 11 in sporadic gastrinomas. *Hum. Genet.* **89,** 445–449.

33. Vortmeyer, A. O., Boni, R., Pak, E., Pack, S., and Zhuang, Z. (1998) Multiple endocrine neoplasia 1 gene alterations in MEN1-associated and sporadic lipomas. *J. Natl. Cancer Inst.* **90,** 398–399.
34. Teh, B. T., Esapa, C. T., Houlston, R., Grandell, U., Farnebo F., Nordenskjold, M., Pearce, C. J., Carmichael, D., Larsson, C., and Harris, P. E. (1998) A family with isolated hyperparathyroidism segregating a missense MEN1 mutation and showing loss of the wild-type alleles in the parathyroid tumors. *Am J. Hum. Genet.* **63,** 1544–1549.
35. Zhuang, Z., Ezzat, S. Z., Vortmeyer, A. O., et al. (1997) Mutations of the MEN1 tumor suppressor gene in pituitary tumors. *Cancer Res.* **57,** 5446–5451.
36. Korf, B. R. and Pagon, R. A. (1998) Overview of molecular genetic diagnosis (Unit 9.1), in *Current Protocols in Human Genetics* (Dracopoli N. C., Haines, J. L., Korf, B. R., et al., eds.), John Wiley & Sons, New York, pp. 9.1.1–9.1.9.
37. Smooker, P. M. and Cotton, R. G. (1993) The use of chemical reagents in the detection of DNA mutations. *Mutat. Res.* **288,** 65–77.
38. Bottema, C. D. and Sommer, S. S. (1993) PCR amplification of specific alleles: rapid detection of known mutations and polymorphisms. *Mutat. Res.* **288,** 93–102.
39. Hayashi, K. (1991) PCR-SSCP: a simple and sensitive method for detection of mutations in the genomic DNA. *PCR Methods Appl.* **1,** 34–38.
40. Loda, M. (1994) Polymerase chain reaction-based methods for the detection of mutations in oncogenes and tumor suppressor genes. *Human Pathol.* **25,** 564–571.
41. Sidransky, D. (1997) Nucleic acid-based methods for the detection of cancer. *Science* **278,** 1054–1058.
42. Liu, Q., Feng, J., and Sommer, S. S. (1996) Bi-directional dideoxy fingerprinting (Bi-ddF): a rapid method for quantitative detection of mutations in genomic regions of 300–600 bp. *Hum. Mol. Genet.* **5,** 107–114.
43. Ben-Ezra, J. (1995) Amplification methods in the molecular diagnosis of genetic diseases. *Clin. Lab. Med.* **15,** 795–815.
44. McPherson, R. (1995) Molecular basis of genetic disease and molecular methods. *Clin. Lab. Med.* **15,** 779–794.
45. Wagener, C., Epplen, J. T., Erlich, H., Peretz, H., and Vihko, P. (1994) Molecular biology techniques in the diagnosis of monogenic diseases. *Clin. Chim. Acta* **225,** S35–S50.
46. Grompe, M. (1993) The rapid detection of unknown mutations in nucleic acids. *Nat. Genet.* **5,** 111–117.
47. Blaszyk, H., Hartmann, A., Schroeder, J. J., McGovern, R. M., Sommer, S. S., and Kovach, J. S. (1995) Rapid and efficient screening for p53 gene mutations by dideoxy fingerprinting (ddF). *BioTech* **18,** 256–260.
48. Warren, W., Hovig, E., Smith-Sorensen, B., Borresen, A. L., Fujimura, F. K., Liu, Q., Feng, J., and Sommer, S. S. (1997) Detection of mutations by single-strand conformation polymorphism (SSCP) analysis and SSCP-hybrid methods (Unit 7.4), in *Current Protocols in Human Genetics* (Dracopoli, N. C., Haines, J. L., Korf, B. R., et al., eds.), John Wiley & Sons, New York, pp. 7.4.1–7.4.23.

49. Mashal, R. D., Koontz, J., and Sklar, J. (1995) Detection of mutations by cleavage of DNA heteroduplexes with bacteriophage resolvases. *Nat. Genet.* **9,** 177–183.
50. Sekiya, T. (1993) Detection of mutant sequences by single-strand conformation polymorphism analysis. *Mutat. Res.* **288,** 79–83.
51. Dracopoli, N., ed. (1994) *Current Protocols in Human Genetics*, John Wiley & Sons, New York.
52. Cotton, R.G. (1993) Current methods of mutation detection. *Mutat. Res.* **285,** 125–144.
53. Thierfelder, L. (1998) Mutation detection by cycle sequencing (Unit 7.7), in *Current Protocols in Human Genetics* (Dracopoli, N. C., Haines, J. L., Korf, B. R., et al., eds.), John Wiley & Sons, New York, pp. 7.7.1–7.7.6.
54. Shuldiner, A. R., LeRoith, D., and Roberts, C. T. (1995) DNA sequence analysis, in *Molecular Endocrinology: Basic Concepts and Clinical Correlations* (Weintraub, B. D., ed.), Raven Press, New York, pp. 13–21.

19

Molecular Detection of Multiple Endocrine Neoplasia Type 2

Edward H. Rowsell and Myra J. Wick

1. Introduction

1.1. Overview

Multiple endocrine neoplasia type 2 (MEN2) comprises three autosomal dominant disorders: MEN2A, familial medullary thyroid carcinoma (FMTC), and MEN2B. Clinical features common to both MEN2A and MEN2B include C-cell hyperplasia, medullary thyroid cancer (MTC), and pheochromocytoma. Other features of MEN2B are ocular and mucosal neuromas, gastrointestinal ganglioneuromatosis, and skeletal abnormalities. FMTC is characterized by MTC in the absence of parathyroid or adrenal disease.

Germline mutations within the RET proto-oncogene are definitively associated with MEN2A, FMTC, and MEN2B. RET encodes a member of the tyrosine kinase receptor family. The RET protein contains an extracellular cadherin-like domain, a cysteine-rich domain, a transmembrane domain, and two intracellular tyrosine kinase domains (**Fig. 1**). The RET-encoded protein is activated by interaction with the glial cell line-derived neurotropic factor GDFN/GDFN receptor-α complex *(1)*. This interaction results in RET dimerization, autophosphorylation, and phosphorylation of intracellular substrates.

Approximately 95% of MEN2A and 85% of FMTC patients have a germline point mutation within one of five cysteine residues in exon 10 (codons 609, 611, 618, and 620) or exon 11 (codon 634) of the RET gene. Rare noncysteine mutations have been identified in exons 11 (codon 631), 13 (codon 768), and 14 (codons 804 and 844) of patients with FMTC/MEN2A, each of these mutations accounts for <1% of MEN2A/FMTC families *(2)*. Recently, two addi-

From: *Methods in Molecular Medicine, vol. 49: Molecular Pathology Protocols*
Edited by: A. A. Killeen © Humana Press Inc., Totowa, NJ

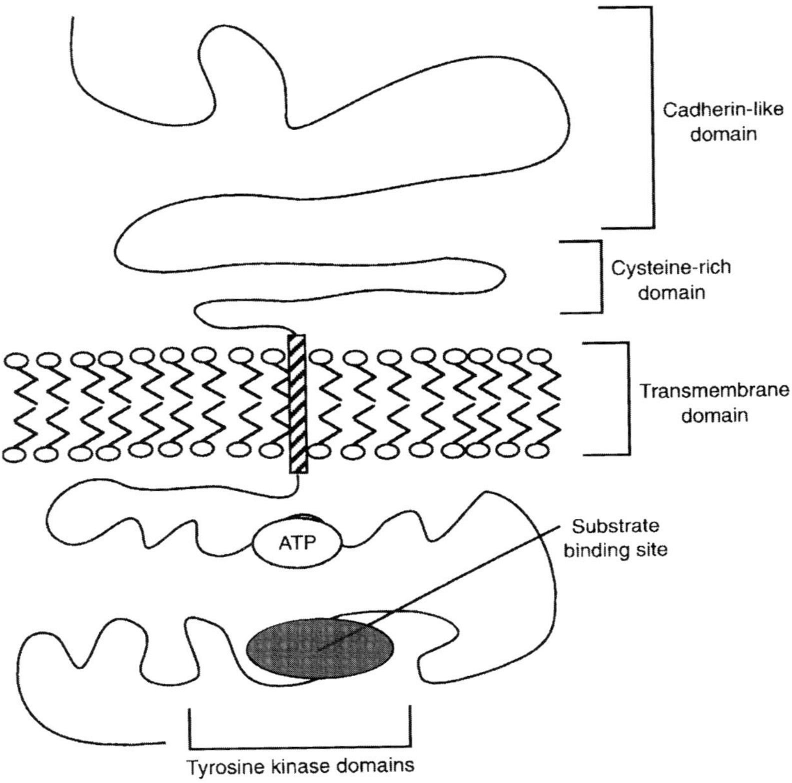

Fig. 1. The RET proto-oncogene–encoded tyrosine kinase. The protein contains extracellular cadherin-like and cysteine-rich domains, a transmembrane domain, and intracellular tyrosine kinase domains. ATP, adenosine triphosphate binding site.

tional germline mutations within codons 790 and 791 (exon 13) were identified in 1.6 and 1.1%, respectively, of German MEN2A/FMTC families ***(2)***. In contrast to the variety of mutations associated with MEN2A/FMTC, a single point mutation within exon 16 (codon 918, ATG→ACG) is detected in 95% of MEN2B patients. Current data indicate that these MEN2/FMTC-associated RET mutations are dominant gain-of-function mutations, resulting in increased kinase activity of the mutant RET-encoded protein ***(3)***.

The MEN literature includes numerous articles with guidelines for evaluation and testing of MEN2/FMTC family members as well as for patients presenting with apparently sporadic cases of MTC ***(4–6)***. The laboratory director should be aware of these guidelines to assist physicians who might be unfamiliar with the evaluation process. Therefore, we briefly summarize these guidelines here. For MEN2A/FMTC families, mutational analysis should initially be performed on an affected family member. Once the mutation has been identified, testing should be offered to at-risk family members. Molecular-based testing should be done at an early age, because thyroidectomy by age 6 is indicated in individuals carrying mutations ***(7)***. It is also recommended that all patients with apparent sporadic MTC be screened for MEN2A/FMTC mutations, because approx 24% of such cases will demonstrate a germline RET mutation ***(8)***. Phenotypic features of MEN2B usually enable the clinician to make an accurate diagnosis in the absence of molecular testing. However, molecular-based testing is useful for individuals who lack some of the phenotypic features of MEN2B, or in very young children who are presymptomatic ***(3)***. Also note that although *de novo* MEN2A/FMTC-associated mutations are rare, as many as 50% of MEN2B cases are the result of *de novo* germline mutations in codon 918 ***(9)***.

1.2. Choice of Methods

A variety of methods have been developed for the molecular diagnosis of MEN2A/FMTC in the clinical molecular genetics laboratory, including sequencing, denaturing gradient gel electrophoresis ***(10)***, single-strand conformation polymorphism (SSCP) analysis ***(11,12)***, heteroduplex (HET) formation ***(13,14)***, and restriction enzyme (RE) analysis ***(14,15)***. Included in this chapter are protocols for manual sequencing of exons 10 and 11; SSCP analysis of exons 10 and 11; HET analysis for mutations in exons 10, 11, and 13; and RE analysis for the codon 918 mutation associated with MEN2B.

Each of the methods for MEN2A/FMTC mutation detection has inherent advantages and disadvantages. Sequencing allows for definitive identification of the mutation, without the need for additional confirmatory testing. The sequencing protocol described herein, however, is relatively time- and labor-intensive (compared to screening methods such as HET) and involves the use of radioisotopes. Adaptation of this sequencing protocol to a semiautomated system such as the Li-Cor Model 4200 or PE Applied Biosystems Model 377 system would increase efficiency and eliminate the use of radioisotopes. Sequencing of exons 10 and 11 results in a detection rate of approx 95% of MEN2A patients and 85% of FMTC families.

The SSCP protocol described herein has the advantage of utilizing a kit and SSCP equipment, both of which can be purchased from Pharmacia Biotech, Piscataway, NJ. The kit includes premade SSCP gels and the silver staining reagents. This SSCP protocol was reported to detect 20 of 21 different mutations that represent approx 90% of known exon 10 and 11 mutations ***(12)***.

The HET protocol ***(14)*** utilizes a modified Mutation Detection Enhancement matrix enabling efficient screening for MEN mutations without the use of radioisotopes. Although this method simultaneously detects at least 16 different RET mutations, the specific mutation must be confirmed by RE analysis or sequencing (in cases in which a mutation has previously been identified in a family member, HET analysis alone is adequate). HET analysis of exons 10, 11, and 13 results in detection rates of 95% and slightly greater than 85% for MEN2A and FMTC patients, respectively.

2. Materials

2.1. Samples

Peripheral blood is the sample type most frequently submitted for molecular genetic analysis of RET mutations, although other specimen types containing nucleated cells may also be used (e.g., buccal swabs, amniocytes, cord blood). It is preferable that peripheral blood be collected in tubes containing EDTA or acid citrate dextrose as the anticoagulant.

The Puregene® DNA Isolation Kit (nos. D-5500, D-5500A, and D-7000A; Gentra Systems, Minneapolis, MN) allows rapid isolation of high-quality genomic DNA from whole blood, cultured cells, and tissue, respectively. It is based on published salting-out procedures, thus eliminating the use of toxic organic solvents.

2.2. Reagents and Equipment for Sequencing (MEN2A)

1. Purified specimen DNA in water or 1X TE buffer (pH 8.0) at 250 µg/mL.
2. Gene Amplification Kit (no. N801-0043; PE Applied Biosystems, Foster City, CA) containing 5 U/µL of AmpliTaq® *Taq* DNA polymerase; 10 m*M* dATP, dCTP, dGTP, and dTTP; and GeneAmp® 10X PCR Buffer (500 m*M* KCl, 100 m*M* Tris-HCl, pH 8.3, 15 m*M* $MgCl_2$, and 0.01% [w/v] gelatin, in a volume of 1.5 mL).
3. 5X reaction buffer with dNTPs. This buffer is made in-house as follows: 100 µL of dATP (10 m*M*), 100 µL of dCTP (10 m*M*), 100 µL of dGTP (10 m*M*), 100 µL of dTTP (10 m*M*), 100 µL of sterile water, and 500 µL of GeneAmp 10X PCR Buffer total volume of 1000 µL). The 5X buffer can be stored at –70°C for up to 6 mo. Thus, it is convenient to make batches of the 5X buffer and to store them as 1-mL aliquots.
4. Previously prepared primers stored (–70°C) at a concentration of 20 µ*M*. Refer to **Table 1** for primer sequences.
5. High-Strength Analytical Grade Agarose (no. 162-0125; Bio-Rad, Hercules, CA).
6. NuSieve® GTG® Agarose (no. 50081; FMC BioProducts, Rockland, ME).
7. TAE buffer, prepared as 50X TAE (2 *M* Tris-acetate, 50 m*M* EDTA): 968.0 g of Tris base, 228.4 g of glacial acetic acid, 400.0 mL of 0.5 *M* EDTA, pH 8.0. Dilute to 4 L with sterile water. The 50X buffer is stable at room temperature for 3 mo. Dilute the appropriate quantity of 50X buffer with sterile water to 1X before use.

Table 1
RET Oligonucleotide PCR Primers

Sequencing analysis	
Locus-specific amplification: ~1000-bp amplicon (amplicon contains exons 10 and 11)	
Forward (RET A2, 21mer):	5′-CAA CAT TTG CCC TCA GGA CTG-3′
Reverse (CRT 19A, 20mer):	5′-CTT GAA GGC ATC CAC GGA GA-3′
Sequencing	
Exon 10 (RET D, 22mer):	5′-TTG GGA CCT CAG ATG TGC TGT T-3′
Exon 11 (CRT 19B, 19mer):	5′-GCA TAC GCA GCC TGT ACC C-3′
HET analysis	
Exon 10: 232-bp amplicon	
Forward (RET I, 19mer):	5′-CGC CCC AGG AGG CTG AGT G-3′
Reverse (RET I, 22mer):	5′-TTG GGA CCT CAG ATG TGC TGT T-3′
Exon 11: 150-bp amplicon	
Forward (CRT 19B, 19mer):	5′-GCA TAC GCA GCC TGT ACC C-3′
Reverse (CRT 2C, 20mer):	5′-GAC AGC AGC ACC GAG ACG AT-3′
Exon 13: 296-bp amplicon	
Forward (CRT 4F, 22mer):	5′-GCA GGC CTC TCT GTC TGA ACT T-3′
Reverse (CRT 4E, 20mer):	5′-GGA GAA CAG GGC TGT ATG GA-3′
SSCP analysis	
Exon 10	
Forward (21mer):	5′-GGG GCA GCA TTG TTG GGG GAC-3′
Reverse (19mer):	5′-CGT GGT GGT CCC GGC CGC C-3′
Exon 11	
Forward (20mer):	5′-CCT CTG CGG TGC CAA GCC TC-3′
Reverse (21mer):	5′-GAA GAG GAC AGC GGC TGC GAT-3′
RFLP analysis	
Exon 16: 195-bp amplicon	
Forward (Ret 16F, 20mer):	5′-AGG GAT AGG GCC TGG GCT TC-3′
Reverse (Ret 16R, 20mer):	5′-TAA CCT CCA CCC CAA GAG AG-3′

8. 6X Sample buffer for agarose gel electrophoresis: 0.125 g of bromophenol blue, 7.5 g of Ficoll® 400 (no. 17-0400-01; Pharmacia Biotech), in sufficient quantity to 50 mL in deionized, distilled water. This buffer is stable for 1 yr at room temperature.
9. Ethidium bromide (EtBr).
10. pGEM® DNA markers (no. G1741; Promega, Madison, WI).
11. Exonuclease I (10 U/mL) (no. E 70073Z; Amersham, Arlington Heights, IL).
12. Shrimp Alkaline Phosphatase (no. E 70092Y; Amersham).
13. ThermoSequenase™ cycle sequencing kit (no. US 78500; Amersham). The kit includes ^{33}P-radiolabeled terminators.
14. 40% Acrylamide/*bis*-acrylamide solution (19:1) (no. 161-0144; Bio-Rad).

15. TBE buffer (5X stock): 216.0 g of Tris base, 110.0 g of boric acid, 80.0 mL of 0.5 *M* EDTA, pH 8.0. Add deionized water to a final volume of 4 L. The 5X stock is stable at room temperature for 1 yr. Dilute the appropriate quantity of 5X buffer to 1 L with deionized water before use.
16. 6% Polyacrylamide/7 *M* urea gel mix (for sequencing gels): 150 mL of 40% acrylamide/bis stock, 200 mL of 5X TBE stock, 420 g of urea. Add water to a total volume of 1 L, and degas under vacuum when freshly made. Store refrigerated in the dark for up to 6 mo.
17. Urea.
18. TEMED.
19. Ammonium persulfate (APS), prepared as a 10% (w/v) solution: 0.1 g of APS diluted to a final volume of 1.0 mL. This may be stored in the refrigerator for 1 wk.
20. Sequencing gel-loading buffer: 45% formamide, 20 m*M* EDTA, 0.05% bromophenol blue, 0.05% xylene cyanol. Bring to a final volume of 10 mL with deionized water.
21. Camera and Polaroid® Polapan® 667 film (Polaroid, Cambridge, MA).
22. Kodak X-Omat AR5 X-ray film (35 × 43 cm) (no. 165 1512; Eastman Kodak Co., Rochester, NY).
23. Thermocycler and polymerase chain reaction (PCR) tubes (*see* **Note 1**).
24. Submarine gel electrophoresis system such as the Bio-Rad Wide Mini-Sub Cell GT System (no. 170-4405).
25. Sequencing gel apparatus with required accessories (plates, spacers, sharkstooth combs, clamps). The sequencing described in this protocol was performed with a Gibco-BRL Model S2 Sequencing Gel Electrophoresis Apparatus (no. 21105-010; Life Technologies, Gaithersburg, MD).
26. Electrophoresis power supplies for submarine gel electrophoresis and sequencing gel electrophoresis.
27. UV transilluminator.
28. Gel dryer, such as Bio-Rad Model 583 Gel Dryer (no. 165 1745).

2.3. Reagents and Equipment for HET Analysis (MEN2A and FMTC)

1. Purified specimen DNA in water or 1X TE buffer (pH 8.0) at 250 µg/mL.
2. *Taq* DNA Polymerase in Storage Buffer A Kit (nos. M2861–M2868; Promega) including *Taq* DNA polymerase (5 U/µL) and 10X Reaction Buffer A with 15 m*M* $MgCl_2$ (500 m*M* KCl; 100 m*M* Tris-HCl, pH 9.0, at 25°C; 1.0% Triton X-100; and 15 m*M* $MgCl_2$).
3. Bulk dNTPs (no. U1330; Promega) containing 100 m*M* dATP, dCTP, dGTP, and dTTP each in water at pH 7.5.
4. 5X Reaction Buffer A with dNTPs. This buffer is made in the lab as follows: 12.5 µL of 100 m*M* bulk dNTPs, 487.5 µL of sterile water, and 500.0 µL of 10X Reaction Buffer A (total volume of 1000 µL). The 5X buffer may be stored at –70°C for up to 6 mo. Thus, it is convenient to make batches of the 5X buffer and store them as 1-mL aliquots.

5. Working primers (10 μ*M*) prepared in water from 100 μ*M* stock primer solutions and stored at –70°C. Refer to **Table 1** for primer sequences.
6. 0.5 *M* EDTA (pH 8.0).
7. MDE™ gel-loading buffer (50% [w/v] sucrose, 0.6% [w/v] bromophenol blue, 0.6% [w/v] xylene cyanol in 1X TE buffer, pH 8.0): Dissolve 25.0 g of sucrose, 0.3 g of bromophenol blue, 0.3 g of xylene cyanol, and 5 mL of 10X TE buffer (pH 8.0) in about 30 mL of deionized water. Dilute with deionized water to a 50-mL final volume. This buffer is stable for 1 yr at room temperature.
8. pGEM DNA markers (no. G1741; Promega).
9. MDE™ gel solution (2X concentrate) (no. 50620; FMC BioProducts).
10. 10X TBE stock solution: 216.0 g of Tris base, 110.0 g of boric acid, 80.0 mL of 0.5 *M* EDTA (pH 8.0). Add deionized water to a final volume of 2.0 L. The 10X stock is stable at room temperature for 1 yr.
11. Urea.
12. Formamide.
13. TEMED.
14. APS, prepared as a 10% (w/v) solution: 0.1 g of APS diluted to a final volume of 1.0 mL. Prepare fresh each time.
15. Ethidium bromide.
16. Camera and Polaroid Polapan 667 film.
17. Thermocycler and PCR reaction tubes.
18. Heating block.
19. Gel electrophoresis apparatus with accessories, including spacer sets, combs, and glass plates. A power supply is also required.
20. UV transilluminator box.

2.4. Reagents and Equipment for SSCP Analysis

1. Purified specimen genomic DNA in water or 1X TE buffer at 10 μg/mL.
2. 5X Reaction Buffer N from PCR Optimization Kit (no. K1220-01; Invitrogen, San Diego, CA).
3. GeneAmp® dNTP mix (no. N808-0007; PE Applied Biosystems) including 10 m*M* each of dATP, dCTP, dGTP, and dTTP.
4. AmpliTaq *Taq* DNA polymerase (5 U/μL) (no. N801-0060; PE Applied Biosystems).
5. Working primers (10 μ*M*) prepared in water from 100 μ*M* stock primer solutions and stored at –70°C. Refer to **Table 1** for primer sequences.
6. Thermocycler and PCR reaction tubes.
7. Heating block.
8. PhastSystem™ gel electrophoresis system (no. 18-1018-23; Pharmacia Biotech), consisting of the Separation and Control Unit (electrophoresis chambers, power supply, microprocessor) and the Development Unit.
9. PhastGel™ sample applicators: either 6/4 (6 samples, 4 μL each) or 8/1 (8 samples, 1 μL each) (nos. 18-0012-29 and 18-1618-01, respectively; Pharmacia Biotech).

10. PhastGel™ Homogeneous 20: native 20% polyacrylamide gel media (no. 17-0624-01; Pharmacia Biotech).
11. PhastGel™ native buffer strips (no. 17-0517-01; Pharmacia Biotech).
12. PhastGel™ Silver Kit gel-staining kit (no. 17-0617-01; Pharmacia Biotech).

2.5. Reagents and Equipment for MEN2B Analysis (PCR and RE Digestion)

1. Purified specimen genomic DNA in water or 1X TE buffer at 10 µg/mL.
2. Gene Amplification Kit (no. N801-0043; PE Applied Biosystems) containing 5 U/µL *Taq* DNA polymerase; 10 m*M* dATP, dCTP, dGTP, and dTTP; and GeneAmp 10X PCR Buffer (500 m*M* KCl, 100 m*M* Tris-HCl, pH 8.3, 15 m*M* $MgCl_2$ and 0.01% [w/v] gelatin, in a volume of 1.5 mL).
3. 5X Reaction buffer with dNTPs. This buffer is made in-house as follows: 100 µL of dATP, 100 µL of dCTP, 100 µL of dGTP, 100 µL of dTTP, 100 µL of sterile water, and 500 µL of GeneAmp 10X PCR Buffer (total volume of 1000 µL). The 5X buffer may be stored at –70°C for up to 6 mo. Thus, it is convenient to make batches of the 5X buffer and store them as 1-mL aliquots.
4. Previously prepared primers stored (–70°C) at a concentration of 20 µ*M*. Refer to **Table 1** for primer sequences.
5. *Fok*I and NEB Buffer 4 (no. 109; New England Biolabs, Beverly, MA).
6. High-Strength Analytical Grade Agarose (no. 162-0125; Bio-Rad).
7. NuSieve GTG Agarose (no. 50081; FMC BioProducts).
8. TAE buffer, prepared as 50X TAE (2 *M* Tris acetate, 50 m*M* EDTA): 968.0 g of Tris base, 228.4 g of glacial acetic acid, 400.0 mL of 0.5 *M* EDTA, pH 8.0. Dilute to 4 L with sterile water. The 50X buffer is stable at room temperature for 3 mo. Dilute the appropriate quantity of 50X buffer with sterile water to 1X before use.
9. 6X Sample buffer for agarose gel electrophoresis: 0.125 g of bromophenol blue, 7.5 g of Ficoll 400 (no. 17-0400-01; Pharmacia Biotech), in sufficient quantity to 50 mL in deionized, distilled water. This buffer is stable for 1 yr at room temperature.
10. EtBr.
11. Camera and Polaroid Polapan 667 film.
12. Thermocycler and PCR reaction tubes (*see* **Note 1**).
13. Submarine gel electrophoresis system such as Bio-Rad Wide Mini-Sub Cell GT System (no. 170-4405).
14. Electrophoresis power supplies for submarine gel electrophoresis.
15. UV transilluminator.

3. Methods

3.1. Sequencing of RET Exons 10 and 11

3.1.1. PCR Amplification of Exons 10 and 11

1. Label PCR reaction tubes for patient specimens, positive controls, and the no-DNA control.
2. Prepare the PCR reaction master mix. It is advisable to prepare a slight excess of master mix to allow for pipetting error. Typically, allowing for a 10% error is

Table 2
PCR Master Mix for PCR Amplification of RET Exons 10 and 11

	Volume/sample (does not include pipetting error) (μL)	Volume/10 samples (includes 10% pipetting error) (μL)
Sterile water	17.75	195.25
5X PCR buffer	5.00	55
Forward primer RET A2	0.5	5.5
Reverse primer CRT 19A	0.5	5.5
Taq DNA polymerase (5 U/μL)	0.25	2.75
Total volume	24.0	264.0

adequate (e.g., the total master mix volume prepared for 10 samples [24 μL of master mix/sample] would be 264 μL rather than 240 μL) (*see* **Table 2**). All reagents should be kept on ice. Mix gently and aliquot 24 μL of the master mix into each of the PCR reaction tubes.

3. Using a clean pipet tip for each specimen, aliquot 1 μL of DNA (at a concentration of 250 μg/mL) into the appropriate PCR reaction tube. Thermocycling reaction conditions are as follows: an initial denaturation step for 2 min at 95°C; and an amplification step consisting of 30 cycles of denaturation for 30 s at 94°C, annealing for 30 s at 65°C, extension for 30 s at 72°C and a final extension step for 10 min at 72°C. After PCR amplification, samples may be stored indefinitely at 5°C.
4. PCR products are detected by agarose gel electrophoresis. Run samples on either a 20 × 14 cm or 20 × 20 cm 2% agarose gel (1% agarose/1% NuSieve). Prepare the gel by mixing 1.2 g each of agarose and NuSieve with 300 mL of 1X TAE. Heat the resulting slurry in a microwave until the agarose is dissolved. Cool to approx 50°C (just cool enough to touch), and add 30 μL of EtBr.
5. Pour the agarose into the gel mold. Use a comb to form the appropriate number of sample wells.
6. To prepare the samples for electrophoresis, combine 2 μL of 6X sample buffer and 10 μL of PCR product in a microcentrifuge tube. Load approx 10 μL of each sample (including the positive control, the no-DNA control, and the pGEM ladder) into the gel. Run the gel for 2 h at 90 V.
7. Following electrophoresis, take a Polaroid picture of the gel by placing the gel on the UV transilluminator. Use the camera setting of f8 at 1 s. The template size is approx 997 bp.

3.1.2. Sequencing of Exons 10 and 11

Refer to **Fig. 2** for a diagram of the protocol.

1. Prepare the DNA template in a microcentrifuge tube by mixing 5 μL of each PCR product with 1 μL of Exonuclease I (10 U/mL) and 1 μL of shrimp alkaline phos-

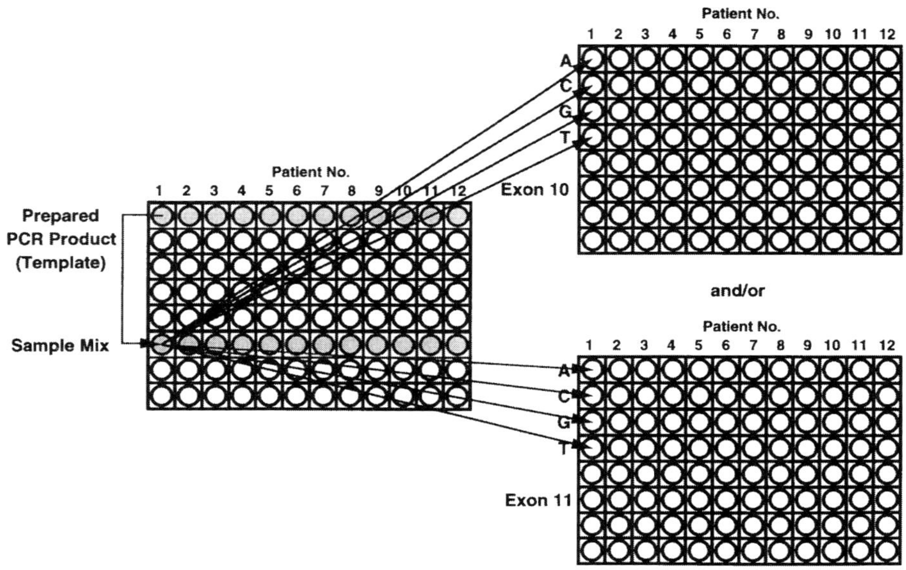

Fig. 2. Diagram of the MEN2A sequencing protocol. (**Left**) Preparation of a sample mix (*see* **Subheading 3.1.2., step 4c**) for each patient by mixing the prepared DNA template *see* **Subheading 3.1.2., step 1**) with the sequencing master mix (*see* **Subheading 3.1.2, step 3**); (**Right**) Aliquoting of the patient sample mix into each of the individual sequencing reactions (A, C, G, T) for exons 10 and 11 of the RET gene (*see* **Subheading 3.1.2., step 4d**).

phatase. Incubate the mixture at 37°C for 15 min, and then heat the sample to 80°C for 15 min. Store the samples at 4°C or on ice until the remainder of the sequencing reagents are prepared.

2. Prepare batches of each of the four termination mixes (α-^{33}P-ddATP mix, α-^{33}P-ddCTP mix, α-^{33}P-ddGTP mix, and α-^{33}P-ddTTP mix) by mixing 2 µL of dGTP nucleotide master mix (from the Amersham kit) with 0.5 µL of each of the four α-^{33}P-ddNTPs. Each individual sequencing reaction requires 2.5 µL of the termination mix. Thus, it is more convenient to prepare enough of each of the four termination mixes for the entire sequencing run. Termination mixes should be prepared on ice.
3. Prepare a sequencing master mix for each sequencing reaction with the following reagents (all volumes in microliters/reaction). As with the PCR master mix, it is advisable to prepare a 10% excess of sequencing master mix; the volumes given do not include the 10% pipetting error volume. Prepare the reactions on ice. Add the ThermoSequenase last: 12.8 µL of sterile water, 2.0 µL of reaction buffer, 0.2 µL of sequencing primer—Ret D or CRT 19B (20 µ*M*), 2.0 µL of ThermoSequenase DNA polymerase (total volume of 17.0 µL/reaction).

4. Prepare the sequencing reactions on ice as follows:
   a. For each specimen (including the positive control) and for each exon to be sequenced, label four PCR tubes with the specimen number (or identifier) and either A, C, G, or T.
   b. Add 2.5 µL of the appropriate d/ddNTP termination mix (*see* **step 2**) to the appropriate tube.
   c. Prepare a sample mix for each patient specimen (and the positive control) by placing 3 µL of treated template (*see* **step 1**) into a microcentrifuge tube labeled with the patient identifier. Then add 17 µL of the sequencing master mix (*see* **step 3**) to each tube to create a sample mix. Vortex gently and spin briefly in the microcentrifuge.
   d. Add 4.5 µL of each sample mix (*see* **step 3**) to the appropriate A-, C-, G-, and T-labeled tubes. Mix by repeatedly pipetting up and down.
5. Thermocycling conditions for the cycle sequencing reactions (both exons 10 and 11) are as follows (do not place samples into the thermocycler until the machine has reached 95°C): an initial denaturation step for 2 min at 95°C; an amplification step consisting of 30 cycles of denaturation for 30 s at 94°C and annealing and extension for 30 s at 70°C; there is no final extension. After thermocycling, the reactions should be stored at –20°C.
6. Prepare the sequencing gel plates and apparatus as recommended by the manufacturer.
7. Prepare the acrylamide gel mixture by mixing 60 mL of 6% polyacrylamide (at room temperature) with 0.6 mL of 10% APS and 10.2 µL of TEMED. The APS and TEMED should be added immediately prior to pouring the gel; a plastic bottle with a nozzle works well for mixing and pouring the gel. The manufacturer of the gel apparatus should provide instructions for pouring the gel. The gel should polymerize within 1 h.
8. Conduct gel electrophoresis of sequencing reaction products as follows:
   a. Prepare the samples for gel analysis by diluting 7 µL of each sample with 4 µL of loading buffer; mix by pipetting up and down.
   b. Heat the samples in the thermocycler for 2 min at 72°C. Quickly cool the samples in an ice/water slurry and keep them on ice until ready for loading. Load the gel within 1 h of heating the samples.
   c. It is important to flush the urea from the wells before loading the specimens. Load 4 µL of each specimen into each well. To detect mutations more easily, load all of the A reactions in adjacent wells, followed by all C reactions, all G reactions, and all T reactions (**Fig. 3**).
   d. Run the gel at 70 W for approx 100 min (about 15 min after the bromophenol blue dye runs off the end of the gel).
   e. Transfer the gel to blotting paper. Dry the gel on the gel dryer for 1 h.
   f. Place the gel in an X-ray cassette, expose an X-ray film overnight at room temperature, and develop the film.

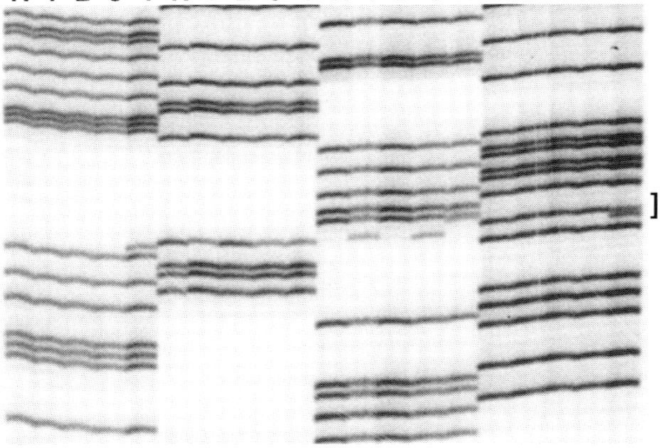

Fig. 3. Sequencing analysis of MEN2A. PCR amplification and sequencing of exon 10 demonstrates mutations in codon 618. (Note that exon 10 was sequenced in the reverse direction from 3′→5′. The base designations have been modified to reflect the sequence of the sense strand.) Lanes N and 2, a normal control and a normal patient, respectively; lanes 1 and 3, the codon 618 TGC→AGC mutation; lane 4, the codon 618 TGC→CGC mutation. The "extra" band in lane C4 (denoted by the bracket on the right of the gel) is a sequencing artifact; it is thought to arise from mutation-induced secondary structural changes in the DNA. (**Figure 3** was provided by S. Thibodeau.)

3.1.3. Interpretation of Results

Mutations within exon 10 of the RET gene will appear as new bands on the sequencing gel at codon 609, 611, 618, or 620; mutations within exon 11 will appear as new bands at codon 634. Because patients are heterozygous for the mutation, the intensity of the corresponding normal band will be decreased (**Fig. 3**).

3.2. Heteroduplex Analysis of RET Exons 10, 11, and 13

3.2.1. PCR Amplification of Exons 10, 11, and 13

1. Set up the appropriate number of PCR reaction tubes, including a positive control for each RET exon being analyzed, a negative control, and a blank (no DNA) control.
2. Prepare a PCR master mix containing the following (in microliters per tube): 78.5 μL of sterile water, 20.0 μL of 5X PCR Reaction Buffer with dNTPs, 0.5 μL of exon 10/11/13 forward primer, 0.5 μL of exon 10/11/13 reverse primer, 0.5 μL of *Taq* DNA polymerase (total master mix volume per tube of 99.5 μL). It is

advisable to prepare a slight excess of master mix to allow for pipetting error. Typically, allowing for a 10% error is adequate (e.g., if there are 10 samples, prepare adequate master mix for 11). All reagents should be kept on ice. Mix gently and aliquot 99.5 µL of the master mix into each PCR reaction tube.

3. Using a clean pipet tip for each specimen, aliquot 0.5 µL of patient, positive control, and negative control template DNA (at a concentration of 250 µg/mL) into the appropriate separate PCR reaction tubes. Aliquot 0.5 µL of sterile water instead of template DNA into the blank tube.
4. Thermocycling reaction conditions are as follows: an initial denaturation step for 5 min at 94°C; an amplification step consisting of 35 cycles of denaturation for 1 min at 94°C, annealing for 1 min at 56°C, extension for 2 min at 72°C, and a final extension step for 10 min at 72°C.
5. After PCR amplification, add 1 µL of 0.5 *M* EDTA (pH 8 0) to each tube to inactivate the *Taq* DNA polymerase. PCR products may be stored indefinitely at 5°C.

3.2.2. MDET Gel Electrophoresis of PCR Products

1. Prepare and pour the 1.2X MDET gel as follows:
   a. MDE gel solution is supplied as a 2X concentrate. A 40 cm × 20 cm × 1 mm gel requires about 80 mL of 1.2X gel solution. Prepare the correct amount for your plates by adjusting each of the following components proportionally: 60 mL of MDE gel solution (2X), 6 mL of 10X TBE, 15 g of urea, 15 mL of formamide, 100 mL of deionized water (fill to), 40 µL of TEMED, 400 µL of 10% APS (prepared fresh).
   b. Mix the first five components in a clean beaker by gently swirling.
   c. After the urea has dissolved, filter the solution through Whatman No. 1 filter paper.
   d. Add the specified amounts of TEMED and fresh 10% APS; mix the solution by gently swirling.
   e. Pour the gel solution into the plates using the standard procedure for acrylamide. Insert a comb. Allow the gel to polymerize for at least 60 min at room temperature.
2. Enhance heteroduplex formation by denaturing the PCR products for 5 min at 94°C and then annealing for 30 min at room temperature.
3. Mix 5 µL of PCR product with 1 µL of MDE gel loading buffer in a microcentrifuge tube. Load the PCR product/buffer mixture onto the 1.2X MDE gel.
4. Run the gel at 20 V/cm for 35,000 V-h (the power supply should be set at 800 V and run 43.75 h for a 40-cm plate).
5. After the run is completed, remove one of the glass plates. Leave the gel attached to the other plate to ease handling during the staining and destaining steps.
6. Stain the gel for 10–15 min at room temperature in 1 µg/mL of EtBr solution (made in 0.6X TBE buffer) (*see* **Note 3**). Adjust the staining, destaining, and photography steps as necessary to achieve the desired results.

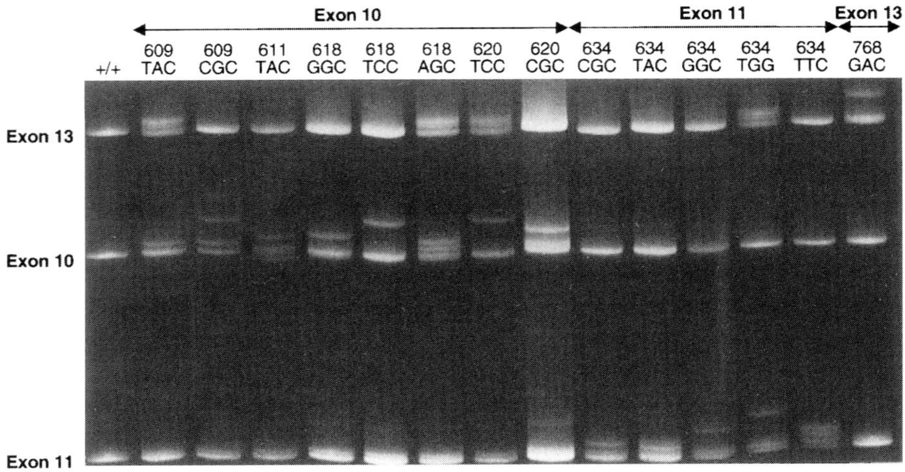

Fig. 4. HET analysis of MEN2A by multiplex PCR amplification of RET proto-oncogene exons 10, 11, and 13. Normal individuals (+/+) have single homoduplex bands for all three exons. Additional bands represent chimeric HETs generated by the presence of MEN2A-, MTC-, and FMTC-associated mutations in exons 10, 11, and 13. A normal polymorphism in exon 13 is present in a number of individuals. Mutations are indicated by codon number and altered nucleotide sequence. (Reprinted from **ref.** ***14*** with permission by John Wiley & Sons, Inc. © 1996 Wiley-Liss, Inc.)

7. Destain the gel for 15–20 min in 0.6X TBE buffer. Destaining for up to an hour may be necessary to eliminate background fluorescence, which may obscure faint bands.
8. Invert the plate (gel side down) on a UV transilluminator to visualize the DNA bands. (For easier handling, cut out the area of the gel containing the DNA bands of interest, and then place the gel onto the UV transilluminator.)
9. Photograph the gel using Polaroid Polapan 667 film.

3.2.3. Interpretation of Results

The HET control DNA lane should contain two bands: a slower moving HET DNA band and a faster moving homoduplex band (HET bands often run as a single band) (**Fig. 4**). Homozygous normal or mutant samples are expected to migrate as a single band (homoduplex). Depending on the mutation, the PCR products of heterozygous DNA will form up to four bands: mutant/mutant, normal/normal homoduplexes, plus two mutant/normal HETs. When using EtBr staining, bands may appear broader because this staining technique requires more DNA to be loaded onto the gel.

3.3. SSCP Analysis of RET Exons 10, 11, and 13

3.3.1. PCR Amplification of Exons 10 and 11

1. Set up the appropriate number of PCR reaction tubes, including a positive control for each RET exon being analyzed, a negative control, and a blank (no DNA) control.
2. Prepare a PCR master mix containing the following (in microliters per tube): 11.25 μL of sterile water, 5.00 μL of 5X Reaction Buffer N, 2.00 μL of dNTPs, 0.625 μL of exon 10/11 forward primer, 0.625 μL of exon 10/11 reverse primer, 0.50 μL of AmpliTaq DNA polymerase (total master mix volume per tube of 20.00 μL). *Do not* add the template DNA at this time. It is advisable to prepare a slight excess of master mix to allow for pipetting error. Typically, allowing for a 10% error is adequate (e.g., if there are 10 samples, prepare adequate master mix for 11). All reagents should be kept on ice. Mix gently and aliquot 20 μL of the master mix into each of the PCR reaction tubes.
3. Using a clean pipet tip for each specimen, aliquot 5 μL of patient, positive control, and negative control template DNA (at a concentration of 250 μg/mL) into the appropriate separate PCR reaction tubes. Aliquot 5 μL of sterile water instead of template DNA into the blank tube.
4. Thermocycling reaction conditions are as follows: an initial denaturation step for 2 min at 94°C; an amplification step consisting of 35 cycles of denaturation for 1 min at 94°C, annealing for 1 min at 65°C, extension for 1 min at 72°C, and a final extension for 10 min at 72°C. After PCR amplification, PCR products may be stored indefinitely at 5°C.
5. To check amplification quality, analyze the PCR products by nondenaturing polyacrylamide electrophoresis. Mix 10 μL of PCR product with 3 μL of gel-loading buffer and run in 1X TBE on an 8% polyacrylamide gel.
6. Photograph the gel using Polaroid Type 667 film.

3.3.2. SSCP Gel Electrophoresis of PCR Products

1. Make a 1 : 10 dilution of each PCR product by mixing 1 μL of product with 10 μL of sterile deionized water. Denature the diluted PCR products for 5 min at 95°C in either a boiling water bath or a thermocycler and then quickly chill them on ice for at least 15 min.
2. While the samples are on ice, prepare the PhastSystem.
3. Turn the instrument on and program it to cool down to ~10°C.
4. Clean the platform and place a dime-sized drop of water (approx 200 μL) on each side of the separation beds.
5. Using forceps, place a 20% homogeneous polyacrylamide native PhastGel over the drops of water. Make sure that no air bubbles are trapped under the gel.
6. Lower the applicator arm over the gel and place two PhastGel buffer strips in the slots at each end of the gel.
7. Program the unit to cool down to 3 ± 1°C and start the programmed pre-run.

8. After the unit has prerun ~50 V-h, prepare the samples for automatic loading as follows.
   a. Either of two sample applicator sizes can be used: the 6/4 (6 samples, 4 mL each per gel) or the 8/1 (8 samples, 1 mL each per gel).
   b. Lay the applicator down on a piece of Parafilm® laboratory film (American National Can™, Neenah, WI) and place ~1 mL of loading dye in alignment with each applicator sample well.
   c. Pipet the diluted, denatured, quick-chilled PCR product (11 mL) onto each microliter of dye and gently mix. Take care not to introduce air bubbles into the drop or mix the drop with adjacent drops.
   d. Lift the applicator and place it vertically over each sample until the sample is picked up.
   e. Place the sample applicator with the loaded sample into the appropriate slot on the separation unit.
   f. After 100 V-h of prerunning, the sample will be automatically applied to the gel.
   g. Actual electrophoresis conditions must be determined empirically and programmed into the unit. Example conditions are as follows:
      a. Prerun: 400 V/5.0 mA/1.0 W/3°C for 100 V-h.
      b. Application: 25 V/5.0 mA/1.0 W/3°C for 2 V-h.
      c. Separation: 400 V/5.0 mA/1.0 W/3°C for 350–390 V-h.
9. After electrophoresis, wearing gloves and using only forceps, place the gel into the PhastSystem Developing Unit (*see* **Note 3**).
10. Silver stain the gel using the PhastGel Silver Kit staining reagents and predetermined conditions.
11. Air-dry the gel for several hours at room temperature before mounting it in a Kodachrome™ slide holder.

3.3.3. Interpretation of SSCP Gel Electrophoresis Results

The positive control DNA lane should contain bands with altered mobility, as should the homozygous mutant and heterozygous patient sample lanes. By contrast, homozygous normal patient lanes should have no bands with altered mobility (**Fig. 5**).

3.4. RFLP-Based Detection of MEN2B

3.4.1. PCR Amplification of Exon 16

1. Set up the appropriate number of PCR tubes, including a positive control, a normal control, and a blank (no DNA) control.
2. Prepare a PCR master mix containing the components in **Table 3**. It is advisable to prepare a slight excess of master mix to allow for pipetting error. Typically, allowing for a 10% error is adequate (e.g., the total master mix volume prepared for 10 samples [24 µL of master mix/sample] would be 264 µL rather than 240 µL). All reagents should be kept on ice. Mix gently and aliquot 24 µL of the master mix into each of the PCR reaction tubes.

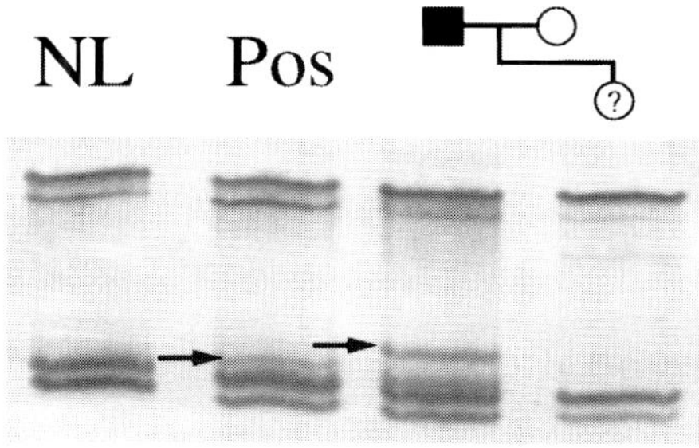

Fig. 5. SSCP analysis of MEN2A by PCR amplification, denaturation, and gel electrophoresis (Phast system) of exon 11. The gel illustrates the wild-type SSCP pattern in a normal control (NL), an abnormal SSCP pattern in a positive control (Pos), an affected father (■), and his affected daughter (?). Arrows indicate the abnormal conformer.

Table 3
Master Mix for PCR Amplification of RET Exon 16

	Volume/sample (does not include pipetting error) (μL)	Volume/10 samples (includes 10% pipetting error) (μL)
Sterile water	14.25	156.75
50% glycerol	2.5	27.5
5X PCR buffer	5.00	55
Primer Ret 16F	1.0	11
Primer Ret 16R	1.0	11
Taq polymerase (5 U/μL)	0.25	2.75
Total volume	24.0	264.0

3. Using a clean pipet tip for each specimen, aliquot 1 μL of DNA (250 μg/mL) into the appropriate tube.
4. Thermocycling reaction conditions are as follows: an initial denaturation step for 2 min at 95°C; an amplification step consisting of 35 cycles of denaturation for 30 s at 94°C, annealing for 30 s at 65°C, extension for 30 s at 72°C, and a final extension for 10 min at 72°C. After PCR amplification, PCR products may be stored indefinitely at 5°C.

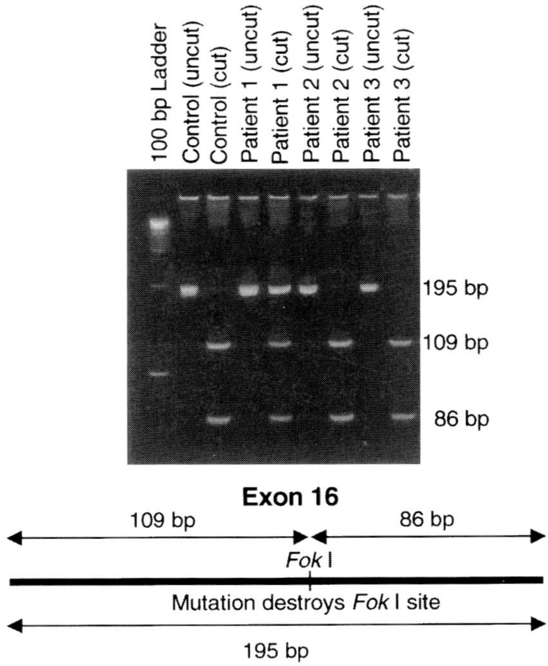

Fig. 6. RE analysis of MEN2B. PCR amplification of exon 16 results in a 195-bp fragment (uncut control), which is restricted by *Fok*I into 109- and 86-bp fragments (cut control). The *Fok*I site is destroyed by the MEN2B mutation in codon 918. Affected individuals (patients) demonstrate a 195-bp fragment, which represents the abnormal allele, and 109- and 86-bp fragments, which represent the normal allele.

3.4.2. RE Digestion

1. Prepare a RE master mix containing the following (in microliters/per/sample) 3.0 μL of sterile water, 1.5 μL of 10X NEB Buffer 4, 0.5 μL of *Fok*I. Mix gently and aliquot 5 μL of the master mix into each of the reaction tubes. (As previously noted, it is advisable to prepare a volume of master mix that allows for a 10% pipetting error.)
2. Using a clean pipet tip for each specimen, aliquot 10 μL of amplified DNA into the appropriate tube.
3. Carry out the digestion reaction at 37°C for a maximum of 2 h; longer digestion may result in a decreased signal.

3.4.3. Agarose Gel Electrophoresis

1. To detect the PCR products by agarose gel electrophoresis, run the samples on either a 20 × 14 cm or 20 × 20 cm 3% agarose gel (1% agarose/2% NuSieve).

Prepare the gel by mixing 1.2 g of agarose and 2.4 g of NuSieve with 300 mL of 1X TAE. Heat the resulting slurry in the microwave until the agarose is dissolved; cool to ~50°C (just cool enough to touch) and add 30 μL of EtBr.

2. Pour the agarose into the gel mold; use a comb to form the appropriate number of sample wells.
3. To prepare the samples for gel loading, mix 15 μL of digest with 3 μL of 6X sample buffer. Load the entire volume (18 μL) onto the gel.
4. Run the gel at 80 V for 2 to 3 h.
5. After electrophoresis, place the gel on a UV transilluminator. Take a Polaroid picture of the gel using a camera setting of f11 and 1 s.

3.4.4. Interpretation of Results

PCR amplification (*see* **Subheading 3.4.1.**) results in a 195-bp amplicon. *Fok*I digestion of the amplicon in normal individuals results in two restriction fragments of 109 and 86 bp. Because affected individuals are heterozygous, all three bands will be present on the gel (**Fig. 6**).

4. Notes

1. The PCR and sequencing protocols described here were optimized with the PE Applied Biosystems GeneAmp® PCR System 9600 and MicroAmp® Reaction Tubes with Caps (nos. N801-0001 and N801-0540, respectively; PE Applied Biosystems). The use of other systems may require reoptimization.
2. Other DNA stains may be used (and may be more sensitive).
3. Rinse the gloves with water prior to handling the gel. Glove powder can leave artifacts on gels that appear after silver staining.

References

1. Trupp, M., Arenas, E., Fainzilber, M., et al. (1996) Functional receptor for GDFN encoded by the c-ret proto-oncogene. *Nature* **381,** 785–789.
2. Berndt, I., Reuter, M., Saller, B., Frank-Raue, K., Groth, P., Grussendorf, M., Raue, M., Ritter, M., and Höppner, W. (1998) A new hot spot for mutations in the ret proto-oncogene causing familial medullary thyroid carcinoma and multiple endocrine neoplasia type 2A. *J. Clin. Endocrinol. Metab.* **83,** 770–774.
3. Marsh, D. J., Mulligan, L. M., and Eng, C. (1997) RET Proto-oncogene mutations in multiple endocrine neoplasia type 2 and medullary thyroid carcinoma. *Horm. Res.* **47,** 168–178.
4. Decker, R. A. and Peacock, M. L. (1997) Update of the Profile of Multiple Endocrine Neoplasia Type 2a RET Mutations. *Cancer* **80(Suppl.),** 557–568.
5. Eng, C., Mulligan, L. M., Smith, D. P., et al. (1995) Mutations of the RET Proto-oncogene in sporadic medullary thyroid carcinoma. *Genes Chrom. Cancer* **12,** 209–212.
6. Heshmati, H. M. and Hofbauer, L. (1997) Multiple endocrine neoplasia type 2: recent progress in diagnosis and management. *Eur. J. Endocrinol.* **137,** 572–578.

7. Wells, S. A. Jr., Chi, D. D., Toshima. K., Dehner, L. P., Coffin, C. M., Dowton, S. B., Ivanovich, I. L., DeBenedetti, M. K., Dilley, W. G., Moley, J. F., et al. (1994) Predictive DNA testing and prophylactic thyroidectomy in patients at risk for multiple endocrine neoplasia type 2A. *Ann. Surg.* **220,** 237–247.
8. Decker, R. A., Peacock, M. L., Borst, M. J., Sweet, J. D., and Thompson, N. W. (1995) Progress in genetic screening of multiple endocrine neoplasia type 2A: is calcitonin testing obsolete? *Surgery* **118,** 257–264.
9. Carlson, K. M., Bracamontes, J., Jackson, C. E., et al. (1994) Parent of origin effects in multiple endocrine neoplasia type 2B. *Am. J. Hum. Genet.* **55,** 1076–1082.
10. Schuffenecker, I., Billuad, M., Calendar, A., Chambe, B., Ginet, N., Calmettes, C., Modigliani, E., and Lenoir, G. M. (1994) Ret Proto-Oncogene mutations in French MEN2A and FMTC families. *Hum. Mol. Genet.* **3,** 1939–1943.
11. Ceccherini, I., Hofstra, R. M. W., Luo, Y., et al. (1995) DNA polymorphisms and conditions for SSCP analysis of the 20 exons of the RET proto-oncogene. *Oncogene* **9,** 3025–3029.
12. Siegelman, M. S., Mohabcer, A. J., Fahey, T., Tomlinson, G., Mayambala, C., Jafari, S., Noil, W. W., Thibodeau, S. N., and Dawson, D. B. (1997) Rapid, non-radioactive SSCP analysis for mutations in exons 10, 11, and 15 of the RET proto-oncogene associated with inherited medullary thyroid carcinoma. *Clin. Chem.* **43,** 453–457.
13. Anonymous. (1998) Heteroduplex Analysis with MDE™ solution. FMC BioProducts Catalog, FMC BioProducts, ME, pp. 93–98.
14. Kambouris, M., Jackson, C. E., and Feldman, G. L. (1996) Diagnosis of Multiple Endocrine Neoplasia [MEN] 2A, 2B and Familial Medullary Thyroid Cancer [FMTC] by multiplex PCR and heteroduplex analyses of RET proto-oncogene mutations. *Human Mutat.* **8,** 64–70.
15. Feldman, G. L., Kambouris, M., Talpos, G. B., Mulligan, L. M., Ponder, B. A. J., and Jackson, C. E. (1994) Clinical value of direct DNA analysis of the RET proto-oncogene in families with multiple endocrine neoplasia type 2A. *Surgery* **116,** 1042–1047.

20

Assay for Detecting the I1307K Susceptibility Allele within the *Adenomatous Polyposis Coli* Gene

Stephen B. Gruber

1. Introduction

Most germline mutations of the *adenomatous polyposis coli* (*APC*) tumor suppressor gene result in a classic inherited cancer syndrome called familial adenomatous polyposis (FAP). FAP is characterized by thousands of colonic polyps, well-defined extracolonic manifestations that may include pigmented lesions of the ocular fundus, supernumerary teeth, osteomas, odontomas, desmoid tumors and epidermoid cysts, and a 100% lifetime risk of developing colorectal cancer. Shortly after the *APC* gene was cloned in 1991 ***(1,2)*** the molecular basis of an attenuated form of FAP was recognized to be related to germline mutations within *APC* that were most likely to be found in the 5′ and 3′ ends of the gene ***(3,4)***. The truncating mutations leading to classic FAP and attenuated FAP are quite rare, but recently a polymorphism of the *APC* gene was found among 6 to 7% of Ashkenazi Jews that approximately doubles the risk of colorectal cancer ***(5)***.

The *APC* I1307K allele confers an increased risk of colorectal cancer by creating a hypermutable tract of eight contiguous A residues, in contrast to the wild-type (WT) sequence $(A)_3T(A)_4$. This poly-A tract functions as a premutation that makes the surrounding DNA sequence especially vulnerable to subsequent somatic mutations. Furthermore, this enhanced somatic mutation rate is completely restricted to the mutant (MU) allele, and the somatic mutations are almost always insertions ***(6)***. It is clear that I1307K increases the carrier's risk of colorectal cancer ***(7)***, but recent evidence suggesting that this allele also increases the risk of breast cancer remains controversial ***(8,9)***.

From: *Methods in Molecular Medicine, vol. 49: Molecular Pathology Protocols*
Edited by: A. A. Killeen © Humana Press Inc., Totowa, NJ

Together these findings suggest that the I1307K allele may have relevant implications for genetic counseling and risk prediction, even though the positive predictive value for this test is relatively low.

Several techniques have been described for detecting the presence of the *APC* I1307K allele ***(9)***. Allele-specific oligonucleotide (ASO) hybridization is used most commonly, because the technique permits MU and WT alleles to be accurately distinguished at low cost for many samples ***(10)***. Some laboratories prefer to screen samples with single-strand conformation polymorphism or conformation-sensitive gel electrophoresis ***(11)*** followed by sequencing in order to detect the I1307K allele, but in our experience each of these techniques is more time-consuming and expensive than ASO hybridization. Variations of the radiolabeled ASO technique using chemiluminescent enzymatic detection are also relatively straightforward to set up, but are more expensive than the radioactive assay.

2. Materials

2.1. General Reagents

1. MilliQ purified, autoclaved double-distilled H_2O (ddH_2O).
2. 10X PCR Buffer: 500 m*M* KCl, 0.1% gelatin, 1% Triton X-100, 100 m*M* Tris-HCl, pH 9.0, 15 m*M* $MgCl_2$.
3. dNTP mix: final concentration of 25 m*M* dATP, 25 m*M* dCTP, 25 m*M* dGTP, 25 m*M* dTTP.
4. *Taq* polymerase (Perkin-Elmer).
5. 50X TAE buffer: 242 g of Tris base, 57.1 mL glacial acetic acid, 100 mL of 0.5 *M* EDTA, pH 8.0, in 1 L of distilled water.
6. Loading buffer for agarose gels: 6X buffer consisting of 15% Ficoll, 60 m*M* EDTA, 3% sodium dodecyl sulfate (SDS), 0.25% bromophenol blue, 0.25% xylene cyanol (1.5 g of Ficoll, 1.2 mL 0.5 *M* EDTA, 3 mL 10% SDS, 25 mg of bromophenol blue, 25 mg of xylene cyanol, in 10 mL of distilled water).
7. 2X saline sodium citrate (SSC): Diluted from a 20X SSC stock solution consisting of 175.3 g of NaCl and 88.2 g of sodium citrate in 800 mL of water. Adjust the pH to 7.0 with a few drops of a 10 *N* solution of NaOH. Adjust the volume to 1 L with H_2O and autoclave).
8. 20X SSPE: 175.3 g of NaCl, 27.6 g of $NaH_2PO_4 \cdot H_2O$ and 7.4 g of EDTA in 800 mL of water. Adjust the pH to 7.4 with NaOH (approx 6.5 mL of 10 *N* solution), in 1 L of distilled water.

2.2. Sample Preparation

1. Lymphocyte separation media (LSM®; ICN Pharmaceuticals, Aurora, OH).
2. Phosphate-buffered saline (PBS) (Sigma, St. Louis, MO).
3. Puregene DNA Isolation kit (Gentra Systems).
4. Isopropanol stored at –20°C.
5. 70% Ethanol.
6. LoTE: 3 m*M* Tris-HCl, 0.2 m*M* EDTA, pH 7.6.

2.3. ASO Hybridization

1. 10X Polynucleotide kinase (PNK) buffer (New England Biolabs); store at –20°C.
2. PNK (New England Biolabs); store at –20°C.
3. γ ^{32}P-ATP (Amersham Pharmacia).
4. 50X DET: DET is Denhardt's with 10 m*M* EDTA and 10 m*M* Tris pH 8.0. 50X Denhardt's is made with 5 g of Ficoll (Type 400; Pharmacia), 5 g of polyvinylpyrrolidone, 5 g of bovine serum albumin (Fraction V; Sigma), and water to 500 mL.
5. 10% SDS.
6. Sheared, single-stranded salmon sperm DNA.
7. 0.4 *M* NaOH, 25 m*M* EDTA.
8. Hybond N+ nylon membrane (Amersham Pharmacia).
9. Trichloroacetic acid (TCA).
10. Metricel membrane filter (P/N 63068; Gelman Sciences).
11. Scintillation fluid (Beckman-Coulter).

2.4. Equipment

1. Centrifuge.
2. Thermocycler.
3. Agarose gel-running aparatus.
4. Dot-blot apparatus.
5. Adjustable temperature water bath with shaker.
6. Scintillation counter.
7. Heat sealer.

3. Methods

The technique for detecting the I1307K allele follows four steps:

1. Sample preparation.
2. Polymerase chain reaction (PCR) amplification of the relevant region of the APC gene.
3. Allele-specific hybridization of oligonucleotide probes to PCR products that have been immobilized on nylon membranes.
4. Washes at a critical temperature and stringency.

The ASO technique takes advantage of the difference in melting temperatures of oligonucleotides with differing sequences. Even a single nucleotide change is sufficient to distinguish two variant alleles at a critical hybridization temperature, and nonspecific hybridization is typically avoided by using oligonucleotide primers between 16 and 20 nucleotides long ***(10)***. The performance of oligonucleotide probes can sometimes be enhanced by designing probes corresponding to the noncoding strand; the probes we use for the I1307K assay are noncoding (L. Brody, personal communication).

3.1. Sample Preparation

1. Transfer 3 mL of defibrinated or heparinized blood into a 15-mL conical tube containing 3 mL of PBS and mix gently by inverting or pipetting.
2. Gently mix LSM by inverting. Then transfer 3.5 mL of LSM to a 15-mL conical tube.
3. Carefully layer the blood/PBS solution onto the LSM, keeping a sharp interface between the dilute blood and the LSM.
4. Centrifuge the tube at 400*g* at room temperature for 15–30 min.
5. Aspirate the top layer of clear plasma to within 2 to 3 mm above the lymphocyte layer.
6. Transfer the lymphocyte layer and about half of the LSM layer below it to a centrifuge tube. Add an equal volume of PBS to the tube and centrifuge for 10 min at 200*g*, in order not to damage the cells. Remove the supernatant.
7. Wash the cells a second time by resuspending in PBS and centrifuge for 10 min at 200*g*. Aspirate the supernatant, and vortex briefly in the small remaining amount of residual supernatant to resuspend the cells.
8. For an average-sized cell pellet, add 3 mL of Cell Lysis Solution (Gentra Systems) to the lymphocytes and pipet up and down to lyse the cells.
9. Add 1 mL of Protein Precipitation Solution and vortex for 20 s.
10. Centrifuge at 13,000–16,000*g* for 3 min.
11. Pour off the supernatant into ice-cold isopropanol.
12. Invert the tube about 40 times until the DNA precipitates. The DNA precipitate should be visible as a white precipitate and can be collected by spooling the DNA on a glass Pasteur pipet. Wash in 70% ethanol and resuspend the DNA in 200 µL of LoTE.
13. If no precipitate can be seen, centrifuge for 1 min at 13,000*g*, pour off the isopropanol, let the tube dry, and then add 150 µL of LoTE.
14. Measure the concentration of the DNA by removing an aliquot and measuring the absorbance at 260 and 280 nm. Dilute an aliquot of DNA in ddH_2O to a concentration of 4 ng/µL.

3.2. PCR Amplification of APC

The oligonucleotide primers that are used to amplify the segment of APC containing the I1307K polymorphism cover a larger region of the *APC* gene than was originally reported by Laken et al. *(5)*. The primers shown in **Table 1** give a single 372-bp PCR product visible as a single band on a 1% agarose gel. Although the originally published primers work quite well by amplifying a 110-bp product, the primers shown in **Table 1** provide a longer product for those investigators who are interested in using one set of primers to study somatic mutations in a larger region surrounding the hypermutable tract of I1307K.

1. Aliquot 5 µL of DNA sample (4 ng/µL) into each well of a 96-well plate.
2. Make a PCR reaction mix for the appropriate multiple of PCR reactions (add the *Taq* polymerase last, and keep reactions on ice prior to loading on a thermocycler) using the following protocol (for each 20-µL individual reaction):

Table 1
Primer and Oligonucleotide Probe Sequences for APC I1307K ASO Hybridization Assay

Primer/probe	Sequence	Product length/ hybridization temperature
APC forward	TCC ACA CCT TCA TCT AAT GCC	372 bp
APC reverse	TAA ACT AGA ACC CTG CAG TCT GC	
Wild type	CTT TTC TTT TAT TTC TGC	44°C
Mutant	CTT TTC TTT TTT TTC TGC	44°C

a. PCR buffer: 2 µL of 10X PCR buffer for a 1X final concentration.
b. dNTP: 0.16 µL of 25 m*M* dNTP mix.
c. Forward primer: 0.2 µL of 50 ng/µL primer for a total of 10 ng per reaction.
d. Reverse primer: 0.2 µL of 50 ng/µL primer for a total of 10 ng per reaction.
e. *Taq* polymerase: 0.2 µL of 5U/µL *Taq* polymerase for a total of 1 U/reaction.
f. ddH_2O: 12.24 µL ddH_2O brings the total volume of the reaction to 20 µL when 5 µL of sample DNA is used.

3. Distribute 15 µL of the PCR mix to each sample and cover with mineral oil.
4. Program the thermocycler to denature at 95°C for 5 min; followed by 35 cycles of denaturing at 95°C for 1 min; annealing at 53°C for 1 min, and extension at 72°C for 1 min; and ending with a final extension at 72°C for 10 min.
5. Visualize an aliquot of the PCR product on 1% agarose/TAE gel to ensure adequate amplification. The product is visualized as a single band at ~370 bp.

3.3. ASO Hybridization

Figure 1 summarizes the general technique for ASO hybridization. PCR-amplified DNA products are denatured and immobilized on a nylon membrane, usually in duplicate in order to make it more convenient to hybridize with WT and MU probes at the same time. The membrane is prehybridized with solution that contains a blocking agent such as Denhardt's or BLOTTO (5% nonfat dried milk in water with 0.02% sodium azide) to prevent nonspecific binding of probes to the membrane. Radiolabeled oligonucleotide probes are hybridized to the immobilized DNA fragments at a temperature that permits specific nucleotide pairing. Excess probe is removed by washing each membrane at a carefully titrated stringency to eliminate nonspecific binding.

1. Denature 10 µL of PCR product in 93 µL of 0.4 *M* NaOH and 25 m*M* EDTA.
2. Transfer the PCR product to a nylon membrane (Hybond N+) using a dot-blot apparatus, rinsing each well twice with 50 µL of 2X SSC. Disassemble the apparatus and neutralize the membrane for 5 min in 2X SSC.
3. Crosslink the DNA to the membrane with 1200 J of UV irradiation.

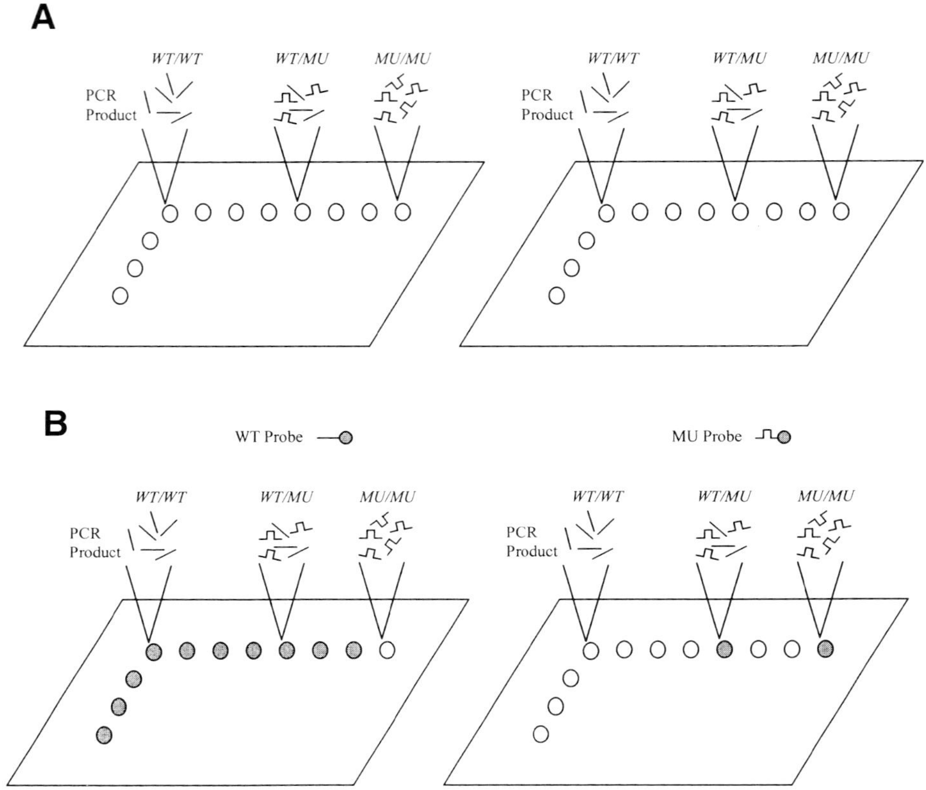

Fig. 1. **(A)** PCR products immobilized on nylon membranes in duplicate; **(B)** ASO hybridization performed separately with WT and MU probes.

4. Prepare a prehybridization solution with 25 mL of 20X SSPE, 10 mL of 50X DET, 5 mL of 10% SDS, 1 mL of single-stranded salmon sperm denatured DNA, and add ddH_2O to bring the total volume to 100 mL.
5. Heat the prehybridization solution to exactly 44°C, reserving 15 mL of the prehybridization solution for hybridization.
6. Prehybridize at exactly 44°C for 1 h.
7. While the membranes are in the prehybridization solution, end-label the wild-type and mutant probes with $\gamma\,^{32}$P-ATP. Label each probe by incubating a 25-µL labeling reaction containing 16.5 µL of ddH_2O, 2.5 µL of 10X PNK buffer, 2 µL of oligonucleotide probe (WT or MU), 1 µL of PNK, and 3 µL of $\gamma\,^{32}$P-ATP at 37°C for 30 min. Quench the reaction at 68°C for 10 min.
8. Determine the activity of each probe to ensure adequate incorporation of ^{32}P and comparability of WT and MU probes. This is done by adding 1 µL aliquots of WT and MU probes to separate tubes containing 1 mL of 10% TCA on ice, and

then slowly pouring this over a Metricel membrane filter (Gelman Sciences). The filter is rinsed several times with TCA and transferred to a scintillation vial containing Beckman scintillation cocktail. The activity is counted using a scintillation counter. Activities >500,000 cpm are acceptable. Lower counts may give weaker signals. The labeled oligonucleotide probes may also be separated from unbound label using spin columns or other techniques.

9. Heat the reserved 15 mL of prehybridization solution to exactly 44°C before adding WT and MU probes to equal aliquots of this solution.
10. Hybridize at exactly 44°C for 1 h.

3.4. Washes and Detection of Mutation

1. Wash membranes briefly with 1X SSC/0.05% SDS at room temperature, and then wash again in 1X SSC/0.05% SDS at 44°C for 20 min.
2. Wrap membranes in plastic wrap and expose to film for 2–4 h at –80°C, depending on the activity of the probe.
3. Read the genotypes by visual inspection. Genotypes are generally not difficult to interpret in the presence of adequate controls, but it is important to make sure that the signal intensity of the WT and MU blots are comparable for known samples before proceeding with interpretation. WT/WT homozygotes are recognized by a strong signal on the WT blot and the absence of a signal on the MU blot. WT/MU heterozygotes are detectable by observing signals on both blots. I1307K homozygotes are rare, but this genotype is recognized by a signal on only the MU blot.

4. Notes

1. The sample preparation technique is not critical to this assay, and virtually any method of isolating genomic DNA is sufficient.
2. Resuspending the isolated lymphocytes in the small amount of residual PBS that remains after aspiration makes the cell lysis much more efficient. Vortexing for 5–10 s is adequate.
3. There are simpler ways to lyse erythrocytes and isolate white cells for DNA preparations, but we prefer this method because it yields a clean fraction of lymphocytes that can be frozen for future transformation or harvested immediately.
4. Treating the cell lysate with RNase is not necessary, and eliminating the RNase treatment saves the expense of a costly reagent.
5. Some investigators prefer to store genomic DNA in ddH_2O because EDTA can chelate magnesium in the buffer for PCR reactions. We prefer to use LoTE in order to preserve the DNA stock solutions for long-term storage, and dilute aliquots for analysis in ddH_2O. This does not interfere with PCR reactions.
6. The membrane transfer is not difficult and can be performed with many different apparatuses and conditions. Some laboratories prefer using a slot-blot apparatus rather than a dot-blot apparatus; we prefer to use a 96-well dot blot to facilitate simultaneous analysis of many samples. Neutralizing the membranes and DNA following the denaturing reaction is recommended but is not critical because the assay does not appear to be sensitive to whether the neutralization step is performed.

7. Prehybridization of both membranes can be performed in the same solution, but it is important for the DNA sides of the membranes to be exposed to the solution. Keeping one membrane faceup and the other facedown permits excellent prehybridization.
8. The hybridization temperature is critical to the success of the assay. Lower temperatures permit nonspecific hybridization, and higher temperatures may lower the sensitivity of the test by making the hybridization conditions too stringent. Washing at the correct stringency is the second most important aspect of the assay, and for this ASO a temperature of 44°C is appropriate for both hybridization and washing.
9. Membranes that are sealed in plastic wrap (and have not dried out completely) can be stripped and reprobed many times.

References

1. Groden, J., Thliveris, A., Samowitz, W., et al. (1991) Identification and characterization of the familial adenomatous polyposis coli gene. *Cell* **66,** 589–600.
2. Kinzler, K. W., Nilbert, M. C., Su, L. K., et al. (1991) Identification of FAP locus genes from chromosome 5q21. *Science* **253,** 661–665.
3. Spirio, L., Olschwang, S., Groden, J., Robertson, M., Samowitz, W., Joslyn, G., Gelbert, L., Thliveris, A., Carlson, M., and Otterud, B. (1993) Alleles of the APC gene: an attenuated form of familial polyposis. *Cell* **75,** 951–957.
4. Soravia, C., Berk, T., Madlensky, L., Mitri, A., Cheng, H., Gallinger, S., Cohen, Z., and Bapat, B. (1998) Genotype-phenotype correlations in attenuated adenomatous polyposis coli. *Am. J. Hum. Genet.* **62,** 1290–1301.
5. Laken, S. J., Petersen, G. M., Gruber, S. B., et al. (1997) Familial colorectal cancer in Ashkenazim due to a hypermutable tract in APC. *Nat. Genetics* **17,** 79–83.
6. Gryfe, R., Di Nicola, N., Gallinger, S., and Redston, M. (1998) Somatic instability of the APC I1307K allele in colorectal neoplasia. *Cancer Res.* **58,** 4040–4043.
7. Gruber, S. B., Petersen, G. M., Kinzler, K. W., and Vogelstein, B. (1999) Cancer, crash sites, and the new genetics of neoplasia. *Gastroenterology* **116,** 210–212.
8. Woodage, T., King, S. M., Wacholder, S., Hartge, P., Struewing, J. P., McAdams, M., Laken, S. J., Tucker, M. A., and Brody, L. C. (1998) The APCI1307K allele and cancer risk in a community-based study of Ashkenazi Jews. *Nat. Genet.* **20,** 62–65.
9. Redston, M., Nathanson, K. L., Yuan, Z. Q., et al. (1998) The APCI1307K allele and breast cancer risk. *Nat. Genetics* **20,** 13–14.
10. Nollau, P. and Wagener, C. (1997) Methods for detection of point mutations: performance and quality assessment. *Clin. Chem.* **43,** 1114–1128.
11. Ganguly, A., Rock, M. J., and Prockop, D. J. (1993) Conformation-sensitive gel electrophoresis for rapid detection of single-base differences in double-stranded PCR products and DNA fragments: evidence for solvent-induced bends in DNA heteroduplexes. *Proc. Natl. Acad. Sci. USA* **90,** 10,325–10,329.

21

Detection of Human Papillomaviruses by Polymerase Chain Reaction and *In Situ* Hybridization

Elizabeth R. Unger and Suzanne D. Vernon

1. Introduction

The clinical utility of human papillomavirus (HPV) testing continues to be the focus of much debate. The clear epidemiologic link of HPV infection with the development of cervical intraepithelial neoplasia and invasive cervical cancers *(1)* leads to widespread expectation that testing for HPV could improve cervical cancer screening or aid in the triage of patients with abnormal cytology. The results of clinical trials of HPV testing are contradictory *(2)*, and widespread implementation of HPV testing is currently not recommended. However, HPV testing is important in epidemiologic studies of cervical and anogenital disease, and a large National Cancer Institute trial is currently evaluating HPV as an adjunct to cytology in cervical cancer screening.

Methods for diagnosing HPV are all dependent on detection of viral DNA, because the agent cannot be cultivated in routine tissue culture and antibody methods lack sensitivity. Detection of HPV DNA therefore requires analysis of cellular material from the viral lesion. Methods for HPV detection are complicated by the fact that HPV is not a single virus, but a group of more than 75 closely related viruses. Typing is based on the viral genomic sequence and at least 30 types infect the genital area. The types are considered high or low risk, based on the frequency of their association with malignant lesions. The assay format and sampling method both influence how often HPV will be detected. The many variations of testing and sampling that have been and are being used make comparisons among studies problematic.

From: *Methods in Molecular Medicine, vol. 49: Molecular Pathology Protocols*
Edited by: A. A. Killeen © Humana Press Inc., Totowa, NJ

Southern blot hybridization was considered the gold standard for HPV detection; however, this technique is no longer frequently employed. More rapid methods that can easily accommodate limited patient samples are favored. In this chapter, we include protocols for an L1 consensus polymerase chain reaction (PCR) assay, as the most commonly used amplification assay, and colorimetric *in situ* hybridization (ISH) assay, as a nonamplified method that yields complementary information to PCR. ISH and PCR assays are both applicable to DNA analysis in formalin-fixed archival tissues. Both assay formats require small amounts of tissue and thus conserve material essential for clinical management. In addition, both formats tolerate some degradation of target nucleic acids and can utilize nonradioactive detection methods ***(3)***.

The HybridCapture HPV test (Digene Diagnostics) is Food and Drug Administration approved and was designed for clinical laboratories. The assay is a solution phase hybridization of sample DNA with an RNA probe. The specific hybrids are selected ("captured") using an antibody bound to a tube or microtiter plate that specifically recognizes DNA-RNA hybrid molecules. The same antibody linked to an enzyme is then used for detection with a chemiluminescent substrate. Although there is no control for input DNA, the assay yields semiquantitative values for the amount of HPV DNA. As currently marketed, the assay groups multiple HPV probes into high- and low-risk groups, so type-specific of information is not obtained. The manufacturer supplies detailed instructions with the kit and trains laboratories in the proper use of the kit on request. Therefore, despite its clinical applicability, the HybridCapture assay is not discussed in this chapter.

1.1. L1 Consensus PCR Assay

Laboratories are increasingly using PCR to detect HPV. Since there are more than 75 different types of HPV ***(4)***, primers designed to amplify the conserved L1 region have become the most widely used in clinical and epidemiologic studies. The MY09 and MY11 primers contain several degenerate nucleotides and amplify a 450-bp region of L1 of at least 25 different types of anogenital HPV ***(5)***. The GP5+-GP6+ primers are a mixture of fixed nucleotide oligonucleotides that amplify a 150-bp region of L1 of a wide range of HPV types by lowering the annealing temperature during PCR ***(6)***. The utility of both primer sets has been compared and contrasted with each set having advantages or disadvantages over the other ***(7–9)***. The protocol described herein is an optimized method for amplifying HPV DNA from fresh cervical swab specimens, cervical lavage specimens, or formalin-fixed paraffin-embedded tissues using the MY09/MY11 primer set. The most reproducible results are achieved when DNA is extracted from samples, and for this reason, sample preparation is described in this protocol. Type-specific PCR assays are described in the literature and for specific applications may have advantages.

1.2. ISH for HPV

Colorimetric ISH is applicable to routinely processed, formalin-fixed paraffin-embedded tissue sections. The chief advantage of the method is that HPV DNA is demonstrated within a morphologic context, allowing the tissue distribution of virus to be evaluated. In addition, the integration status of HPV correlates with the pattern of signal produced in the assay ***(3,10)***. The methods of colorimetric detection and interpretation are the same as those used for immunohistochemistry, making ISH the molecular technique with the greatest potential for ready incorporation into diagnostic histopathology laboratories.

ISH is labor-intensive and requires extensive optimization of conditions in order to achieve maximum sensitivity. The method described herein uses capillary gap technology to introduce and remove reagents, minimizing the individual handling of slides ***(11–13)***. Empirical adjustment of conditions is required if other methods of reagent application, slide denaturation, and incubation are used.

ISH is conceptually straightforward, requiring tissue pretreatment (to allow for probe penetration), denaturation of probe and tissue nucleic acids, hybridization, washes, and detection. The method described is for formalin-fixed paraffin-embedded tissues. Methods of preparation of cell block controls and probe labeling are also included, because these are essential to obtaining optimal results on a routine basis.

2. Materials

2.1. L1 Consensus PCR Assay

2.1.1. Preparation of Samples

1. Pro-par clearant (Anatech, Battle Creek, MI).
2. Proteinase K buffer: 50 m*M* Tris-HCl, pH 8.3, 1 m*M* EDTA, 0.5% Tween-20, 200 µg/mL of proteinase K.
3. MµlTI-Lid-Locs (cat. nos. C5000 and C6000; Marsh Biomedical).
4. Phenol/chloroform/isoamyl alcohol (25:24:1) (v/v/v).
5. Phase Lock Gel I Light (5 Prime-3 Prime, Boulder, CO).
6. 100% Ethanol (4°C).
7. 10 *M* Ammonium acetate.

2.1.2. HPV L1 Consensus and β-Globin PCR

1. Sterile double-distilled H_2O (ddH_2O).
2. 10X $MgCl_2$-free PCR buffer (Roche).
3. 25 m*M* $MgCl_2$ (*see* **Note 1**).

Table 1
Oligonucleotide Primer Information

Primer	Origin	Sequence (5′–3′)	Amplicon size	Reference
MY09	HPV	CGT CCM ARR GGA WAC TGA TC[a]	approx 450	**5**
MY11		GCM CAG GGW CAT AAY AAT GG[a]		
PC04	β-Globin	GAA GAG CCA AGG ACA GGT AC	286	
GH20		CAA CTT CAT CCA CGT TCA CC		

[a]M = A or C, R = A or G, W = A or T, Y = C or T.

4. 10 m*M* dNTPs.
5. 50 μ*M* Working oligonucleotide primers (*see* **Table 1**).
6. Template DNA (test samples, HPV-positive and -negative control DNA).
7. *Taq* DNA polymerase (5 U/μL).
8. Mineral oil.
9. DNA-Erase™ (ICN Biomedicals, Aurora, OH).

2.1.3. Typing of HPV L1 Consensus Amplicons

2.1.3.1. Probe Labeling

1. Reagents for PCR (*see* **Subheading 2.2.**).
2. Template HPV DNA: Clones of HPV-6, -11, -16, -18, -31, and -35 are available from American Type Culture Collection. Other clones are available by request from investigators.
3. PCR DIG Labeling Mix (cat. no. 1 585 550; Boehringer Mannheim).
4. Positively charged nylon membrane (cat. no. 1 417 240; Boehringer Mannheim).
5. 20X saline sodium citrate (SSC): 3 *M* NaCl, 0.3 *M* sodium citrate, pH 7.0.

2.1.3.2. Preparation and Hybridization of Amplicon Dot Blots

1. 10X Denaturation solution: 4 *M* NaOH, 100 m*M* EDTA.
2. 0.4 *M* NaOH.
3. 2X SSC.
4. Nylon membrane.
5. DIG-Easy Hyb (cat. no. 1 603 558; Boehringer Mannheim).
6. 2X Wash solution (2X SSC, 0.1% sodium dodecyl sulfate [SDS]).
7. 0.5X Wash solution (0.5X SSC, 0.1% SDS).

2.1.3.3. Chemiluminescent Detection

1. DIG Wash and Block Buffer Set (cat. no. 1 585 762; Boehringer Mannheim).
2. Antidigoxigenin-conjugated with alkaline phosphatase (cat. no. 1 093 274; Boehringer Mannheim).
3. CDP-Star (cat. no. 1 759 051; Boehringer Mannheim).
4. Lumi-film (cat. no. 1 666 657; Boehringer Mannheim).

2.2. *In Situ Hybridization*

Cervical cancer cell lines with well-defined characteristics and a known copy number of HPV are suggested as a dependable and consistent control for many HPV assays. When prepared as formalin-fixed paraffin-embedded cell blocks, the cell lines form quite effective tissue controls for monitoring the sensitivity of the ISH reaction. Suggested lines include Caski, 400–600 copies HPV-16/cell; Hela, 10–50 copies of HPV-18/cell; SiHa, 1 to 2 copies of HPV-16/cell; HTB-31, HPV negative. The HPV-16 in SiHa cells is near the limits of detection of the assay, and results on this cell block clearly demonstrate when any component of the assay is failing.

2.2.1. Preparation of Cell Block

1. Dulbecco's phosphate-buffered saline (D-PBS).
2. 10% Neutral buffered formalin.
3. Collodion (no. 4560-1; Mallinckrodt).

2.2.2. Probe Labeling

1. 10X Nick translation buffer: 500 m*M* Tris, pH 8.0, 50 m*M* $MgCl_2$, 100 m*M* β-mercaptoethanol, 100 µg/mL of nuclease-free bovine serum albumin (BSA). Filter sterilize (0.2-µ filter) and store in 0.5-mL aliquots at –20°C.
2. DNase activation buffer: 10 m*M* Tris-HCl, pH 7.6, 5 m*M* $MgCl_2$, 1 mg/mL of nuclease-free BSA. Store at –20°C.
3. DNase I (10 µg/µL (Gibco-BRL, Gaithersburg, MD).
4. DNA Polymerase I/DNase I (0.4 U of polymerase and 40 pg of DNase/µL (Gibco-BRL).
5. Nucleotide buffer solution: 0.5 mL of 10X nick translation buffer; 0.5 mL of sterile ddH_2O, 10 µL each of 10 m*M* solutions of dATP, dCTP, dGTP (Gibco-BRL). Store in 100-µL aliquots at –20°C.
6. Bio-11-dUTP (1.0 m*M*) (Enzo).

2.2.3. Verification of Probe Size and Labeling

1. Biotinylated DNA ladder (Gibco-BRL).
2. Agarose, Sigma Type 2 (Sigma, St. Louis, MO).
3. 10X Running buffer: 0.3 *M* NaOH, 30 m*M* EDTA (store at room temperature).
4. 10X Gel buffer: 0.3 *M* NaCl, 30 m*M* EDTA (store at room temperature).
5. Ficoll dye solution: 50 m*M* Tris-HCl, pH 7.5, 20% Ficoll, 5 m*M* EDTA, 0.9% bromophenol blue, 0.9% xylene cyanole FF (store at room temperature).
6. 20X SSC: 3 *M* NaCl, 0.3 *M* sodium citrate.
7. TS Brij 7.5: 0.1 *M* Tris-HCl, pH 7.5, 0.1 *M* NaCl, 5 m*M* $MgCl_2$, 2.5 mL of 30% Brij 35/L.
8. TS Brij 9.5: 0.1 *M* Tris-HCl, pH 9.5, 0.1 *M* NaCl, 50 m*M* $MgCl_2$, 2.5 mL of 30% Brij 35/L.
9. ddH_2O.

10. Neutralizing buffer: 3 *M* NaCl, 0.5 *M* Tris-HCl, pH 7.5.
11. Nitroblue tetrazolium chloride (NBT) stock: 50 mg of NBT (grade III, no. N6876; Sigma), 0.5 mL of sterile dH_2O, 0.5 mL of *N,N*-dimethylformamide (DMF). Store at room temperature.
12. 5-Bromo-4-chloro-3-indolyl phosphate *p*-toluidine salt (BCIP) stock: 50 mg of BCIP (no. 0885; Amresco) and 1.0 mL DMF. Store at 4°C.
13. Avidin–alkaline phosphatase conjugate (Dako). Store at 4°C.
14. 1% BSA/TS Brij 7.5: 1 g of BSA fraction V (no. A4503; Sigma) and 0.1 g of sodium azide to a final volume of 100 mL in TS Brij 7.5. Filter sterilize and store at 4°C.
15. McGadey reagent: 67 µL of NBT stock, 33 µL of BCIP stock, 10 mL of TS 9.5 Brij. Prepare within 4 h of use.

2.2.4. ISH Assay

1. 0.01 *N* HCl, 2.5 mL of 35% Brij 35/L.
2. TS Brij 7.5: *see* **Subheading 2.2.3, item 7**.
3. TS Brij 9.5: *see* **Subheading 2.2.3, item 8**.
4. ddH_2O Brij: 2.5 mL of 30% Brij 35 to 1 L with ddH_2O (store at room temperature).
5. 2X SSC SDS/Brij: 2X SSC, 0.1% SDS, 2.5 mL of 35% Brij 35/L.
6. 0.2X SSC SDS/Brij: 0.2X SSC, 0.1% SDS, 2.5 mL of 35% Brij 35/L.
7. 0.1X SSC SDS/Brij: 0.1X SSC, 0.1% SDS, 2.5 mL of 35% Brij 35/L.
8. Nuclear Fast Red counterstain: 0.1 g of Nuclear Fast Red (Sigma) dissolved with heating and stirring in 5% aluminum sulfate. Cool and filter through Whatman no. 1 filter paper. Add one crystal of Thymol (Sigma). Store at room temperature.
9. Cytoseal 60 mounting media (cat. no. 48212-154; VWR Scientific).
10. CrystalMount (no. M02; Biomeda).
11. NBT stock: *see* **Subheading 2.2.3, item 11**.
12. BCIP stock: *see* **Subheading 2.2.3, item 12**.
13. McGadey reagent: *see* **Subheading 2.2.3, item 15**.
14. Pepsin (no. P7012; Sigma)
15. Xylene (histologic grade).
16. Absolute alcohol.
17. 95% Alcohol.
18. Avidin–alkaline phosphatase conjugate (Dako). Store at 4°C.
19. HPV Probe set: All probes are nick translated with biotin (*see* **Subheading 2.2.2**) and mixed in 1 mL of 45% formamide hybridization cocktail (Amresco). Store at –20°C. Other HPV probe mixtures or single HPV probes may be prepared as required. Final probe concentration is 1–1.5 µg/mL.
    a. HPV-6/11 probe: 0.5 µg each of biotinylated HPV-6 and HPV-11.
    b. HPV-16/18 probe: 0.5 µg each of biotinylated HPV-16 and HPV-18
    c. HPV-31/33/35 probe: 0.5 µg each of biotinylated HPV-31, HPV-33, and HPV-35.

20. Control probe set: All probes are nick translated with biotin (*see* **Subheading 2.2.2**) and mixed in 1 mL of 45% formamide hybridization cocktail (Amresco). Store at –20°C. Final probe concentration is 1 µg/mL.
    a. HG probe (endogenous positive control probe): 1.0 µg of biotinylated human placental DNA (Sigma).
    b. pBR probe (negative control probe): 1.0 µg of biotinylated pBR322 DNA (Gibco-BRL).

2.3. Equipment

2.3.1. L1 Consensus PCR Assay

1. Thermal cycler.
2. Horizontal gel electrophoresis apparatus.
3. UV transilluminator and camera for gel image documentation.
4. Heat block.
5. SpeedVac.
6. Microcentrifuge.
7. Bio-Dot Apparatus (cat. no. 170-6545; Bio-Rad, Hercules, CA).
8. UV crosslinker.
9. X-ray film developer.
10. Hybridization bags or roller bottles.

2.3.2. ISH Assay

1. MicroProbe Slide Stainer and accessories (reagent buckets, rubber and glass isolons, and blotting pads) or Fisher Codon Automated Slide Stainer (*see* **Fig. 1**).
2. TissueTek slide carrier, staining rack, and buckets.
3. Convection oven.
4. Water bath, 37°C, with test tube rack.

3. Methods

3.1. L1 Consensus PCR Assay Methods

3.1.1. Preparation of Samples: Formalin-Fixed Paraffin-Embedded Tissues

To monitor the histology of the lesion assayed in the PCR reaction, it is good practice to request that serial 5-µ sections be cut, with levels 1 and 4 mounted on a glass slide and stained with hematoxylin and eosin (H&E) and levels 2 and 3 combined into one sterile microcentrifuge tube for PCR analysis. To prevent carryover between cases, a new disposable microtome blade should be used for each case, and the sections for PCR analysis should be transferred from the microtome directly to the tube using sterile disposable sticks. Sections cut for PCR are stored at room temperature until ready for processing.

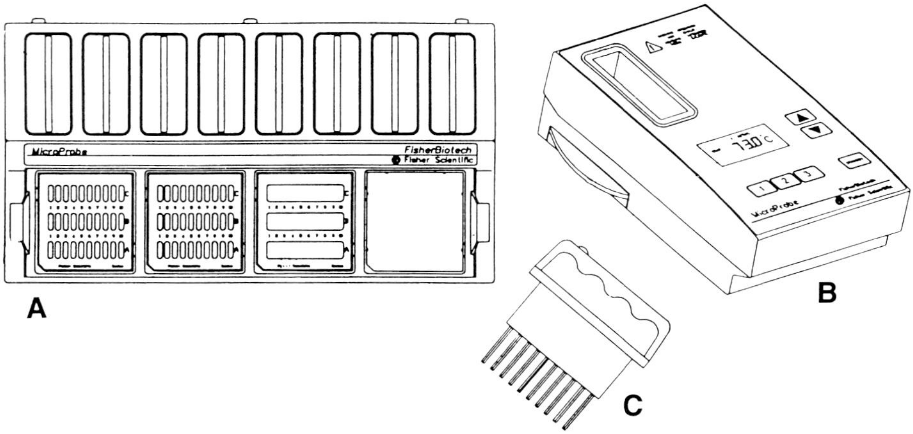

Fig. 1. Schematic drawing of **(A)** the MicroProbe system demonstrating the staining station, **(B)** programmable temperature-controlled incubation chamber, and **(C)** the slide holder. (From **ref. *17*** with permission.)

1. Add 1 mL of Pro-par clearant to each sample and incubate for 5 min at 55°C.
2. Centrifuge at 10,000*g* in a microfuge for 5 min at room temperature. Remove the Pro-par clearant and discard into an organic waste container. Repeat **steps 1** and **2** twice to remove all paraffin.
3. To remove traces of Pro-par clearant, wash the pellet twice with 1 mL of ethanol, followed by centrifugation at 10,000*g* in a microfuge for 5 min at room temperature.
4. Dry the pelleted cellular material briefly in a speed vac and resuspend in 200 µL of proteinase K buffer.
5. Place a lid-loc on each tube and incubate overnight in a heat block at 55°C. Inactivate the proteinase K by heating at 100°C for 10 min.
6. Store the samples at –20°C until ready for amplification. Prior to PCR, centrifuge each sample briefly to pellet any remaining cellular material. An aliquot (usually 5–10 µL) of the clarified sample is used in the amplification.

3.1.2. Preparation of Samples: Swabs or Cervicovaginal Lavage

1. Place cervical samples collected on dacron swabs or cytobrushes in 1 mL of collection fluid and transport to the laboratory. Briskly agitate or vortex the tubes for several minutes to dislodge material from the collection device. Press and swirl the swab or brush against the side of the tube to remove excess fluid. Discard the collection device into biohazard waste. Use a 100 µL aliquot of the fluid for DNA extraction and store the remainder at –20°C.
2. For cervical vaginal lavage samples, collect the cellular material by low-speed centrifugation. Discard the supernatant into biohazard waste. Resuspend the pellet at a 1 : 10 dilution (v/v) in PBS or a minimum volume of 450 µL. Use 100 µL for DNA extraction and store the remainder at –20°C.

3. Add 200 µL of proteinase K buffer to each 100-µL sample, mix, and digest for 1 h at 55°C in a heat block.
4. Transfer the digested samples to a Phase-Lock tube and add an equal volume of phenol : chloroform : isoamyl alcohol. Vortex to mix thoroughly and centrifuge at 10,000*g* for 10 min to separate the phases.
5. Transfer the aqueous (upper) phase containing the DNA to a clean sterile microfuge tube and add 2 vol of ice-cold 100% ethanol and 1/10 vol of 10 *M* ammonium acetate. Allow the DNA to precipitate at –20°C for at least 1 h. Pellet the DNA at 10,000*g* for 15 min in a microcentrifuge. Remove the alcohol supernatant and allow the pellets to air-dry briefly.
6. Resuspend the precipitated DNA in 100 µL of sterile distilled deionized water. Use 5–10 µL in the amplification reaction.

3.1.3. HPV L1 Consensus and β-Globin PCR

Excellent technique is required to avoid contamination of PCR samples and the possibility of false-positive results. At least three distinct sites within the laboratory should be used for the different steps of routine PCR. All surfaces should be thoroughly cleaned with a DNA contaminant removal solution. The initial PCR preparation including reagent master mixes is completed in the first location. Test samples are added in a second location (we routinely use a laminar flow hood without the airflow on and turn on the UV lamp when complete). Amplified samples are handled and analyzed in the third location. Each location should have a dedicated set of micropipettors, and sterile, disposable, aerosol block tips should be used. Finally, talking should be minimal when setting up the reactions.

A set of positive, negative, and contamination controls should be included for every 12 samples. For the HPV consensus PCR, an HPV-containing cell line such as SiHa or CaSki (both containing HPV-16, described in **Subheading 2.2.**) are good controls. Avoid the use of cloned HPV DNA unless used at a very high dilution, because the high copy number easily results in cross contamination of samples. Human placental DNA is used as the negative control. A tube that contains all the reagents, with water in place of the test sample, serves as the contamination control. Another important control performed on all samples in parallel with the HPV consensus PCR is a PCR that amplifies a normal gene such as β-globin. These reactions test for inhibitors or insufficient quantity of test sample.

1. Prepare a work sheet for the appropriate number of 50-µL reactions. (An example worksheet is shown in **Fig. 2**.)
2. At the designated setup location, label the lid of the PCR tube (0.5-mL Eppendorf tubes) with the sample number from the work sheet and the date.
3. Following the formula shown in **Table 2**, prepare two separate reagent master mixes in 1.5-mL Eppendorf tubes, one for the HPV primers and the other for the

HPV L1 Consensus PCR Worksheet

Date:

Samples:

1.________	7.________	13. CaSki
2.________	8.________	14. water
3.________	9.________	15. Placental DNA
4.________	10.________	
5.________	11.________	
6.________	12.________	

Consensus HPV Master Mix

Reagent	μL(X n xns) = tot μL	
10 X Buffer	5	___
25 mM $MgCl_2$	5	___
dNTPs (each)	1	___
50 μM MY09	0.5	___
50 μM MY11	0.5	___
1.25 U Taq	0.25	___
water	29.75	___

β-Globin Master Mix

Reagent	μL(X n rxns) = tot μL	
10 X Buffer	5	___
25 mM $MgCl_2$	5	___
dNTPs (each)	1	___
50 μM PC04	0.5	___
50 μM GH20	0.5	___
1.25 U Taq	0.25	___
water	29.75	___

Results:

Gel Lane	Sample ID	MY09/11	PC04/GH20	Comment
1,17				
2, 18				
3, 19				
4, 20				
5, 21				
6, 22				
7, 23				
8, 24				
9, 25				
10, 26				
11, 27				
12, 28				
13, 29	CaSki			
14, 30	water			
15, 31	placental DNA			

Fig. 2. An example worksheet for HPV L1 consensus PCR that allows calculation of reagent volumes, prompts inclusion of required controls, directs loading of agarose gel, and documents PCR results. A Polaroid photograph of the ethidium bromide (EtBr)–stained gel (*see* **Fig. 3**) should be attached to the worksheet.

Table 2
Master Mixes for 16 Reactions Each of MY09/MY11 and β-Globin Primer Sets

Components	Final concentration	Volume per reaction (μL)	Master mix (μL)	
			HPV	β-Globin
10X PCR buffer	1X	5	80	80
25 m*M* $MgCl_2$	2.5 m*M*	5	80	80
dNTP (each)	0.2 m*M*	1	16 (each)	16 (each)
50 μ*M* MY09	0.5 μ*M*	0.5	8	—
50 μ*M* MY11	0.5 μ*M*	0.5	8	—
50 μ*M* PC04	0.5 μ*M*	0.5	—	8
50 μ*M* GH20	0.5 μ*M*	0.5	—	8
Taq Polymerase	1.25 U	0.25	4	4
H_2O	—	29.75	476	476

globin primers (the calculations are based on 12 test samples, 3 control samples, plus one extra).

4. Dispense 45 μL of each master mix into the appropriate set of 0.5-mL microfuge tubes.
5. Add two drops of mineral oil to each tube. (This step can be omitted if the thermocycler has a condenser lid.)
6. Move to the designated area for handling patient samples. As directed on the worksheet, add 5 μL of each test DNA to the appropriate tubes Also add positive and negative control samples and water blank to the appropriate tubes. (The concentration of positive control DNA needs to be determined during optimization of the protocol so that the resulting product is clearly detectable but does not overwhelm the system, leading to cross contamination. We use 100 ng of CaSki DNA as the positive control sample.)
7. Tightly cap the tubes and mix gently. Place the samples in the thermocycler (should be located in a separate room) and program for the following thermocycling profile: hold at 95°C for 5 min then cycle with 94°C to denature for 1 min, ramp 10 s to 55°C to anneal for 1 min, ramp 10 s to 72°C to elongate for 1 min, ramp 10 s back to 94°C; repeat the cycle profile 30 times. Follow the 30 cycles with a "topping off" elongation step at 72°C for 5 min.
8. After amplification, take the sealed sample tubes to the location designated for analysis. Samples may be frozen at –20°C until needed.
9. Electrophorese 10 μL of each sample in a 1.5% agarose gel along with an appropriate marker. Stain briefly in an EtBr solution containing 1 mg/L EtBr.
10. Examine the stained gel on a UV transilluminator and photograph for documentation.

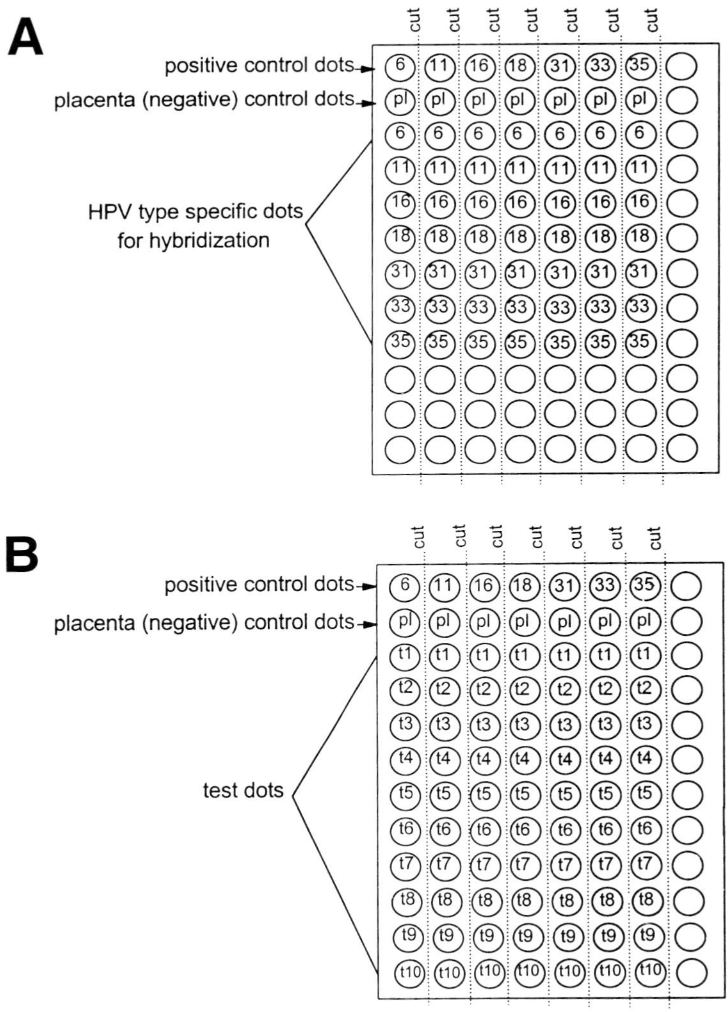

Fig. 3. Arrangement of dot-blot assay. The dot blot uses the 96-well format. **(A)** The dot blot for probe and hybridization optimization can be arranged as shown. **(B)** Template for evaluating test samples. Ten samples (t1–t10) can be placed on each strip. Each strip is hybridized with the probe corresponding to the positive control dot at the top of the strip.

3.1.4. Typing of HPV L1 Consensus Amplicons

The advantage of an HPV consensus reaction is that all (or most) types of HPV will yield a positive result; thus, one reaction may be used to determine whether a sample has HPV DNA. However, further testing is required to determine the type(s) of HPV in the sample. There are several different approaches for typing the amplicon, such as restriction fragment length polymorphism ***(14)***, single-strand conformation polymorphism ***(15)***, solid-phase or solution hybridization (SHARP Signal System, Digene Diagnostics) with either probe cocktails or single type-specific probes, and, finally, direct sequencing of the PCR product (Advanced Biotechnologies Inc.).

This section presents a solid-phase dot-blot hybridization assay with type-specific hybridization and chemiluminescent detection. This format permits detection of multiple types of HPV present in a single sample, and because of the chemiluminescent detection, it is highly sensitive. The limitation is that a separate hybridization must be performed for each type. The following sections include the protocols for synthesis of digoxigenin-11-dUTP-labeled HPV probes, synthesis of the HPV DNA positive control PCR products, preparation and hybridization of dot blots, and chemiluminescent detection.

At least one company is developing a simplified approach to typing L1 consensus PCR products. A reverse dot-blot format, called a line probe assay, has HPV type-specific DNA immobilized as lines on a plastic strip ***(16)***. The patient sample is amplified and labeled during the consensus PCR reaction (modified to include biotinylated primers). The labeled patient material is then directly hybridized to the strip to detect the types of HPV present in the assay.

3.1.5. Probe Labeling

To make HPV-specific probes, known HPV templates are amplified and labeled with MY09/MY11 primers using a modified nucleotide mix that includes digoxigenin-dUTP (DIG-dUTP). Include one PCR tube for each HPV DNA template, plus a negative control and no-template control reaction for every 10 tubes. The following procedure is designed for 100-µL reactions.

1. Add the components listed in **Table 3** to a sterile 0.5-mL microfuge tube.
2. Move to the designated location for addition of template and add 5 µL (100 ng) of the appropriate HPV DNA template to its respective tube.
3. Follow the PCR protocol outlined in **Subheading 3.1.3.**
4. Analyze 10 µL of each reaction by agarose gel electrophoresis and visualize the products after EtBr staining. The molecular size of the products will be considerably larger than 450 bp because of the DIG-dUTP incorporation.

Table 3
DIG-Labeled Probe Synthesis PCR Mix

Reagent	Final concentration	Volume per reaction (μL)
10X PCR buffer	1X	10
25 m*M* $MgCl_2$	2.5 m*M*	10
DIG dNTP mix	0.2 m*M*	10
50 μ*M* MY09	0.5 μ*M*	1
50 μ*M* MY11	0.5 μ*M*	1
Taq polymerase	2.5 U	0.5
H_2O	—	62.5
Total volume		100

5. After gel documentation, retain the gel. This gel is used to determine the efficiency of DIG-dUTP incorporation.
6. Blot DIG-labeled PCR products from the gel by downward capillary transfer to a positively charged nylon membrane using 20X SSC. Allow the transfer to proceed overnight.
7. After the transfer, rinse the membrane in 2X SSC and UV-crosslink the DNA to the membrane.
8. Detect the DIG-labeled probes (as described in **Subheading 3.1.7.**) to estimate the efficiency of the DIG-dUTP incorporation during the PCR.

3.1.6. Preparation and Hybridization of Amplicon Dot Blots

The sensitivity and specificity of the dot-blot assay using the DIG-labeled probes must be validated before testing patient samples. The assay optimization dot-blot format should include unlabeled HPV type-specific amplicons prepared from known HPV templates in the MY09/MY11 protocol. The optimized dot-blot assay should not allow cross hybridization between HPV types to be detected, and type-specific hybridization should be easily detected. **Figure 3A** gives an example of how to set up an optimization dot-blot assay.

1. Prepare the sample for alkaline transfer to the membrane. The sample is either 100 ng of control DNA (positive HPV type of control amplicons or negative control placental DNA) or 10 μL of test PCR reaction (unknown amplicons to be typed). Mix the sample with 10 μL of 10X denaturing solution and bring to a final volume of 100 μL with sterile ddH_2O. Incubate for 10 min at room temperature.
2. Wet the nylon membrane in a dish of water, and assemble the nylon membrane in the dot-blot apparatus according to the manufacturer's instructions.

3. Transfer the denatured DNA solution to the appropriate well in the assembled apparatus. Use gentle vacuum to suck the solution through the membrane. Turn the vacuum off after the solution is through to avoid drying the membrane.
4. Add 500 µL of 0.4 *M* NaOH to each well to rinse, and use gentle vacuum to suck the solution through the membrane.
5. While maintaining the vacuum, disassemble the apparatus and mark the columns with a waterproof ink pen for ease in cutting at a later point. Maintaining the vacuum allows the wells to be visualized as depressions.
6. After the membrane is marked, release the vacuum and remove the membrane. Rinse the membrane in 2X SSC and UV-crosslink the DNA to the membrane.
7. Use a ruler and pencil to draw a line between the columns of dots and cut the strips as illustrated in **Fig. 3A,B**. Each strip will be approx 0.5 × 15 cm.
8. Prehybridize the membranes for 1 h at 70°C with 2 mL of DIG-Easy Hyb per strip. The membrane strips can be hybridized in glass trays, small roller bottles, or hybridization bags, but care should be taken to ensure that the strips do not stick to one another.
9. Dilute each probe to a final concentration of 5 ng/mL of DIG-Easy Hyb, boil for 10 min, and place on ice.
10. Remove and discard the prehybridization fluid, and replace with the same volume of hybridization solution containing the probe. Hybridize overnight at 70°C.
11. Remove the hybridization solution and save at –20°C. (We have found that these probe solutions can be used at least one more time without significant loss of signal.)
12. Remove the strips from the hybridization vessel, and rinse in excess 2X SSC 0.1% SDS to remove adherent hybridization cocktail. Add the strips into a plastic dish containing 200 mL of 2X SSC and 0.1% SDS and wash twice for 5 min at room temperature with gentle rocking. All the strips can be put into the same container for washes.
13. Wash twice with 200 mL of 0.5X SSC and 0.1% SDS for 15 min each at 68°C with gentle rocking.
14. Proceed to the chemiluminescent detection (*see* **Subheading 3.1.7.**).

3.1.7. Chemiluminescent Detection

Chemiluminescent detection is extremely sensitive, but requires careful technique to keep the background reproducibly low. Membranes need to be handled gently with forceps. Gloves should be worn for all steps. The dishes used for washing, blocking, and detection steps should be rinsed with 0.1 *N* HCl, washed with a soap solution, and rinsed with water. The acid wash inactivates any "environmental" or carryover alkaline phosphatase that could contribute to high background. Several membranes may be handled in the same dish provided that they are not allowed to overlap (*see* **Note 2**).

1. Equilibrate the membrane in wash buffer (supplied in the DIG Wash and Block Buffer Set) for 1 min.

2. Transfer the membrane into a clean plastic dish and add sufficient blocking solution to soak and cover the membrane completely. Cover and incubate at 37°C for 30–60 min.
3. During the blocking step, prepare the conjugate. Centrifuge the tube of conjugate in a microcentrifuge at top speed for 5 min (this step pellets any aggregates that may have formed).
4. Dilute the conjugate 1 : 10,000 in blocking solution (i.e., 5 μL of anti-DIG-alkaline phosphatase in 50 mL of 1X blocking solution) and mix gently by inversion. Pour the conjugate solution into a "dedicated" conjugate dish (this will help minimize the alkaline phosphatase carryover). Make enough diluted conjugate to cover the membrane (e.g., a 10 × 14 cm nylon membrane requires about 50 mL of diluted conjugate).
5. Drain the blocking solution from the membrane and transfer the membrane to the dish with diluted conjugate solution. Ensure that the membrane is covered evenly with conjugate, cover the dish, and incubate at 37°C for 30 min.
6. Pour off the conjugate solution from the membrane and rinse the membrane with wash buffer. Transfer the membrane to a fresh dish, and wash twice in 200 mL of wash buffer at room temperature with gentle agitation, 15 min each wash.
7. Drain the final wash and transfer the membrane to a fresh dish with detection buffer. Equilibrate for 5 min at room temperature.
8. Prepare 10 mL of a 1 : 100 dilution of CDP-Star in detection buffer.
9. Drain the detection buffer, add the 1 : 100 CDP-Star (chemiluminescent substrate for alkaline phosphatase), and incubate for 5 min at room temperature.
10. Remove the membrane from the CDP-Star, and blot off excess CDP-Star by sandwiching the membrane between blot paper.
11. Place the membrane into a plastic bag and expose to film. It is likely that a 1-min exposure or shorter will be sufficient to determine the efficiency of DIG-dUTP incorporation during the probe synthesis. Longer times will be required for detection of dot-blot results.

3.1.8. Interpretation of L1 Consensus PCR Assay

All samples, except the water blank (contamination control), should amplify the 286-bp region of β-globin and the DNA product of that size should be visible in each lane. The HPV positive control should amplify the 450-bp HPV consensus product, and the negative control (human placental DNA) should not produce any product. If the positive and negative controls give the expected results, the assay may interpreted. Test samples that amplify β-globin and have no HPV product visible are considered HPV negative. Those with an HPV product are considered HPV positive, whether or not β-globin is amplified. Test samples failing to amplify both β-globin and HPV cannot be interpreted. These samples require further optimization or purification as described in **Notes 3–6**. **Figure 4** is a photograph of an EtBr-stained gel and shows the results of an HPV consensus and β-globin PCR.

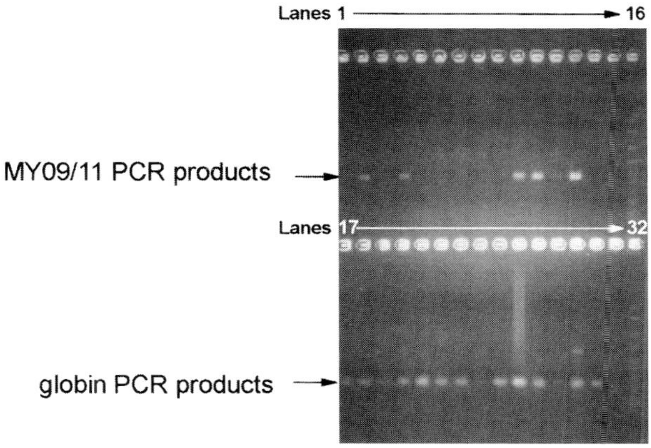

Fig. 4. EtBr gel. Ten microliters of each PCR product is analyzed by gel electrophoresis. The MY09/MY11 products are in the top half of the gel, and the corresponding β-globin PCR product for each sample is in the bottom half of the gel. Samples are placed to correspond to the worksheet. Lanes 1–12 and 17–28 are clinical samples. Lanes 13 and 29 are amplimers from Caski DNA, lanes 14 and 30 are amplimers from placental DNA, and lanes 15 and 31 are water in place of DNA template. Lanes 16 and 32 contain molecular size markers. In this example, HPV-positive products are visible in samples 2, 4, 10, 11, 12, as well as in the Caski control (lane 13). The water blank is negative. All samples have amplifiable DNA except sample 8 (lane 24).

3.1.9. Interpretation of Typing of HPV Consensus Amplicons

After chemiluminescent detection, the dot-blot optimization experiment should result in specific hybridization to the positive control position dots and to the HPV type-specific dot in the column (**Fig. 5**). There should be no hybridization signal detected in the negative control and little to no cross hybridization to the other types of HPV. If conditions are satisfactory, dot blots can be made for testing clinical samples using template as shown in **Fig. 3B**.

3.2. ISH Methods

3.2.1. Preparation of Cell Block

1. Harvest cells and wash two times with D-PBS. Check cell viability and adjust cell concentration to 5×10^6 cells/mL by resuspending in 10% neutral buffered formalin.
2. Allow the cell suspension to fix at room temperature for 1 h.
3. Using a labeling pencil, label the cassette with the name of the cell line, block number, and year. Place one piece of Histowrap with each cassette.

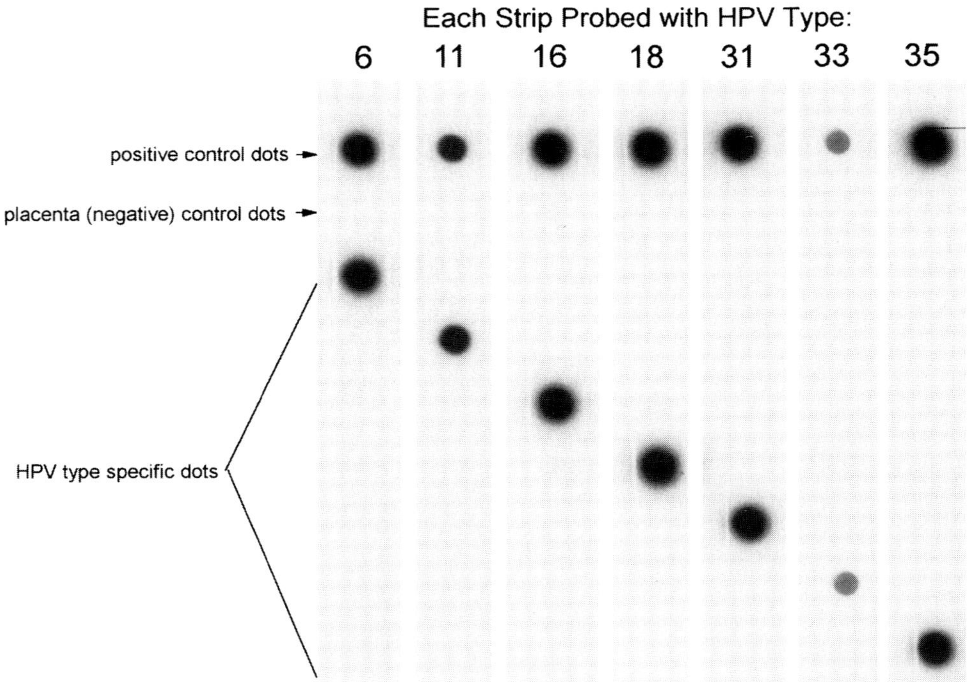

Fig. 5. Chemiluminescent detection of digoxigenin-labeled HPV probes hybridized to strips dotted with specific types of HPV. The format of the strips is exactly as shown in **Fig. 3A** (i.e., 9 dots per strip). There is no cross hybridization between types of HPV. This result indicates satisfactory optimization of probe labeling and hybridization conditions.

4. Near the end of the fixation period, prepare collodion bags in a chemical fume hood. Completely fill a clean 15-mL glass conical centrifuge tube with undiluted collodion. Immediately pour the collodion back into the reagent bottle, rotating the tube while pouring (collodion is reusable). Place the tube upside down in the test tube rack and allow to dry approx 10–15 min. Touch the inside of the tube to determine whether the bag is dry. Once prepared, the bag must be used within 10 min.
5. Pour the formalin-cell suspension into the bag and obtain the pellet by centrifuging for 5 min at 400–500*g* in a tabletop centrifuge.
6. Carefully decant the supernatant. Remove the bag from the tube by cutting around the top edge with sharp-nosed tweezers. Twist the bag gently using the tweezers and carefully lift and pull the bag away from the bottom of the tube.
7. Cut off the excess bag and fold down the top of the bag close to the surface of the pellet.

8. Place the folded bag in the center of the Histowrap. Wrap the Histowrap around the pellet and bag to form a closed envelope. Place the wrapped pellet in the cassette and close the lid.
9. Place the cassette in a 10% formalin container and take to the histology laboratory for processing into paraffin block.

3.2.2. Probe Labeling

1. On ice, thaw the DNA to be labeled, Bio-11-dUTP, and one aliquot each of nucleotide buffer solution and DNase activation buffer.
2. Prepare an appropriate dilution of DNase I. (Lot-to-lot variation will require adjustment of this dilution, but a final dilution of 80 pg/µL is a good starting point.) Remove the DNase I from the freezer and place on ice. Using a sterile micropipet tip, remove 2 µL and place in a sterile microcentrifuge tube. Replace the DNase I stock solution into the freezer. Add 250 µL of DNase activation buffer to the 2-µL aliquot and mix gently. Transfer 2 µL of this dilution to a fresh sterile tube using a clean sterile micropiet tip. Add 200 µL of DNase activation buffer and mix gently. This last tube is the working dilution of DNase I. Discard the other tubes.
3. For each DNA to be labeled, calculate the volume that equals 1 µg. Label one sterile microcentrifuge tube for each reaction with identification of DNA, date, and concentration and place on ice.
4. To the labeled tubes on ice add the following: 1–2 µL of diluted DNase I, __ µL of DNA to be labeled (volume to equal 1 µg), 10.0 µL of nucleotide buffer solution, 1.0 µL of Bio-11-dUTP, 5.0 µL of DNA Polymerase I/DNase I mixture, and __ µL of sterile distilled water (to yield a final reaction volume of 50 µL). Return the enzymes and Bio-11-dUTP to the freezer.
5. Close the lids of the tubes and mix gently. Briefly centrifuge to concentrate the reagents in the bottom of the tube. Incubate in a 14°C ice/water bath for 1 h and 15 min.
6. Stop the reaction by transferring the tubes to a 70°C water bath for 10 min. Store the labeled probes at –20°C until size and incorporation of label is verified (*see* **Subheading 3.2.3.**). Once the size is verified, add 5 µL of EDTA solution to each 50-µL reaction and mix. Probes are stable at –20°C for at least 2 yr.

3.2.3. Verification of Probe Size and Labeling

Alkaline gel electrophoresis of nick-translated probes, followed by transfer to nitrocellulose membrane and colorimetric detection, allows monitoring of the incorporation of label and evaluation of the final size of the products. For efficient tissue penetration, probes should be less than 300 bases. Because of the strong alkaline environment, this procedure will not work for probes with alkali-labile linkages of the affinity label.

1. Prepare a 2% agarose gel in 1X gel buffer in a minihorizontal gel electrophoresis apparatus. Fill the buffer reservoirs and cover the gel with 1X running buffer.

2. For each sample, label a microcentrifuge tube and add 7 μL of 1X running buffer, 1 μL of Ficoll dye solution and 1–3 μL of DNA (6–180 ng). Treat end-labeled markers as sample. Mix and briefly centrifuge to collect liquid.
3. Run electrophoresis at 25 V for about 20 min to allow the samples to enter the gel. Then increase to 75 V and run until the bromophenol blue dye front is about three fourths of the way down the gel (approx 2.5 h).
4. Soak the gel in neutralization solution until the pH is <9.0. Monitor the pH of the gel by touching the surface with pH paper. Neutralization will require about four changes of 30 mL of buffer, 10 min/change. Rinse the gel in ddH_2O.
5. Set up Southern blot with nitrocellulose filter using 20X SSC. Blot at room temperature for 2 h. (Overnight blotting can be done if more convenient.)
6. Wash the filter in 2X SSC for 5 min, air-dry, and UV-crosslink (Stratalinker). Bake in an 80°C oven between filter paper for 1 h to overnight (at this point the filter may be stored in the refrigerator).
7. Float the nitrocellulose membrane in a clean plastic tray filled with 1% BSA/TS Brij 7.5. Once the membrane is wet, incubate with 1% BSA/TS Brij 7.5 for 10–30 min in a 37°C water bath.
8. Add 40 μL of avidin-alkaline phosphatase conjugate to 20 mL of 1% BSA/TS Brij 7.5 and mix gently. Using forceps, transfer the nitrocellulose to a fresh plastic dish and cover with diluted conjugate. Incubate at room temperature for 10 min.
9. Remove the filter from the conjugate and transfer to a clean plastic dish with TS Brij 7.5. Wash the nitrocellulose filter four times in TS Brij 7.5, 3 min/wash.
10. Wash the filter in TS Brij 9.5 and transfer the membrane to a clean plastic dish with McGadey reagent. Incubate at 37°C until the signal reaches the desired intensity. Remove the nitrocellulose, rinse in water, and air-dry. Keep the membrane as a record of the results.

3.2.4. ISH Assay

Formalin-fixed paraffin-embedded tissue sections for ISH should be cut at 5 μm and mounted from a protein-free tap water histobath on silanized or positively charged glass (such as Fisher Plus). Tissue should be mounted within 0.2 mm of the end of the slide opposite the label. Slides are air-dried and stored unmelted in a clean dust-free box until ready for use (*see* **Note 7**).

1. Select test and control slides for the assay: five slides of each specimen and control are required for the complete probe set (HPV-6/11, HPV-16/18, HPV-31/33/35, positive control [HG], negative control [pBR322]). Complete the work sheet (*see* **Fig. 6**) with the proper pairing of slides to ensure that each tissue is matched with respect to the digestion conditions and probe that will be used. Label the frosted or painted end of each slide with alcohol/xylene stable marker, identifying the position it occupies in the MicroProbe slide holder and verify that the work sheet matches this position.

MicroProbe Worksheet

Date________________________ **Technologist** ____________________________________

Hybridization Protocol ____________________________

Probes: (types and lot numbers)____

Comments:

Position	Slide ID	Digestion	Probe
1			
2			
3			
4			
5			
6			
7			
8			
9			
10			

Fig. 6. An example ISH work sheet that allows for appropriate pairing of slides to receive the same reagents, and directing of appropriate placement of digestion reagent and probes for each slide. Positions of the holder correspond to positions in the isolons (individual wells) in the staining station of the MicroProbe system.

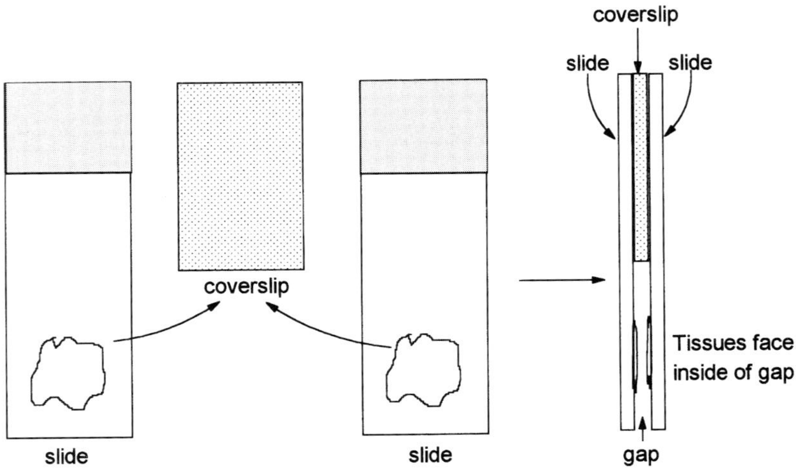

Fig. 7. Placement of slides to produce capillary gap. A "sandwich" is made using two slides and a no. 2 cover slip. The cover slip keeps a narrow gap between the slides. Slides are placed so that the tissues face the inside of the gap. The gap will draw fluid up to cover the inside surface of the glass. Fluid is removed from the gap by blotting onto absorbent material (pad).

2. Place the test and control slides vertically (label at top, tissue at bottom) in a TissueTek slide carrier and place the carrier upright in a 65–80°C convection oven. Allow the slides to melt a minimum of 20 min. Air-dry the slides in the carrier under the chemical fume hood.
3. Prepare a Tissue-Tek staining rack under the chemical fume hood for dewaxing of slides. Fill three green solvent-resistant buckets with fresh xylene and two white buckets with fresh absolute alcohol. Dewax the slides in TissueTek slide carrier at room temperature. Perform three 10-min incubations in xylene and two 5-min incubations in absolute alcohol. Remove the slide carrier and slides from the last alcohol wash and air-dry under the fume hood. Discard the xylene in a xylene waste container (*see* **Notes 8–9**).
4. Match up the slide position number on the slide with the position on the work sheet. Form capillary gaps with slide pairs and a 40 × 22 mm no. 2 cover slip by sandwiching the cover slip between the frosted (label) ends of the slides with the tissues facing each other (**Fig. 7**). Load the slides into the proper position in the MicroProbe slide holder. Make sure the slide pairs are flush against the base of the holder.
5. Add water to the reservoir of the incubator and set the temperature to 37°C. Fill the MicroProbe reagent buckets with appropriate buffers as designated on the work sheet. Insert the reagent isolons and blotting pad in the MicroProbe workstation.

6. Prepare the digestion reagent. Weigh 8 mg of pepsin and transfer into a clean test tube. Add 2 mL of 0.01 *N* HCl/Brij (final concentration of 4 mg/mL). The digestion reagent should be made up fresh prior to each run and placed in a 37°C water bath for 15 min to ensure that the enzyme has dissolved. Make less concentrated solutions of digestion reagent as needed by dilution with 0.01 *N* HCl/Brij. Digestion reagent is varied empirically to achieve optimal signal with endogenous positive control probe. Suggested starting concentrations are as follows: 4 mg/mL for cell blocks, 2 mg/mL for biopsy tissue, 3 mg/mL for surgical resection, 4 mg/mL for autopsy tissue.
7. Fill the reagent isolons with the appropriate concentration of protease. Isolons may be filled with a transfer pipet; approximately 200 μL is required for each position. The position of the well determines which slide pair will receive the reagent. Verify reagent placement by consulting the work sheet.
8. Wash the slides with 95% alcohol, by placing the holder in the reagent bucket with 95% alcohol and allowing the reagent to completely fill the gaps between the slides by capillary action (*see* **Note 10**). Remove the holder and transfer to a blotting pad to remove the reagent from the gaps by absorption of fluid. Make sure the entire surface of each tissue is covered with each reagent at each step of the assay and that the blotting steps completely drain each capillary gap. This cycle of reagent pickup and removal by capillary action is repeated throughout the assay. The term *gap* refers to the capillary gap between the slides. Washing the gaps, or adding reagent to the gaps, is synonymous with adding reagent or washing the tissues on the slides.
9. Wash the gaps with ddH_2O Brij and blot. Pick up the digestion reagent from the isolon, aligning the well and slide gaps. Transfer the holder to a 37°C incubator. Set the timer for 30 min.
10. While the slides are in the digestion step, remove the probe set from the freezer and allow them to reach room temperature.
11. Fill the appropriate wells of the glass isolon with 155 μL of probe, as indicated on the work sheet.
12. At the end of 30 min of digestion, remove the holder and change the temperature of the incubator to 105°C. Blot to remove protease reagent and wash the gaps four times with TS Brij 7.5. For each wash, allow the reagent to cover the area of gap briefly and then blot to completely remove all the reagent.
13. Wash the gaps twice with 95% alcohol and twice with 100% alcohol. Allow the gaps to air-dry briefly.
14. Pick up the probe from the glass isolon. Make sure the holder and isolon are properly aligned so that each gap receives the appropriate reagent. The probe enters the gap slowly because of the viscosity of the hybridization cocktail. Watch carefully during this process to be sure that the probes do not mix. Make sure each capillary gap is filled at least 2 mm above the height of each tissue. Add additional probe if needed.
15. After the incubator has reached 105°C, transfer the holder to the incubator and set the timer for 20 min. After 20 min, change the incubator temperature to 37°C.

Add water to the reservoir to ensure that the chamber is moist, and let the slides hybridize for 2 h.

16. After the hybridization time is complete, remove the holder from the incubator and change the incubator temperature to 42°C. Remove the cocktail from the gaps by blotting. The solution is usually difficult to remove, so after some has come out in the blotting pad, transfer the slides to 2X SSC SDS/Brij to dilute the cocktail. Repeat this procedure several times until the gaps are completely emptied of cocktail. Then start stringency washes.
17. Wash the gaps three times with 2X SSC SDS/Brij and three times with 0.2X SSC SDS/Brij. Pick up the 0.1X SSC SDS/Brij and transfer the holder to the incubator for 5 min (42°C). Repeat three times. Change the incubator temperature to 37°C.
18. Fill the gaps with blocking reagent and remove by blotting. Repeat addition of block to the gaps and transfer the holder to the incubator (37°C) for 5 min.
19. Make up the detection reagent using a 1:400 dilution of Dako avidin-alkaline phosphatase in 1% BSA TS7.5/Brij. Fill each isolon well with 200 µL of the diluted detection reagent.
20. Remove the block by blotting and pick up the conjugate. Transfer the holder to the incubator (37°C) for 20 min.
21. Remove the conjugate by blotting and wash the gaps four times with TS Brij 7.5 and then twice with TS Brij 9.5.
22. Fill two reagent wells with 5 mL of freshly prepared McGadey reagent.
23. Wash the gaps with McGadey reagent and blot. Then refill the gaps with McGadey reagent and transfer the holder to incubator (37°C) for 1 h.
24. Toward the end of the incubation, fill the reagent isolons with approx 200 µL of Nuclear Fast Red counterstain.
25. At the end of incubation, remove the McGadey reagent by blotting and wash the gaps twice with TS Brij 7.5 and three times with ddH$_2$O Brij.
26. Fill the gaps with stain and keep in place for 2 min. Then remove the stain by blotting and wash the gaps twice with ddH$_2$O Brij.
27. Carefully remove the slides from the holder and place them flat, tissue side up, on a metal tray. Put a small thin layer of CrystalMount over each tissue section and bake for 10 min at 60°C, to harden the CrystalMount. (Alternatively, the slides can be air-dried overnight.) Allow the slides to cool to room temperature and cover slip each tissue with Cytoseal 60.
27. Label the slides with the date and the type of probe. Review the slides with the pathologist and record the quality control data.

3.2.5. Interpretation of ISH

3.2.5.1. Probe Labeling and Verification

Color development should result in dark purple where biotinylated DNA is localized. DNA in the marker lane should be visible as distinct bands with good resolution. If the DNA ladder is not resolved, the procedure must be repeated.

Nick-translated probes appear as a smear in the lane as the probes are randomly sized. To be acceptable for use, the probe should be less than 300 bases and average about 200 bases. Probes that are not clearly visible after this process or that are too large cannot be used. If probes are too large, attempts can be made to renick them by incubation with DNase. Once probe size is verified, EDTA is added to stabilize the probes and inhibit any residual DNase. If EDTA is added prior to verifying the size, renicking cannot be achieved because of inhibition of DNase by EDTA.

3.2.5.2. *In Situ* Hybridization

The control blocks Caski and Hela should be positive with HPV 16/18 and negative with the other probe groups. SiHa cells are at the limit of sensitivity of the assay and should be weakly positive with HPV 16/18. Assays in which Caski or Hela controls do not give appropriate results must be repeated. A negative result with SiHa is acceptable but indicates that one or more components of the assay could be failing.

The positive control probe (human placental DNA; HG) demonstrates whether the assay conditions allow hybridization of DNA in the test tissue. Tissues hybridized with the HG probe should have an even dark blue-black signal over every nucleus. Hybridization with the negative control probe (pBR322) should result in no detectable signal. If these two conditions are met, the hybridization with the HPV probes may be interpreted (**Fig. 8**). Signal with the HPV probe is seen as blue-black primarily over the nuclei of infected cells containing the target DNA. Some samples may demonstrate reaction with more than one group of HPV probes. This is most often owing to cross hybridization among the probe groups, and the sample should be typed as the group giving the strongest signal. In some instances, the intensity of multiple probe groups is identical, indicating the presence of more than one type of HPV. The assay may be repeated with more stringent washes if the type of HPV is questionable.

The ISH assay must be interpreted within the context of the histologic lesion and the clinical setting. It is not intended to replace routine histopathologic diagnosis, but to provide additional information in a manner analogous to immunohistochemical assays. Interpretation must be made by a pathologist. The H&E slide of the original lesion must be reviewed by the pathologist to verify that the recut sections assayed by ISH are representative of the lesion.

4. Notes

1. This protocol uses a final $MgCl_2$ concentration of 2.5 m*M*, found to be optimal for the HPV MY09/MY11 consensus PCR in our hands. The optimal $MgCl_2$ concentration may vary depending on the primer synthesis and should be tested by assaying control samples with low (1.5 m*M*), moderate (2.5–3.5 m*M*), and high (5 m*M*) $MgCl_2$ concentrations.

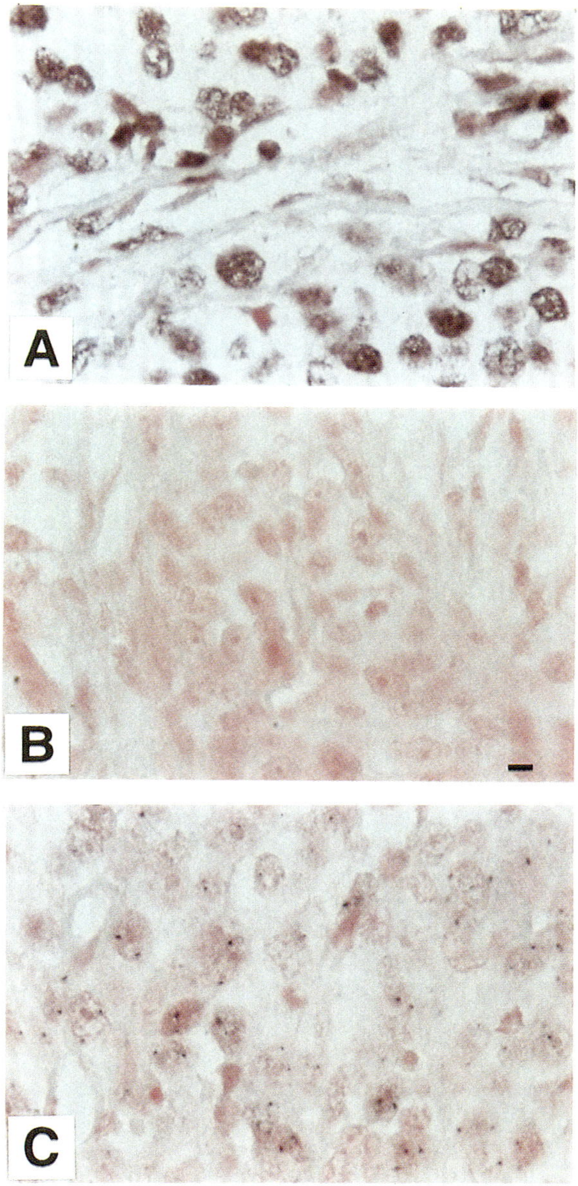

Fig. 8. Appropriate controls for ISH. Probe labeling, hybridization and detection are as described in the text. Results are for serial sections of the same tissue (nuclear fast red counterstain, BCIP/NBT substrate, bar = 5 μm). **(A)** Human placental DNA. The positive control probe results in a dark even signal over all nuclei, indicating that the tissue DNA is preserved and that tissue is adequately treated to allow hybridization **(B)** pBR322. The negative control probe shows no signal, indicating no apparent problems with nonspecific reactions of probe and detection reagents. **(C)** HPV probe. Results can be interpreted as indicative of HPV. (Modified from **ref. *3*** with permission.)

2. Boehringer Mannheim's guide to the use of digoxigenin affinity labels in filter hybridizations includes an extensive trouble-shooting guide.
3. Patient samples that fail to amplify globin may have insufficient intact DNA, may require a different $MgCl_2$ concentration, or may contain an inhibitor of the *Taq* polymerase. Adjusting the input DNA by increasing or decreasing the sample volume, or varying the $MgCl_2$ concentration, may result in successful amplification.
4. The heme component of blood is a potent inhibitor of *Taq* polymerase. Visible blood in clinical samples should be recorded in the notes during purification, because failure to amplify the globin control in these samples may be owing to residual heme. Although the digestion and extraction of DNA described in **Subheadings 3.1.1.** and **3.1.2.** is frequently sufficient for DNA amplification, occasionally further steps must be taken to remove blood components. Several commercially available DNA purification kits are effective in purifying DNA from blood or blood-containing samples (e.g., from QIAGEN, Santa Clarita, CA). Alternatively, hydrogen peroxide treatment of blood-containing samples has been shown to be effective in decomposing the heme compound ***(17)***.
5. Degradation of template DNA can affect amplification of larger amplicons. The 450-base MY09/MY11 amplicon is nearing the size limit of 500 bp recommended for formalin-fixed paraffin-embedded archival tissues. If degradation of sample DNA is a problem, other HPV consensus primers that amplify smaller fragments may be tried; for example, the GP5+-GP6+ amplifies a 155-bp region of HPV DNA ***(6)***.
6. Contamination is detected when the "no template reaction" has an amplicon. The fastest remedy is to discard all open reagents and begin again with fresh reagents. All PCR locations should be thoroughly cleaned with a DNA contaminant-removal solution, such as DNA Erase. The exterior of all micropipets should be wiped with a DNA contaminant-removal solution and exposed to UV light for 15 min on each side.
7. The importance of good histologic sectioning is often overlooked. Sections must be of uniform thickness without folds or tears, and the thickness must be uniform from section to section to allow even and reproducible penetration of reagents. Tissue adherence to glass is also crucial. Conditions for the hybridization assay are drastic, and the loss of tissue may occur during the assay if steps are not taken to improve tissue adherence. Treatment of the glass slides with 3-aminopropyltriethoxysilane has largely replaced other techniques such as coating the glass with poly-L-lysine or glue. When tissue sections are cut and floated on a protein-free tap water bath, the silane-treated glass will form a covalent bond with the tissue section. This "silanized glass" is available commercially and greatly minimizes the problem of tissue adherence. The quality of silanization may be monitored by the behavior of tissue sections during cutting. If the glass is properly treated, the tissue will not be able to be "refloated" or moved around on the slide once it has been lifted from the surface of the water. Difficulties with the procedure can be attributed to poorly treated glass, dirty glass, or protein in the

Table 4
Controls for ISH[a]

Control	Requirement	Purpose
Positive control tissue (handle as additional tissue sample)	1. Processed in manner identical to test tissue. 2. Known to contain target that hybridizes to test probe.	Positive results verify reaction of probe and detection reagents.
Positive control probe (use on each tissue)	1. Hybridizes with a target present in all tissues. 2. Labeled in similar manner to test probe and used at similar concentration.	Positive result verifies preservation of nucleic acid and availability to probe.
Negative control probe (use on each tissue)	1. Probe of similar base pair composition to test probe that should not hybridize to test and control tissues. 2. Labeled in similar manner to test probe and used at similar concentration.	Negative results monitor specificity of hybridization and detection.

[a]Modified from **ref.** ***18***. Used with permission.

water bath. Once the section is picked up on the microscope slide, the slide is placed vertically and allowed to air-dry. The paraffin should be retained on the section (i.e., section not melted) until just before the assay is begun.

8. The paraffin must be completely removed for efficient reagent penetration. Xylene is the most efficient clearing agent, but xylene substitutes may be used if care is taken to ensure that dewaxing steps are efficient. Several changes of dewaxing agents are recommended. Deparaffinization conditions that are satisfactory for routine staining may not be adequate for ISH. Overtreatment with dewaxing agents has not been observed.
9. Ideally, the time and temperature of fixation should be standardized and when processing to the paraffin block fresh reagents should be used. These ideal conditions are seldom met. Significant variations in fixation and processing that dramatically influence nucleic acid preservation may go unnoticed by standard light microscopic examination. Until histology laboratories develop methods to ensure standardization of fixation and processing, ISH assays on diagnostic samples must include controls that will detect and adjust for variations in tissue preservation. The purpose of controls is to ensure that tissues without signal are devoid of the target nucleic acid and that tissues with signal do contain the target. Interpretation of a precipitated product as evidence of a particular nucleic acid

sequence requires that all other explanations be eliminated. Controls also allow problems in any assay to be detected so that appropriate corrective measures can be instituted. There are many different kinds of controls that can be included, but the three essential controls are listed in **Table 4**. These three are the minimum required by the College of American Pathologists' Checklist for Molecular Pathology.

10. Brij 35 is added to most buffers used in the ISH protocol to lower surface tension and improve flow through the capillary gap. Flow of reagents must be efficient. Occasional variations in glass thickness or the use of a cover slip of different thickness may cause problems with flow. When slides are first assembled in the holder, flow of the reagent should be evaluated for each slide pair. Readjusting the position of the slide or changing the cover slip usually corrects problems with flow.

Acknowledgments

We gratefully acknowledge Donna L. Miller and Daisy R. Lee for their expert technical contributions to standardization of the protocols.

References

1. Schiffman, M. H. and Burk, R. D. (1998) Human papillomaviruses, in *Viral Infections of Humans: Epidemiology and Control*, 4th ed. (Evans, A. S. and Kaslow, R. A., eds.), Plenum, New York, pp. 983–1022.
2. Jenkins, D., Sherlaw-Johnson, C., and Gallivan, S. (1998) Assessing the role of HPV testing in cervical cancer screening. *Papillomavirus Rep.* **9,** 89–101.
3. Unger, E. R., Vernon, S. D., Lee, D. R., Miller, D. L., and Reeves, W. C. (1998) Detection of human papillomavirus in archival tissues: comparison of in situ hybridization and polymerase chain reaction. *J. Histochem. Cytochem.* **46,** 535–540.
4. De Villiers, E. M. (1994) Human pathogenic papillomaviruses: an update. *Curr. Top. Microbiol. Immunol.* **186,** 1–12.
5. Ting, Y. and Manos, M. (1990) Detection and typing of genital human papillomaviruses, in *PCR Protocols: A Guide to Methods and Applications* (Innis, M. A., Gelfand, D. H., Sninsky, J. J., and White, T. J., eds.), Academic, New York, pp. 356–367.
6. De Roda Husman, A. M., Walboomers, J. M., Van Den Brule, A. J. C., Meijer, C. J., and Snijders, P. J. (1995) The use of general primers GP5 and GP6 elongated at their 3′ ends with adjacent highly conserved sequences improves human papillomavirus detection by PCR. *J. Gen. Virol.* **76,** 1057–1062.
7. Qu, W., Jiang, G., Yvette, C., Chang, C. J., Ho, G. Y. F., Klein, R. S., and Burk, R. D. (1997) PCR detection of human papillomavirus: comparison between MY09/MY11 and GP5+/GP6+ primer systems. *J. Clin. Microbiol.* **35,** 1304–1310.
8. Zehbe, I. and Wilander, E. (1996) Two consensus primer systems and nested polymerase chain reaction for human papillomavirus detection in cervical biopsies: a study of sensitivity. *Hum. Pathol.* **27,** 812–815.

9. Baay, M., Quint, W., Koudstaal, J., Hollema, H., Duk, J. M., Burger, M., Stolz, E., and Herbrink, P. (1996) Comprehensive study of several general and type-specific primer pairs for detection of human papillomavirus DNA by PCR in paraffin-embedded cervical carcinomas. *J. Clin. Microbiol.* **34,** 745–747.
10. Cooper, K., Herrington, C. S., Strickland, J. E., Evans, M. F., and McGee, J. O. (1991) Episomal and integrated human papillomavirus in cervical neoplasia shown by non-isotopic in situ hybridization. *J. Clin. Pathol.* **44,** 990–996.
11. Unger, E. R., Hammer, M. L., and Chenggis, M. L. (1991) Comparison of ^{35}S and biotin labels for in-situ hybridization: use of an HPV model system. *J. Histochem. Cytochem.* **39,** 145–150.
12. Unger, E. R., Brigati, D. J., Chenggis, M. L., Budgeon, L. R., Koebler, D., Cuomo, C., and Kennedy, T. (1988) Automation of in-situ hybridization: application of the capillary action robotic workstation. *J. Histotechnol.* **11,** 253–258.
13. Chenggis, M. L. and Unger, E. R. (1993) Application of a manual capillary action workstation to colorimetric in-situ hybridization. *J. Histotechnol.* **16,** 33–38.
14. Lungu, O., Wright, T. C., and Silverstein, S. (1992) Typing of human papillomaviruses by polymerase chain reaction amplification with L1 consensus primers and RFLP analysis. *Mol. Cell. Probes* **6,** 145–152.
15. Rubben, A., Traidl, C., Baron, J. M., and Grussendorf-Conen, E. I. (1995) Evaluation of non-radioactive temperature gradient SSCP analysis and of temperature gradient gel electrophoresis for the detection of HPV 6-variants in condylomata acuminata and Buschke-Loewenstein tumors. *Eur. J. Epidemiol.* **11,** 501–506.
16. Gravitt, P. E., Peyton, C. L., Apple, R. J., and Wheeler, C. M. (1998) Genotyping of 27 human papillomavirus types by using L1 consensus PCR products by a single-hybridization, reverse line blot detection method. *J. Clin. Microbiol.* **36,** 3020–3027.
17. Akane, A. (1996) Hydrogen peroxide decomposes the heme compound in forensic specimens and improves the efficiency of PCR. *Biotechniques* **21,** 392–394.
18. Unger, E. R. and Lee, D. R. (1995) In situ hybridization: principles and diagnostic applications in infection. *J. Histotechnol.* **18,** 203–209.

22

Molecular Methods for Detecting Epstein-Barr Virus (Part I)

In Situ *Hybridization to Epstein-Barr Virus–Encoded RNA (EBER) Transcripts*

Hongxin Fan and Margaret L. Gulley

1. Introduction

In situ hybridization (ISH) to Epstein-Barr virus (EBV)–encoded RNA (EBER) is considered the "gold standard" for detecting and localizing latent EBV in biopsy samples. Transcripts from the EBER1 and EBER2 genes are an appropriate target because they are the most abundant viral RNA in latently infected cells, exceeding 1 million transcripts per cell. Furthermore, EBERs are consistently expressed in virtually all EBV-infected tumors and in the lymphoid tissues of infectious mononucleosis ***(1–5)***. As a result, EBERs represent a naturally amplified target for detecting and localizing latent EBV in histologic samples. The only EBV-related disorder in which EBER is consistently absent is oral hairy leukoplakia, an infection of squamous epithelial cells in which the virus undergoes lytic viral replication rather than latent infection ***(6)***.

EBER ISH relies on the use of riboprobes ***(7,8)***, oligonucleotide probes ***(9)***, or peptide nucleic acid probes (Dako, Carpinteria, CA) to identify EBER1 or EBER2 transcripts in histologic samples. Even though EBER transcripts are abundantly expressed, these and other species of RNA are subject to degradation by ubiquitous RNase enzymes, potentially causing loss of signal in all or part of the tissue. To avoid false-negative EBER results, and to properly interpret the morphologic and cytologic distribution of EBER in human tissues, it is imperative that a control stain be run alongside every EBER stain to ensure that RNA is preserved and available for hybridization. Some investigators

From: *Methods in Molecular Medicine, vol. 49: Molecular Pathology Protocols*
Edited by: A. A. Killeen © Humana Press Inc., Totowa, NJ

target poly-A tails of mRNA as a control, whereas others target cellular U6 transcripts because they are similar in copy number to EBERs and are likewise localized to the nucleus.

There are several clinical situations in which EBER ISH imparts diagnostic or prognostic information. In transplant recipients with lymphoproliferative lesions, the assay is used to help distinguish EBV-driven posttransplant lymphoproliferative disorder from organ rejection or other inflammatory conditions ***(10)***. The assay is also helpful in confirming a diagnosis of infectious mononucleosis or nasopharyngeal carcinoma. EBERs are sometimes detected within tumor cells of Hodgkin disease, AIDS-related lymphoma, and lymphoepithelioma-like carcinomas arising in various anatomic sites such as the stomach; however, the clinical utility of EBER testing is limited because only a fraction of these tumors harbor EBV, and clinical management does not depend on whether EBV is present.

The procedure described herein is a 1-d ISH assay targeting EBER1 and U6 control RNA using digoxigenin (DIG)-labeled riboprobes, a procedure adapted from one first introduced by Wu et al. ***(1)*** and Barletta et al. ***(7)***. Types of samples amenable to EBER ISH include paraffin-embedded tissues, frozen sections, and cytology preparations.

2. Materials

2.1. Preparation of Probes

1. *Hind*III, *Eco*RI, *Bam*HI restriction endonuclease.
2. RNase-free TE buffer: 10 m*M* Tris-HCl, pH 8.0, 0.1 m*M* EDTA. (*see* **Note 1**).
3. Diethylpyrocarbonate (DEPC)-treated H_2O (*see* **Note 1**).
4. 25X labeling reaction buffer: 1 *M* Tris and 150 m*M* $MgCl_2$ made with DEPC-H_2O.
5. 100 m*M* Spermidine.
6. 100 m*M* Dithiothreitol (DTT).
7. Acetylated bovine serum albumin (BSA) (10 mg/mL).
8. RNasin® Ribonuclease inhibitor (40 U/µL) (Promega, Madison, WI).
9. 100 m*M* each of r-ATP, r-GTP, r-CTP, and r-UTP.
10. Digoxigenin-11-UTP (250 nmol/25 µL) (Boehringer-Mannheim, Mannheim, Germany).
11. T3 and T7 RNA polymerase (Promega).
12. RNase-free DNase (Promega).
13. 0.4 *M* EDTA, pH 8.0.
14. RNase-free tRNA (10 mg/mL).
15. 4 *M* LiCl.
16. 100% Ethanol.
17. 70% Ethanol made with DEPC-H_2O.

18. Buffer 1: 100 m*M* Tris-HCl, 150 m*M* NaCl, pH 7.5.
19. Blocking reagent (Boehringer-Mannheim).
20. Blocking buffer: 1% (w/v) blocking reagent, dissolved in buffer 1.
21. Anti-DIG-alkaline phosphatase (Boehringer-Mannheim), stored at 4°C.
22. Buffer 2: 100 m*M* Tris-HCl, 100 m*M* NaCl, 50 m*M* $MgCl_2$, pH 9.5. (The proper pH is critical to the color reaction. Filter before each use.)
23. Buffer 3: 10 m*M* Tris-HCl, 1 m*M* EDTA, pH 8.0.
24. Labeled control RNA (Boehringer Mannheim).
25. Template DNA for EBER1 and U6 (plasmid available from Richard Ambinder, MD, PhD, Johns Hopkins University).
26. Nitroblue tetrazolium chloride (NBT) solution: 75 mg/mL in 70% *N,N*, dimethylformamide (DMF) (*see* **Note 2**).
27. 5-Bromo-4-chloro-3-indolyl phosphate *p*-toluidine salt (BCIP) solution: 50 mg/mL in 100% DMF (*see* **Note 3**).

2.2. In Situ *Hybridization*

1. Xylene.
2. Graded ethanol solutions: 50, 70, 80, and 95% made with DEPC-H_2O.
3. 10X phosphate-buffered saline (PBS) made with DEPC-H_2O
4. Proteinase K (10 mg/mL) in RNase-free 100 m*M* Tris-HCl, 50 m*M* EDTA, pH 7.5.
5. Digestion buffer: 100 m*M* Tris-HCl, 50 m*M* EDTA, pH 8.0, 0.3% Triton X-100.
6. Formamide (molecular biology grade); store at 4°C in the dark.
7. 20X saline sodium citrate (SSC): 3 *M* NaCl, 0.3 *M* sodium citrate, pH 7.4.
8. 100X Denhardt's reagent made with DEPC-H_2O: 2% Ficoll 400 (type 400), 2% polyvinylpyrrolidon), 2% BSA (Fraction V).
9. 20% sodium dodecyl sulfate (SDS) solution.
10. 0.4 *M* EDTA, pH 7.5.
11. Sonicated salmon sperm DNA (10 mg/mL); boil before use.
12. Yeast tRNA, RNase-free (10 mg/mL) (Sigma, St. Louis, MO).
13. 75% Dextran sulfate made with DEPC-H_2O.
14. Hybridization solution: 50% formamide, 5X SSC, pH 7.4, 5X Denhardt's reagent, 1% SDS, 1 m*M* EDTA, pH 7.5, 100 µg/mL of boiled sonicated salmon sperm DNA, 460 µg/mL of tRNA, 7% dextran sulfate, made using RNase-free stock solutions.
15. RNase A (Sigma; concentration varies by lot number).
16. Sheep serum.
17. Triton X-100.
18. Wash solution: 2X SSC + 0.1% SDS.
19. Wash solution: 0.1X SSC + 0.1% SDS.
20. Methyl green counterstain: 1% in H_2O.
21. Permount.
22. Rubber cement.

2.3. Equipment

1. Silane-coated slides (or slides otherwise treated to promote tissue adherence).
2. 55°C Water bath.
3. 80°C Vacuum oven.
4. Vacuum centrifuge.
5. Microscope.
6. Cover slips.
7. PAP PEN™ (Daido Sangyo, Japan).
8. Moist chamber (RNase-free).
9. Microcentrifuge.
10. Slide-staining baths (Tissue-Tek®II, Sakura Finetek).

3. Methods

3.1. Preparation of Probes

Single-stranded RNA probes (riboprobes) complementary to target RNA transcripts are generated by transcribing cloned DNA sequences using T3 or T7 RNA polymerases in the presence of DIG-labeled UTP. Transcription and labeling are accomplished using commercial kits or by the following method.

3.1.1. General Comments

Gloves should be worn during probe preparation procedures to avoid RNase contamination. All solutions should be RNase-free (*see* **Note 1**) as well as all glassware and plasticware (*see* **Note 4**).

3.1.2. Preparation of DNA Templates

The DNA constructs that serve as templates for probe production are RA386 (EBER1) and RA390 (U6). The RA386 construct represents the full-length 458-bp EBER1 gene in a 2746-bp M13BS + pBS vector (Strategene, La Jolla, CA), and the U6 construct represents U6 sequences in the BS-SK vector.

1. Digest each construct with an appropriate restriction enzyme (*see* **Note 5**).
2. Purify the digested construct by phenol/chloroform extraction and ethanol precipitation, and then resuspend in 20 µL of RNase-free TE buffer at a concentration of 1 µg/µL. This purified DNA is used as a template for producing DIG-labeled riboprobes.

3.1.3. Labeling of Probes

1. For each labeling reaction, prepare 41.25 µL of labeling reaction mixture on ice by combining the following reagents: 15.25 µL of DEPC-H_2O, 2 µL of 25X labeling reaction buffer; 1 µL of 100 m*M* spermidine; 0.5 µL of 100 m*M* DTT; 2.5 µL of 10 mg/mL acetylated BSA; 2 µL of RNasin; 5 µL of each 10 m*M* r-ATP, r-GTP, r-CTP; 3 µL of 10 m*M* r-UTP.

2. To each reaction tube, add 1.75 µL of DIG-UTP, 1 µg of linearized template DNA brought up to 5 µL with DEPC-H_2O, and 2 µL of RNA polymerase (either T3 or T7 RNA polymerase per **Note 5**) for a total reaction volume of 50 µL.
3. Incubate at 37°C for 2 h, adding another 1 µL of the appropriate RNA polymerase after the first hour.
4. Digest the residual DNA template by adding 1 µL of 1 U/µL RNase-free DNase and incubating at 37°C for 10 min.
5. Stop the reaction by adding 1 µL of 0.4 *M* EDTA, pH 8.0.
6. To precipitate the labeled RNA probe, add 2 µL of 10 mg/mL tRNA, mix, and then add 0.1 vol of 4 *M* LiCl and 2.5–3.0 vol of chilled 100% ethanol. Mix and incubate at –70°C overnight.
7. Remove the reaction from the freezer and centrifuge at 12,000*g* at 4°C for 15 min.
8. Decant the ethanol supernatant and wash the pellet with 100 µL of 70% cold ethanol, centrifuge at 12,000*g* at 4°C for 5 min, and then remove as much ethanol supernatant as possible.
9. Spin the tube in a vacuum centrifuge until the pellet is completely dry. Add 50 µL of DEPC-H_2O and mix well by pipetting up and down a few times. Take out 2 µL to test for adequacy of labeling (see **Subheading 3.1.4.**), and immediately store the rest of labeled RNA probe at –70°C. (**Note**: Minimize freeze/thaw cycles and always use appropriate tissue controls to ensure probe integrity.)

3.1.4. Probe-Labeling Test

Estimate the incorporation of DIG label into the RNA probe using the following "spot test" protocol, which is essentially the same as that described in the Boehringer-Mannheim package inserts accompanying the probe labeling and detection reagents.

1. Pipette 1 µL of each reaction and dilutions thereof (1:10, 1:100, and 1:1000 in DEPC-H_2O) onto a small nylon membrane, along with equivalent dilutions of control-labeled RNA.
2. Bake the membrane at 80°C for 20 min in a vacuum oven.
3. Wash the membrane 1 min in buffer 1 with shaking.
4. Incubate the membrane for 30 min in blocking buffer with shaking at room temperature.
5. Wash the membrane for 1 min in buffer 1 with shaking.
6. Dilute the antibody conjugate 1:5000 in buffer 1 (20 mL of buffer 1, 4 µL of anti-DIG-alkaline phosphatase) and use immediately.
7. Incubate the membrane in antibody diluent for 30 min with shaking.
8. Wash two times in 100 mL of buffer 1 for 15 min with shaking. Equilibrate in 20 mL of buffer 2 for 2 min with shaking.
9. Place the membrane in a bag and prepare the color reaction buffer in a darkened room (10 mL of filtered buffer 2, 45 µL of NBT solution, 35 µL of BCIP solution).

10. Add the color reaction buffer to the bag and seal; do not shake. Store in the dark for about 20–40 min or until the color is adequate.
11. Wash the membrane for 5 min with shaking in 50 mL of buffer 3 to stop the reaction. If desired, store in a sealed bag containing buffer 3 to preserve color.
12. To interpret probe labeling, each probe should be labeled at least as strongly as a 1:10 dilution of the control probe, as judged by comparing the intensity of spot colors. If not, the probe labeling reaction should be rerun using half or twice the volume of linearized template DNA. Probe specificity and adequacy of labeling are further verified by actual ISH to control tissues.

3.2. In Situ *Hybridization*

3.2.1. General Comments

All steps through the hybridization procedure must be RNase free (*see* **Notes 1** and **4**). The following incubations are at room temperature unless otherwise stated. Before starting, prepare eight slide baths, each 200 mL in volume, containing xylene; graded ethanols (100, 95, 80, 70, and 50%); 1X PBS; and 20 μg/mL of proteinase K solution (200 mL of digestion buffer prewarmed to 37°C; when ready for use, add 400 μL of proteinase K stock solution and mix well).

3.2.2. Preparation of Specimens for Hybridization

1. From a fixed, paraffin-embedded tissue block, cut 4-μm sections onto silane-coated slides using a sterile water bath and gloves to reduce RNA degradation. (Tissues fixed in 10% buffered formalin more consistently retain RNA than do those fixed in B5 or subjected to decalcification.) To prepare cytology specimens, *see* **Note 6** and then go directly to **step 4**. For frozen sections, go directly to **step 4**.
2. Place paraffin section slides in an RNase-free staining rack for **steps 2–4**. Each experiment should include appropriate controls including positive and negative tissue controls, and sense as well as antisense probes (*see* **Note 7**). Bake the slides at 80°C for 40 min under a vacuum if recently cut, or 20 min if thoroughly dry. Immediately (while the paraffin is still hot) immerse the slides in fresh xylene for 6 min to deparaffinize.
3. Rehydrate the slides for 1 min each through graded ethanols (100, 95, 80, 70, and 50%) and then DEPC-PBS.
4. Digest the protein by immersing the slides in 20 μg/mL of proteinase K in digestion buffer at 37°C for 6 min (*see* **Note 8**).
5. Dip in 1X DEPC-PBS for 1 min to diminish proteinase K activity. Dab the slides on Kimwipes to remove excess proteinase K, and lay them flat in an RNase-free chamber in preparation for hybridization.

3.2.3. Hybridization

1. Add DIG-labeled EBER1 or U6 riboprobe to the hybridization solution at a 1:20 dilution. (The precise dilution may vary with each new batch of probe and is

determined empirically by running known control tissues and examining stain intensity. It is recommended that EBER stains be slightly more intense than U6 stains to avoid false-negative EBER results.)

2. Use a pipet to dispense the probe hybridization solution over each tissue section, using about 20 µL/slide or enough to cover the tissue completely. The pipet tip can be used to help spread the solution over the section, but avoid scraping the tissue. Cover slip with parafilm squares that are cut larger than the tissue dimensions, and remove any bubbles from under the parafilm using a clean pipet tip. If using more than one probe on a slide, rubber cement can be applied as a dam to prevent carryover from one area to another.
3. Lay the slides flat and allow them to hybridize in a covered, barely humid RNase-free chamber at 55°C for 3 h. Longer hybridization times produce stronger signals but will also increase background. Beyond this step, there is no need to use RNase-free solutions or glassware.

3.2.4. Washing and Detection of Antibody

1. Prewarm the 2X SSC to 37°C in preparation for **step 4**, and prewarm the 0.1X SSC + 0.1% SDS to 55°C in preparation for **step 5**.
2. Remove the parafilm cover slip using a scalpel blade to facilitate lifting but taking care not to scratch the tissue. To remove excess probe, blot the slides on clean Kimwipes. Insert the slides into a rack, in which they will remain for the next several wash steps. Dip the slides in a bath containing 200 mL of 2X SSC + 0.1% SDS.
3. Wash the slides in a bath of 2X SSC + 0.1% SDS for 10 min.
4. To remove excess unbound probe, incubate the slides at 37°C for 5 min in 2X SSC into which you have freshly mixed 0.3 U/mL of RNase A. (If high background is a problem, the RNase concentration may be doubled.) **Caution:** All reagents and plasticware used in this and subsequent steps should be labeled "RNase-contaminated," and should not be allowed to come in contact with any materials used in the prehybridization steps.
5. Dab the slides on Kimwipes, and wash in 0.1X SSC + 0.1% SDS for 5 min at 55°C. (It is in this step that the tissue is most susceptible to falling off the slide; the likelihood of this occurring is diminished by blotting the slide on dry Kimwipes prior to this wash.)
6. Rinse in 2X SSC for 1 min.
7. Prepare the anti-DIG antibody solution. This solution represents a 1:500 dilution of anti-DIG antibody linked to alkaline phosphatase, 1% sheep serum, and 0.3% Triton X-100 in buffer 1. (To make this solution, combine 2.8 mL of buffer 1, 28 µL of sheep serum, 84 µL of 1:10 Triton X-100, and 5.6 µL of anti-DIG-alkaline phosphatase.)
8. Dab the slides on Kimwipes and place in a horizontal staining tray. Circle each section using a PAP PEN to form a dam. Apply only enough antibody solution to each slide to cover the tissue completely, but not to overrun the dam, usually around 100 µL per section.

9. Incubate for 1 h at room temperature in a humid chamber. Add extra antibody solution as needed to prevent the sections from drying out; dried antibody results in nonspecific staining.
10. Dab the slides on Kimwipes, and then transfer slides to a staining rack for the duration of washes.
11. Immediately wash in buffer 1 for 1 min with shaking.
12. Wash in filtered buffer 2 for 1 min with shaking.
13. Immerse the slides into freshly prepared color reaction buffer (180 mL of filtered buffer 2, 810 μL of NBT solution, 630 μL of BCIP solution), and incubate in the dark for 90 min or until the positive control is strongly blue.
14. Wash the slides in a bath of buffer 3 for 5 min to stop the reaction.

3.2.5. Counterstaining and Cover Slipping

1. Dip the slides for 1 min in methyl green (1% in H_2O), dehydrate by dipping for 2 s each through four baths of 100% ethanol, followed by two dips in xylene. (Do not use the same ethanol baths that are used for prehybridization because of the risk of RNase contamination.) Let the slides sit in the xylene while you proceed with cover slipping the individual slides.
2. Remove each slide from the xylene and place onto absorbent paper towels to allow excess xylene to run off, but do not let the xylene dry completely. Mount with Permount under a 50-mm cover slip.

3.2.6. Interpretation of Results

A pathologist should examine the slides microscopically in conjunction with routine hematoxylin and eosin (H&E) stains to evaluate tissue architecture and cytomorphology. EBV EBER1 and U6 transcripts are visualized as multiple and often confluent blue specks localized to the nucleus, except in dividing cells in which cytoplasmic extension of the signal is seen (*see* **Fig. 1**).

Examine the U6 stain to determine whether RNA is well preserved in the target cells. Then proceed to look for EBER1 signal in these cells. If both are positive, then the target cells are interpreted as positive for latent EBV infection. (Because U6 contamination of EBER1 slides is feasible, be wary of positivity in inappropriate cell types.) If U6 is negative but EBER1 is positive in a particular case, use your discretion regarding the appropriate cytomorphology of the EBER1-positive cells, and consider whether U6 might be below the threshold for detection.

If EBER1 and U6 stains are both negative in a particular case, repeat with a shorter (i.e., 2 min) proteinase K incubation, or reduce the RNase concentration and duration of treatment. If both stains are still negative, then the results are not interpretable owing to insufficient RNA preservation. Lack of adequate RNA is especially prevalent in salivary gland and in any small biopsy that was not fixed immediately on collection.

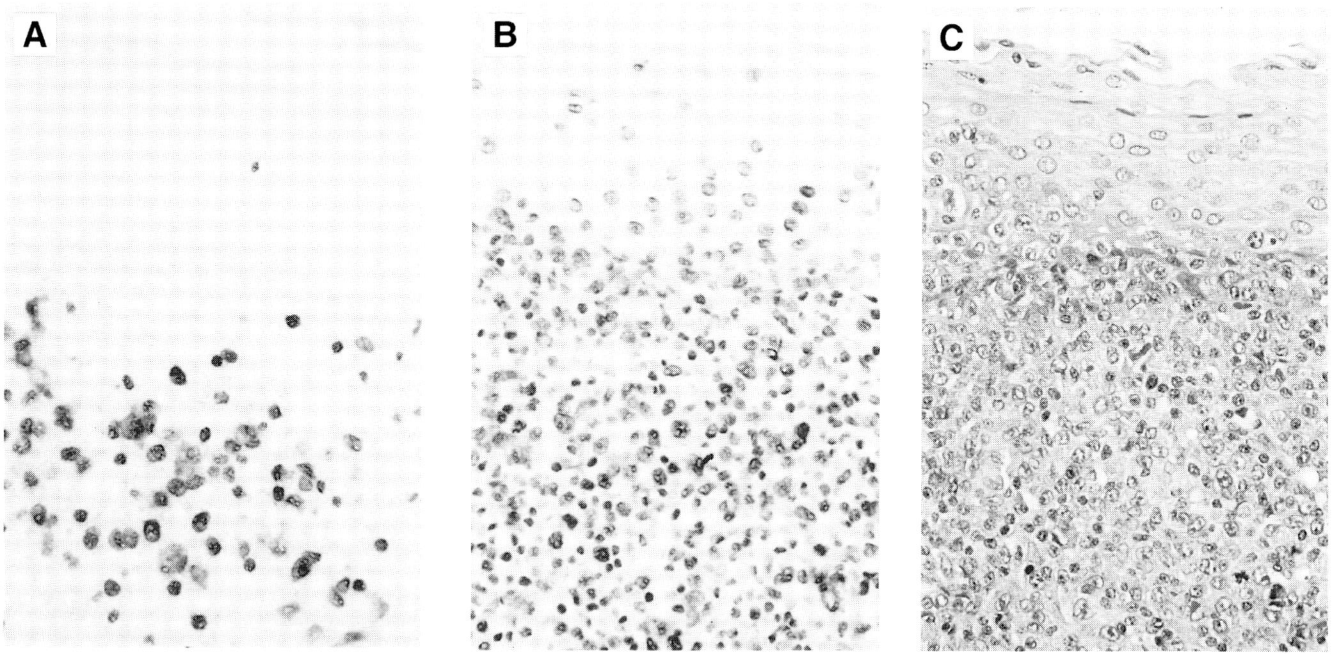

Fig. 1. (**A**) ISH to EBER1 transcripts in a paraffin section of PTLD reveals EBER1 localization to the nucleus of many lymphoid cells. (**B**) The presence of U6 transcripts in virtually all cells within the tissue confirms that RNA is preserved and available for hybridization. (**C**) The same tissue stained with standard H&E reveals normal squamous epithelium overlying a dense atypical lymphoid infiltrate.

4. Notes

1. To make a solution RNase-free, add 0.1% DEPC, mix well, incubate at 37°C overnight (or stir vigorously for at least 2 h), and then autoclave for 20 min on liquid cycle. Be aware that DEPC cannot be relied on to eliminate RNase activity in solutions containing Tris, because Tris inactivates DEPC. Instead, crystalline Tris can be dissolved in RNase-free H_2O. We have not tested rapid commercial RNase inactivators.
2. NBT is reconstituted from powder (Boehringer-Mannheim) to a concentration of 75 mg/mL in 70% DMF/water. Make the 70% DMF in a polypropylene tube before adding the NBT. (Polystyrene tubes and pipets react with DMF.) The resulting solution is stable when stored in the dark at 4°C for 1 mo, or at –20°C for at least 4 mo.
3. BCIP (previously called X-phos) is made from powder (Boehringer-Mannheim). Bring the BCIP to a concentration of 50 mg/mL in 100% DMF, avoiding polystyrene tubes and pipets.
4. All glassware and plasticware used in the steps leading to hybridization should be RNase free. To make them RNase free, bake glassware at 250°C for at least 4 h, or soak glassware and plasticware in 0.1% DEPC for a few minutes, wrap in aluminum foil, and autoclave for 20 min. Plastic items can be soaked in 0.5 *M* NaOH for 10 min, rinsed thoroughly with DEPC water, and autoclaved. Disposable pipets are preferred, and they need not be treated prior to onetime use. Be aware that some laboratories claim that extensive precautions against RNA degradation are unnecessary if proper controls for RNA degradation are included. We recommend a cautious approach in which RNase-free reagents are used in addition to appropriate controls.
5. The RA386 and RA390 plasmids can be transfected into *Escherichia coli* and propagated in ampicillin-containing broth. Abundant plasmid is then isolated, cut by the appropriate restriction enzyme to linearize the DNA template, and transcribed to produce riboprobes. To make antisense EBER1 riboprobe, cut the RA386 construct with *Hin*dIII and use T7 polymerase. To make sense EBER1 probe, cut RA386 with *Eco*RI and use T3 polymerase. To make antisense U6 probe, cut RA390 with *Eco*RI and use T3 polymerase. To make sense U6 probe, cut RA390 with *Bam*HI and use T7 polymerase. Antisense EBER1 probe recognizes a nonpolyadenylated pol III transcript characteristic of latent EBV infection that is not translated to protein, whereas sense EBER1 probe serves as a control of nonspecific hybridization. Antisense U6 probe recognizes an ubiquitously transcribed human small nuclear pol III transcript that serves as an indicator of RNA preservation.
6. Cytospins can be prepared from suspensions of mononuclear cells including blood, body fluids, or cell cultures. Wash cultured cells twice in RNase-free PBS before suspending about 2×10^6 cells in 400 µL of RNase-free PBS. Add an equal volume of 10% buffered formalin (Polysciences, Warrington, PA), vortex gently, and incubate at 4°C for 30 min. Prepare several cytospins on silane-coated slides, using about 2.5×10^5 cells per slide. Air-dry at room temperature and hybridize as soon as possible, or store in an RNase-free box at 4°C for up to 2 d before hybridization.

7. EBV-related Hodgkin disease makes a good positive control because Hodgkin cells are easily distinguished from uninfected small background lymphocytes on microscopic examination.
8. Proteinase K digestion facilitates probe penetration into paraffin-embedded tissues. Less digestion produces a weaker hybridization signal, whereas overdigestion destroys tissue morphology. Optimal digestion time can be determined empirically for each tissue.

References

1. Wu, T. C., Mann, R. B., Epstein, J. I., MacMahon, E., Lee, W. A., Charache, P., Hayward, S. D., Kurman, R. J., Hayward, G. S., and Ambinder, R. F. (1991) Abundant expression of EBER1 small nuclear RNA in nasopharyngeal carcinoma: a morphologically distinctive target for detection of Epstein-Barr virus in formalin-fixed paraffin-embedded carcinoma specimens. *Am. J. Pathol.* **138,** 1461–1469.
2. Wu, T. C. and Kuo, T. T. (1993) Study of Epstein-Barr virus early RNA-1 (EBER1) expression by in situ hybridization in thymic epithelial tumors of Chinese patients in Taiwan. *Hum. Pathol.* **24,** 235–238.
3. Gulley, M. L., Eagan, P. A., Quintanilla-Martinez, L., Picado, A. L., Smir, B. N., Childs, C., Dunn, C. D., Craig, F. E., Williams, J. W., and Banks, P. M. (1994) Epstein-Barr Virus DNA is abundant and monoclonal in the Reed-Sternberg cells of Hodgkin's disease: association with mixed cellularity subtype and Hispanic American ethnicity. *Blood* **83,** 1595–1602.
4. Reynolds, D. J., Banks, P. M., and Gulley, M. L. (1995) New characterization of infectious mononucleosis and a phenotypic comparison with Hodgkin's disease. *Am. J. Pathol.* **146,** 379–388.
5. Ambinder, R. F. and Mann, R. B. (1994) Epstein-Barr encoded RNA in situ hybridization: diagnostic applications. *Hum. Pathol.* **25,** 602–605.
6. Gilligan, K., Rajadurai, P., Resnick, L., and Raab-Traub, N. (1990) Epstein-Barr virus small nuclear RNAs are not expressed in permissively infected cells in AIDS-associated leukoplakia. *Proc. Natl. Acad. Sci. USA* **87,** 8790–8794.
7. Barletta, J. M., Kingma, D. W., Ling, Y., Charache, P., Mann, R. B., and Ambinder, R. F. (1993) Rapid in situ hybridization for the diagnosis of latent Epstein-Barr virus infection. *Mol. Cell. Probes* **7,** 105–109.
8. Ambinder, R. F., Browning, P. J., Lorenzana, I., et al. (1993) Epstein-Barr virus and childhood Hodgkin's disease in Honduras and the United States. *Blood* **81,** 462–467.
9. Randhawa, P. S., Jaffe, R., Demetris, A. J., Nalesnik, M., Starzl, T. E., Chen, Y. Y., and Weiss, L. M. (1992) Expression of Epstein-Barr virus-encoded small RNA in liver specimens from transplant recipients with post-transplantation lymphoproliferative disease. *N. Engl. J. Med.* **327,** 1710–1714.
10. Montone, K. T., Friedman, H., Hodinka, R. L., Hicks, D. G., Kant, J. A., and Tomaszewski, J. E. (1992) In situ hybridization for Epstein-Barr virus NotI repeats in posttransplant lymphoproliferative disorder. *Mod. Pathol.* **5,** 292–302.

23

Molecular Methods for Detecting Epstein-Barr Virus (Part II)

Structural Analysis of Epstein-Barr Virus DNA as a Marker of Clonality

Hongxin Fan and Margaret L. Gulley

1. Introduction

The Southern blot technique can be used to determine the clonality of Epstein-Barr virus (EBV) infected cells *(1,2)*. This clonality assay capitalizes on measurable polymorphisms in EBV genomic structure, namely, the variable number of tandem repeats lying at either end of the linear viral genome. Thus, the size of genome varies from virion to virion depending on the number of terminal repeat sequences. When a particular virion infects a cell, its linear genome circularizes by fusing the terminal repeats to form an episome containing from 1–20 tandem repeat sequences. If an infected cell undergoes malignant transformation, the viral DNA replicates along with cell DNA during mitosis, and the same terminal repeat structure is inherited by all tumor cell progeny. Therefore, Southern blot analysis of the EBV terminal restriction fragment serves as a marker of cellular clonality.

The EBV clonality assay presented herein, which is adapted from a procedure first described by Raab-Traub and Flynn *(1)*, begins by preparing a Southern blot using *Bam*HI-restricted DNA extracted from patient tissue. The blot is hybridized to a probe targeting the terminal restriction fragment, such as the *Xho*1a probe that recognizes unique DNA adjacent to the terminal repeat sequences on the right end of the EBV genome. The resultant band pattern reflects the clonality of the lesion with respect to the structure of EBV DNA (**Fig. 1**).

From: *Methods in Molecular Medicine, vol. 49: Molecular Pathology Protocols*
Edited by: A. A. Killeen © Humana Press Inc., Totowa, NJ

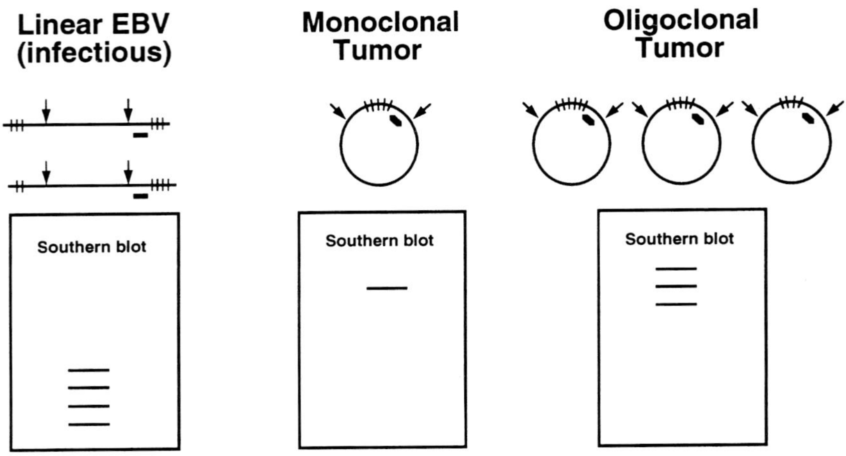

Fig. 1. Southern blot analysis of EBV DNA structure can be used to determine whether viral DNA is derived from monoclonal or oligoclonal cells, or whether it is a product of infectious viral replication. First, DNA is cut with the *Bam*HI restriction enzyme (arrows), size fractionated by gel electrophoresis, and transferred to a membrane by the Southern blot method. The probe most commonly used to detect the EBV terminal restriction fragment is the 1.9-kb *Xho*1a probe (bar), which targets unique sequences adjacent to the right terminal repeats. Infectious virions have variably sized terminal restriction fragments resulting in a ladder array of bands on the Southern blot. In monoclonal tumors, a single fused terminal restriction fragment is seen. In oligoclonal tumors, several discrete restriction fragments are seen, reflecting the presence of multiple separate clones.

Distinguishing polyclonal from monoclonal lymphoid tumors may have prognostic and therapeutic implications in immunosuppressed patients. In addition, latent (episomal) viral DNA may be distinguished from replicative (linear) viral DNA in this assay; only linear viral DNA is inhibited by acyclovir or related nucleoside analogs.

2. Materials

2.1. DNA Digestion and Southern Blot

1. *Bam*HI restriction endonuclease.
2. 10X Restriction enzyme *Bam*HI buffer.
3. 10X Gel-loading buffer: 0.25% bromophenol blue, 0.25% xylene cyanol, 15% Ficoll (type 400) in 10X TAE buffer.
4. Agarose.
5. 1X TAE buffer: 40 m*M* Tris-acetate, 1 m*M* EDTA.
6. Ethidium bromide (10 mg/mL).
7. 20X Saline sodium citrate (SSC): 3 *M* NaCl, 0.3 *M* sodium citrate, pH 7.4.

8. Nylon membrane.
9. Whatman 3MM paper.
10. Paper towels.

2.2. Preparation of RNA Probe from DNA Template

Preparation and use of RNA probes requires that all solutions be RNase free (*see* **Note 1**).

1. *Hind*III, *Eco*RI restriction endonuclease.
2. 10X Restriction enzyme *Hind*III, *Eco*RI buffer.
3. RNase-free TE buffer: 10 m*M* Tris-HCl, pH 8.0, 0.1 m*M* EDTA.
4. 100 m*M* Dithiothreitol (DTT), RNase free.
5. RNasin® ribonuclease inhibitor (40 U/μL) (Promega, Madison, WI).
6. Bovine serum albumin (BSA), nuclease-free (1 mg/mL).
7. 10 m*M* NTP stock.
8. ^{32}P-UTP (10 mCi/mL) (3000 Ci/mmol) (New England Nuclear, Boston, MA).
9. SP6 or T7 RNA polymerase (Promega).
10. 5X Transcription buffer (Promega).
11. RNase-free DNase (Promega).
12. G-50 Sephadex (RNA) Quick Spin™ columns (Boehringer Mannheim, Mannheim, Germany).

2.3. Hybridization

1. Formamide (molecular biology grade); store at 4°C in the dark.
2. Diethylpyrocarbonate (DEPC)-treated H_2O.
3. 20X SSC: 3 *M* NaCl, 0.3 *M* sodium citrate, pH 7.4.
4. Sonicated salmon sperm DNA (10 mg/mL).
5. 20% sodium dodecyl sulfate (SDS).
6. 1 *M* PIPES, (piperazine-1,4-diethanesulfonic acid), pH 6.5.
7. 100X Denhardt's reagent made with DEPC-H_2O: 2% Ficoll 400 (type 400), 2% PVP (polyvinylpyrrolidone), 2% BSA (Fraction V).
8. Hybridization solution made from RNase-free stock solutions: 50% formamide, 5X SSC, pH 7.4, 1X Denhardt's reagent, 0.2% SDS, 100 μg/mL of boiled sonicated salmon sperm DNA, 50 m*M* PIPES, pH 6.5.
9. Washing solutions (no. 1, 2, 3, and 4): 0.2% SDS, 0.01% sodium pyrophosphate, and sequential dilutions of 2X SSC (2, 1, 0.5, and 0.25X SSC).
10. RNase A (Sigma, St. Louis, MO; concentration varies by lot number).
11. RNase buffer: 2X SSC in 20 m*M* Tris, 5 m*M* EDTA, pH 8.0.

2.4. Equipment

1. Vacuum oven.
2. Hybridization oven.
3. Centrifuge.
4. Water bath.
5. Scintillation counter.

3. Methods

3.1. Preparation of DNA

Biopsy tissue is snap-frozen and stored at –70°C until analysis. Intact genomic DNA is isolated by SDS-proteinase K lysis and phenol-chloroform extraction (*see* Chapter 2).

3.2. DNA Digestion and Southern Blot

1. Restriction endonuclease digestion: Mix 10 μg of genomic DNA, 100 μ of *Bam*HI restriction enzyme, and 5 μL of 10X *Bam*HI reaction buffer. Add double-distilled H_2O (ddH_2O) to a total volume of 50 μL, mix well, and incubate at 37°C for 4 h to overnight. Add 5 μL of gel-loading buffer to stop the reaction.
2. Load the sample onto a 0.7% agarose gel in 1X TAE buffer containing 0.5 μg/mL of ethidium bromide. Electrophorese for about 16 h at 1.5 V/cm until the dye reaches the end of the gel.
3. Denature the DNA and transfer to a nylon membrane using 10X SSC, pH 7.4, by the Southern blot method.
4. To immobilize the DNA, place the nylon membrane between two sheets of Whatman 3MM paper and bake under vacuum at 80°C for 1 to 2 h. Keep the membrane dry until hybridization, or put it in a sealed plastic bag at –20°C for long-term storage.

3.3. Preparation of RNA Probes from DNA Template

3.3.1. Linearizing Plasmid Vector Containing Template DNA

1. Set up a restriction endonuclease digestion reaction using one of the following vectors containing template DNA (*see* **Note 2**):
   a. *Xho*1a probe in pGEM2 vector: To 20 μg of vector DNA, add 20 μL of 10X *Hind*III reaction buffer, 100 U of *Hind*III restriction endonuclease, and ddH_2O to 200 μL.
   b. *Eco*R1I probe in pGEM2 vector: To 20 μg of vector DNA, add 20 μL of 10X *Eco*RI reaction buffer, 100 U of *Eco*RI restriction endonuclease, and ddH_2O to 200 μL.
2. Incubate the digests at 37°C for 4 h to overnight.
3. Electrophorese a small aliquot of undigested vector/insert alongside the digested vector/insert in an agarose gel to check for completeness of digestion. Only one band of the appropriate size should be evident in the linearized template.
4. Purify the linearized DNA by phenol/chloroform extraction and ethanol precipitation, and resuspend it in 20 μL of RNase-free TE buffer at a concentration of 1 μg/μL. This purified linear DNA is used as a template for producing ^{32}P-labeled riboprobes.

3.3.2. Labeling of RNA Probes with ^{32}P-UTP

Preparation of probes must be carried out in an RNase-free environment. Gloves should be worn during all steps to avoid RNase contamination (*see*

Note 1). RNA is transcribed in the presence of radionucleotides to produce a labeled riboprobe. Transcription initiates in vector sequences containing RNA polymerase recognition sites ***(3)***.

1. For each 20-µL transcription reaction, mix 4 µL of 5X transcription buffer; 2 µL of 100 m*M* DTT; 2 µL of 1 mg/mL BSA; 0.8 µL of 40 U/µL RNasin; 1 µL each of 10 m*M* rATP, rGTP, and rCTP; 1.5 µL of freshly made 1:100 dilution of 10 m*M* rUTP; 5 µL of 10 mCi/mL ^{32}P-UTP; 1 µL of linearized template DNA; and 1 µL of appropriate RNA polymerase (SP6 for *Xho*1a, T7 for *Eco*R1I).
2. Incubate the reaction at 37°C for 30 min, add another 1 µL of the appropriate RNA polymerase, and incubate at 37°C for another 30 min.
3. Add 1.25 µL of RNasin to stablilize the product, and 1 µL of 1 U/µL DNase (RNase free) to degrade the template DNA. Incubate the reaction at 37°C for 10 min.
4. Isolate the ^{32}P-labeled RNA probe on a G-50 Sephadex (RNA) Quick Spin column according to the manufacturer's protocol. Collect the probe in a microfuge tube for hybridization.
5. Measure the labeling activity of the RNA probe by assaying 1 µL in a scintillation counter. Counts should be between 1–3 million cpm/µL.

3.4. Hybridization

Southern blot hybridization to either the *Xho*1a or the *Eco*R1I riboprobe yields visible bands on autoradiographs. Nonspecific hybridization is avoided by pretreating the membrane with prehybridization solution, and by removing excessive unbound probe by RNase treatment. DNA from the Raji Burkitt's lymphoma cell line (American Type Culture Collection, Rockville, MD) is recommended as a positive control. Any EBV-negative tissue can serve as a negative control.

1. Prepare 40 mL of fresh hybridization solution at room temperature; then prewarm to 45°C.
2. To prehybridize, pour half of the hybridization solution (20 mL) over the membrane and incubate at 45°C while shaking for at least 2 h. Then discard the prehybridization solution.
3. Add about 30 µL of ^{32}P-UTP-labeled *Xho*1a or *Eco*R1I RNA probe to 20 mL of fresh hybridization solution and mix well. Incubate with the membrane at 45°C while shaking overnight. (Because the probe is single stranded, it need not be boiled prior to use.)
4. Prepare the four wash solutions (no. 1, 2, 3, and 4) and warm them to 68°C for at least 1 h or overnight.
5. Wash at 68°C for 30 min each in wash solution no. 1 and wash solution no. 2.
6. Rinse the membrane several times in ddH$_2$O, then once with RNase buffer.
7. Digest the unbound probe by incubating the membrane while shaking it in 20 mL of prewarmed RNase buffer containing 0.3 U/mL of RNase A at 37°C for exactly

5 min. Then rinse the blot several times with ddH_2O to remove excess RNase. Be careful to contain the RNase solution so that it does not contaminate RNase-free materials in the laboratory.
8. Wash at 68°C for 30 min each in wash solution no. 3 and wash solution no. 4.
9. Place the membrane in an envelope of Whatman 3MM paper or air-dry for at least 30 min.
10. Set up autoradiography by exposing the blot to X-ray film overnight.

3.5. Interpretation of Results

In this procedure, total DNA was extracted from patient tissues, digested with *Bam*HI restriction endonuclease, electrophoresed through an agarose gel to size fractionate the fragments, and transferred to a nylon membrane. The immobilized DNA fragments were hybridized to a ^{32}P-radiolabeled RNA probe targeting the terminal restriction fragment of the EBV genome. Unbound probe was washed away, and the membrane was exposed to X-ray film to detect hybridized bands. Positive and negative control samples, and a molecular weight size marker, should be run in adjacent lanes.

Raji control DNA produces a single band of about 23 kb, confirming that monoclonal EBV DNA is present. In patient samples, the presence of a single band larger than 6 kb is interpreted as monoclonal EBV DNA, implying the presence of a monoclonal population of infected cells. Two bands larger than 6 kb represent biclonal EBV DNA, and additional bands over 6 kb represent oligoclonal EBV DNA (*see* **Fig. 1**). A ladder of bands smaller than 6 kb is indicative of linear EBV DNA, which is the product of viral replication. Viral replication may coexist in the same tissue as latent infection, potentially yielding both small and large bands.

4. Notes

1. To make any solution RNase free, add 0.1% DEPC, mix well, incubate at 37°C overnight (or stir vigorously for at least 2 h), and then autoclave for 20 min on liquid cycle. Be aware that DEPC cannot be relied on to eliminate RNase activity in solutions containing Tris, because Tris inactivates DEPC. Instead, Tris solutions are made using RNase-free H_2O. We have not tested commercial RNase inactivators. Glassware and plasticware used in all steps through hybridization should be RNase free. To make them RNase free, bake glassware at 250°C for at least 4 h, or soak glassware and plasticware in 0.1% DEPC for a few minutes, wrap in aluminum foil, and autoclave for 20 min. Plastic items can also be soaked in 0.5 *M* NaOH for 10 min, rinsed thoroughly with water, and autoclaved. Disposable pipets are preferred, and they need not be treated prior to onetime use.
2. The probes most commonly used to detect the terminal restriction fragment of EBV DNA are the 1.9-kb *Xho*1a probe or the 4.0-kb *Bam*H1 subfragment of the *Eco*R1I fragment ***(1,4)***. The templates for making these probes are available in

plasmid vectors from Nancy Raab-Traub, PhD, University of North Carolina at Chapel Hill. The plasmid can be transfected into *Escherichia coli* and propagated in ampicillin-containing LB broth. Then abundant plasmid can be isolated and cut with an appropriate restriction enzyme to linearize the DNA immediately downstream of the cloned insert. The insert can then serve as a template for RNA transcription in the presence of radionucleotides to produce "riboprobes" labeled with ^{32}P. Instead of making RNA probe as described in this procedure, an alternative approach is to make a labeled DNA probe from the same plasmid insert previously mentioned, or to use another probe such as the 5.2-kb *Bam*HI/*Eco*RI fused terminal repeat probe labeled by random priming *(5)*.

References

1. Raab-Traub, N. and Flynn, K. (1986) The structure of the termini of the Epstein-Barr virus as a marker of clonal cellular proliferation. *Cell* **47,** 883–889.
2. Gulley, M. L. and Raab-Traub, N. (1993) Detection of Epstein-Barr virus in human tissues by molecular genetic techniques. *Arch. Pathol. Lab. Med.* **117,** 1115–1120 (review).
3. McCracken, S. (1985) Preparation of RNA transcripts using SP6 RNA polymerase. *Focus* (Bethesda Research Laboratories) **7,** 5.
4. Gulley, M. L., Raphael, M., Lutz, C. T., Ross, D. W., and Raab-Traub, N. (1992) Epstein-Barr virus integration in human lymphomas and lymphoid cell lines. *Cancer* **70,** 185–191.
5. Weiss, L. M., Strickler, J. G., Warnke, R. A., Purtilo, D. T., and Sklar, J. (1987) Epstein-Barr viral DNA in tissues of Hodgkin's disease. *Am. J. Pathol.* **129,** 86–91.

24

Molecular Methods for Detecting Epstein-Barr Virus (Part III)

EBV Viral Load by Competitive Polymerase Chain Reaction

Hongxin Fan and Margaret L. Gulley

1. Introduction

Epstein-Barr virus (EBV) viral load testing is rapidly gaining acceptance in the diagnosis and monitoring of patients with EBV-related neoplasia, including transplant recipients, autoimmune deficiency syndrome (AIDS) patients with brain lymphoma, and patients with nasopharyngeal carcinoma. In transplant recipients, several studies have shown that EBV viral load in blood is a useful marker of EBV-driven posttransplant lymphoproliferative disease (PTLD), both in terms of predicting disease and in monitoring efficacy of therapy ***(1–4)***. In AIDS patients, high EBV viral load in cerebrospinal fluid (CSF) is so characteristic of brain lymphoma that the assay has been touted as sufficient for making that diagnosis without the need for brain biopsy, assuming that there is also clinical and radiographic support for the diagnosis ***(5)***. In nasopharyngeal carcinoma patients, a recent study showed that plasma EBV viral load is nearly always elevated, and the degree of elevation is higher in those with distant metastases ***(6)***. Additional studies are needed to more completely define the utility of EBV viral load measurement in monitoring residual disease following therapy, and to evaluate clinical utility in other EBV-associated diseases.

EBV viral load can be measured by several methods including quantitative culture, counting the proportion of EBV-encoded RNA (EBER)-stained cells in tissue specimens, and quantitative polymerase chain reaction (PCR) ***(7–10)***. Quantitative PCR is recommended because it is sensitive, specific, quantita-

From: *Methods in Molecular Medicine, vol. 49: Molecular Pathology Protocols*
Edited by: A. A. Killeen © Humana Press Inc., Totowa, NJ

tive across a wide dynamic range, and semiautomated to reduce labor costs. Furthermore, several studies have suggested that blood or CSF is amenable for testing, thus avoiding invasive biopsy procedures.

Several protocols have been described for quantitative PCR, including real-time measurement of PCR products in a thermocycler ***(6,11,12)***. or post-PCR quantitation of products using commercial detection kits (DiaSorin, Stillwater, MN; Digene Diagnostics, Silver Spring, MD; BioSource International, Camarillo, CA). The EBV viral load protocol presented here is a competitive PCR assay modified from a commercial kit (Viral Quant™ EBV kit, BioSource International). This assay relies on competition between EBV genomic sequences in the patient sample and an internal calibration standard (ICS) that is spiked into the sample prior to extraction. Following coamplification using biotinylated primers, PCR products are detected in an automated enzyme-linked immunosorbent assay (ELISA) plate system using a 96-well plate washer and reader. The spiked standard contains the same primer recognition sequences as the EBV genomic target (the EBER gene), but has different interim sequences that are distinguished by specific internal probes coating the inside of the microwells. Comparison between the amount of EBV product and the amount of internal standard product permits calculation of EBV viral load in the patient specimen.

In our modified procedure, DNA is extracted using a commercial kit (QIAmp Viral RNA kit, Qiagen, Valencia, CA), and dUTP replaces dTTP in the PCR reaction so that uracil *N*-glycosylase (UNG) enzyme can be used to diminish the risk of amplicon contamination ***(13)***. Sample types include plasma, serum, blood mononuclear cells, or CSF.

2. Materials

2.1. Reagents

1. QIAamp Viral RNA kit (Qiagen) (*see* **Note 1**).
2. AE buffer (Qiagen).
3. 100% Ethanol.
4. GeneAmp dNTPs with dUTP (PE Applied Biosystems, Foster City, CA).
5. *Taq* DNA polymerase (Gibco-BRL, Gaithersburg, MD).
6. Uracil-DNA glycosylase, heat labile (heat labile UNG; Boehringer Mannheim, Mannheim, Germany).
7. Viral Quant EBV kit (BioSource International).
8. 1X TAE buffer: 40 m*M* Tris-acetate, 1 m*M* EDTA.
9. Agarose.
10. Ethidium bromide (10 mg/mL).
11. 10X Gel-loading buffer: 0.25% bromophenol blue, 0.25% xylene cyanol, 15% Ficoll (type 400) in 10X TAE buffer.
12. Nuclease-free H_2O.

2.2. Equipment

1. Centrifuge.
2. Microcentrifuge.
3. Thermocycler (GeneAmp PCR system 9700; PE Applied Biosystems).
4. ELP-40 Microplate Strip Washer (Bio-Tek, Winooski, VT).
5. Elx 800 Automated Microplate Reader (Bio-Tek).

3. Methods

3.1. General PCR Precautions

Precautions are necessary to prevent contamination of PCR reactions. Clean work areas, physical separation of pre- and postamplification laboratories, and appropriate controls are essential. Most important is meticulous care by well-trained personnel. UNG is used to further ensure that amplicons from previous reactions are not amplified.

3.2. Preparation of Samples

Plasma, serum, and blood mononuclear cells are all potential sources of virus in transplant recipients. Plasma and serum are recommended in nasopharyngeal carcinoma patients, whereas blood mononuclear cells have not yet been studied. CSF is the preferred sample type in AIDS patients with suspected brain lymphoma. For comparability purposes, serial samples from patients followed over time should always be analyzed using the same sample type and laboratory procedure.

1. Plasma: Collect whole blood in EDTA anticoagulant. Centrifuge at 1800*g* for 10 min. Recover the plasma, aliquot, and freeze at –20°C.
2. Serum: Recover the serum from the whole blood following centrifugation at 1800*g* for 10 min. Aliquot and store at –20°C.
3. CSF: Collect 1 mL of fresh specimen, aliquot, and store at –20°C. (If the CSF is reddish or cloudy, indicating high probability of red cells or leukocytes, centrifuge it and recover the supernatant for testing.)
4. Peripheral blood mononuclear cells: Isolate the DNA using your standard protocol, such as the Puregene DNA isolation kit (Gentra Systems, Minneapolis, MN). Quantitate the DNA, and then proceed directly to to PCR, or store the DNA at –20°C.

3.3. Isolation of Viral DNA

Viral DNA is isolated from plasma, serum, or CSF using the QIAamp Viral RNA kit. Although the name of this kit implies that its purpose is to isolate RNA, we found it effective in isolating EBV DNA from patient samples. The kit is supplied with carrier RNA to improve sample recovery. (Alternatively, the QIAmp Blood kit can be used as described in **Note 1.**)

1. Pipet 140 µL of plasma, serum, or CSF into a 1.5-mL microfuge tube.
2. Add 5000 copies of ICS (supplied in the Viral Quant EBV kit) to each tube, including the positive and negative controls.
3. Follow the manufacturer's instructions provided in the QIAmp viral RNA kit, and at the last step elute the DNA into 50 µL of AE buffer or nuclease-free H_2O. Of this, only 5 µL is typically used in subsequent PCR reactions.

3.4. Polymerase Chain Reaction

PCR is performed using primers targeting the EBV EBER gene. One of these primers is biotinylated, and both are provided in the Viral Quant EBV kit (5′-CCCGCCTACACACCAACTAT-3′; 5′-AGTCTGGGAAGACAACCA-CA-3′). The manufacturer's procedure has been modified to accommodate the UNG system of hindering amplicon contamination (*see* **Note 2**).

1. Prepare the PCR master mix in a 1.5-mL microfuge tube on ice, and aliquot 95 µL into each 0.2-mL thin-walled tube for PCR. Per reaction, the master mix should include 69.5 µL of nuclease-free H_2O, 10 µL of 10X PCR buffer, 2 µL of 25 pmol/µL primer set, 1 µL of heat-labile UNG, 8 µL of dNTPs with dUTP (2.5 m*M* of each dATP, dCTP, and dGTP; 5.0 m*M* of dUTP), 4 µL of 50 m*M* $MgCl_2$, and 0.5 µL of 5 U/µL of *Taq* polymerase (*see* **Note 3**).
2. For DNA isolated from plasma, serum, or CSF, add 5 µL of template DNA (which contains 500 copies of spiked ICS) to the aliquot of master mix. For DNA extracted from blood mononuclear cells, add 1 µg of template DNA to the aliquot of master mix, and since ICS has not already been spiked into this sample, add 500 copies of ICS directly to the PCR mixture, adjusting the total PCR volume to 100 µL.
3. Controls: Use the plasmid construct containing EBER1 sequences and the carrier DNA in the Viral Quant EBV kit to serve as a positive and a negative control, respectively. In addition, it is wise to include high and low patient controls in each run, and additional negative controls for every 10 patient samples.
4. Run the thermocycler program as follows: 20°C for 10 min (to allow heat-labile UNG to act); 95°C for 3 min (to inactivate heat-labile UNG); and then 34 PCR cycles consisting of denaturation at 94°C for 30 s, annealing at 60°C for 30 s, and extension at 72°C for 1 min. Run the final extension step at 72°C for 15 min, and then hold briefly at 72°C until the PCR tubes are removed for immediate detection or storage at –20°C (*see* **Note 4**). According to the Viral Quant EBV kit protocol, these thermocycler conditions allow detection of about 25 copies per amplification reaction. To detect lower copy numbers, *see* **Note 5**.

3.5. Confirmation of PCR Products by Agarose Gel Electrophoresis

3.5.1. Agarose Gel Electrophoresis

Viewing the size and relative proportion of ICS and EBV products is useful for quality assurance purposes and for troubleshooting. It is also used to confirm PCR productivity prior to proceeding with the relatively expensive ELISA plate detection steps.

1. Prepare a 2% agarose gel in 1X TAE buffer containing 0.5 µg/mL of ethidium bromide.
2. Mix 25 µL of the PCR product with 3 µL of 10X gel-loading buffer and load into the wells. Load one lane with a molecular weight marker.
3. Electrophorese at 5 V/cm until the dye has migrated about three fourths the length of the gel.
4. Photograph the gel under a UV transilluminator.

3.5.2. Interpretation of Gel Electrophoresis

Amplified ICS produces a 260-bp product, whereas amplified EBV produces a 210-bp product. Bands at 210 and 260 bp indicate coamplification of EBV and ICS. The relative amount of EBV and ICS in each sample reflects the proportion of starting templates in the PCR reaction.

ICS at 260 bp should be visible in all patient samples. If only the ICS band is seen, then EBV DNA is below the threshold for visualization, and generally will also be near or below the threshold for reporting following the ELISA plate detection steps. If the ICS band is absent but a strong EBV 210-bp band is seen, this probably indicates that abundant EBV DNA is present and has overwhelmed the ICS amplification. In this circumstance, dilute an aliquot of the original patient sample 1 : 10 with H_2O, then spike with ICS, extract the DNA, and amplify again. Be sure to document the dilution so that the final results will not underestimate the amount of EBV.

If no bands are detected in the patient lane but the controls are as expected, a PCR inhibitor may be the culprit. If this is the case, consider repeating the PCR reaction using less template DNA, and document this so that calculations can be adjusted accordingly. Alternatively, further purify the original template DNA by phenol/chloroform extraction and ethanol precipitation before repeating the assay.

3.6. ELISA Plate Detection System

3.6.1. Microplate Detection

Microtiter plates precoated with ICS or EBV capture oligonucleotide probes are provided in the Viral Quant EBV kit. All detection reagents are prepared according to the manufacturer's instructions.

1. If frozen, thaw the PCR product immediately before use. Make serial dilutions and follow the Viral Quant EBV kit instructions for detection of products (*see* **Note 6**).
2. Proceed with the detection procedure and wash steps according to the Viral Quant EBV kit instructions. Measure the OD_{450} on an ELISA plate reader.

3.6.2. Calculation of Results

For each sample, calculate the EBV viral load as instructed in the Viral Quant EBV kit protocol (*see* **Note 7**). Remember to adjust the copy number by any dilution factor used prior to amplification (*see* **Note 8**). Assay results are objective; however, medical use of these results requires clinicopathologic correlation.

3.6.3. Clinicopathologic Interpretation of Results

The "normal" range for this assay depends on the clinical status. Each laboratory is encouraged to validate the assay on its own patient populations. Healthy nonimmunosuppressed patients generally have undetectable viral loads, i.e., less than about 1000 copies/mL of plasma or serum. For clinical evaluation of immunosuppressed transplant recipients, serial samples are encouraged rather than a onetime test. In serial samples analyzed over time, 10-fold differences in viral load are considered to be clinically significant. Baseline values are encouraged in healthy transplant recipients so that future values may be judged in comparison. Baseline values may be higher in patients who were seronegative at the time of transplant, compared with seropositive recipients who harbor prior immunity. In general, patients with EBV-driven PTLD have plasma or serum values higher than 5000 copies/mL. Undetectable EBV viral loads are consistent with the absence of EBV-driven PTLD. Values in the gray zone, as well as onetime values at any level, should be interpreted in the context of clinicopathologic findings.

Although few studies of nasopharyngeal carcinoma have been conducted, our own experience suggests that these patients have relatively low EBV viral loads until the disease becomes widely metastatic.

4. Notes

1. An alternate kit for isolating DNA from these samples is the QIAamp Blood kit (Qiagen). It has the advantage of slightly higher sensitivity since it samples 200 rather than 140 μL of patient specimen; however, the kit is not supplied with carrier DNA. Therefore, carrier nucleic acid, such as Poly-deoxy-adenylic-thymidylic acid (Boehringer Mannheim), must be added to the AE buffer at a final concentration of 20 μg/mL. The amount of spiked ICS remains the same at 5000 copies/sample, and target DNA is eluted off the column into 50 μL of AE buffer. Calculation of viral load must be adjusted to accommodate the higher initial sample volume.
2. We recommend heat-labile rather than conventional UNG. The problem with conventional UNG is that it may not be completely inactivated by heating for 10 min at 95°C, and therefore it may degrade newly formed PCR products ***(14)***. By contrast, heat-labile UNG is more rapidly and efficiently inactivated ***(15)***, and we have confirmed that it works better in this protocol. Be aware that some

laboratories use an alternate strategy: UNG is not used on a routine basis, but dUTP is routinely incorporated into PCR products so that UNG will be effective should a contamination problem occur.

3. Although the PCR conditions have been carefully optimized in this protocol, it might be necessary to further optimize this protocol in your own laboratory's thermocycler, considering the dUTP and magnesium concentrations, and verifying that UNG activity is ablated during the 95°C preincubation.
4. Following amplification, immediately proceed to the detection procedure or freeze the products at –20°C. Attention to timeliness will minimize the possibility of residual UNG activity destroying the PCR products ***(14)***.
5. Lower EBV copy numbers can be detected by using 40 rather than 34 cycles; however, if 40 cycles are used, begin by spiking with 100 rather than 500 copies of ICS per reaction. For routine clinical use in transplant recipients, we have found 34 cycles to be adequate.
6. The manufacturer's instructions recommend making two- or fivefold dilutions of the PCR products prior to detection. These dilution factors can be adjusted according to your experience with the patient samples in your own facility. In our laboratory, we found that fourfold dilutions produced more definitive values. To make fourfold serial dilutions in wells B–D, add 100 µL of hybridization buffer to wells B, C, and D of both the ICS and EBV strips. Add 133.3 µL of the suggested starting dilution (1:20) of EBV or ICS to well A. Transfer 33.3 µL from row A to B and mix up and down six times by pipeting with plugged tips. Continue this process through row D. After mixing row D, remove and discard 33.3 µL.
7. The manufacturer's instructions state that an OD_{450} of 0.3–1.5 is the acceptable range for proceeding, but we often visualize an electrophoretic EBV band in samples with an OD_{450} as low as 0.1. Therefore, we recommend that if a weak EBV band is visualized on the gel, and the OD_{450} is between 0.1 and 0.3, you may still calculate a result.
8. To clarify the adjustments that must be made to accommodate dilution factors, remember that the starting volume of patient plasma, serum, or CSF is typically 140 µL (QIAamp Viral kit) or 200 µL (QIAamp Blood kit). This gets eluted into 50 µL of diluent following column extraction. Then 5 µL of that is used in PCR. Therefore, to report EBV copies/mL of patient specimen, the raw result should be adjusted as follows. For 140-µL samples, multiply the raw result by 71.4. For 200-µL patient samples, multiply the raw result by 50. For DNA extracted from blood mononuclear cells and later spiked with ICS, results are reported in copies/µg of DNA, so raw results need not be adjusted, as 1 µg of template DNA was used in the PCR reaction. Finally, round off all results to the first two digits (e.g., 5397 becomes 5400; 236,000 becomes 240,000).

References

1. Savoie, A., Perpete, C., Carpentier, L., Joncas, J., and Alfieri, C. (1994) Direct correlation between the load of Epstein-Barr virus-infected lymphocytes in the

peripheral blood of pediatric transplant patients and risk of lymphoproliferative disease. *Blood* **83,** 2715–2722.

2. Rooney, C. M., Loftin, S. K., Holladay, M. S., Brenner, M. K., Krance, R. A., and Heslop, H. E. (1995) Early identification of Epstein-Barr virus-associated post-transplantation lymphoproliferative disease. *Br. J. Haematol.* **89,** 98–103.
3. Rowe, D. T., Qu, L., Reyes, J., Jabbour, N., Yunis, E., Putnam, P., Todo, S., and Green, M. (1997) Use of quantitative competitive PCR to measure Epstein-Barr virus genome load in the peripheral blood of pediatric transplant patients with lymphoproliferative disease. *J. Clin. Microbiol.* **35,** 1612–1615.
4. Riddler, S. A., Breinig, M. C., and McKnight, J. L. (1994) Increased levels of circulating Epstein-Barr virus (EBV)-infected lymphocytes and decreased EBV nuclear antigen antibody responses are associated with the development of posttransplant lymphoproliferative disease in solid-organ transplant recipients. *Blood* **84,** 972–984.
5. Cingolani, A., De Luca, A., Larocca, L. M., Ammassari, A., Scerrati, M., Antinori, A., and Ortona, L. (1998) Minimally invasive diagnosis of acquired immunodeficiency syndrome-related primary central nervous system lymphoma. *J. Natl. Cancer Inst.* **90,** 364–369.
6. Lo, Y. M., Chan, L. Y., Lo, K. W., Leung, S. F., Zhang, J., Chan, A. T., Lee, J. C., Hjelm, N. M., Johnson, P. J., and Huang, D. P. (1999) Quantitative analysis of cell-free Epstein-Barr virus DNA in plasma of patients with nasopharyngeal carcinoma. *Cancer Res.* **59,** 1188–1191.
7. Randhawa, P. S., Jaffe, R., Demetris, A. J., Nalesnik, M., Starzl, T. E., Chen, Y. Y., and Weiss, L. M. (1992) Expression of Epstein-Barr virus-encoded small RNA (by the EBER-1 gene) in liver specimens from transplant recipients with post-transplantation lymphoproliferative disease. *N. Engl. J. Med.* **327,** 1710–1714.
8. Stevens, S. J., Vervoort, M. B., van den Brule, A. J., Meenhorst, P. L., Meijer, C. J., and Middeldorp, J. M. (1999) Monitoring of Epstein-Barr virus DNA load in peripheral blood by quantitaive competitive PCR. *J. Clin. Microbiol.* **37,** 2852–2857.
9. Laroche, C., Drouet, E. B., Brousset, P., Pain, C., Boibieux, A., Biron, F., Icart, J., Denoyel, G. A., and Niveleau, A. (1995) Measurement by the polymerase chain reaction of the Epstein-Barr virus load in infectious mononucleosis and AIDS-related non-Hodgkin's lymphomas. *J. Med. Virol.* **46,** 66–74.
10. Bai, X., Hosler, G., Rogers, B. B., Dawson, D. B., and Scheuermann, R. H. (1997) Quantitative polymerase chain reaction for human herpesvirus diagnosis and measurement of Epstein-Barr virus burden in posttransplant lymphoproliferative disorder. *Clin. Chem.* **43,** 1843–1849.
11. Swinnen, L. J., Gulley, M. L., Hamilton, E., and Schichman, S. A. (1998) EBV DNA quantitiation in serum is highly correlated with the development and regression of post-transplant lymphoproliferative disorder (PTLD) in solid organ transplant recipients. *Blood* **92(Suppl. 1),** 314a,315a.

12. Kimura, H., Morita, M., Yabuta, Y., Kuzushima, K., Kato, K., Kojima, S., Matsuyama, T., and Morishima, T. (1999) Quantitative analysis of Epstein-Barr virus load by using a real-time PCR assay. *J. Clin. Microbiol.* **37,** 132–136.
13. Longo, M. C., Berninger, M. S., and Hartley, J. L. (1990) Use of uracil DNA glycosylase to control carry-over contamination in polymerase chain reactions. *Gene* **93,** 125–128.
14. Thornton, C. G., Hartley, J. L., and Rashtchian, A. (1992) Utilizing uracil DNA glycosylase to control carryover contamination in PCR: characterization of residual UDG activity following thermal cycling. *Biotechniques* **13,** 180–184.
15. Sobek, H., Schmidt, M., Frey, B., and Kaluza, K. (1996) Heat-labile uracil-DNA glycosylase: purification and characterization. *FEBS Lett.* **388,** 1–4.

25

Molecular Detection of Kaposi's Sarcoma–Associated Herpesvirus/ Human Herpesvirus-8

Ethel Cesarman

1. Introduction

Kaposi's sarcoma–associated herpesvirus (KSHV), also called human herpesvirus-8 (HHV-8), is the most recently identified human herpesvirus *(1)*. It has been found to be invariably present in Kaposi's sarcoma (KS) lesions, whether these are associated with AIDS (epidemic KS), therapeutic immunosuppression (iatrogenic KS), or high-incidence regions in Africa (endemic KS), or in its "classic" form (sporadic KS) (for reviews see **refs.** ***2*** and ***3***). By contrast, with few reported exceptions, it has not been found to be present in a variety of other vascular tumors and reactive conditions. A seroepidemiologic association of this virus and KS has been well documented, and it is currently accepted that KSHV plays a necessary, although not sufficient, role in the development of KS. Although diagnosis of KS is usually not difficult based on clinical and histologic features, some cases may have unusual morphology, with features overlapping those of other vascular and spindle cells proliferations. In these instances, molecular detection is useful to confirm or rule out a diagnosis of KS.

This virus has also been found to be present in a subset of malignant lymphomas called primary effusion lymphomas (PELs) or body cavity–based lymphomas *(4)*. These lymphomas have an unusual set of features that in conjunction with the presence of KSHV suggest that they represent a distinct disease entity *(5,6)*. Among these features are a morphology bridging that of anaplastic large-cell lymphoma and immunoblastic lymphoma, and the frequent lack of expression of B-cell-associated antigens in spite of a B-cell geno-

From: *Methods in Molecular Medicine, vol. 49: Molecular Pathology Protocols*
Edited by: A. A. Killeen © Humana Press Inc., Totowa, NJ

type. However, other types of lymphomas can involve body cavities as malignant effusions, either primarily or secondarily, and do not contain this virus. This is particularly frequent in the case of Burkitt lymphomas. Furthermore, PELs can have an "extracavitary" presentation. In these cases, the detection of KSHV may be important for their subclassification.

A third disease in which the presence of KSHV has been convincingly demonstrated is multicentric Castleman's disease (MCD). When occurring in association with AIDS, KSHV is present in the vast majority of cases, whereas it is seen in close to 50% of cases of MCD in human immunodeficiency virus (HIV)-negative individuals. Thus far no studies have suggested that the KSHV-positive cases of MCD are different from the negative ones in terms of disease behavior, outcome, or potential treatment. However, it is possible that as more information is gathered, assessment of the status of KSHV in MCD may be useful clinically.

The easiest and by far the most common method used so far for the detection of KSHV is polymerase chain reaction (PCR). However, extreme care must be taken, as always with this method, to avoid contamination. Many published studies have suggested that this virus is present in a variety of conditions or in the general population, creating extensive controversy in the literature, and mostly being unconfirmed. Most of these studies have used techniques that increase the sensitivity of detection, such as nested PCR. In our hands a single-step PCR, followed by hybridization with a radiolabeled internal oligonucleotide, detects between 1 and 10 copies of the virus in 100 ng of DNA, and has been found to be sensitive and specific (*see* **Note 1**). Using this method, we can detect every case of KS and PEL, 50% of cases of MCD, close to 30% of tissues from HIV-positive patients, and <10% of non-KS tissues. However, to exclude the possibility of contamination, we strongly recommend performing PCR with at least three independent sets of primers. A wide variety of primer sets have been published. In this chapter, we provide the sequences and protocol for three sets with which we have the most extensive experience in our laboratory. One of these sets, called $KS330_{233}$, is the first reported method for detection of KSHV, and the most extensively used ***(1)***. The other two sets were developed in our laboratory, and we have found the sequences they recognized to be well conserved among the various KSHV isolates we have examined and those reported in the literature.

A second method, which we believe to be important in the diagnosis of PEL, is Southern blot analysis on genomic DNA. Because these lymphomas occur most frequently in HIV-positive patients, detection by PCR may mean systemic infection with KSHV, rather than a specific association with this lymphoma. Furthermore, PELs contain 40–80 copies of the viral genome per cell, making its detection using this method quite easy. A full protocol for Southern

Table 1
Oligonucleotides for PCR detection of KSHV

Region	Size of amplicon (bp)	Primer	Primer
ORF 26 ($KS330_{233}$)	233	Forward	5′-AGCCGAAAGGATTCCACCAT-3′
		Reverse	5′-TCCGTGTTGTCTACGTCCAG-3′
		Probe	5′-TGCAGCAGCTGTTGGTGTACCACATC-3′
K9 (vIRF1)	184	Forward	5′-CCCTTTCGCGGATATACACA-3′
		Reverse	5′-AGTGAGGGGAAAGCGTCAAT-3′
		Probe	5′-GTCTCTGCGCCATTCAAAAC-3′
ORF 74 (vGPCR)	492	Forward	5′-CCGTGGTGCCTTACACGTGG-3′
		Reverse	5′-CAGTCTGCAGTCATGTTTCC-3′
		Probe	5′-TGTGTGCGTCAGTCTAGTGAG-3′
β-Actin	540	Forward	5′-GTGGGGCGCCCCAGGCACCA-3′
		Reverse	5′-CTCCTTAATGTCACGCACGATTTC-3′

blotting is not provided, because any standard method can be used, but the details specific for KSHV detection are given in **Note 2**. If Southern blot analysis is not possible, approximate quantitation to document high viral copy numbers is necessary before a diagnosis of PEL is made. This can be performed by serially diluting the DNA and comparing to known standards.

2. Materials

2.1. Oligonucleotide Primers and Probes

Primers and internal oligonucleotide probes for open reading frame 26 (ORF 26) (Capsid protein), K9 (vIRF1), and ORF 74 (vGPCR). Sequences are provided in **Table 1**. Any primer set can be used as a control for integrity of DNA and absence of inhibitors. One of these control primers sets, shown in **Table 1**, is for the β-actin gene.

2.2. Controls

As a positive control, any PEL cell line can be used. One of these is BC-3, which contains KSHV but lacks EBV. This cell line can be obtained from the American Type Culture Collection (ATCC) (Rockville, MD; ATCC designation CRL-2277). This cell line contains approx 30 copies of the viral genome/cell, so it can be diluted 100- to 1000-fold to be used as a control for PCR. Alternatively, DNA extracted from a KS lesion can be used as a positive control. DNA from a KS cell line should not be used, because these "lose" the

KSHV genome after a few passages in culture. As a negative control, DNA from peripheral blood mononuclear cells of healthy individuals, or a KSHV-negative cell line (any lymphoblastoid or myeloid cell line), can be used.

2.2. Polymerase Chain Reaction

1. 10X PCR buffer containing 15 m*M* $MgCl_2$ (Perkin-Elmer, Norwalk, CT).
2. *Taq* DNA polymerase (5 U/µL) (Perkin-Elmer).
3. Primers (10 pmol/µL).
4. dNTP mixture of 10 pmol/µL of each nucleotide (Boehringer Mannheim, Indianapolis, IN).

2.3. Analysis of PCR Products

1. 2% Agarose gel in 1X TAE buffer: 40 m*M* Tris-acetate, 1 m*M* EDTA, 0.0001% ethidium bromide.

2.4 Transfer and Hybridization

1. Oligonucleotide probe at 10 pmol/µL (**Table 1**).
2. [γ-^{32}P]ATP (3000 Ci/mmol; NEN).
3. T4 polynucleotide kinase (10 U/µL) (Boehringer Mannheim).
4. 10X T4 polynucleotide kinase buffer (Boehringer Mannheim).
5. Sephadex G25 spin column (Amersham-Pharmacia).
6. Salmon sperm DNA (10 mg/mL) (Boehringer Mannheim).
7. 20X SSPE: 3 *M* NaCl, 0.2 *M* NaH_2PO_4, 0.5 *M* EDTA, pH 7.4.
8. 20% Sodium dodecyl sulfate (SDS).
9. 50X Denhardt's solution: 1% Ficoll 400 (Sigma, St. Louis, MO), 1% polyvinylpyrrolidone (Sigma), and 1% bovine serum albumin, (Pentax fraction V; Sigma).
10. X-ray film (Kodak).

3. Methods

3.1. Isolation of Nucleic Acid

PCR can be performed on DNA extracted from fresh, frozen, or paraffin-embedded tissue using standard methodology. It is important to extract the DNA in a physical area that is separate from that used for amplification and manipulation of PCR products.

3.2. Polymerase Chain Reaction

1. Prepare a master mix in a plastic microfuge tube. This mix should be prepared in a "clean" area that is separate from those where the DNA is extracted and where the amplification is performed and PCR products are analyzed. Calculate the amount of solution to be used by multiplying by the number of samples (*n*) to be

analyzed plus one (n + 1). Per sample add and mix the following: 14.05 mL of H_2O, 1.25 µL of 2m*M* dNTP, 2.5 µL of 10X buffer, 1 µL of each forward and reverse primer at a concentration of 10 pmol/µL, and 0.2 µL of *Taq* polymerase.
2. Aliquot 20 µL of master mix in each sample tube.
3. Add 100 ng of DNA previously diluted in a total volume of 5 µL.
4. Perform PCR on a thermocycler starting with a denaturation step at 94°C for 3.5 min, followed by 30 cycles of denaturation (1 min at 94°C), annealing (1 min at 58°C), and extension (1.5 min at 72°C).

3.3. Analysis of PCR Products

1. Withdraw 10 µL from each sample tube. Add 1 µL of 10X loading dye containing bromophenol and xylene-cyanol blue, and mix.
2. Load onto a 2% agarose gel and electrophorese for approx 2 h at 80 V.
3. Visualize in a UV transilluminator and photograph the gel.

3.4. Transfer and Hybridization

1. Transfer of PCR products onto a nitrocellulose filter or nylon membrane should be performed according to standard procedures as first described by Southern *(7)*.
2. Prehybridize the filters for 2 h at 37°C in a hybridization solution containing 5X SSPE, 5X Denhardt's solution, and 0.5% SDS.
3. Label the internal oligonucleotide probe as follows: In a plastic tube mix 2.5 µL of probe (25 pmol), 5 µL of [γ-^{32}P]ATP, 1 µL of 10X kinase buffer, and 1 µL of T4 polynucleotide kinase. Incubate for 90 min at 37°C. Stop the reaction by adding 90 µL of TE (10 m*M* Tris-HCl/1 m*M* EDTA) and 1 µL 0.5 *M* EDTA. Remove free label by centrifugation in a G25 spin column.
4. Hybridize the filters for 5 h to overnight at 37°C in hybridization solution containing 100 µg/mL of salmon sperm DNA and radiolabeled probe at approx 2×10^6 cpm/mL.
5. Wash the filters twice for 15 min at room temperature in 2X SSPE and 1% SDS, followed by washing for 10 min at 60°C ($KS330_{233}$), 55°C (vIRF1), or 57°C (vGPCR), using a preheated solution of 5X SSPE, and 0.1% SDS. Rinse the filters in 2X saline sodium citrate.
6. Expose on an autoradiograph film.

3.5. Interpretation of Results

Cases should be considered positive only when at least two sets of primers detect a clearly positive signal. In negative cases, it is important to make sure that the DNA is amplifiable using a control set of primers.

4. Notes

1. In our hands, the PCR products can be visualized without the need for hybridization, even when very low copy numbers (10–100) are present. With the vIRF1 primers we can detect 1–5 copies without the need for hybridization. However, hybridization is useful to confirm the specificity of the amplified products.

2. Southern blot using genomic DNA for detection of KSHV should be performed for distinction of PEL and circumstantial presence of KSHV owing to disseminated viremia in an AIDS-associated lymphoma. For this, 5 µg of DNA may be digested with *Bam*HI, electrophoresed, and transferred using standard procedures ***(7)***. We recommend hybridization with a probe to ORF 26 as described ***(1)***. If a plasmid containing this insert is not available, this probe can be made by PCR amplification of the ORF 26 ($KS330_{233}$) fragment, using a PEL positive control as template. A hybridization band of 330 bp will be obtained in positive cases. This method also detects approx 75% of cases of KS.

References

1. Chang, Y., Cesarman, E., Pessin, M. S., Lee, F., Culpepper, J., Knowles, D. M., and Moore, P. S. (1994) Identification of herpesvirus-like DNA sequences in AIDS-associated Kaposi's sarcoma. *Science* **266,** 1865–1869.
2. Cesarman, E. and Knowles, D. M. (1997) Kaposi's sarcoma-associated herpesvirus: a lymphotropic human herpesvirus associated with Kaposi's sarcoma, primary effusion lymphoma, and multicentric Castleman's disease. *Semin. Diagn. Pathol.* **14,** 54–66.
3. Ganem, D. (1997) KSHV and Kaposi's sacroma: the end of the beginning? *Cell* **91,**157–160.
4. Cesarman, E., Chang, Y., Moore, P. S., Said, J. W., and Knowles, D. M. (1995) Kaposi's Sarcoma-associated Herpesvirus-like DNA sequences in AIDS-related body cavity-based lymphomas. *N. Engl. J. Med.* **332,** 1186–1191.
5. Nador, R. G., Cesarman, E., Chadburn, A., Dawson, D. B., Ansari, M. Q., Said, J., and Knowles, D. M. (1996) Primary effusion lymphoma: a distinct clinicopathologic entity associated with the Kaposi's sarcoma-associated herpesvirus. *Blood* **88,** 645–656.
6. Cesarman, E. and Knowles, D. M. (1999) The role of Kaposi's sarcoma-associated herpesvirus (KSHV/HHV-8) in lymphoproliferative diseases. *Semin. Cancer Biol.* **9,** 165–174.
7. Southern, E. M. (1975) Detection of specific sequences among DNA fragments separated by gel electrophoresis. *J. Mol. Biol.* **98,** 503–517.

26

Diagnostic Applications of Quantitative Polymerase Chain Reaction for Cytomegalovirus

Richard H. Scheuermann and Xin Bai

1. Introduction

Eight viruses in the herpes family have been identified that infect humans: herpes simplex viruses 1 and 2, varicella-zoster virus, Epstein-Barr virus, cytomegalovirus (CMV), human herpesviruses 6 and 7 and the Kaposi sarcoma–associated herpesvirus *(1)*. In immunocompetent individuals, primary infections are usually handled effectively by the host immune system without therapeutic intervention. However, these viruses are never completely eradicated by the immune response, probably because these viruses have the capacity to enter a latent state in a subset of infected cells. However, this does not normally pose a problem since the host immune system has been primed to handle any subsequent reactivation. Thus, human herpesviruses rarely cause serious problems in immunocompetent individuals.

By contrast, individuals who are immunocompromised owing to congenital abnormalities, therapeutic immunosupression, or human immunodeficiency virus infection frequently experience life-threatening complications due to primary infection or reactivation by these viruses. For example, bone marrow allograft recipients receiving immunosupressive therapy have a high risk of developing several complications related to CMV infection, including encephalitis, esophagitis, hepatitis, and pneumonitis; the latter is associated with a high mortality rate *(2,3)*.

In normal patients, diagnosis of viral infection is usually made based on serology, i.e., the detection of antibodies to the virus in question in the blood (e.g. *[4]*). However, the interpretation of serology for herpesviruses in immuno-

From: *Methods in Molecular Medicine, vol. 49: Molecular Pathology Protocols*
Edited by: A. A. Killeen © Humana Press Inc., Totowa, NJ

compromised patients is difficult owing to the high seroprevalence of herpesviruses in the normal population, and the variable effects of immunosuppression on antibody titers. For CMV, viral culture methods have been developed for the direct detection of infectious viral particles. However, these methods suffer from relatively low sensitivity and are very sensitive to sample-handling conditions. These culture techniques have largely been replaced by an antigenemia test for the detection of CMV infection in the management of immunosuppressed patients ***(5–8)***.

More recently, the polymerase chain reaction (PCR) has been applied to the detection of CMV in these patients. However, it appears that simple PCR is not useful in the detection of clinically relevant disease since CMV can be detected in a significant subset of normal, healthy individuals, presumably owing to the presence of latently infected cells in the diagnostic sample ***(9–15)***. Therefore, this simple PCR procedure has been adapted to include an internal calibration standard (ICS) in such a way as to provide clinically useful information ***(16)***. ICS-PCR has two major advantages over simple PCR. First, it provides quantitative determination of CMV levels that allows the distinction between latent and active infection. Second, the use of an internal control helps rule out false-negative results occasionally seen in PCR reactions when using DNA isolated from patient samples. Thus, ICS-PCR provides an accurate, objective, and sensitive technique for diagnosing and monitoring CMV disease in immunosuppressed patients.

2. Materials

2.1. Isolation of DNA

QIAamp Blood Kit (PN 29104; QIAGEN, Santa Clara, CA) (*see* **Note 13** for an important update). For 50 isolations, the kit includes the following components:

1. Lyophilized QIAGEN Protease (28 mg).
2. Reagent AL1 (12 mL).
3. Reagent AL2 (3 mL).
4. Buffer AW concentrate (17 mL).
5. Buffer AE (12 mL).
6. Fifty QIAamp spin columns.
7. One hundred fifty 2-mL Microfuge collection tubes.

2.1.1. Preparation of Reagents from Kit

1. Protease solution: Add 1.4 mL of double-distilled H_2O (ddH_2O) to 28 mg of QIAGEN protease and dissolve. Store in aliquots at –20°C.
2. AL buffer: Mix 12 mL of reagent AL1 with 3 mL of reagent AL2. Store in the dark at room temperature.

3. AW buffer: Add 40 mL of 100% ethanol to 17 mL of buffer AW concentrate. Store at room temperature.
4. Sterile ddH_20.
5. Microfuge tubes (1.5 mL).
6. 100% Ethanol.
7. Extra AL buffer (PN 19075; QIAGEN).
8. TE: 10 m*M* Tris-HCl, 1 m*M* EDTA, pH 8.0.

2.2. Polymerase Chain Reaction (*see* Note 1)

1. 10X AmpliTaq Buffer (PN N808-0006; Perkin-Elmer, Branchburg, NJ).
2. 10 m*M* each of dATP, dCTP, and dGTP, and 20 m*M* dUTP (*see* **Note 2**) (PN N808-0095; Perkin-Elmer).
3. AmpliTaq DNA polymerase (5 U/µL) (PN N801-0060; Perkin-Elmer).
4. 5′ CMV primer resuspended in ddH_2O at 100 pmol/µL (TACCCCTATCG-CGTGTGTTC) ***(16)***.
5. 3′ CMV primer resuspended in ddH_2O at 100 pmol/µL (ATAGGAGGCGC-CACGTATTC) ***(16)***.
6. HHVQ-1 Internal Calibration Standard (available from authors; ***[16]***) or another ICS incorporating CMV-specific primer sequences (10 molecules/µL TE). *See* **Note 3** for the characteristics of an effective ICS.
7. Microamp reaction tubes and caps.
8. Thermocycler with heated lid, e.g., Perkin-Elmer GeneAmp PCR System 9600 (*see* **Note 1**).

2.3. Detection of Product

1. 5X DNA sample buffer: 200 m*M* Tris-HCl acetate, 10 m*M* EDTA, 50% glycerol, 0.25% (w/v) bromophenol blue.
2. Agarose (molecular biology grade, e.g., Seakem GTG Agarose, FMC, Rockland, ME).
3. 50X TAE buffer: 2.0 *M* Tris-HCl acetate, 50 m*M* EDTA. Dissolve 242 g of Tris base in 600 mL of ddH_2O while adding 57.1 mL of glacial acetic acid and 100 mL of 0.5 *M* EDTA, pH 8.0. Bring up the volume to 1.0 L with ddH_2O.
4. DNA molecular weight marker, e.g., 123-bp DNA ladder (PN 15613-011; Gibco-BRL, Gaithersburg, MD) at 0.1 µg/µL in 1X DNA sample buffer.
5. Sybr Gold nucleic acid gel stain (PN S-11494; Molecular Probes, Eugene, OR) (*see* **Note 4**), or ethidium bromide (EtBr) (PN E8751; Sigma, St. Louis, MO) at 10 mg/mL in ddH_2O.
6. Gel-casting tray, electrophoresis apparatus, and DC power supply.
7. Imaging hardware (*see* **Note 5**): For analysis of gels stained with SYBR Gold, illumination with a 488-nm laser and a fluorescence imaging system is used (e.g., Fluorimager SI; Molecular Dynamics, Sunnyvale, CA). For analysis of gels stained with EtBr, illumination with UV light at a 254-nm wavelength and analysis using a UV imaging system is used (e.g., AlphaImager 2000; Alpha Innotech, San Leandro, CA).

3. Methods

3.1. Isolation of DNA

In the early days of molecular analysis, DNA was isolated from cell sources using organic extraction methods. The cells were first lysed with detergent, proteins removed by phenol extraction, and the DNA purified and concentrated by alcohol precipitation. Although this technique is effective, it is also somewhat time-consuming and involves the use of hazardous chemicals. More recently, several companies have developed DNA isolation kits based on a number of nonorganic methods for DNA purification. These kits provide a cost-effective means of isolating high-quality DNA without the use of organic solvents. We have evaluated many of these kits for their suitability in the isolation of viral DNA from patient samples, especially whole blood, and found that three give high-quality material suitable for most PCR applications: the QIAamp Blood Kit (QIAGEN), the Puregene DNA Isolation Kit (GENTRA Systems, Minneapolis, MN), and the Isoquick Nucleic Acid Extraction Kit (ORCA Research, Bothell, WA). In this section, we describe a modification of the QIAamp Blood Kit that we use for the analysis of CMV levels in patient samples. Regardless of the method used, the key point is that the DNA material isolated should allow sensitive and specific target amplification. In **Subheading 3.4.1.**, we provide an example of how one can evaluate any DNA isolation procedure to determine whether the performance characteristics are optimal.

The isolation method employed in the QIAamp Blood Kit relies on the preferential binding of nucleic acids to silica gel surfaces in the presence of chaotropic salts. The bound nucleic acids are washed to remove contaminants and eluted in small volumes using a low-salt buffer (AE buffer). The silica gel matrices are provided in a spin column format to facilitate rapid isolation. This procedure can be applied to a wide variety of patient samples. Here we describe the isolation of DNA from whole blood; for isolation from other sample sources, one should refer to the product guide for specifics (*see* **Note 13** for an important update):

1. Place 200 µL of blood in a sterile 1.5-mL microfuge tube.
2. Add 25 µL of protease solution.
3. Add 200 µL of AL buffer. Mix immediately by vortexing for 15 s.
4. Incubate the cell lysate at 70°C for 10 min.
5. Add 210 µL of 100% ethanol and mix by vortexing.
6. Apply the mixture to a QIAamp spin column seated in a 2-mL microfuge tube.
7. Centrifuge at 6000*g* (8000 rpm in a standard Eppendorf microfuge) for 1 min.
8. Discard the flowthrough.
9. Wash the column twice with 500 µL of AL buffer. (This step is a modification of the original procedure that was developed in our laboratory to further improve the quality of the isolated DNA specifically for PCR applications; *see* **Subheading 3.4.1.**)

10. Wash the column twice with 500 µL of AW buffer. For the last wash, centrifuge the column for 3 min at 20,000*g* (14,000 rpm) to remove as much of the wash solution as possible.
11. Place the column in a clean 1.5-mL microfuge tube.
12. Elute DNA by adding 200 µL of AE buffer that has been preheated to 70°C to the column. Incubate at 70°C for 5 min. Centrifuge the column 1 min to collect eluted DNA. At this stage the purified DNA can be used directly in PCR reactions, further concentrated by alcohol precipitation (*see* **Note 6**), or stored at –20°C for later use.

3.2. Polymerase Chain Reaction

The PCR reaction involves a variety of components and conditions that can vary depending on the specific primer-template combination used. Rather than trying to optimize these factors for every target we wish to analyze, we have taken a different approach to the issue of optimization. When we are developing a new procedure to amplify a new target, we evaluate a panel of primers and select only the ones that work well under standard PCR reaction conditions. This approach has greatly simplified all PCR protocols in our laboratory because they all work well under essentially the same amplification conditions. For a detailed discussion on primer selection in general and the primers used here for detection and quantification of CMV, see Bai et al. ***(16)***. The following protocol is for 50-µL PCR reactions:

1. Place purified DNA into individual microfuge tubes. For maximum sensitivity (i.e., low limits of detection), we routinely use DNA isolated from 10 µl of blood in 10 µL of AE elution buffer (*see* **Note 7**).
2. Add 2 µL of HHVQ-1 standard (10 molecules/µL) to each tube (*see* **Note 8**).
3. Determine the number of samples to be analyzed in a given experiment.
4. Design a master mix containing all the PCR components except the purified sample DNA (*see* **Table 1**). A mix is prepared for 10% more than the required number of samples. For example, for 10 samples prepare enough master mix for 11 samples; for 20 samples, prepare a master mix for 22 samples. In this example, the analysis of 10 samples is described.
5. In a 1.5-mL microfuge tube prepare the PCR master mix as described in **Table 1**. Mix by vortexing.
6. Add 38 µL of master mix to each tube containing purified blood DNA/standard mixture. Vortex briefly.
7. Seal the tubes carefully with caps and place in a thermocycler.
8. Amplify under the following cycling conditions: 1 cycle of 94°C for 2 min; 34 cycles of 94°C for 0.4 min, 60°C for 0.4 min, 72°C for 1.0 min; 1 cycle of 72°C for 9.0 min; and hold at 8°C. After amplification is complete, the samples can be stored for several hours at 4°C. For longer storage, –20 or –70°C is recommended. (N.B. The optimal conditions may vary depending on the thermocycler used. *See* **Note 1** for a discussion of how this can be evaluated. The conditions described here work well for the Perkin-Elmer GeneAmp PCR System 9600.)

Table 1
Preparation of PCR Master Mix

Component	Volume for 11 reactions (μL)	Volume/ reaction (μL)	Final concentration
ddH_2O	310.2[a]	28.2[a]	—
10X PCR buffer	55	5	1X
10 m*M* dATP	11	1	200 μ*M*
10 m*M* dCTP	11	1	200 μ*M*
10 m*M* dGTP	11	1	200 μ*M*
20 m*M* dUTP	11 (*see* **Note 2**)	1	400 μ*M*
5′ CMV primer (100 pmol/μL)	2.2	0.2	20 pmol
3′ CMV primer (100 pmol/μL)	2.2	0.2	20 pmol
AmpliTaq polymerase 5 U/μL)	4.4	0.4	2 U

[a]The amount of ddH_2O to include in the reaction depends on the volume of sample to be analyzed. In this example, we are analyzing a sample containing 10 μL of blood DNA and 2 μL of internal standard in a final reaction volume of 50 μL. This means that 38 μL of the master mix will need to be added to the DNA mixture. To calculate the amount of ddH_2O to include in the master mix, multiply 38 μL × 11 samples to give a final volume of 418 μL for the total master mix. Then subtract the volumes of all the other master mix components to give the volume of ddH_2O required (418 – 55 – 11 – 11 – 11 – 11 – 2.2 – 2.2 – 4.4 = 310.2 μL). The volumes of the other components are determined by the concentrations of the stock solutions used and the final concentrations required in the PCR reaction.

3.3. Detection of PCR Product

Two methods are commonly used to detect and quantify specific PCR products following amplification: staining following gel electrophoresis or product capture and detection on a solid support (e.g., microtiter plate wells). The advantages to these two detection methods are that each offers an additional layer of specificity to the PCR reaction. In gel electrophoresis, the size of the DNA product is evaluated and should correspond to the size predicted for the DNA target in question. In the microtiter plate approach, capture and/or detection involves the hybridization of a probe to specific sequences contained in the specific PCR product. A method for the detection and quantification of CMV using the microtiter/capture approach has been developed by BioSource International, Inc. (Camarillo, CA) ***(17)***. Here we describe detection and quantification of PCR products following gel electrophoresis. Although we give specific details of a procedure that works well for this analysis, many other systems can also be used, including polyacrylamide gels and real-time PCR.

1. Add 2 g of agarose to 100 mL of 1X TAE buffer in a 500-mL Erlenmeyer flask. Heat in a microwave on high setting for 2 to 3 min until all of the agarose is dissolved. (The amount of agarose solution may be adjusted based on the size of the gel to be used.)
2. Pour molten agarose into a gel-casting tray with a well comb in position. Allow it to cool until solidified (~1 h at room temperature).
3. Place the gel in an electrophoresis apparatus. Cover with 1X TAE buffer.
4. Add 12 µL of 5X DNA sample buffer to each 50-µL PCR reaction sample. Mix by vortexing.
5. Carefully load 20–30 µL of each sample into separate wells of the gel using a micropipettor.
6. After all the samples are loaded, load an appropriate molecular weight marker (e.g., 123-bp DNA ladder) into the next adjacent well.
7. Close the electrophoresis apparatus. Connect the cables to the power supply and apparatus with the positive cathode positioned at the bottom end of the gel in the direction of migration.
8. Electrophorese for 1.5 h at 100 V or until the bromophenol blue tracking dye is within 1 cm of the end of the gel.
9. Turn off the power supply, remove the gel, and place in a staining solution containing either ethidium bromide (1 µg/mL) or Sybr Gold (1 : 10,000 dilution of stock) for 30–60 min.
10. Examine EtBr-stained gels using UV wavelength illumination; examine Sybr Gold–stained gels using 488 nm illumination.

3.4. Experimental Results

3.4.1. Quality of DNA Isolation Procedure

The quality of the DNA for PCR amplification can be evaluated in reactions that contain a relatively large amount of material with a small number of specific targets. The experiment presented in **Fig. 1** shows an example of this kind of analysis. In this case, a constant amount of ICS has been added to each PCR reaction with increasing amounts of DNA isolated from whole blood using the standard and modified QIAamp procedure. (The standard procedure lacks **step 9** in **Subheading 3.1.**) In reactions containing DNA isolated by the standard procedure, the addition of 0.1 or 1.0 µL of this DNA had no effect on the ability to amplify the ICS (compare lanes 9 and 10 with lane 8). However, if 10 or 20 µL of this DNA was added (lanes 11 and 12), inhibition of ICS amplification was observed. On the other hand, even 20 µL of blood DNA isolated by the modified procedure could be added without affecting amplification efficiency of the ICS (lane 6). This indicates that DNA isolated by the standard procedure contains a PCR inhibitor that reaches significant levels when 10 µL of this DNA is used under these conditions. However, with a simple modification, these inhibitors can be largely removed and more DNA included in the reaction. (*See* **Note 13** for an important update on the DNA isolation procedure.)

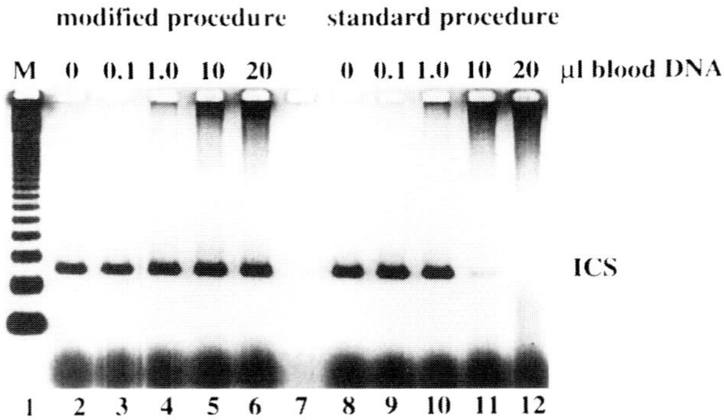

Fig. 1. Efficient PCR amplification from blood samples using a modified DNA isolation protocol. DNA was isolated from 200 µL of whole blood from a healthy volunteer using the standard QIAamp Blood Kit protocol (lanes 8–12) that does not include **step 9** in **Subheading 3.1.** or by a modification of this procedure (lanes 2–6) that includes **step 9**. PCR reactions were set up with CMV-specific primers, 300 molecules of the HHVQ-1 ICS, and varying amounts of this purified DNA (from 0 to 20 µL) as indicated. Reactions were amplified under standard conditions and products analyzed following agarose gel electrophoresis and Sybr Gold staining. A 123-bp DNA ladder (M) is included to determine product sizes (lane 1).

The use of a standard molecule as an amplification target allows one to assess amplification efficiency under the conditions used. In this case, we used this approach to evaluate the quality of the DNA isolation procedure used. However, a similar approach can be used to evaluate any of the components of the PCR reaction. For example, if one is considering the use of an alternative polymerase for amplification, it should be able to generate product when a limiting amount of target is mixed with DNA isolated from a patient sample.

3.4.2. Determination of CMV Viral Burden in Patient Samples

CMV viral burden can be determined by using serial dilutions of patient sample DNA amplified with a constant quantity of ICS. For analysis of whole blood, DNA is isolated as described in **Subheading 3.1.** from 200 µL of blood collected in acid citrate dextrose (ACD), EDTA, or even heparin tubes (*see* **Note 9**). To achieve low limits of detection, as much of this purified DNA is included in the first PCR reaction. In our experience, 10-µL samples can be reproducibly used in these PCR reactions without adverse effects of inhibitors. Additional reactions are also prepared using 1.0 µL and 1.0 µL of a 1/10 dilution of this purified DNA. Each reaction contains a constant amount of ICS; when conditions are optimal, 20 molecules of ICS can be routinely amplified. Thus, for each patient sample, three PCR reactions are prepared with 10-fold serial dilutions of purified patient DNA and a constant amount of ICS.

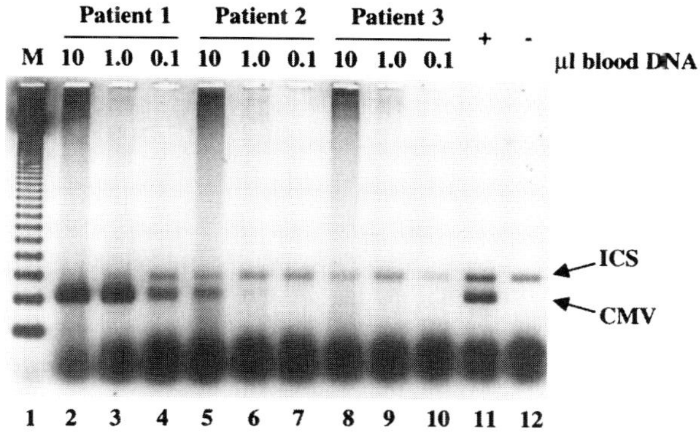

Fig. 2. Analysis of CMV viral burden in whole blood from three different patient samples. DNA was isolated from whole blood of three patient samples by the modified QIAamp procedure. PCR reactions were set up with CMV-specific primers, 20 molecules of the HHVQ-1 ICS, and varying amounts of this purified DNA (from 0.1 to 10 µL) as indicated. Samples were also prepared that contained 67 molecules of purified CMV DNA (lane 11) or no DNA (lane 12) as target. Reactions were amplified under standard conditions and products analyzed following agarose gel electrophoresis and Sybr Gold staining. The upper band derived from the ICS standard and the lower band derived from the CMV viral genome are indicated with arrows. A 123-bp DNA ladder (M) is included to determine product sizes (lane 1).

Figure 2 presents results of this type of analysis for three different patient samples. Using 10 µL of DNA isolated from patient 1, a single intense band is observed derived from the CMV viral DNA (lane 2). In this case, no ICS-specific band is found owing to competition from the large amount of viral target present in the reaction. Even with 1.0 µL of DNA, the ICS-specific band is very faint when compared with the CMV-specific band (lane 3). Only with 0.1 µL of blood DNA from this patient can both bands be observed clearly (lane 4). Quantification of the intensities of these two bands gives a virus : ICS ratio of 2 (*see* **Note 10**). Since 20 molecules of ICS were included in this reaction, this indicates that 40 viral targets were present in 0.1 µL of blood, or a viral burden of 400,000 viral genomes/mL of blood.

For patient 2, clear bands from both the ICS and the CMV targets were observed only when 10 µL of blood DNA was included in the PCR reaction (lane 5). Quantification of the band intensities gives a virus : ICS ratio of 1.5, in a reaction containing 20 molecules of ICS. Thus, patient 2 has a viral burden of 3000 viral genomes/mL of blood.

Finally, no CMV-specific bands were observed in any of the samples with DNA from patient 3. Using this procedure, we can estimate the limits of detection in this experiment because we could have expected to see a CMV band one fourth the intensity of the ICS-specific band in the 10 µL DNA sample (lane 8). This would give a viral burden of <500 viral genomes/mL of blood for patient 3. In addition, the importance of detecting an ICS-specific band in the reactions using DNA from patient 3 is discussed in **Note 11**.

Lanes 11 and 12 contain positive and negative control samples, respectively, which should always be included at the end of each set of reactions. The positive sample contained 67 copies of CMV, and the ratio of intensities is approx 3, as expected. The absence of a CMV-specific band in the negative control sample indicates that contamination of these PCR reactions during reaction setup has not occurred in this experiment.

3.4.3. Conclusion

CMV viral monitoring can be used to improve the management of solid organ and bone marrow transplant recipients. Sensitive techniques to identify patients with high CMV levels before clinical manifestations of viral disease allow the application of preemptive therapeutic approaches rather than prophylactic therapy of high-risk patients. This reduces the risk of clinical complications associated with the antiviral therapies used and promises to reduce the overall patient cost associated with these therapies ***(18–22)***.

One of the challenges in using a sensitive method such as PCR for the detection of CMV in the transplant population is to distinguish between clinically relevant and latent infection. Growing evidence indicates that this distinction can be made based on the differences in CMV levels in these two populations (***[23]***; our unpublished data). The use of ICSs allows quantitative measurement of CMV levels in patient samples.

From our studies, it appears that the cutoffs for clinically relevant detection are levels above 10,000 viral targets/mL of blood, at least for cmv in the pediatric solid organ transplant population. The numbers for the adult solid-organ transplant population appear to be similar. With this information in hand, it may be possible to simplify the analysis described in **Subheading 3.4.2.** so that only a single PCR reaction would need to be evaluated for each patient sample (*see* **Note 12**).

In addition to its ability to facilitate quantification, ICS-PCR also provides another important use in clinical diagnostic laboratories. By serving as an internal positive control in every reaction, amplification of the ICS helps rule out false-negative results.

4. Notes

1. We have found that the source of reagents and polymerase used in the PCR reaction and the thermocycler used for amplification can have dramatic effects on the

results when low limits of detection are sought in a complex nucleic acid mixture. Using an evaluation strategy similar to the one described in **Fig. 1**, the suitability of other reagents and cycling parameters can be evaluated easily by performing PCR reactions containing small amounts of ICS target (e.g., 20–50 molecules) in DNA isolated from relatively large amounts of blood (5–10 µL). If the reagents give strong, specific product without nonspecific amplification, they can be substituted for the ones recommended here.

2. In clinical laboratories, dUTP is routinely used in place of dTTP in the PCR reactions. This is done to facilitate the elimination of PCR product carryover from one experiment to another. Because PCR generates a large amount of specific product and because it is also able to detect a small number of targets, product carryover is an important problem. To avoid this problem, it is important to physically separate different steps in the amplification process, i.e., DNA isolation from PCR reaction setup from postamplification sample handling. In addition, if dUTP is incorporated into the PCR products during amplification, these molecules can be eliminated during subsequent reaction setup using uracil *N*-glycosylase (PN N808-0068; Perkin-Elmer) which hydrolyzes DNA containing uracil. Although we do not routinely include this step in our PCR analyses, we include a negative control at the end of each experiment (*see* **Fig. 2**, lane 12) to determine whether contamination has occurred. If contamination is evident, the glycosylase step can then be included to allow clean results.
3. Because reaction components can have dramatic effects on amplification efficiency, it is essential to use an internal standard for accurate quantification. The most critical characteristic of this internal standard is that it is amplified with the same PCR primers as the target in the sample. The ICS is designed to give product that differs in size from product derived from the specific target in order to distinguish them following gel electrophoresis. Here we describe the use of HHVQ-1, which can be used as an ICS for all HHVs ***(16)***. However, any DNA molecule that incorporates the specific primers to be used for amplification and can be distinguished from the specific target can be used. The advantage of using HHVQ-1 is that the CMV primers incorporated into this ICS were selected after screening more than 20 different primer pairs for specificity and low limits of detection, and quantification using this ICS has been extensively validated.
4. The advantage of SYBR Gold over other DNA-binding dyes is that it gives extremely low background fluorescence in agarose when it is not bound to DNA.
5. The key aspect of the imaging hardware used is that it allows the accurate quantification of the amount of PCR product generated following gel electrophoresis.
6. Purified DNA can be concentrated by ethanol precipitation. Add 20 µL of 3 *M* sodium acetate to 200 µL of eluted DNA. Then add 600 µL of 100% ethanol. Vortex briefly. Centrifuge at maximum speed in a microfuge for 10 min at room temperature. Decant the supernatant. Briefly air-dry the DNA pellet and resuspend in 10–20 µL of TE. However, keep in mind that this procedure may also concentrate PCR inhibitors carried over during DNA isolation.

7. Using DNA isolated by the modified version of the QIAamp procedure, we find that we can routinely use 10 µL of blood DNA in PCR reactions without evidence of inhibition. Although blood collected in EDTA is preferable for maximum sample stability, ACD and heparin blood samples can also be used with satisfactory results. See **Subheading 3.4.1.** for further discussion.
8. Under the conditions described here, 20 ICS molecules can be routinely amplified to give enough product to be visualized by standard gel electrophoresis and staining protocols. However, for diagnostic use it appears that this level of detection is probably not necessary. The most important criteria for determining the amount of ICS to use is that it can be amplified reproducibly when mixed with patient DNA. A discussion of the clinically relevant limits of detection is in **Subheading 3.4.2**.
9. Many groups have found that DNA isolated from heparin blood samples is difficult to amplify. We have found that by using the modified QIAamp isolation procedure, these samples can be amplified with only small effects on amplification efficiency.
10. For reasons that are not entirely clear, quantification is most accurate when the intensity ratio of the two products is close to 1, i.e., within a factor of 3 of a 1:1 ratio. Using three 10-fold serial dilutions, one of the reactions usually gives results within these parameters.
11. It is difficult to overemphasize the value of using internal standards for identifying false-negative results in clinical PCR analysis. Many factors can have adverse effects on amplification efficiency, not only inhibitors carried over during DNA isolation, but even effects of lot-to-lot difference in reagent compositions. Although the effects may be small, their impact is amplified with each PCR cycle. For example, a reduction of 20% in amplification efficiency results in a 36-fold reduction in the amount of PCR product after 34 cycles. The use of an ICS is critical to verify that amplification was achieved with acceptable efficiency in each sample analyzed.
12. Although this procedure was established to maximize the limits of detection, it may not be necessary to detect clinically relevant disease. For example, if one uses 10,000 viral targets/mL of blood for the clinically relevant cutoff, a single PCR reaction containing 2.0 µL of blood DNA and 20 molecules of ICS standard could be used. A clinically relevant positive result would be indicated if the CMV-specific band were more intense than the ICS-specific band, regardless of the exact quantification. This approach could be used for routine patient monitoring. For positive samples, more accurate quantification using a series of DNA dilutions would be useful to help monitor therapeutic responses.
13. Since this chapter was written, QIAGEN has replaced the QIAamp Blood Kit with a second-generation kit (same part number) that incorporates the modifications described in this chapter based on these findings. The new kit and protocol can now be used as suggested by the manufacturer to give DNA with low levels of PCR inhibitors without further modification.

References

1. Zuckerman, A. J., Banatvala, J. E., and Pattison, J. R., eds. (1994) Principles and Practice of Clinical Virology, John Wiley & Sons, West Sussex, England.
2. Zaia, J. A. (1994) Cytomegalovirus infection, in *Bone Marrow Transplantation* (Forman, S. J., Blume, K. G., and Thomas, E. D., eds.), Blackwell Scientific, Boston, MA, pp. 376–403.
3. Couriel, D., Canosa, J., Engler, H., Collins, A., Dunbar, C., and Barrett, A. J. (1996) Early reactivation of cytomegalovirus and high risk of interstitial pneumonitis following T-depleted BMT for adults with hematological malignancies. *Bone Marrow Transplant.* **18,** 347–353.
4. Arvin, A. M. (1992) Human cytomegalovirus, in *Laboratory Diagnosis of Viral Infections* (Lennette, E. H., ed.), Marcel Dekker, New York, pp. 333–350.
5. Niubo, J., Perez, J. L., Martinez-Lacasa, J. T., Garcia, A., Roca, J., Fabregat, J., Gil-Vernet, S., and Martin, R. (1996) Association of quantitative cytomegalovirus antigenemia with symptomatic infection in solid organ transplant patients. *Diagn. Microbiol. Infect. Dis.* **24,** 19–24.
6. Salzberger, B., Franzen, C., Fatkenheuer, G., Cornely, O., Schwenk, A., Rasokat, H., Diehl, V., and Schrappe, M. (1996) CMV-Antigenimia in peripheral blood for the diagnosis of CMV disease in HIV-infected patients. *J. Acquir. Immune Defic. Syndr. Hum. Retrovirol.* **11,** 365–369.
7. Wetherill, P. E., Landry, M. L., Alcabes, P., and Friedland, G. (1996) Use of a quantitative cytomegalovirus (CMV) antigenemia test in evaluating HIV+ patients with and without CMV disease. *J. Acquir. Immune Defic. Syndr. Hum. Retrovirol.* **12,** 33–37.
8. Murray, B. M., Amsterdam, D., Gray, V., Myers, J., Gerbasi, J., and Venuto, R. (1997) Monitoring and diagnosis of cytomegalovirus infection in renal transplantation. *J. Am. Soc. Nephrol.* **8,** 1448–1457.
9. Patel, R., Smith, T. F., Espy, M., Portela, D., Wiesner, R. H., Krom, R. A. F., and Paya, C. V. (1995) A prospective comparison of molecular diagnostic techniques for the early detection of cytomegalovirus in liver transplant recipients. *J. Infect. Dis.* **171,** 1010–1014.
10. Peiris, J. S. M., Taylor, C. E., Main, J., Graham, K., and Madeley, C. R. (1995) Diagnosis of cytomegalovirus (CMV) disease in renal allograft recipients: the role of semiquantitative polymerase chain reaction (PCR). *Nephrol. Dial. Transplant.* **10,** 1198–1205.
11. Abecassis, M. M., Koffron, A. J., Kaplan, B., Buckingham, M., Muldoon, J. P., Cribbins, A. J., Kaufman, D. B., Fryer, J. P., Stuart, J., and Stuart, F. P. (1997) The role of PCR in the diagnosis and management of CMV in solid organ recipients; What is the predictive value for the development of disease and should PCR be used to guide antiviral therapy? *Transplantation* **63,** 275–279.
12. Lo, C. Y., Ho, K. N., Yuen, K. Y., Lui, S. L., Li, F. K., Chan T. M., Lo, W. K., and Cheng, K. P. (1997) Diagnosing cytomegalovirus disease in CMV seroposi-

tive renal allograft recipients: a comparison between the detection of CMV DNAemia by polymerase chain reaction and antigenemia by CMV pp65 assay. *Clin. Transplant.* **11,** 286–293.
13. Imbert-Marcille, B.-M., Cantarovich, D., Ferre-Aubineau, V., Richet, B., Soulillou, J.-P., and Billaudel, S. (1997) Usefulness of DNA viral load quantification for cytomegalovirus disease monitoring in renal and pancreas/renal transplant recipients. *Transplantation* **63,** 1476–1481.
14. Lao, W. C., Lee, D., Burroughs, A. K., Lanzini, G., Rolles, K., Emery, V. C., and Griffiths, P. D. (1997) Use of polymerase chain reaction to provide prognostic information on human cytomegalovirus disease after liver transplantation. *J. Med. Virol.* **51,** 152–158.
15. Stephan, F., Fajac, A., Grenet, D., Honderlick, P., Ricci, S., Frachon, I., Friard, S., Caubarrere, I., Bernaudin, J.-F., and Stern, M. (1997) Predictive value of cytomegalovirus DNA detection by polymerase chain reaction in blood and broncoalveolar lavage in lung transplant patients. *Transplantation* **63,** 1430–1435.
16. Bai, X., Hosler, G., Rodgers, B. B., Dawson, D. B., and Scheuermann, R. H. (1997) Quantitative PCR for human herpes viruses and measurement of Epstein Barr virus burden in post-transplant lymphoproliferative disorder. *Clin. Chem.* **43,** 1843–1849.
17. Reagan, K. J., Cabradilla, C., Shuman, B., Stollar, N., Laudemann, J., Bai, X., Hosler, G., and Scheuermann, R. H. (1998) Analytical performance of a quantitative CMV DNA detection method, in *CMV-Related Immunopathology*. Monographs in Virology, vol. 21 (Scholz, M., Rabenau, H. F., Doerr, H. W., and Cinatl, J. Jr., eds.), Karger, Basel, Switzerland, pp. 252–261.
18. Einsele, H., Ehninger, G., Hebart, H., Wittkowski, K. M., Schuler, U., Jahn, G., Mackes, P., Herter, M., Klingebiel, T., Loffler, J., Wagner, S., and Muller, C. A. (1995) Polymerase chain reaction monitoring reduces the incidence of cytomegalovirus disease and the duration and side effects of antiviral therapy after bone marrow transplantation. *Blood* **86,** 2815–2820.
19. Brennan, D. C., Garlock, K. A., Lippmann, B. A., Buller, R. S., Gaudreault-Keener, M., Lowell, J. A., Miller, S. B., Shenoy, S., Howard, T. K., and Storch, G. A. (1997) Control of cytomegalovirus-associated morbidity in renal transplant patients using intensive monitoring and either preemptive or deferred therapy. *J. Am. Soc. Nephrol.* **8,** 118–125.
20. Gotti, E., Suter, F., Baruzzo, S., Perani, V., Moioli, F., and Remuzzi, G. (1996) Early ganciclovir therapy effectively controls viremia and avoids the need for cytomegalovirus (CMV) prophylaxis in renal transplant patients with cytomegalovirus antigenemia. *Clin. Transplant.* **10,** 550–555.
21. Egan, J. J., Lomax, J., Barber, L., Lok, S. S., Martyszcuzuk, R., Yonan, N., Fox, A., Deiraniya, A. K., Turner, A. J., and Woodcock, A. A. (1998) Preemptive treatment for the prevention of cytomegalovirus disease in lung and heart transplant recipients. *Transplantation* **65,** 747–752.

22. Hebart, H., Kanz, L., Jahn G., and Einsele, H. (1998) Management of cytomegalovirus infection after solid-organ or stem-cell transplantation; current guidelines and future prospects. *Drugs* **55,** 59–72.
23. Drouet, E., Colimon, R., Michelson, S., Fourcade, N., Neveleau, A., Ducerf, C., Boibieux, A., Chevallier, M., and Denoyel, G. (1995) Monitoring levels of human cytomegalovirus DNA in blood after liver transplantation. *J. Clin. Microbiol.* **33,** 389–394.

27

A Colorimetric Microtiter Plate Polymerase Chain Reaction System That Detects Herpes Simplex Virus in Cerebrospinal Fluid and Discriminates Genotypes 1 and 2

Yi-Wei Tang

1. Introduction

Herpes simplex virus (HSV) is an ubiquitous agent responsible for a wide variety of human infections. In addition to epithelial infections such as gingivostomatitis, pharyngitis, genital herpes, whitlow, conjunctivitis, and keratitis, HSV is an important cause of central nervous system (CNS) infections and accounts for 2–19% of human encephalitis cases *(1,2)*. The clinical spectrum of CNS diseases has been recently expanded; for example, most cases of benign recurrent aseptic meningitis (Mollaret meningitis) are caused by HSV *(3)*, especially HSV-2 *(4)*. Because specific antiviral therapy is available, the rapid, definitive laboratory diagnosis of HSV is important to support clinical findings. Moreover, in the setting of possible HSV encephalitis, patients are often managed as inpatients while awaiting test results.

Although cell culture is considered the standard method for laboratory diagnosis of ulcerative HSV infections, HSV is rarely recovered in cell cultures inoculated with cerebrospinal fluid (CSF). Brain biopsy specimens may yield culturable virus, but this invasive surgical procedure is controversial when performed solely to collect specimens for the laboratory diagnosis of infectious disease. The sensitivity of HSV antigen and antibody assays for CNS infections is very low *(5)*. In addition, antibodies may appear in the CSF as the consequence of a breakdown in the blood-brain barrier, leading to false-positive results *(6)*.

From: *Methods in Molecular Medicine, vol. 49: Molecular Pathology Protocols*
Edited by: A. A. Killeen © Humana Press Inc., Totowa, NJ

The diagnosis of HSV CNS infections has recently been facilitated by the development of polymerase chain reaction (PCR) technology. As an alternative to the aforementioned techniques, the detection of HSV DNA in the CSF of patients with suspected HSV encephalitis or meningitis allows rapid and noninvasive confirmation of the diagnosis. With the utilization of primers from an HSV DNA sequence that was common to both HSV-1 and HSV-2, several investigators ***(7–13)*** have reported successful identification of HSV DNA in the CSF. Further studies have shown that PCR detection of HSV DNA in CSF should be considered the new standard for laboratory diagnosis of CNS disease caused by this virus ***(14–18)***.

Although the technology underlying PCR is relatively rapid, the PCR product (amplicon) must be identified definitively as the sequence of interest to provide adequate diagnostic specificity. The conventional technique for this is the hybridization of a specific probe to a Southern blot, increasing both sensitivity and specificity of the test. This step, however, takes an additional 12–24 h to complete, delaying the use of test results for clinical intervention. The ideal postamplification detection system would combine the increased sensitivity and specificity of the Southern blot with rapid turnaround time. For this purpose, enzyme-linked adsorbent microtiter plate systems have been adapted for amplicon identification ***(15,19–21)***.

2. Materials

2.1. Special Instruments

1. Thermal cycler (PE 9600 or 9700 is preferred).
2. Enzyme-linked immunosorbent assay (ELISA) automatic washer and reader.
3. Shaking incubator.
4. Positive displacement pipettor.
5. Multichannel pipettor.

2.2. Extraction of DNA

1. RNase-free water.
2. Isopropanol.
3. Ethanol.
4. Pellet Paint Co-Precipitant (Novagen, Madison, WI).
5. IsoQuick DNA Extraction Kit (Orca Research, Bothell, WA).

2.3. PCR Amplification

1. RNase-free water.
2. GeneAmp 10X PCR Buffer II (Perkin-Elmer, Foster City, CA).
3. Deoxynucleotide mixture (dNTPs) (Roche Diagnostics, Indianapolis, IN).

Table 1
Characteristics of Primers Used to Detect HSV DNA in CSF

Primer	Description	Genbank accession no. (reference)	Sequence (5' → 3')[a]
TK-A	Upstream PCR primer	X03764 *(22)* and X01712 *(23)*	GAC MAG CGC CCA GAT AAC AA
TK-B	Downstream PCR primer	X03764 *(22)* and X01712 *(23)*	MCA GCA TRG CCA GGT CAA GC
TK-G	HSV-1-specific probe	X03764 *(22)*	ACA AAC ATC GTG TTG GGG GC
TK-H	HSV-2-specific probe	X01712 *(23)*	ACG AAC CTG GTC CTG GGT GT

[a]M = A or C; R = A or G.

4. Primers for PCR, (polyacrylamide gel electrophorisis (PAGE) purified. Sequences are listed in **Table 1**.
5. Digoxigenin-11-2′deoxyuridine-5′-triphosphate (DIG-dUTP) (Roche Diagnostics).
6. Glycerol.
7. Ampli *Taq* polymerase (Perkin-Elmer).
8. Uracil *N*-glycosylase (UNG) (Epicentre Technologies, Madison, WI).

2.4. Reagents for Colorimetric Detection

1. PCR ELISA (DIG detection) Kit (Roche Diagnostics) (*see* **Note 1**).
2. Capture probe sequences are listed in **Table 1**. These are PAGE purified and 5′ biotinylated.

3. Methods

The protocol is divided into three stages: nucleic acid extraction, PCR amplification, and amplicon identification.

3.1. Extraction of Nucleic Acid by IsoQuick Extraction Kit

A modified solvent-extraction procedure (IsoQuick) is used for DNA extraction. The procedure described here is slightly modified from the instructions provided by Ocra Research (*see* **Note 2**).

1. Prepare lysate by mixing an equal volume (200 μL) of reagent 1 (lysis solution) to a CSF sample in a 2.0-mL microcentrifuge tube. Mix the tube.
2. Shake reagent 2 (extraction matrix) vigorously. Add 750 μL to sample lysate.
3. Add 500 μL of reagent 3 (extraction buffer) to the sample. Vortex thoroughly.
4. Centrifuge at 12,800*g* for 5 min.

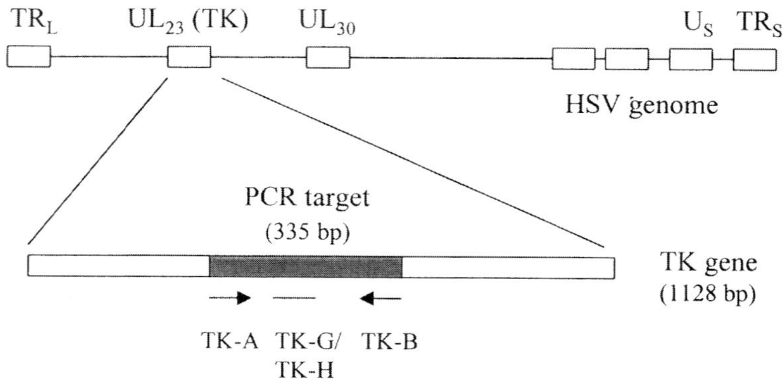

Fig. 1. Gene location and nucleotide base position of primers and probes designed to detect HSV DNA and differentiate genotypes 1 and 2.

5. Transfer the upper aqueous phase (about 500 µL) to a new 1.5-mL microcentrifuge tube.
6. Add 0.1 vol (50 µL) of reagent 4 (sodium acetate) to the aqueous-phase sample.
7. Add 2.0 µL of Pellet Paint Co-Precipitant to the aqueous-phase sample.
8. Add an equal volume (500 µL) of isopropanol to the aqueous-phase sample. Mix gently by inversion to precipitate nucleic acid. Precipitate for 30 min at –20°C. A visible pink pellet should be seen on the bottom of the tube.
9. Centrifuge at 12,800*g* for 30 min.
10. Discard the supernatant by aspirating the alcohol without disturbing the pink nucleic acid pellet.
11. Add 1 mL of 70% ethanol to the pellet. Mix gently by inverting the tube several times.
12. Centrifuge at 12,800*g* for 5 min.
13. Discard the supernatant by aspirating the alcohol without disturbing the nucleic acid pellet. Allow the DNA pellet to air-dry at room temperature.
14. Resuspend the DNA pellet in 25 µL of reagent 5 (RNase-free water). Allow the pellet to dissolve at room temperature with occasional gentle mixing.

3.2. PCR amplification

A specific 335-bp DNA sequence encoding a portion of the thymidine kinase (TK) gene (**Fig. 1**) is amplified by PCR ***(22,23)*** (*see* **Note 3**).

1. Prepare the PCR master mix as follows: 1X PCR Buffer II; 1.5 m*M* $MgCl_2$; 200 µ*M* each dATP, dCTP, and dGTP; 100 µ*M* dTTP; 90 µ*M* dUTP; 10 µ*M* DIG-dUTP; 1 µ*M* each primer TK-A and TK-B; 10% glycerol; 0.01 U/µL of UNG; 0.025 U/µL Ampli *Taq* polymerase.
2. Aliquot 45 µL of master mix into 0.2-mL MicroAmp tubes using a positive displacement pipettor.

3. Add 5 µL of sample extract to the master mix.
4. Transfer the tubes to the DNA thermal cycler.
5. Run the PCR thermal profile using the following parameters: 50°C for 5 min, 94°C for 3 min, 50 cycles of 94°C for 15 s and 60°C for 30 s, 72°C for 10 min, 4°C soak. Approximate run time is 2.2 h on the PE thermocycler 9600. PCR reactions may be left in the thermocycler overnight at 4°C to soak.
6. After the profile is completed, remove the tubes from the thermocycler. If amplicon identification is not to be completed the same day, store the tubes at –20°C.

3.3. Identification of Amplicon

Identification of amplicon is performed using an ELISA microtiter format. Denatured amplicon is mixed with a hybridization solution containing a biotin-labeled DNA capture probe specific for HSV-1 or HSV-2. The probes hybridize to the corresponding target DNA sequence if present, and the resulting complexes are captured on the streptavidin-coated microtiter plate wells. HSV-specific DNA complexes are detected by anti-DIG-peroxidase conjugate, and the peroxidase substrate is added (**Fig. 2**). Determination of the presence of HSV-1 or HSV-2 is then made based on the color production *(21)*.

The following procedure is slightly modified from the instructions provided by Roche Diagnostics:

1. Complete the HSV PCR ELISA tray map using the work sheet provided in the kit. Calculate the amount of each reagent required for the batch run. Prepare an excess of each reagent to allow for multichannel pipetting losses. As a rule of thumb, prepare enough reagent for at least eight extra wells.
2. Reconstitute the lyophilized anti-DIG-peroxidase stock (vial 7) with 250 µL of sterile water.
3. Dispense the calculated volume of hybridization buffer (vial 4) to two 50-mL conical tubes, and add the calculated volume of HSV capture probes TK-G and TK-H (final concentration of 7.5 pmol/mL) to the appropriate tubes. Mix gently and avoid foaming.
4. Prepare the anti-DIG-peroxidase working solution by diluting 1 vol of the reconstituted solution from vial 7 (**step 3**) with 99 vol of conjugate dilution buffer (vial 6) in a 50-mL conical tube using the calculated values on the work sheet.
5. Prepare an adequate volume of 2,2′-azinobis (3-ethylbenzothiazoline-6-sulfonic acid), diammonium salt (ABTS) substrate solution for the number of wells being detected. Dissolve one tablet of ABTS (vial 9) per 5 mL of substrate buffer (vial 8) in a 50-mL conical tube using the calculated values on the work sheet. **Steps 4** and **5** should be done at least 1 h prior to use. Mix gently and avoid foaming. Store the solution away from light at room temperature. Prepare a fresh reagent each day of use.
6. Prepare a wash solution by dissolving one wash tablet (vial 5) in 2 L of distilled water. Mix thoroughly prior to use.

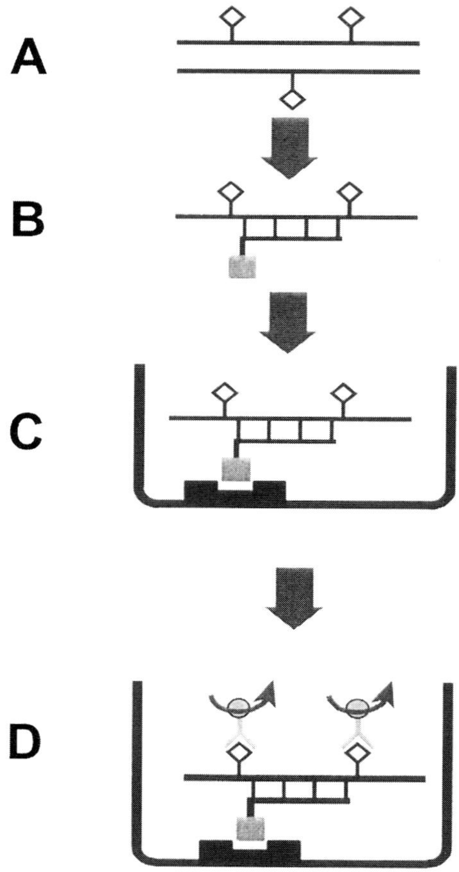

Fig. 2. Detection of DIG-labeled PCR amplicon with the Roche PCR ELISA (DIG detection) Kit. **(A)** During PCR amplification, *Taq* DNA polymerase incorporates DIG-dUTP into the target DNA. **(B)** A biotin-labeled oligonucleotide probe "captures" the DIG-labeled PCR amplicon. **(C)** The probe-amplicon hybrid is immobilized on a streptavidin-coated microtiter plate. **(D)** The immobilized probe-amplicon hybrid is detected with peroxidase-conjugated anti-DIG antibody and ABTS colorimetric substrate.

7. Add 10 μL of reconstituted DIG-labeled Control PCR product to a 1.5-mL tube. Add 40 μL of denaturation solution to the tube. Mix the contents up and down five times, and allow the reaction to incubate 10 min at room temperature.
8. Add 40 μL of denaturation solution to each 50-μL PCR reaction tube using a multichannel pipettor. Mix the contents up and down five times and allow the reactions to incubate for 10 min at room temperature.
9. Just prior to the end of the 10-min incubation, add 180 μL of the two hybridization solutions containing 7.5 pmol/mL of capture probe (TK-G or TK-H) to the

alternating rows of the detection wells according to the tray map using a multichannel pipettor. Well A1 is designated as the reagent control. Add 180 µL of hybridization buffer (vial 4) to the well. All the reagents should be added with the exception of target DNA throughout the procedure. Well B1 is designated as the kit positive control well. Add 180 µL of the hybridization buffer/control capture probe mixture prepared earlier. Add 20 µL of denatured DIG-labeled Control PCR product to this well.

10. Add 20 µL of denatured amplicon to the appropriate wells. Mix up and down five times using a multichannel pipettor. Seal the plate with a mylar sheet provided in the kit. Each specimen is detected in duplicate; that is, 20 µL of denatured amplicon is added to a well containing TK-G and to a well in the parallel row containing probe TK-H.
11. Place the plate containing the microtiter strips into the 37°C rotary incubator for 3 h at 60 rpm in the dark.
12. Remove the plate and wash each well five times on the automatic plate washer with the wash solution prepared previously.
13. Add 200 µL of freshly prepared anti-DIG-peroxidase working solution to each well using a multichannel pipettor. Seal the plate and incubate the solution in the 37°C rotary incubator for 30 min at 60 rpm in the dark.
14. Remove the plate and wash each well five times on the automatic plate washer with the wash solution prepared previously.
15. Add 200 µL of freshly prepared ABTS substrate to each well using a multichannel pipettor.
16. Seal the plate and incubate the solution in the 37°C rotary incubator for 30 min at 60 rpm in the dark.
17. Remove the mylar sheet cover and immediately read the plate on the plate reader using dual wavelengths (405/490 nm) with blank correction.

3.4. Interpretation of Results

The results are strictly qualitative. The presence of HSV DNA is determined by relating the absorbance of the specimen well to the intrinsic extinction of the ABTS solution well. A clinical specimen with an $OD_{405/490} \geq 0.1$ should be interpreted as positive for the presence of HSV DNA. A clinical specimen with an $OD_{405/490} < 0.1$ should be interpreted as negative for the presence of HSV DNA. If positive, the specimen is identified as being positive for HSV-1 or HSV-2 or both. The results should be interpreted with consideration of other clinical laboratory findings. A negative result does not eliminate the possibility of infection. Reliable results depend on an adequate specimen collection and the absence of inhibitory substances in the specimens.

4. Notes

1. Although only one colorimetric microtiter plate PCR system is described for the detection of HSV in the CSF, several equivalent systems are commercially avail-

able. They include the PrimeCapture™ from ViroMed Laboratories, QuantiPATH™ from CPG, and GEN-ETI-K™ from DiaSorin. Our evaluation indicated that the majority of those systems, including the one described herein, have a comparable sensitivity and specificity in comparison to the conventional Southern blot followed by probe hybridization *(21)*.

2. Ideally, separate rooms are designed for nucleic acid extraction, PCR amplification, and amplicon identification in order to avoid cross contamination. However, laboratories with limited space can separate these functions by established separate workstations in two rooms, one for preamplification steps and another for amplification and postamplification steps. In addition, a UNG-based inactivation system was adapted to control possible contamination by amplicon carryover *(21,24)*.
3. Additional advantages of the described system include the recognition of polymorphisms in the TK gene that may be responsible for drug resistance. Several point mutations in the TK gene may also be responsible for acyclovir resistance *(25–27)*. The determination of acyclovir resistance by detection of these point mutations may be important in patients undergoing long-term therapy and in immunocompromised hosts *(27,28)*. Acyclovir resistance could be determined by direct sequencing of the amplicon based on clinical management.

Acknowledgment

This chapter contains information presented in the *Molecular Microbiology Laboratory Procedure Manual* used at the Mayo Clinic. I acknowledge the contributions to this manual from Paul N. Rys, Mark J. Espy, Shawn P. Mitchell, Dr. Thomas F. Smith, and Dr. David H. Persing.

References

1. Skoldenberg, B., Forsgren, M., Alestig, K., Bergstrom, T., Burman, L., Dahlqvist, E., Forkman, A., Fryden, A., Lovgren, K., and Norlin, K. (1984) Acyclovir versus vidarabine in herpes simplex encephalitis: randomised multicentre study in consecutive Swedish patients. *Lancet* **2,** 707–711.
2. Whitley, R. J., Alford, C. A., Hirsch, M. S., Schooley, R. T., Luby, J. P., Aoki, F. Y., Hanley, D., Nahmias, A. J., and Soong, S. J. (1986) Vidarabine versus acyclovir therapy in herpes simplex encephalitis. *N. Engl. J. Med.* **314,** 144–149.
3. Yamamoto, L. J., Tedder, D. G., Ashley, R., and Levin, M. J. (1991) Herpes simplex virus type 1 DNA in cerebrospinal fluid of a patient with Mollaret's meningitis. *N. Engl. J. Med.* **325,** 1082–1085.
4. Tedder, D. G., Ashley, R., Tyler, K. L., and Levin, M. J. (1994) Herpes simplex virus infection as a cause of benign recurrent lymphocytic meningitis. *Ann. Intern. Med.* **121,** 334–338.
5. Kohl, S. (1988) Herpes simplex virus encephalitis in children. *Pediatr. Clin. North Am.* **35,** 465–483.

6. Nahmias, A. J., Whitley, R. J., Visintine, A. N., Takei, Y., and Alford, C. A. Jr. (1982) Herpes simplex virus encephalitis: laboratory evaluations and their diagnostic significance. *J. Infect. Dis.* **145,** 829–836.
7. Powell, K. F., Anderson, N. E., Frith, R. W., and Croxson, M. C. (1990) Non-invasive diagnosis of herpes simplex encephalitis. *Lancet* **335,** 357,358.
8. Rowley, A. H., Whitley, R. J., Lakeman, F. D., and Wolinsky, S. M. (1990) Rapid detection of herpes-simplex-virus DNA in cerebrospinal fluid of patients with herpes simplex encephalitis. *Lancet* **335,** 440,441.
9. Puchhammer-Stockl, E., Popow-Kraupp, T., Heinz, F. X., Mandl, C. W., and Kunz, C. (1990) Establishment of PCR for the early diagnosis of herpes simplex encephalitis. *J. Med. Virol.* **32,** 77–82.
10. Klapper, P. E., Cleator, G. M., Dennett, C., and Lewis, A. G. (1990) Diagnosis of herpes encephalitis via Southern blotting of cerebrospinal fluid DNA amplified by polymerase chain reaction. *J. Med. Virol.* **32,** 261–264.
11. Kimura, H., Futamura, M., Kito, H., Ando, T., Goto, M., Kuzushima, K., Shibata, M., and Morishima, T. (1991) Detection of viral DNA in neonatal herpes simplex virus infections: frequent and prolonged presence in serum and cerebrospinal fluid. *J. Infect. Dis.* **164,** 289–293.
12. Aurelius, E., Johansson, B., Skoldenberg, B., Staland, A., and Forsgren, M. (1991) Rapid diagnosis of herpes simplex encephalitis by nested polymerase chain reaction assay of cerebrospinal fluid. *Lancet* **337,** 189–192.
13. Aslanzadeh, J., Osmon, D. R., Wilhelm, M. P., Espy, M. J., and Smith, T. F. (1992) A prospective study of the polymerase chain reaction for detection of herpes simplex virus in cerebrospinal fluid submitted to the clinical virology laboratory. *Mol. Cell. Probes* **6,** 367–373.
14. Lakeman, F. D. and Whitley, R. J. (1995) Diagnosis of herpes simplex encephalitis: application of polymerase chain reaction to cerebrospinal fluid from brain-biopsied patients and correlation with disease. *J. Infect. Dis.* **171,** 857–863.
15. Vesanen, M., Piiparinen, H., Kallio, A., and Vaheri, A. (1996) Detection of herpes simplex virus DNA in cerebrospinal fluid samples using the polymerase chain reaction and microplate hybridization. *J. Virol. Methods* **59,** 1–11.
16. Tang, Y. W., Espy, M. J., Persing, D. H., and Smith, T. F. (1997) Molecular evidence and clinical significance of herpesvirus coinfection in central nervous system. *J. Clin. Microbiol.* **35,** 2869–2872.
17. Mitchell, P. S., Espy, M. J., Smith, T. F., Toal, D. R., Rys, P. N., Berbari, E. F., Osmon, D. R., and Persing, D. H. (1997) Laboratory diagnosis of central nervous system infections with herpes simplex virus by PCR performed with cerebrospinal fluid specimens. *J. Clin. Microbiol.* **35,** 2873–2877.
18. Tang, Y. W., Mitchell, P. S., Espy, M. J., Smith, D. H., and Persing, D. H. (1999) Molecular diagnosis of herpes simplex virus infections in the central nervous system [minireview]. *J. Clin. Microbiol.* **37,** 2127–2136.
19. Mantero, G., Zonaro, A., Albertini, A., Bertolo, P., and Primi, D. (1991) DNA enzyme immunoassay: general method for detecting products of polymerase chain reaction. *Clin. Chem.* **37,** 422–429.

20. Loeffelholz, M. J., Lewinski, C. A., Silver, S. R., Purohit, A. P., Herman, S. A., Buonagurio, D. A., and Dragon, E. A. (1992) Detection of *Chlamydia trachomatis* in endocervical specimens by polymerase chain reaction. *J. Clin. Microbiol.* **30,** 2847–2851.
21. Tang, Y. W., Rys, P. N., Rutledge, B. J., Mitchell, P. S., Smith, T. F., and Persing, D. H. (1998) Comparative evaluation of colorimetric microtiter plate systems for detection of herpes simplex virus in cerebrospinal fluid. *J. Clin. Microbiol.* **36,** 2714–2717.
22. Graham, D., Larder, B. A., and Inglis, M. M. (1986) Evidence that the 'active centre' of the herpes simplex virus thymidine kinase involves an interaction between three distinct regions of the polypeptide. *J. Gen. Virol.* **67,** 753–758.
23. Swain, M. A. and Galloway, D. A. (1983) Nucleotide sequence of the herpes simplex virus type 2 thymidine kinase gene. *J. Virol.* **46,** 1045–1050.
24. Longo, M. C., Berninger, M. S., and Hartley, J. L. (1990) Use of uracil DNA glycosylase to control carry-over contamination in polymerase chain reactions. *Gene* **93,** 125–128.
25. Englund, J. A., Zimmerman, M. E., Swierkosz, E. M., Goodman, J. L., Scholl, D. R., and Balfour, H. H. Jr. (1990) Herpes simplex virus resistant to acyclovir. A study in a tertiary care center. *Ann. Intern. Med.* **112,** 416–422.
26. Palu, G., Gerna, G., Bevilacqua, F., and Marcello, A. (1992) A point mutation in the thymidine kinase gene is responsible for acyclovir-resistance in herpes simplex virus type 2 sequential isolates. *Virus Res.* **25,** 133–144.
27. Gaudreau, A., Hill, E., Balgour, H. H. Jr., Erice, A., and Boivin, G. (1998) Phenotypic and genotypic characterization of acyclovir-resistant herpes simplex viruses from immunocompromised patients. *J. Infect. Dis.* **178,** 297–303.
28. Pease, A. C., Solas, D., Sullivan, E. J., Cronin, M. T., Holmes, C. P., and Fodor, S. P. (1994) Light-generated oligonucleotide arrays for rapid DNA sequence analysis. *Proc. Natl. Acad. Sci. USA* **91,** 5022–5026.

28

Detection and Typing of Hepatitis C Virus

Frederick S. Nolte

1. Introduction

For more than two decades prior to the discovery of the hepatitis C virus (HCV), posttransfusion non-A, non-B (NANB) hepatitis was thought to have a viral etiology. In 1989, the virus was finally identified through a unique application of molecular cloning techniques by investigators at the Centers for Disease Control, and the Chiron Corporation *(1)*. In a reversal of the usual sequence of events, HCV was identified and defined before its existence was substantiated through tissue culture growth, electron microscopic observation, or serologic detection. Molecular cloning of HCV preceded the use of any of the conventional methods of viral identification and serologic detection then evolved from the blind immunoscreening of millions of clones with serum from a patient who had NANB hepatitis *(2)*. The peptide expressed in a single reactive clone (5-1-1) served as the basis for the first Food and Drug Administration (FDA)–licensed diagnostic test for detection of antibodies to HCV *(3)*.

HCV is now recognized as the cause of most cases of posttransfusion NANB hepatitis and more than half of sporadic NANB hepatitis. About half of all infected individuals develop chronic hepatitis and about 20% of these may develop cirrhosis. It is estimated that nearly 4 million people are chronically infected with HCV in the United States. End-stage liver disease owing to chronic HCV infection is the leading reason for liver transplantation in the United States.

The entire genome of HCV has been cloned and sequenced. It is a single-stranded, positive sense RNA virus composed of approx 10,000 nucleotides coding for 3000 amino acids. The genome consists of a single open reading frame that is translated to yield a polyprotein from which viral proteins are

From: *Methods in Molecular Medicine, vol. 49: Molecular Pathology Protocols*
Edited by: A. A. Killeen © Humana Press Inc., Totowa, NJ

derived by posttranslational cleavage. HCV exists as a heterogeneous group of viruses showing about 70% homology overall with six distinct major genotypes and a number of subtypes ***(4)***. The virus is related to the *Flaviviridae* and *Pestiviridae* and has a high spontaneous mutation rate (10^{-2} mutations/[nucleotide · yr]) ***(5,6)***. As a result of this high spontaneous mutation rate, individual patients are infected with a heterogeneous population of virus having closely related yet heterogeneous genomes termed *quasispecies*. The extensive genetic heterogeneity of HCV has important diagnostic and clinical implications.

Detection of HCV RNA in serum by nucleic acid amplification methods has become important in confirming the diagnosis of hepatitis C and in assessing response to antiviral therapy ***(7)***. Many different qualitative and quantitative assays for HCV RNA have been described. These assays have employed reverse transcriptase polymerase chain reaction (RT-PCR), nucleic acid sequence-based amplification, and branched DNA as amplification methods ***(7)***. Standardization of in-house-developed RT-PCR assays for HCV RNA has been difficult, as demonstrated by the results of a recent international collaborative proficiency testing study ***(8)***. In this performance survey of 86 laboratories, only 16% of the laboratories performed faultlessly, with 29% missing only a weak positive specimen, and 55% reporting false-positive or false-negative results. An RT-PCR test for HCV RNA for only research use is available from Roche Molecular Systems (AMPLICOR HCV Test) ***(9)***. The test has undergone several preclinical evaluations and is currently used in FDA clinical trials in the United States ***(9–11)***. Because this test will likely become the first standardized HCV RNA test marketed to clinical laboratories in the United States, it is the method described in detail in this chapter.

The AMPLICOR test is based on five major processes: specimen preparation, reverse transcription of target RNA to generate complementary DNA (cDNA), PCR amplification of target cDNA using HCV-specific complementary primers, hybridization of the amplified products to oligonucleotide probes specific to the target(s), and detection of the probe-bound amplified products by color formation.

HCV RNA is isolated from serum or plasma by lysis of virus particles with a chaotropic agent followed by precipitation of the RNA with alcohol. An internal control (IC) RNA is introduced into the specimen with the specimen diluent and serves as an amplification control for each processed specimen. The HCV IC is an in vitro RNA transcript with primer-binding sequences identical to those of the HCV target sequences, a randomized internal sequence of similar length and base composition as the HCV target sequences, and a unique probe-binding region that differentiates the IC from the target amplicon. The IC is introduced into each amplification reaction and is coamplified with target RNA from the clinical specimen.

The appropriate selection of primers and probes is critical to the ability of the test to detect all the HCV genotypes. The 5′ untranslated region (UTR) of the HCV genome is the most conserved RNA sequence among the known HCV genotypes ***(12)***. The AMPLICOR test uses primers KY78 and KY80 to amplify a sequence of 244 nucleotides within the highly conserved 5′ UTR.

The thermostable recombinant enzyme *Thermus thermophilus* DNA polymerase (r*Tth*) has both RT and DNA polymerase activity in the presence of manganese ***(13)***. The processed specimens are added to the amplification mixture in reactions tubes in which both reverse transcription and PCR amplification occur. The antisense primer (KY78) is biotylinated at the 5′ end and the sense primer (KY80) is not. The reaction mixture is heated to allow the antisense primer to anneal to the HCV and IC target RNA. In the presence of excess deoxynucleoside triphosphates (dNTPs), r*Tth* polymerase extends the annealed primer forming cDNA. Following reverse transcription of the target RNA, the reaction mixture is heated to denature the RNA : cDNA hybrids and expose the primer-binding sequences. As the mixture cools, the sense primer binds to the cDNA strand, and the r*Tth* polymerase extends the sense primer to synthesize a second DNA strand. This completes the first cycle of PCR, yielding a double-stranded DNA (dsDNA) copy of the target RNA. The reaction mixture is heated again to separate the dsDNA and expose the primer-binding regions. As the mixture cools, the primers, KY78 and KY80, anneal to the target DNA. r*Tth* extends the annealed primers along the target templates to produce a 244-bp dsDNA product. This process is repeated for 37 cycles, each cycle effectively doubling the amount of amplicon DNA.

Selective amplification of target nucleic acid from the clinical specimen is achieved by the use of uracil-*N*-glycosylase (UNG) (AmpErase). UNG recognizes and catalyzes the destruction of DNA strands containing deoxyuridine, but not DNA containing thymidine ***(14)***. Deoxyuridine is not present in naturally occurring DNA, but it is always present in amplicon owing to the use deoxyuridine triphosphate as one of the dNTPs in the master mix. Therefore, only amplicon contains deoxyuridine. UNG, which is included in the master mix, catalyzes the cleavage of deoxyuridine containing DNA at deoxyuridine residues by opening the deoxyribose chain at the C1 position. When heated in the first thermal cycling step at the alkaline pH of the master mix, the amplicon DNA strand breaks at the position of the deoxyuridine residue, rendering the DNA nonamplifiable. UNG is not active above 55°C (i.e., throughout the thermal cycling steps) and therefore does not destroy newly synthesized amplicon. Following amplification, any residual enzyme is denatured by the addition of the denaturation solution. The use of UNG in the AMPLICOR test helps prevents false-positive results owing to crosscontamination with amplicon.

Following amplification, the HCV and IC amplicons are chemically denatured to form single-stranded DNA by the addition of denaturation solution, and aliquots of the denatured amplicon are added to microwell plates coated with HCV-specific (KY150) and IC-specific (SK535) oligonucleotide probes, respectively. This hybridization increases the overall specificity of the test.

Following hybridization, the microwell plates are washed to remove any unbound material, and an avidin-horseradish peroxidase (Av-HRP) conjugate is added to each well of the microwell plates. The Av-HRP binds to the biotin-labeled amplicon captured by the plate-bound oligonucleotide probe. The microwell plates are washed again to remove unbound Av-HRP, and a substrate solution containing H_2O_2 and 3,3′,5′,5′-tetramethylbenzidine (TMB) is added to the microwell plates. In the presence of H_2O_2, the bound HRP catalyzes the oxidation of TMB to form a color complex. The reaction is stopped by the addition of a weak acid, and the optical density (OD) at 450 nm is measured using an automated microwell plate reader.

The six major genotypes and subtypes of HCV vary in their worldwide distribution. In the United States, type 1 is predominant (75%) and types 2, 3, and 4 comprise the remaining 25% ***(15,16)***. Several studies suggest that genotypes other than 1 are more likely to be associated with a sustained response to interferon alone or in combination with ribavirin ***(17,18)***. Although treatment should not be withheld from patients based on genotype of the virus, this information can help in advising patients on the likelihood of response to treatment and in determining the duration of therapy ***(18)***.

Various methods have been used for HCV genotyping, including genomic amplification and sequencing ***(19–22)***, PCR with genotype-specific primers ***(23,24)***, restriction fragment-length polymorphism of PCR amplicons ***(25)***, differential hybridization ***(26)***, allele-specific oligonucleotide hybridization of PCR amplicon ***(27)***, cleavase fragment length polymorphism ***(28)***, PCR amplicon heteroduplex tracking assay, and detection of genotype-specific antibodies by immunoenzymatic methods ***(29,30)***. Genomic amplification and sequencing, followed by sequence comparison and phylogenetic tree construction for confirmation, is currently the "gold standard." Genomic regions commonly used for this approach include nonstructural region 5, envelope 1 region, and core region. This method is costly, labor-intensive, not standardized from laboratory to laboratory, but does lend itself to large-scale testing.

A line-probe assay (LiPA) employing reverse hybridization of PCR amplicon to type-specific probes on nitrocellulose strips is available commercially (INNO-LiPA HCV II; Innogenetics, Norcross, GA) for HCV genotyping ***(27)***. The LiPA is based on variations found in the 5′ UTR of the different HCV genotypes. It is a simple and quick procedure that has compared favorably with more cumbersome procedures in several recent evaluations ***(31–33)***.

Because the LiPA works well with the amplicon from the AMPLICOR HCV test, laboratories could detect HCV and determine its genotype from a single PCR.

2. Materials

2.1. Detection of HCV RNA Using the AMPLICOR HCV Test, Version 2.0

2.1.1. Collection of Specimens

The AMPLICOR HCV test is for use only with serum or plasma specimens. For serum samples, collect blood in VACUTAINER serum separator tubes (Becton-Dickinson no. 367784 or 367789), and for plasma, collect blood in tubes containing EDTA (lavender top, Becton-Dickinson no. 6454 or equivalent) or acid citrate dextrose (yellow top, Becton Dickinson no 4606 or equivalent) as the anticoagulant. Specimens collected in tubes containing heparin as the anticoagulant are unsuitable for this test.

2.1.2. Preparation of Specimens

The manufacturer provides **items 1–6**. The composition of several reagents is proprietary.

1. Lysis reagent: 68% guanidinium thiocyanate, 3% dithiothreitol, glycogen, Tris-HCl buffer. Warm to 25–37°C and mix thoroughly prior to use.
2. Specimen diluent: synthetic poly rA RNA, EDTA, sodium azide, Tris-HCl buffer.
3. Negative human plasma: nonreactive by antibody tests for HCV, human immunodeficiency virus-1 (HIV-1) and HIV-2, and HBsAg; ProClin 300 (Rohm and Haas).
4. Positive control: noninfectious in vitro transcribed RNA containing HCV sequences, synthetic poly rA RNA, EDTA, sodium azide.
5. Negative control: synthetic poly rA RNA, EDTA, sodium azide.
6. Internal control: noninfectious in vitro transcribed RNA containing HCV primer-binding sequences and a unique probe-binding region, synthetic poly rA RNA, EDTA, sodium azide (*see* **Note 1**).
7. 70% Ethanol: Add 1 vol of deionized water to 2.75 vol of 95% ethanol. Prepare fresh daily.
8. Isopropyl alcohol.

2.1.3. Reverse Transcription and cDNA Amplification

All reagents are provided by the manufacturer.

1. Master mix: primers KY78 and KY80; dATP, dCTP, dGTP, and dUTP; r*Tth* DNA polymerase; UNG; glycerol; potassium acetate; dimethyl sulfoxide; bicine buffer; sodium azide (*see* **Note 2**).
2. Manganese solution: manganese, acetic acid, amaranth dye, sodium azide.

2.1.4. Detection of Amplicon

All reagents are provided by the manufacturer.

1. HCV DNA probe-coated microwell plate: twelve 8-well strips in a resealable pouch with desiccant.
2. Internal control probe-coated microwell plate: twelve 8-well strips in a resealable pouch with desiccant.
3. Denaturation solution: 1.6% NaOH, EDTA, thymol blue.
4. Hybridization buffer: sodium phosphate, sodium thiocynate, solubilizer.
5. Av-HRP conjugate: Av-HRP conjugate, bovine γ-globulin, Emulsit 25 (Dai-ichi Kogyo Seiyaku); 0.1% phenol, 1% ProClin 150 (Rohm and Haas).
6. Substrate A: citrate solution, 0.01% H_2O_2; 0.1% ProClin 150.
7. Substrate B: 0.1% TMB, 40% *N,N*-dimethylformamide (DMF).
8. 10X Wash concentrate: phosphate buffer, NaCl, EDTA, detergent, 0.5% ProClin 300.
9. Stop reagent: 4.9% sulfuric acid.

2.2. Genotyping HCV Using LiPA (INN0-LiPA HCV II)

The most convenient source of amplicons for the LiPA assay is the PCR products from the AMPLICOR HCV 2.0 assay. Alternatively, RT-PCR of HCV can be performed using primers supplied by Innogenetics. The following protocol uses AMPLICOR HCV 2.0 PCR products.

2.2.1. Line-Probe Assay

The following reagents are supplied by the manufacturer. The detailed composition of these reagents is proprietary.

1. Nitrocellulose strips with 19 type-specific probes bound to the surface thorough poly-T tails (**Fig. 1**).
2. Alkaline denaturation solution.
3. Hybridization solution containing saline sodium citrate (SSC) buffer with 0.1% sodium dodecyl sulfate (SDS).
4. Stringent wash solution containing SSC buffer with 0.1% SDS.
5. Concentrated conjugate: streptavidin labeled with alkaline phosphatase. Prior to use, dilute 1 : 100 conjugate diluent.
6. Concentrated 5-bromo-5-chloro-3-indolyl phosphate β-toluidine salt (BCIP) and nitroblue tetrazolium chloride (NBT) substrate solution in DMF. Dilute 1 : 100 in substrate buffer before use.
7. Conjugate diluent containing phosphate buffer containing NaCl, Triton, protein stabilizers, and sodium azide.
8. Substrate buffer containing Tris buffer with NaCl and $MgCl_2$.
9. Concentrated rinse solution: phosphate buffer with NaCl, Triton, and sodium azide. Dilute 1 : 5 in distilled water before use.
10. Incubation trays containing eight troughs.
11. Transparent plastic reading chart for identification of positive lines.

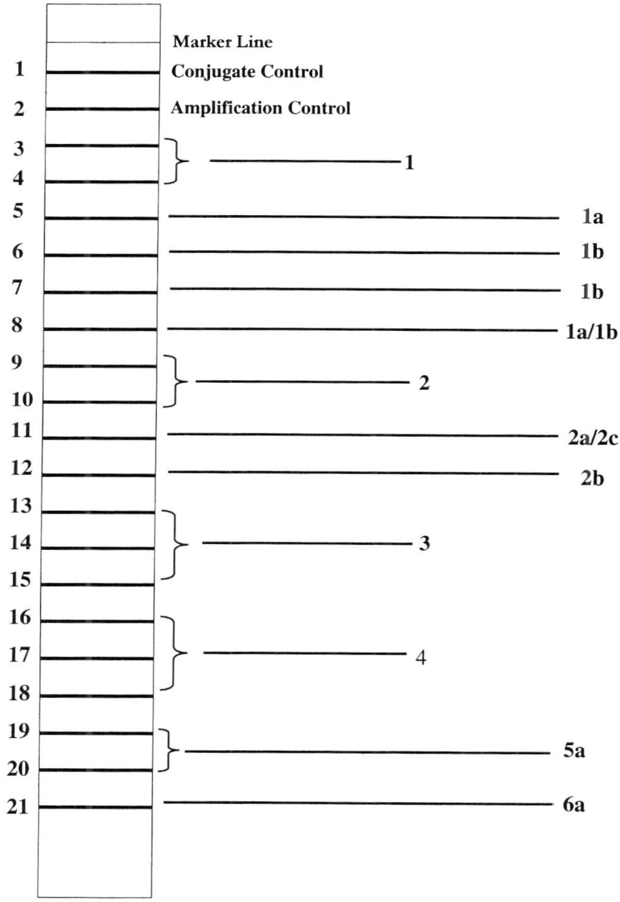

Fig. 1. Type- and subtype-specific probe location on the INNO-LiPA HCV II strip.

The following items are not provided by the manufacturer and must be supplied by the user.

1. Shaking water bath, capable of 80 rpm, with an inclined lid and temperature adjustable to a minimum of 50°C.
2. Liquid aspirator.
3. Tweezers.
4. Vortex mixer.
5. Pipets adjustable to deliver 1–20, 20–200, and 200–1000 μL.
6. Orbital shaker or rocker shaker capable of 160 and 50 rpm, respectively.

3. Methods

3.1. Amplicor HCV Assay

3.1.1. Collection, Transport, and Storage of Specimens

1. Whole blood should be kept at 2–25°C and serum or plasma should be separated within 6 h of collection to avoid degradation of HCV RNA. A minimum of 200 µL of serum or plasma is required for the test.
2. Serum or plasma may be transported at 2–8°C or frozen at –20 to –80°C.
3. Aliquot serum or plasma into appropriately labeled 1.5-mL polypropylene screw-cap tubes (Sarstedt cat. no. 72.692.105).

3.1.2. Preparation of Specimens

1. Label one 1.5-mL polypropylene screw-cap tube for each patient specimen and kit control.
2. Prepare the working lysis reagent by adding 100 µL of IC to one bottle of lysis reagent.
3. Add 400 µL of working lysis reagent to each labeled tube and cap.
4. Prepare plasma controls as follows: To each of three 1.5-mL tubes (two negative and one positive control tubes) add 200 µL of negative plasma. Vortex for 3–5 s. Then add 25 µL of the negative control to each of the two negative control tubes and 25 µL of the positive control to the positive control tube. Vortex the control tube tubes for 3–5 s.
5. Vortex the patient specimens for 3–5 s. Add 200 µL of specimen to the appropriate tube containing the working lysis reagent and vortex again.
6. Incubate all the specimens and control tubes for 10 min at 60°C and vortex.
7. Add 600 µL of isopropyl alcohol (at room temperature) to each tube and vortex.
8. Incubate all the tubes for 2 min at room temperature.
9. Put a mark on each tube and place the tubes into the microcentrifuge with the orientation mark facing outward, so that the resulting pellet will align with the orientation mark. Centrifuge for 15 min at 13,000–16,000*g* at room temperature.
10. Using a new, fine-tip, disposable transfer pipet for each tube, carefully remove and discard the supernatant from each tube, being careful not to disturb the pellet. The pellet may not be visible but should be aligned with the orientation mark.
11. Add 1.0 mL of 70% ethanol to each tube and vortex.
12. Centrifuge the tubes for 5 min as in **step 9**. Use the orientation mark on the tubes to align the pellet.
13. Remove and discard the supernatant as in **step 10**.
14. Pulse centrifuge the tubes for 5 s.
15. Using a P200 pipet fitted with a plugged tip, remove all the residual supernatant from each tube.
16. Pipet 200 µL of specimen diluent into each tube. Resuspend the pellet by scraping the pellet from the side of the tube using a plugged pipet tip and then vortex. Let the particulate matter settle for 5–10 s. The processed specimens and controls can be held at room temperature for up to 3 h or for up to 1 mo at –20 to –80°C prior to amplification (*see* **Note 3**).

3.1.3. Reverse Transcription and cDNA Amplification

1. Place the appropriate number of MicroAmp tubes for patient and control testing in a MicroAmp tray and lock in place with the retainer.
2. Prepare the working master mix by adding 100 µL of manganese solution to one tube of master mix.
3. Recap the master mix tube and mix well by inverting the tube 10–15 times. Discard the remaining manganese solution.
4. Pipet 50 µL of the working master mix solution into each MicroAmp reaction tube using an Eppendorf repeater pipet and an individually wrapped sterile 1.25-mL Combitip reservoir or a micropipet with a plugged tip. One tube of master mix is enough for 12 reactions.
5. Place the MicroAmp tray containing the master mix in a resealable plastic bag without capping the tubes. Seal the bag securely and store the sample tray at 2–8°C until specimen preparation is completed. Amplification must begin within 4 h of preparation of the master mix.
6. Pipette 50 µL of each processed specimen and control into the appropriate MicroAmp reaction tube containing the working master mix.
7. Cap the MicroAmp reaction tubes and move to the amplification and detection area.
8. Place the tray/retainer assembly into the thermal cycler sample block.
9. Program the thermal cycler as follows: hold program, 5 min at 50°C; hold program, 30 min at 62°C; cycle program (37 cycles), 10 s at 90°C, 25 s at 58°C; hold program, 91°C for a maximum of 3 h.
10. Start the thermal cycle program. The program runs approx 1 h and 45 min. Specimens must be removed within 3 h of the start of the final hold program.

3.1.4. Detection of Amplicon

1. Remove the MicroAmp caps carefully to avoid creating aerosols of amplicon. Immediately pipet 100 µL of the denaturation solution into the reaction tubes using a multichannel pipettor. Mix by pipetting up and down. Denatured amplicon can be held at room temperature for no longer than 2 h or at 2–8°C for up to 1 wk.
2. Add 100 µL of hybridization buffer to each well to be tested on the HCV and IC microwell plates.
3. Pipet 25 µL of each denatured amplicon to the appropriate wells of the HCV and IC microwell plates.
4. Cover the microwell plates and incubate for 1 h at 37°C.
5. Wash the microwell plates five times with 1X wash solution using a microwell plate washer.
6. Add 100 µL of av-HRP conjugate to each well. Cover the microwell plates and incubate for 15 min at 37°C.
7. Wash the microwell plates five times with 1X wash solution using a microwell plate washer.
8. Prepare the working substrate reagent by mixing 2.0 mL of substrate A and 0.5 mL of substrate B for each of the 16 tests, no earlier than 3 h prior to use.

9. Pipet 100 µL of the working substrate reagent into each well being tested.
10. Allow color development for 10 min at room temperature in the dark.
11. Add 100 µL of stop reagent to each well.
12. Measure the OD at 450 nm within 30 min of adding the stop reagent. Record the absorbance value for each patient specimen and control tested.

3.1.5. Interpretation of Results

The assay results for the HCV positive and HCV negative controls should be ≥1.5 A_{450} and <0.25 A_{450}, respectively. If the absorbance values are <1.5 for the positive control and ≥0.25 for the negative controls, the run is invalid and the entire test procedure should be repeated. The presence of HCV RNA in a specimen is determined by comparing the absorbance at 450 nm of the unknown specimen to the established cutoff values for the test. The test result interpretation is based on the combination of the HCV and IC results as shown in **Table 1**. If invalid negative test results are obtained, either another aliquot of the original specimen should be processed or a new specimen should be collected. If equivocal test results are obtained, repeat the entire test procedure in duplicate using a new aliquot of the specimen. If both repeat test results are ≥0.3, the specimen should be considered positive. Specimens with one or both repeat test results that are <0.3 should be considered negative. The analytical sensitivity of this test is difficult to determine because of the lack of a recognized "gold standard" HCV RNA preparation. In our hands, it is at least as sensitive as our in-house-developed assay at ≤100 copies/m ***(34)***. Recent progress toward establishing international units for HCV RNA preparations should help to determine the relative sensitivities of the various nucleic acid amplification assays currently in use. The PCR products from the AMPLICOR assay may be used in the LiPA assay ***(35)***.

3.2. LiPA HCV II

3.2.1. Denaturation and Hybridization (*see* **Note 4**)

1. Heat a water bath to 50°C and prewarm the hybridization solution to at least 37°C but not more than 50°C. Mix the hybridization solution before use to dissolve any crystals.
2. Remove the required number of strips and write an identification number above the black line on the strips with a pencil.
3. Place one trough per test in the plastic tray.
4. Pipet 10 µL of denaturation solution into the upper corner of each trough.
5. Add 10 µL of the PCR product to the denaturation solution and carefully mix by pipetting up and down. Allow denaturation to proceed for 5 min at room temperature.
6. Add 2 mL of hybridization solution to the denatured PCR product in each trough. Take care not to contaminate adjacent troughs during pipetting.

Table 1
Interpretation of AMPLICOR HCV Test, Version 2.0 Results

HCV result (A_{450})	IC result (A_{450})	Interpretation
<0.3	≥0.3	HCV RNA not detected
<0.3	<0.3	Invalid negative test result
≥1.0	Any	HCV RNA detected
≥0.3, <1.0	Any	Equivocal

7. Immediately place the strip with the black marker line side up into the trough. The strips must be completely submerged in the solution.
8. Place the tray into the 50°C shaking water, set the speed at 80 rpm, and incubate for 60 min.

3.2.2. Stringent Wash

1. Remove the tray from the water bath, hold the tray at a low angle, and aspirate the liquid from the trough.
2. Add 2 mL of prewarmed stringent wash solution into each trough and rinse by rocking the tray for 10–20 s at room temperature.
3. Repeat **step 2** once more.
4. Incubate each strip in 2 mL of prewarmed stringent wash solution in the shaking water bath at 50°C for 30 min.

3.2.3. Color Development

1. Wash each strip twice for 1 min using 2 mL of the diluted rinse solution.
2. Add 2 mL of diluted conjugate to each trough and incubate for 30 min while agitating the tray on the shaker.
3. Wash each strip twice for 1 min with 2 mL of diluted rinse solution and wash once more using 2 mL of substrate buffer.
4. Add 2 mL of substrate solution to each trough and incubate for 30 min while agitating the tray on the shaker.
5. Stop the color development by washing the strips in 2 mL of deionized water with agitation on the shaker for at least 5 min.
6. Using tweezers, remove the strips from the troughs and place them on absorbent paper. Let the strips dry completely before reading the results. Store the developed strips in the dark.

3.2.4. Interpretation of Results

After hybridization, streptavidin labeled with alkaline phosphatase is added and binds to any biotinylated hybrid previously formed. Incubation with BCIP/NBT chromogen results in a purple/brown precipitate. Consequently, a col-

Table 2
INNO-LiPA HCV II Interpretation Chart

Line	1a			1b						1						2a/2c						2b						2					3a						3b		3c	3	4a	4b	4c/4d	4e		4f	4h	4				5a		6a				10a*	Line
1	x	x	x	x	x	x	x	x	x	x	x	x	x	x	x	x	x	x	x	x	x	x	x	x	x	x	x	x	x	x	x	x	x	x	x	x	x	x	x	x	x	x	x	x	x	x	x	x	x	x	x	x	x	x	x	x	x	x	x	x	1
2	x	x	x	x	x	x	x	x	x	x	x	x	x	x	x	x	x	x	x	x	x	x	x	x	x	x	x	x	x	x	x	x	x	x	x	x	x	x	x	x	x	x	x	x	x	x	x	x	x	x	x	x	x	x	x	x	x	x	x	x	2
3	x	x		x	x		x	x		x	x		x	x																																												x			3
4	x		x	x		x	x		x	x		x	x		x																																									x	x	x	x		4
5	x	x	x													x	x	x				x	x	x				x	x																x	x		x			x	x	x			x	x		x		5
6				x	x	x																																		x		x						x	x				x	x			x		x	6
7							x	x	x																																																				7
8													x	x	x																x																x														8
9																x		x	x		x	x		x	x		x	x	x	x		x																	x			x					x					9
10																x	x		x	x		x	x		x	x		x			x	x																													10
11																x	x	x	x	x	x									x		x																													11
12																						x	x	x	x	x	x																																		12
13																																	x		x	x			x	x		x																			13
14																																	x	x		x	x				x																				14
15																																	x	x	x			x			x																				15
16																																											x	x	x	x	x	x		x	x	x									16
17																																							x					x	x				x	x	x		x								17
18																																							x	x					x				x	x	x	x	x							x	18
19																																																							x							19
20																													x	x																			x						x	x						20
21																																																									x	x	x	x		21

*This pattern is found with some isolates from Indonesia and is provisionally classified as 10a.

ored precipitate forms only when there is a perfect match between the probe and the PCR products. A line is considered positive when a distinct purple/brown band appears at the end of the test procedure.

The first line on the strip is the conjugate control line that controls for the color development steps in the procedure. It should be lined up with the conjugate control line on the transparent plastic reading strip. The second positive line controls the addition of amplified product for hybridization. This line should always be positive if the amplified product form of HCV is present. Inhibition of PCR might be the reason for complete failure of the genotyping test. Record all the line numbers that are positive on the strip and deduce the HCV genotype using the interpretation chart (*see* **Table 2**). Coinfection with different types of HCV may be recognized when lines from two different major types are present.

The INNO-LiPA HCV II test is based on nucleotide variability of the 5′ UTR, and the test yields high concordance with sequences obtained for this region using nucleic acid sequencing techniques. However, subtyping may occasionally not be possible owing to lack of subtype-specific sequence variation in the 5′ UTR.

The INNO-LiPA is effective in identifying HCV genotypes that occur most frequently in North America, Europe, and Japan. However, DNA sequencing is currently the best means of discriminating types endemic to other geographic regions.

4. Notes

1. The IC control not only tests for inhibition of the amplification reaction but also tests for RNA recovery. Therefore, a failed IC reaction may indicate the presence of inhibitors in the specimen or poor recovery of RNA from the specimen. In our experience, most failed IC reactions are resolved by simply processing another aliquot of the original specimens and repeating the test.
2. The presence of UNG and deoxyuridine triphosphate in the PCR master mix reduces the risk of amplicon contamination. UNG has been demonstrated to inactivate a least 1000 copies of deoxyuridine-containing HCV amplicon per PCR (*see* Roche AMPLICOR HCV Test, version 2.0 package insert). However, contamination from HCV positive controls and clinical specimens can be avoided only by good laboratory practices and careful adherence to procedure.
3. Recovery of the often invisible RNA pellet is the most challenging part of this procedure. Careful attention to this step is critical to achieving reproducible results ***(34)***.
4. The hybridization, stringent washing, and color development steps have been automated in the Auto-LiPA instrument.

References

1. Choo, Q. L., Kuo, G., Weiner, A. J., Overby, L. R., Bradley, D. W., and Houghton, M. (1989) Isolation of a cDNA clone derived from a blood-borne non-A non-B viral hepatitis genome. *Science* **224,** 359–362.
2. Alter, H. J. (1991) Descartes before the horse: I clone, therefore I am: the hepatitis C virus in current perspective. *Ann. Intern. Med.* **115,** 644–649.
3. Kuo, G., Choo, Q. L., Alter, H. J., et al. (1989) An assay for circulating antibodies to a major etiologic virus of human non-A, non-B hepatitis. *Science* **244,** 362–364.
4. Simmonds, P., Alberti, A., Alter, H. J., et al. (1994) A proposed system for the nomenclature of hepatitis C viral genotypes. *Hepatology* **19,** 1321–1324 (letter).
5. Miller, R. H. and Purcell, R. H. (1990) Hepatitis C virus shares amino acid sequence similarities with pestiviruses and flaviviruses as well as members of two plant virus supergroups. *Proc. Natl. Acad. Sci. USA* **87,** 2057–2061.
6. Ogata, N., Alter, H. J., Miller R. H., and Purcell, R. H. (1991) Nucleotide sequence and mutation rate of the H strain of hepatitis C virus. *Proc. Natl. Acad. Sci. USA* **88,** 3391–3396.
7. Gretch, D. R. (1997) Diagnostic tests for hepatitis C. *Hepatology* **26,** 43S–47S.
8. Daman, M., Cuypers, H. T. M., Zaaijer, H. L., Reesink, H. W., Schaasberg, W. P., Gerlich, W. H., Miesters, H. G. M., and Lelie, P. N. (1996) International collaborative study on the second EUROHEP HCV-RNA reference panel. *J. Virol. Methods* **58,** 175–185.
9. Young, K. K. Y., Resnick, R. M., and Myers, T. W. (1995) Detection of hepatitis C virus RNA by a combined reverse transcription-polymerase chain reaction assay. *J. Clin. Microbiol.* **31,** 882–886.
10. Zeuzem, S., Ruster, B., and Roth, W. K. (1994) Clinical evaluation of a new polymerase chain reaction assay (Amplicor™ HCV) for detection of hepatitis C virus. *Z. Gastroenterol.* **32,** 342–347.
11. Nolte, F. S., Thurmond, C., and Fried, M. W. (1995) Preclinical evaluation of AMPLICOR hepatitis C virus test for detection of hepatitis C virus RNA. *J. Clin. Microbiol.* **33,** 1775–1778.
12. Bukh, J., Purcell, R. H., and Miller, R. H. (1992) Importance of primer selection for the detection of hepatitis C virus RNA with the polymerase chain reaction. *Proc. Natl. Acad. Sci. USA* **89,** 187–191.
13. Myers, T. W. and Gelfand, D. H. (1991) Reverse transcription and DNA amplification by a thermus thermophilus DNA polymerase. *Biochemistry* **30,** 7661–7666.
14. Longo, M. C., Berninger, M. S. and Hartley, J. L. (1990) Use of uracil DNA glycosylase to control carry-over contamination in polymerase chain reactions. *Gene* **93,** 125–128.
15. Mahaney, K., Tedeschi, V., Maertens, G., Di Bisceglia, A., Vergalia, J., Hoofnagle, J., and Sallie, R. (1994) Genotypic analysis of hepatitis C virus in American patients. *Hepatology* **20,** 1405–1411.

16. Lau, J. Y. N., Mizokami, M., Kolberg, J. A., et al. (1995) Application of six hepatitis C virus genotyping systems to sera from chronic hepatitis C patients in the United States. *J. Infect. Dis.* **171,** 218–289.
17. McHutchison, J. G., Gordon, S., Schiff, E. R., et al. (1998) Interferon alpha-2b alone or in combination of ribavirin as initial treatment for chronic hepatitis C. *N. Engl. J. Med.* **339,** 1485–1499.
18. Poynard, T., Marcellin, P., Lee, S. S., et al. (1998) Randomised trial of interferon α2b plus ribavirin for 48 weeks or for 24 weeks versus interferon α2b plus placebo for 48 weeks for treatment of chronic infection with hepatitis C virus. *Lancet* **352,** 1426–1432.
19. Cha, T. A., Beall, E., Irvine, B., et al. (1992) At least five related, but distinct, hepatitis C viral genotypes exist. *Proc. Natl. Acad. Sci. USA* **89,** 7144–7148.
20. Chan, S. W., McOmish, F., Holmes, E. C., et al. (1992) Analysis of a new hepatitis C virus type and its phyylogenetic relationship to existing variants. *J. Gen. Virol.* **73,** 1131–1141.
21. Bukh, J., Purcell, R. H., and Miller, R. H. (1993) At least 12 genotypes of hepatitis C virus predicted by sequence analysis of the putative E1 gene of isolates collected worldwide. *Proc. Natl. Acad. Sci. USA* **90,** 8234–8238.
22. Simmonds, P., Holmes, E. C., Cha, T.-A., et al. (1993) Classification of hepatitis C virus into six major genotypes and a series of subtypes by phylogenetic analysis of the NS-5 region. *J. Gen. Virol.* **74,** 2391–2399.
23. Okamoto, H., Sugiyama, Y., Okada, S., et al. (1992) Typing hepatitis C virus by polymerase chain reaction with type-specific primers: application to clinical surveys and tracing infectious sources. *J. Gen. Virol.* **73,** 673–679.
24. Chayama, K., Tsubota, A., Arase, Y., et al. (1993) Genotypic subtyping of hepatitis C virus. *J. Gastroenterol. Hepatol.* **8,** 150–156.
25. Nakao, T., Enomoto, N., Tadada, N., Tadada, A., and Date, T., (1991) Typing of hepatitis C virus genomes by restriction fragment length polymorphism. *J. Gen. Virol.* **72,** 2105–2112.
26. Takada, N., Takase, S., Enomoto, N., Takada, A., and Date, T. (1992) Clinical backgrounds of the patients having different types of hepatitis C virus genomes. *J. Hepatol.* **14,** 35–40.
27. Stuyver, L., Rossau, R., Wyseur, A., Duhamel, M., Vanderborght, B., Van Heuverswyn, H., and Maertens, G. (1993) Typing of hepatitis C virus isolates and characterization of new subtypes using a line probe assay. *J. Gen. Virol.* **74,** 1093–1102.
28. Marshall, D. J., Heisler, L. M., Lyamichev, V., Murvine, C., Olive, D. M., Ehrlich, G. D., Neri, B. P., and deArruda, M. (1997) Determination of hepatitis C virus genotypes in the United States by cleavase fragment length polymorphism analysis. *J. Clin. Microbiol.* **35,** 3156–3162.
29. Simmonds, P., Rose, K. A., Graham, S., et al. (1993) Mapping of serotype-specific immunodominant epitopes in the HS-4 region of hepatitis C virus (HCV). Use of type-specific peptides to serologically differentiate infections with HCV type 1, type 2 and type 3. *J. Clin. Microbiol.* **31,** 1493–1503.

30. Bhattacherjee, V., Prescott, L. E., Pike, I., et al. (1995) Use of NS-4 peptides to identify type-specific antibody to hepatitis C virus genotypes 1, 2, 3, 4, 5 and 6. *J. Gen. Virol.* **76,** 1737–1748.
31. Andonov, A. and Chaudhary, R. K. (1995) Subtyping of hepatitis C virus isolates by a line probe assay using hybridization. *J. Clin. Microbiol.* **33,** 254–256.
32. Lau, J. Y. N., Simmonds P., and Urdea, M. S. (1995) Implications of variations of "conserved" regions of hepatitis C virus genome. *Lancet* **346,** 425, 426.
33. Hadziyannis, E., Larsen, N., Thurmond, C., Mauer, D., and Nolte, F. (1997) Genotyping of hepatitis C virus with direct sequencing: comparison with a line probe assay, in *Program and Abstracts of the Annual Meeting of the Association of Molecular Pathology*, San Diego, CA.
34. Nolte, F. S., Thurmond, C., and Mitchell, P. S. (1994) Isolation of hepatitis C virus RNA from serum for reverse transcription-PCR. *J. Clin. Microbiol.* **32,** 519,520.
35. Hadziyannis, E., Fried, M., and Nolte, F. S. (1995) Evaluation of two methods for quantitation of hepatitis C virus RNA, in *Program and Abstracts of the 46th Annual Meeting of the American Association for the Study of Liver Diseases*, Chicago, p. 356A.

29

Detection and Speciation of Mycobacteria in Formalin-Fixed, Paraffin-Embedded Tissue Sections

Diana Mohl and Thomas J. Giordano

1. Introduction

The ability to detect mycobacterial DNA by polymerase chain reaction (PCR)–based methodology in formalin-fixed, paraffin-embedded tissue sections is useful in several clinical scenarios. The major use of this type of assay is in those instances in which infectious disease is not clinically suspected and microbiological cultures are not performed. In these cases, the only tissue available for examination is that present in routinely prepared paraffin blocks after histologic examination. The presence of necrotizing granulomatous inflammation should result in special stains for acid-fast organisms. However, in many such cases the special stains are unsatisfactory, because the number of organisms present is very low (as in *Mycobacterium tuberculosis*). Thus, the tedious examination of multiple serial sections is often necessary to identify the pathogenic organism, and often no organism is found. Therefore, more sensitive detection methods are needed. PCR-based detection of mycobacterial DNA is more sensitive and can be used either to verify the presence of organisms seen on special stains or to identify an occult organism. By combining the PCR assays with restriction analyses of the products, it is often possible to speciate the pathogenic organism.

In addition, given the rapidity of the PCR assays compared to mycobacterial culture, this technology can be used whenever mycobacterial disease is suspected, but the clinical situation precludes waiting for culture results. In these cases, often the determination of typical vs atypical organisms is all the information one needs to provide until culture confirmation and speciation becomes available.

From: *Methods in Molecular Medicine, vol. 49: Molecular Pathology Protocols*
Edited by: A. A. Killeen © Humana Press Inc., Totowa, NJ

A variety of assays has been employed to detect mycobacterial DNA in formalin-fixed, paraffin-embedded tissues ***(1,2)***. Most have used a nested PCR approach to amplify the 65-kDa surface antigen gene ***(3)***, the IS6110 insertion sequence ***(4–6)***, the mtp40 sequence ***(7)***, or the 16S rRNA gene ***(8,9)***. The assays have been shown to be rapid, specific, and sensitive. The assay described herein is based on that of Cook et al. ***(10)*** and employs nested PCR of the 65-kDa surface antigen gene followed by an algorithmic restriction analysis for speciation.

2. Materials

2.1. Slides

1. One positive control slide (*see* **Note 1**).
2. Four to six slides of the case (*see* **Note 2**).

2.2. DNA Extraction

1. 1.5-mL Microfuge tubes.
2. Xylene.
3. Razor blades, single edge.
4. 100% Ethanol.
5. 70% Ethanol.
6. Proteinase K (20 mg/mL) (Gibco-BRL, Gaithersburg, MD).
7. 50 m*M* Tris-HCl, pH 8.3.
8. Dry ice.

2.3. Polymerase Chain Reaction

1. 0.5-mL Microfuge tubes (or 0.2 mL, depending on the type of thermal cycler).
2. *Taq* DNA polymerase and buffer with $MgCl_2$ (Gibco-BRL).
3. dNTPs (10 m*M*) (Gibco-BRL).
4. Sterile H_2O.
5. Oligonucleotides (1 µg/mL stocks). Sequences are shown in **Table 1**.

2.4. Analysis of PCR Products

1. NuSieve agarose (FMC Bioproducts, Rockland, ME).
2. Agarose, multipurpose (Gibco-BRL).
3. DNA size markers, e.g., phi-X174/*Hae*III digest (Gibco-BRL).
4. 10X Gel-loading buffer (Gibco-BRL).
5. 10X Tris-borate EDTA (TBE) buffer (Gibco-BRL).
6. Ethidium bromide (10 mg/mL stock).

2.5. Restriction Analysis of PCR Products

1. Restriction enzymes *Bst*UI, *Cfo*I, *Mbo*I (Gibco-BRL).
2. Reaction buffer provided by manufacturer.
3. Mineral oil (Sigma, St. Louis, MO).

Table 1
Sequences of PCR Primers

Round 1: mycobacteria primers
5′-AAGGAGATCGAGCTGGAGGA-3′ (upstream 1)
5′-AGGCGTTGGTTCGCGAGGG-3′ (upstream 2)
5′-TGATGACGCCCTCGTTGCC-3′ (downstream)
Round 2: mycobacteria primers[a]
5′-GTCTCAAACGCGGCATCG-3′ (upstream)
5′-GTCACCGATGGACTGGTC-3′ (downstream)
Round 1: β-globin primers
5′-CCATAGGCAGAGAGAGTCAGTG-3′ (upstream 1)
5′-TGCCAGAAGAGCCAAGGACAGG-3′ (downstream 1)
Round 2: β-globin primers[a]
5′-CACATAGGCAGAGAGCGTCAGTG-3′ (upstream)
5′-CCTATCAGAAACCCAAGAGTC-3′ (downstream)

[a]Round 2 product sizes are 130 and 322 bp for mycobacteria and β-globin, respectively.

2.6. Equipment

1. Thermal cycler.
2. Pipets with filtered pipet tips.
3. Agarose gel apparatus.
4. Tabletop centrifuge.
5. Tube racks.
6. Shaking incubator.
7. Heat blocks (37 and 60°C).
8. Ice bath.

3. Methods

The following methods are those of Cook et al. ***(10)*** with only minor modifications.

3.1. DNA Extraction

1. Label the appropriate number of 1.5-mL microfuge tubes with the date and sample number (*see* **Note 3**).
2. Pipet 100 µL of xylene into each tube.
3. Using a clean razor blade, scrape the tissue off the glass slide.
4. Place the tissue into the tube containing the xylene and tap to make sure the tissue is submerged.
5. Stand at room temperature for 5–10 min to deparaffinize the tissue.
6. Spin the xylene and tissue at 12,800*g* in a microcentrifuge for 5 min (*see* **Note 4**).
7. Remove the supernatant with a pipet, making sure the tissue pellet remains in the tube (*see* **Note 4**). Blot the excess xylene with a tissue.

8. Add 100 µL of 100% ethanol to the tissue pellet. Gently tap to resuspend.
9. Spin at 14,000 rpm in a tabletop centrifuge for 5 min.
10. Pour off the supernatant and remove the excess liquid with a Kimwipe (*see* **Note 4**).
11. Repeat **steps 8–10** with 70% ethanol.
12. Place the open tubes in a rack and heat in a 60°C oven for 15 min or until the pellets are dry.
13. Prepare fresh proteinase K digestion solution (0.2 mg/mL in 50 m*M* Tris-HCl, pH 8.3) from a stock solution of 20 mg/mL of proteinase K.
14. Add 100 µL of the proteinase K digestion solution to each tube.
15. Tap the tubes to dissolve the pellet quick-spin.
16. Incubate for 6 h to overnight at 37°C in a shaking incubator.
17. Quick-spin the tubes to collect the liquid at the bottom of the tubes.
18. Place the tubes in a dry ice–ethanol bath for 1 min. Remove the tubes and place them into a boiling water bath for 8 min to inactivate the proteinase K.
19. Place the tubes on ice for 5 min, and then spin at 12,800*g* in a tabletop centrifuge for 5 min.
20. Transfer the supernatant, which contains the DNA, to a clean, labeled tube. Alternatively, the DNA can be stored in the same tube; spin again before removing the DNA.

3.2. Polymerase Chain Reaction

1. Prepare PCR master mix for round 1. The master mix contains dNTPS, 1X *Taq* buffer with $MgCl_2$, and oligonucleotide primers. It is prepared in large batches, aliquoted, and stored at –20°C. The master mix for round 1 (makes mix for 200 reactions) contains the following (*see* **Note 5**): 25 µL of mycobacteria primers (three each at 1 µg/µL), 2.5 µL of β-globin primers (two at 1 µg /mL), 20 µL of 10 m*M* dNTPs, 1000 µL of 10X *Taq* buffer with $MgCl_2$, and 2540 µL of H_2O (total of 3700 µL/200 rxn = 18.5 µL/rxn).
2. Label 0.5-mL tubes with the date and sample number.
3. In a 1.5-mL tube, add 18.5 µL of master mix for each reaction plus 1. Thus, if there are nine reactions, add 185 µL (9 + 1 = 10 × 18.5 µL = 185 µL).
4. To the tube with the master mix, add 0.5 µL of *Taq* DNA polymerase (5 U/µL) for each reaction.
5. Mix well by tapping.
6. Pipet 19 µL of the master mix with *Taq* into prelabeled 0.5-mL tubes.
7. Add 31 µL of the DNA to each tube. Mix well and quick-spin.
8. Place the tubes in a thermal cycler and run the following program: initial denaturation for 4 min at 94°C; followed by 36 cycles of 94°C for 1 min, 57°C for 2 min, and 72°C for 2 min; followed by a 10-min extension at 72°C. Bring to 25°C and hold at that temperature. This will take about 4 h.
9. Remove the tubes and quick-spin.

10. Label a new set of 0.5 mL tubes with the same information as in round 1, but specify them as round 2.
11. Prepare the master mix for round 2 (makes mix for 200 reactions): 25 µL of Mycobacteria round 2 primers (two, each at 1 µg/µL) 20 µL of β-globin primers round 2 (two, each at 1 µg/mL) 20 µL of 10 m*M* dNTPs 1000 µL of 10X *Taq* buffer with $MgCl_2$, and 7835 µL of H_2O (total of 8900 µL).
12. In a 1.5-mL tube, add 44.5 µL of master mix for round 2 for each reaction plus 1. Thus, if there are nine reactions, add 445 µL (9 + 1 = 10 × 44.5 µL = 445 µL).
13. To the tube with the master mix, add 0.5 µL of *Taq* DNA polymerase (5 U/µL) for each reaction.
14. Mix well by tapping.
15. Pipet 45 µL of the master mix with *Taq* into prelabeled 0.5 mL tubes.
16. Add 5 µL of the round 1 products to the round 2 tubes (*see* **Note 6**).
17. Place the tubes in the thermal cycler and run the following program: initial denaturation for 4 min at 94°C, followed by 36 cycles of 94°C for 1 min, 52°C for 2 min, and 72°C for 2 min. Finish with a 10-min extension at 72°C.
18. Remove the tubes and quick-spin to collect the solution at the bottom of the tubes.
19. Analyze the products on a 3% agarose gel.

3.3. Agarose Gel Electrophoresis

1. Analyze the products on a 3% agarose/0.5X TBE gel buffer in a submersible apparatus of choice (*see* **Note 7**).
2. Use size markers of choice to cover 100–400 bp.
3. Run 10 µL of PCR products along with 2 µL of 10X gel-loading buffer.
4. Photograph using a UV light box.
5. Proceed to restriction analysis if the duplicate extractions of the case contain the appropriate mycobacterial band (130 bp). The β-globin product (322 bp) should be present in all reactions except the mock extraction (*see* **Fig. 1A**).

3.4. Restriction Analysis of PCR Products

1. Digest 10 µL of each PCR product with three separate restriction enzymes—*Cfo*I, *Bst*UI, and *Mbo*I—according to the supplier's recommendations. Use 5 U of enzyme/10 µL of PCR product (*see* **Note 8**).
2. After digestions are complete, load the entire digestion onto a 3% agarose gel as before and electrophorese until the bromophenol tracking dye has migrated approximately three fourths the length of the gel.
3. Analyze the restriction patterns using the algorithm of Cook et al. *(10)* for patterns that match those of known mycobacterial organisms. The patterns associated with the most important organisms, *M. tuberculosis* and *Mycobacterium avium intracellulare*, are shown in **Table 2**. *See* **Figs. 1B** and **2** for examples (*see* **Note 9**).

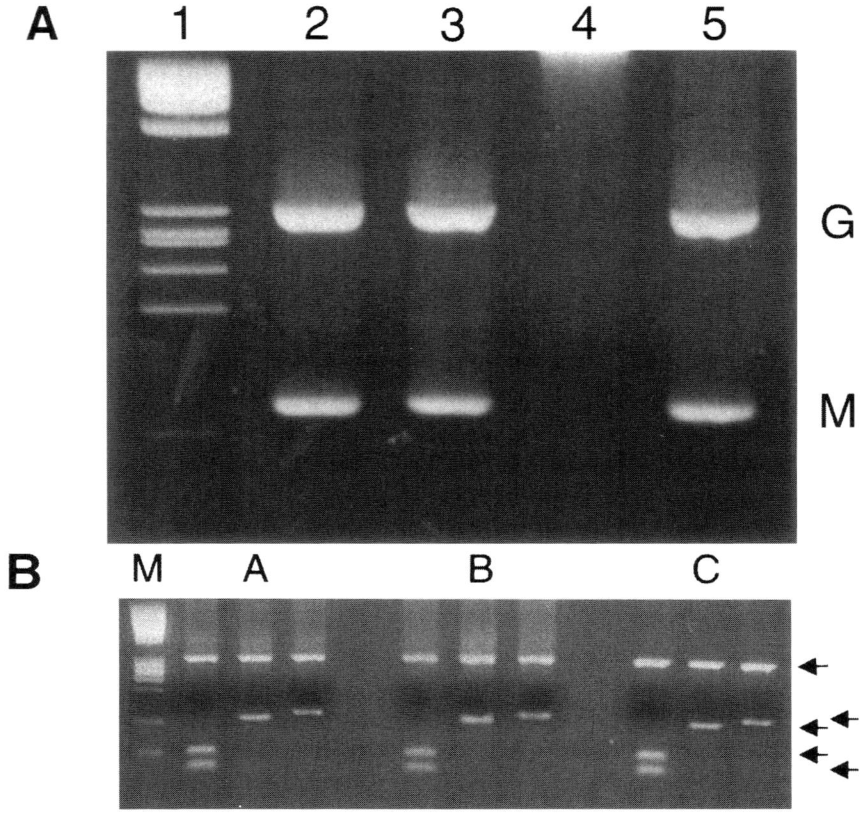

Fig. 1. **(A)** Results of two rounds of nested PCR for mycobacterial DNA. The case is extracted and amplifed in duplicate (lanes 2 and 3). Lane 4, mock extraction; lane 5, positive mycobacterial control; lane M, DNA markers; G, 322-bp β-globin internal control band; M, 130-bp mycobacterial band. **(B)** Restriction analysis of the products from (A). Each PCR product is digested with a panel of restriction enzymes—*Cfo*I, *Bst*UI, and *Mbo*I—and the digests are analyzed as a group. Group A–C represents the restriction digests of the PCR products of lanes 2, 3, and 5 in (A), respectively. The arrows represent 322, 130, 120, 76, and 65 bp. This restriction pattern matches that of *M. tuberculosis*. Lane M: DNA size markers; lanes 2, 5, and 8: = *Cfo*I digest; lanes 3, 6, and 0: *Mbo*I digest; lanes 4, 7, and 10: *Bst*UI digest.

Table 2
Restriction Enzyme Patterns for *M. tuberculosis* and *M. avium-intracellulare*

Enzyme	*M. tuberculosis* (bp)	*M. avium-intracellulare* (bp)
*Cfo*I	75 + 65	130 (uncut)
*Bst*UI	120	85–90
*Mbo*I	130 (uncut)	80–100

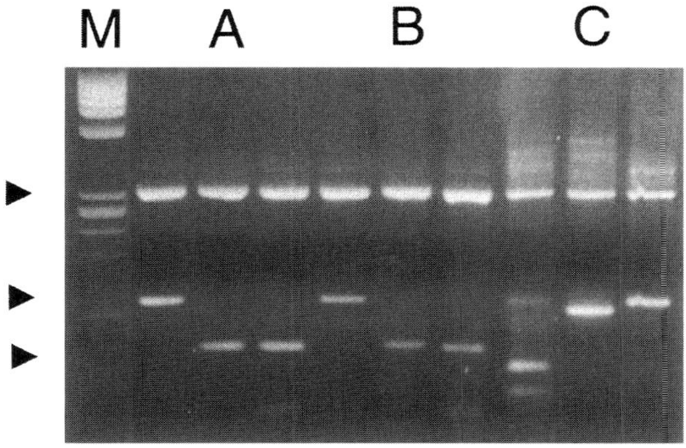

Fig. 2. Restriction analysis of a different positive mycobacterial assay. In this case, the restriction digests do not match those of *M. tuberculosis*. The pattern is that of an atypical organism, most consistent with *M. avium-intracellulare*. A and B represent the restriction digests of duplicate extractions of the case and C represents the digests of an *M. tuberculosis* control. Arrows represent 322, 130, and 100 bp. Lane M: DNA size markers; lanes 2, 5, and 8: *Cfo*I digest; lanes 3, 6, and 0: *Mbo*I digest; lanes 4, 7, and 10: *Bst*UI digest.

4. Notes

1. The best positive control tissues are obtained from culture-proven patients who have evidence of disease at the time of autopsy. Several paraffin blocks from such a case can provide control tissues for a significant period of time. The tissue sections of the control can be cut into batches and stored in a slide box at room temperature.
2. The tissue sections of the case need to be cut with a clean knife and with careful attention not to pick up any tissue bath floaters. The sections should be about 5 µm thick, should placed on plain glass slides (not treated slides), and should not be heated. Use the tissue from multiple sections of the tissue. Tissue fixed in B5 is suboptimal and should be avoided.
3. For each clinical sample and control pair, include a "mock" extraction that contains only the extraction reagents. This is used to monitor contamination in the reagents. Clinical samples should be extracted in duplicate. If more than one block is available, it is possible to combine a section from each block into a single tube. Always wear gloves and handle the tubes from the sides; that is, do not touch the rims of the tubes or the cap. Use filtered pipet tips to prevent contamination of the pipetmen.
4. It is very easy to dislodge and lose the tissue at this step. Remove the samples as soon as the centrifuge stops spinning. If unable to do so, spin again and remove the xylene.

5. Two upstream primers specific to the 65-kDa surface antigen are used to increase the number of amplifyable cases ***(10)***. Because the assay consists of two rounds of nested PCR, the final products are the same regardless of which first-round primer was used in the amplification. Add a drop of mineral oil to the PCR reactions if the thermal cycler does not have a heated lid.
6. This is best performed in a "clean" environment, such as a "template tamer" or a UV biological hood to minimize contamination. Care should be taken not to contaminant any of the round 2 reactions with any round 1 products.
7. We use a mixture of multipurpose and Nusieve agarose when preparing the 3% gels. This agarose boils over easily, so be careful when preparing the gel. Prepare the gel with ethidium bromide by adding 6.5 μL of 10 mg/mL stock per 100 mL of gel.
8. The restriction digests should be set up in a designated "post-PCR" room to avoid contamination by PCR product. We use a 4-h incubation at 37°C for *Cfo*I and *Mbo*I and 60°C for *Bst*UI. Add a drop of mineral oil to the *Bst*UI digest to prevent evaporation.
9. If the restriction patterns of the duplicate extractions of the case are the same but do not match the algorithm of Cook et al. ***(10)***, you may consider sequencing the PCR product to determine the species of origin. If the patterns of the duplicate extractions do not match each other, then contamination is likely the source of the mycobacterial DNA.

References

1. Osaki, M., Adachi, H., Gomyo, Y., Yoshida, H., and Ito, H. (1997) Detection of mycobacterial DNA in formalin-fixed, paraffin-embedded tissue specimens by duplex polymerase chain reaction: application to histopathologic diagnosis. *Mod. Pathol.* **10,** 78–83.
2. Totsch, M., Bocker, W., Brommelkamp, E., Fille, M., Kreczy, A., Ofner, D., Schmid, K. W., and Dockhorn-Dworniczak, B. (1996) Diagnostic value of different PCR assays for the detection of mycobacterial DNA in granulomatous lymphadenopathy. *J. Pathol.* **178,** 221–226.
3. Bascunana, C. R. and Belak, K. (1996) Detection and identification of mycobacteria in formalin-fixed, paraffin-embedded tissues by nested PCR and restriction enzyme analysis. *J. Clin. Microbiol.* **34,** 2351–2355.
4. Ferrara, G., Cannone, M., Guadagnino, A., Nappi, O., and Barberis, M. C. (1999) Nested polymerase chain reaction on vaginal smears of tuberculous cervicitis: a case report. *Acta Cytol.* **43,** 308–312.
5. Salian, N. V., Rish, J. A., Eisenach, K. D., Cave, M. D., and Bates, J. H. (1998) Polymerase chain reaction to detect Mycobacterium tuberculosis in histologic specimens. *Am. J. Respir. Clin. Care Med.* **158,** 1150–1155.
6. Berk, R. H., Yazici, M., Atabey, N., Ozdamar, O. S., Pabuccuoglu, U., and Alici, E. (1996) Detection of Mycobacterium tuberculosis in formaldehyde solution-fixed, paraffin-embedded tissue by polymerase chain reaction in Pott's disease. *Spine* **21,** 1991–1995.

7. Marchetti, G., Gori, A., Catozzi, L., Vago, L., Nebuloni, M., Rossi, M. C., Esposti, A. D., Bandera, A., and Franzette, F. (1998) Evaluation of PCR in detection of mycobacterial tuberculosis from formalin-fixed, paraffin-embedded tissues: comparison of four amplification assays. *J. Clin. Microbiol.* **36,** 1512–1517.
8. Hardman, W. J., Benian, G. M., Howard, T., McGowan, J. E. Jr., Metchock, B., Murtagh, J. J. (1996) Rapid detection of mycobacteria in inflammatory necrotizing granulomas from formalin-fixed, paraffin-embedded tissue by PCR in clinically high-risk patients with acid-fast stain and culture negative tissue biopsies. *Am. J. Clin. Pathol.* **106,** 184–389.
9. Kox, L. F., van Leeuwen, J., Knijper, S., Jansen, H. M., and Kolk, A. H. (1995) PCR assay based on DNA coding for 16S rRNA for detection and identification of mycobacteria in clinical samples. *J. Clin. Microbiol.* **33,** 3225–3233.
10. Cook, S. M., Bartos, R. E., Pierson, C. L., and Frank, T. S. (1994) Detection and characterization of atypical mycobacteria by the polymerase chain reaction. *Diagn. Mol. Pathol.* **3,** 53–58.

30

Ultrasensitive Quantitation of Human Immunodeficiency Virus Type 1 RNA in Plasma by the AMPLICOR and COBAS AMPLICOR HIV-1 MONITOR™ Tests

Steven Herman, James Novotny, and Maurice Rosenstraus

1. Introduction

The measurement of plasma human immunodeficiency virus type 1 (HIV-1) RNA levels has become an important tool for identifying individuals likely to benefit from antiretroviral therapy *(1–7)* as well as monitoring patients on therapy *(1,8–14)*, and is now regarded as standard medical practice for managing the treatment of HIV-1-infected individuals *(15–21)*. Three commercially available assays for measuring HIV-1 RNA levels are available. The first-generation AMPLICOR HIV-1 MONITOR™ Test, which uses reverse transcriptase-polymerase chain reaction (RT-PCR) technology, has a lower limit of quantitation of 400 copies/mL of plasma *(22,23)*. The NucliSens HIV-1 QT Test (Organon Teknika, Boxtel, Netherlands), a second-generation assay based on the nucleic acid sequence–based amplification technique, has a lower limit of quantitation of 100 HIV-1 RNA copies/mL of plasma *(24)*. The Quantiplex HIV-1 Version 2.0 Test (Chiron, Emeryville, CA), which uses the branched-chain DNA signal amplification technique, has a lower limit of quantitation of 500 HIV-1 RNA copies/mL of plasma *(25,26)*.

Recently, the use of combination therapy has resulted in rapid and potent antiretroviral and immunologic effects that lead to a sharp decline in plasma HIV-1 RNA concentration, frequently to an undetectable level *(10,12,14)*. A more sensitive method with a lower detection limit for plasma HIV-1 RNA is therefore required. By employing a modified specimen preparation procedure,

From: *Methods in Molecular Medicine, vol. 49: Molecular Pathology Protocols*
Edited by: A. A. Killeen © Humana Press Inc., Totowa, NJ

which incorporates an ultracentrifugation step to concentrate virus from plasma *(27,28)*, we increased the sensitivity of the AMPLICOR HIV-1 MONITOR Test eightfold, achieving a lower limit of quantitation of 50 HIV-1 RNA copies/mL of plasma (*[29,30]*; N. Michael, personal communication).

Roche Molecular Systems has incorporated the UltraSensitive processing procedure into the first-generation AMPLICOR HIV-1 MONITOR Test; the second-generation AMPLICOR HIV-1 MONITOR Test, Version 1.5; and the fully automated COBAS AMPLICOR HIV-1 MONITOR™ Test, Version 1.5. By offering the option of using either the UltraSensitive or Standard processing method, these tests achieve the wide dynamic range required to measure viral RNA titer throughout the course of HIV-1 infection. The first-generation AMPLICOR HIV-1 MONITOR Test has been cleared by the Food and Drug Administration. The second-generation Version 1.5 tests, which are commercially available outside the United States, are upgraded tests that contain a primer pair and modified thermal cycling conditions designed to yield equivalent quantitation of all group M subtypes of HIV-1.

2. Materials

2.1. AMPLICOR Kits

2.1.1. AMPLICOR HIV-1 MONITOR Test, Version 1.5

1. AMPLICOR HIV-1 MONITOR, Version 1.5 Kit (contains all specimen preparation, amplification, and detection reagents).

2.1.2. COBAS AMPLICOR HIV-1 MONITOR Test, Version 1.5

1. COBAS AMPLICOR HIV-1 MONITOR, Version 1.5 Kit (contains all specimen preparation, amplification, and detection reagents).

2.2. Laboratory Supplies and Equipment

2.2.1. Preamplification: Reagent Preparation Area

2.2.1.1. Common Equipment

1. Plastic resealable bag.
2. Eppendorf® Repeater™ pipet with 1.25-mL Combitip® Reservoir (sterile, individually wrapped).
3. Pipettors (200-µL capacity) with aerosol barrier or positive displacement RNase-free tips.
4. Latex gloves, powderless.

2.2.1.2. AMPLICOR Test

1. Perkin-Elmer MicroAmp® reaction tubes.
2. Perkin-Elmer MicroAmp caps.
3. Perkin-Elmer MicroAmp tray/retainers.
4. Perkin-Elmer MicroAmp tray base.

2.2.1.3. COBAS AMPLICOR Test

1. COBAS AMPLICOR A-ring fitted with 12 A-tubes.
2. COBAS AMPLICOR A-ring holder.

2.2.2. Preamplification: Specimen Preparation Area

1. Microcentrifuge (max. relative centrifugal force [RCF] 16,000*g*, min. RCF 12,500*g*); Eppendorf 5415C, HERMLE Z230M, or equivalent.
2. Refrigerated ultracentrifuge with fixed-angle rotor (45°, capacity for 24 1.5-mL tubes) with an RCF of 23,600*g* (Heraeus Centrifuge 17 RS or Biofuge 28 RS with HFA 22.1 rotor, Heraeus Biofuge Stratos with the 3331 rotor or equivalent). The rotor lid must form an aerosol-tight seal to the rotor to contain aerosols in case of tube failure.
3. 2.0-mL Sterile, nonsiliconized, conical polypropylene screw-cap tubes (Sarstedt 72.694.006 or equivalent).
4. 1.5-mL Sterile, nonsiliconized, conical polypropylene screw-cap tubes (Sarstedt 72.692.105 or equivalent).
5. Tube racks (Sarstedt 93.1428).
6. 70% Ethanol (freshly diluted from 95% using deionized water).
7. Isopropyl alcohol, reagent grade.
8. Sterile fine-tip transfer pipets, RNase-free.
9. Vortex mixer.
10. Latex gloves, powderless.
11. Sterile, disposable, polystyrene serologic pipets (5, 10, and 25 mL).
12. Pipettors (capacity 12.5, 25, 50, 100, 200, 400, 500, 600, 800, and 1000 µL) with aerosol barrier or positive displacement RNase-free tips.

2.2.3. Postamplification Area

2.2.3.1. AMPLICOR Test

1. Perkin-Elmer GeneAmp PCR System 9600 or GeneAmp PCR System 2400 thermal cycler.
2. MicroAmp Base and cap-installing tool for Perkin-Elmer Applied Biosystems GeneAmp PCR System 9600 or GeneAmp PCR System 2400.
3. Multichannel pipettor (25 and 100 µL) or electronic pipettor (Impact® or AMPLICOR®).
4. Aerosol barrier or positive displacement RNase-free pipettor tips (25 and 100 µL) and barrier-free tips (100 µL).
5. Microwell plate washer.
6. Microwell plate reader.
7. Disposable reagent reservoirs.
8. Microwell plate lid (cat. no. 07-200-376; Fisher).
9. Incubator (37 ± 2°C).
10. Graduated vessels.
11. Distilled or deionized water.
12. Latex gloves, powderless.

2.2.3.2. COBAS AMPLICOR Test

1. COBAS AMPLICOR Analyzer and printer.
2. Operator's manual for the COBAS AMPLICOR Analyzer.
3. HIV-1 MONITOR Test Method Manual for the COBAS AMPLICOR Analyzer.
4. COBAS AMPLICOR D-cups.
5. Distilled or deionized water.
6. 5-mL Serologic pipets.
7. Graduated cylinder (minimum 1 L).
8. Vortex mixer.
9. Latex gloves, powderless.

3. Methods

The AMPLICOR and COBAS AMPLICOR HIV-1 MONITOR tests are based on five major processes: specimen preparation, reverse transcription of target RNA to generate cDNA, PCR amplification of target cDNA using HIV-1 specific complementary primers, hybridization of the amplified products (amplicon) to oligonucleotide probes specific to the target(s), and detection of the probe-bound amplified products by colorimetric determination.

Either of two specimen processing methods can be used with the tests. The Standard method has a limit of quantitation of 400 copies of HIV-1 RNA/mL of plasma and a dynamic range of 400–750,000 copies of HIV-1 RNA/mL of plasma. The UltraSensitive method has a limit of quantitation of 50 copies of HIV-1 RNA/mL of plasma and a dynamic range of 50–75,000 copies of HIV-1 RNA/mL of plasma. The user has the option of using either method. The Standard method would be used when a high viral RNA titer is expected, e.g., to obtain titers at baseline. The UltraSensitive method would be used when very low viral titer is expected, e.g., after initiation of therapy or after the viral titer exhibits a substantial decrease.

For the AMPLICOR test, the user programs a thermal cycler to perform reverse transcription and amplification automatically; hybridization, detection, and calculations are performed manually. For the COBAS AMPLICOR HIV-1 test, the user simply enters the test name and specimen identification codes. The COBAS AMPLICOR Analyzer *(31)* then uses preprogrammed parameters to automatically perform reverse transcription, amplification, detection, and calculation of results without user intervention.

To achieve selective amplification of target nucleic acid from the clinical specimen, the amplification reaction mixtures for both HIV-1 MONITOR tests contain AmpErase® and deoxyuridine triphosphate (dUTP) *(32)*. A Quantitation Standard (HIV-1 QS) is utilized as a reference for calculating the HIV RNA concentration in the specimen.

3.1. Selective Amplification

AmpErase (uracil-*N*-glycosylase) recognizes and catalyzes the destruction of DNA strands containing deoxyuridine, but not DNA containing thymidine *(32)*. Deoxyuridine is not present in naturally occurring DNA, but is always present in amplicon owing to the use of dUTP as one of the dNTPs in the master mix reagent; therefore, only amplicon contains deoxyuridine. Deoxyuridine renders contaminating amplicon susceptible to destruction by AmpErase prior to amplification of the target DNA. AmpErase, which is included in the master mix reagent, catalyzes the cleavage of deoxyuridine-containing DNA at deoxyuridine residues by opening the deoxyribose chain at the C1 position. When heated in the first thermal cycling step at the alkaline pH of the master mix, the amplicon DNA chain breaks at the position of the deoxyuridine, thereby rendering the DNA nonamplifiable. AmpErase is inactive at temperatures above 55°C (i.e., throughout the thermal cycling steps) and therefore does not destroy target amplicon. Following amplification, any residual enzyme is denatured by the addition of the denaturation solution, thereby preventing the degradation of target amplicon. AmpErase in the AMPLICOR HIV-1 MONITOR tests has been demonstrated to inactivate at least 10^3 copies of deoxyuridine-containing HIV-1 amplicon per PCR.

3.2. Quantitation Standard

The HIV-1 quantitation standard (QS) is a noninfectious 233 nucleotide in vitro transcribed RNA molecule that contains primer binding sites identical to those of the HIV-1 target. The HIV-1 QS generates an amplification product of the same length and base composition as the HIV-1 target sequence. The HIV-1 QS contains a unique probe binding region that allows amplicon generated from it to be distinguished from HIV-1 amplicon.

In the Standard procedure, a known number of HIV-1 QS copies is added to each individual specimen at the first step of the specimen-processing procedure and is carried through the specimen preparation, reverse transcription, PCR amplification, hybridization, and detection steps along with the HIV-1 target. Levels of HIV-1 RNA in the test specimens are determined by comparing the HIV-1 signal to the HIV-1 QS signal for each specimen. Therefore, the HIV-1 QS compensates for any effects of inhibition and controls variation in the specimen preparation, amplification, and detection processes to allow the accurate quantitation of HIV-1 RNA in each specimen.

In the UltraSensitive procedure, a known number of HIV-1 QS copies is added to each individual specimen immediately after it has been concentrated by ultracentrifugation and is then carried through all the remaining assay steps.

The HIV-1 QS cannot be added to the specimen prior to ultracentrifugation because it is in the form of pure RNA. Whereas HIV-1 RNA associated with viral particles is efficiently recovered during ultracentrifugation, free RNA molecules such as the HIV-1 QS are not. Thus, the HIV-1 QS does not control or compensate for variation in virus recovery during the initial ultracentrifugation step.

3.3. Collection, Transport, and Storage of Specimens

Both the COBAS AMPLICOR and AMPLICOR HIV-1 MONITOR tests are for use with plasma specimens alone. Blood should be collected in sterile tubes using EDTA (lavender top, Becton Dickinson no. 6454 or equivalent) or acid citrate dextrose (ACD) (yellow top, Becton Dickinson no. 4606 or equivalent) as the anticoagulant. Specimens containing heparin as the anticoagulant are unsuitable for this test. Store whole blood at 2–25°C for no longer than 6 h. Specimens containing ACD as the anticoagulant will yield test results that are approx 15% lower than those obtained from specimens containing EDTA as the anticoagulant owing to the dilution effect of the 1.5 mL of ACD anticoagulant present in the blood collection tube. Whole blood may be stored, or transported, at 2–25°C for up to 6 h from the time of collection.

Plasma must be separated from whole blood within 6 h of collection by centrifugation at 800–1600*g* for 20 min at room temperature (*see* **Note 1**). After separation from whole blood, plasma must be transferred to a sterile polypropylene tube. Plasma specimens may be stored, or transported, at 2–8°C for up to 5 d, or frozen at –20°C. It is recommended that specimens be stored in 600 to 700-µL aliquots in sterile, 2.0-mL polypropylene screw-cap tubes (such as Sarstedt 72.694.006). Plasma specimens may be frozen and thawed up to three times.

3.4. Work Flow

Both the COBAS AMPLICOR and AMPLICOR HIV-1 MONITOR tests can be completed in 1 d or over the course of 2 d. If the testing is to be completed in a single workday, perform the procedures in **Subheading 3.5.** first and then proceed to **Subheading 3.6.** If the testing is to be completed over the course of 2 d, perform the procedures described in **Subheadings 3.6.1.** or **3.6.2.** on d 1 and store the processed specimens as described in **step 19** or **14** of the UltraSensitive or Standard specimen-processing procedures, respectively. On d 2, perform the procedures described in **Subheading 3.5.** first and then proceed to **step 20** or **15** of the UltraSensitive or Standard specimen-processing procedures, respectively.

The laboratory should contain two distinct work areas, one for preamplification activities and one for postamplification activities. Within the preamplification area, there should be separate work spaces for preparation of reagents and preparation of specimens (*see* **Note 2**).

3.5. Preparation of Reagents

Each kit contains reagents sufficient for two 12-test runs, which may be performed separately or simultaneously. It is recommended that one replication of the AMPLICOR HIV-1 MONITOR (–) control, AMPLICOR HIV-1 MONITOR low (+) control, and AMPLICOR HIV-1 high (+) control be included in each test run. For the most efficient use of reagents, specimens and controls should be processed in batches that are multiples of 12.

1. Determine the appropriate number of MicroAmp reaction tubes (AMPLICOR) or A-rings (COBAS AMPLICOR) needed for patient specimen and control testing. Place the reaction tubes in the MicroAmp tray and lock into place with the retainer or place the A-ring(s) in the A-ring holder(s).
2. Prepare working master mix by adding 100 µL of HIV-1 Mn^{2+} to one vial of HIV-1 master mix (*see* **Notes 3–6**). Mix by inverting 10–15 times (*see* **Note 7**). The pink dye in the manganese solution is used for visual confirmation that the manganese solution has been added to the master mix. Discard the remaining manganese solution. The working master mix must be stored at 2–8°C and used within 4 h of preparation.
3. Add 50 µL of working master mix to each reaction tube or A-tube using a repeat pipettor or a pipettor with an aerosol barrier or positive displacement tip. Do not cap the reaction tubes or close the covers of the A-tubes at this time. Discard unused working master mix.
4. Place the MicroAmp tray and the appropriate number of reaction tube caps or the A-ring(s) in a resealable plastic bag and seal the bag securely. Move the tray or A-ring(s) to the specimen preparation work space in the preamplification area. Store the reaction tubes or A-ring(s) containing working master mix at 2–8°C until preparation of specimen and control is completed. Working master mix is stable for 4 h at 2–8°C in reaction tubes or A-tubes sealed in the plastic bag.

3.6. Preparation of Specimen

In both the UltraSensitive and Standard specimen-processing methods, HIV-1 RNA is extracted from viral particles with HIV-1 lysis reagent and the extracted RNA is then recovered by alcohol precipitation (*see* **Note 8**). The HIV-1 lysis reagent contains the chaotropic reagent guanidine thiocyanate. The UltraSensitive method differs in two ways from the Standard method. First, viral particles are concentrated from 500 µL of plasma by ultracentrifugation prior to extraction, whereas 200 µL of whole plasma is extracted directly in the

Standard method. Second, the recovered RNA is resuspended in a final volume of 100 μL in the UltraSensitive method compared with 400 μL in the Standard method. Thus, compared to the Standard method, the UltraSensitive method produces a 10-fold (2.5 times more plasma in one fourth the volume) more concentrated processed specimen. This increase in concentration is possible because the ultracentrifugation step eliminates soluble plasma components that potentially interfere with RT-PCR.

3.6.1. UltraSensitive Method

1. Precool the ultracentrifuge and rotor to 2–8°C as described in the operating instructions for the ultracentrifuge.
2. Prepare 70% ethanol (*see* **Notes 9** and **10**). For 12 tests, mix 11.0 mL of 95% ethanol and 4.0 mL of deionized water.
3. Label one 1.5-mL screw-cap tube for each patient specimen and label three additional tubes as HIV-1 (–) C, HIV L(+)C, and HIV H(+)C.
4. Prepare the UltraSensitive working lysis reagent. Vortex HIV-1 QS for at least 10 s before use (*see* **Notes 11** and **12**). For each batch of up to 12 specimens and controls, add 25 μL of HIV-1 QS to one bottle of HIV-1 lysis buffer and mix well. It is not necessary to measure the volume of HIV-1 lysis buffer. The pink dye in the HIV-1 QS is used for visual confirmation that the HIV-1 QS has been added to the lysis reagent. Discard the remaining HIV-1 QS. UltraSensitive working lysis reagent is stable for 4 h at room temperature. If using frozen specimens, thaw the specimens at room temperature and vortex for 3–5 s. Spin the specimen tube briefly to collect the specimen in the base of the tube. Take care to avoid contaminating gloves when manipulating specimens (*see* **Note 13**).
5. Add 500 μL of each patient specimen to the appropriately labeled tubes (*see* **Note 14**).
6. Add 500 μL of normal human plasma to each of the appropriately labeled control tubes (*see* **Note 15**).
7. Put an orientation mark on each tube and place the tubes in the ultracentrifuge with the orientation marks facing outward, so that the pellets will align with the orientation marks. Centrifuge the specimens and controls at 23,600*g* for 60 min at 2–8°C.
8. Using a new, fine-tip disposable transfer pipet for each tube, carefully remove and discard the supernatant from each tube, being careful not to disrupt the pellet (which may not be visible) (*see* **Note 16**). Remove as much liquid as possible without disturbing the pellet. Withdraw the supernatant slowly, allowing the liquid to drain completely off the sides of the tube. Do not use vacuum aspiration.
9. Add 600 μL of working lysis reagent to each of the labeled tubes and cap the tubes. Check that the working lysis reagent is pink to confirm that HIV-1 QS was added to the lysis reagent.
10. Prepare the UltraSensitive controls as follows:
    a. Vortex HIV-1 (–), HIV-1 low (+), and HIV-1 high (+) controls for 3–5 s.

b. Add 12.5 µL of HIV-1 (–) control to the tube labeled HIV-1 (–) C containing UltraSensitive working lysis reagent. Cap the tube and vortex for 3–5 s.
c. Add 12.5 µL of HIV-1 low (+) control to the tube labeled HIV-1 L(+)C containing UltraSensitive working lysis reagent. Cap the tube and vortex for 3–5 s.
d. Add 12.5 µL of HIV-1 high (+) control to the tube labeled HIV-1 H(+)C containing UltraSensitive working lysis reagent. Cap the tube and vortex for 3–5 s.

11. Incubate the specimen and control tubes for 10 min at room temperature.
12. For each specimen and control tube, remove the cap, add 600 µL of 100% isopropyl alcohol (at room temperature), recap the tube, and vortex vigorously for 3–5 s. Do not have more than one tube open at a time.
13. Put an orientation mark on each tube and place the tubes in the microcentrifuge with the orientation marks facing outward, so that the pellets will align with the orientation marks. Centrifuge the specimens and controls at maximum speed (12,500–16,000*g*) for 15 min at room temperature.
14. Using a new, fine-tip disposable transfer pipet for each tube, carefully remove and discard the supernatant from each tube, being careful not to disrupt the pellet (which may not be visible). Remove as much liquid as possible without disturbing the pellet. Withdraw the supernatant slowly, allowing the liquid to drain completely off the sides of the tube. Do not use vacuum aspiration.
15. Add 1.0 mL of 70% ethanol (at room temperature) to each tube, recap, and vortex for 3–5 s.
16. Place the tubes into a microcentrifuge with the orientation marks facing outward and centrifuge the tubes for 5 min at maximum speed (12,500–16,000*g*) at room temperature.
17. Using a new, fine-tip disposable transfer pipet for each tube, carefully remove the supernatant without disturbing the pellet. The pellet should be clearly visible at this step. Remove as much of the supernatant as possible. (**Note:** residual ethanol can inhibit amplification.)
18. Repeat **step 17** to remove as much of the remaining supernatant as possible.
19. Add 100 µL of HIV-1 diluent to each tube. Recap the tubes. Vortex vigorously for 10 s to resuspend the extracted RNA. Some insoluble material may remain. Start the reverse transcription/amplification procedure within 2 h of specimen and control preparation. If amplification cannot be undertaken within 2 h of preparation, the samples can be stored frozen at –20°C or colder for up to 1 wk, with no more than one freeze/thaw. More than one freeze/thaw cycle may result in loss of copy number. If processed specimens and controls were stored frozen prior to amplification, thaw at room temperature and vortex for 5 s before proceeding to **step 20**.
20. Add 50 µL of each processed specimen and control to appropriate reaction tubes or A-tubes containing working master mix using a pipettor with an aerosol barrier or a positive displacement tip. Use a new tip for each specimen and control. Be careful to avoid transferring any precipitated material that may not have gone back into the solution. Cap the reaction tubes and seal the caps using the MicroAmp cap-installing tool or cap the A-tubes (*see* **Notes 17–20**).

21. Record the positions of the controls and specimens. Reverse transcription/amplification must be started within 45 min of the time that the processed specimens and controls were added to the reaction tubes or A-tubes containing working master mix. Move the prepared specimens and controls in the MicroAmp trays or A-rings to the amplification/detection area.

3.6.2. Standard Method

1. Prepare 70% ethanol. For 12 tests, mix 11.0 mL of 95% ethanol and 4.0 mL of deionized water.
2. Label one 2.0-mL screw-cap tube for each patient specimen and label three additional tubes as HIV-1 (–) C, HIV L(+)C, and HIV H(+)C (*see* **Note 13**).
3. Prepare Standard working lysis reagent. Vortex HIV-1 QS for at least 10 s before use (*see* **Notes 11** and **12**). For each batch of up to 12 specimens and controls, add 100 µL of HIV-1 QS to one bottle of HIV-1 lysis reagent and mix well. It is not necessary to measure the volume of HIV-1 lysis reagent. The pink dye in the HIV-1 QS is used for visual confirmation that HIV-1 QS has been added to the lysis reagent. Discard the remaining HIV-1 QS. Standard working lysis reagent is stable for 4 h at room temperature. If using frozen specimens, thaw the specimens at room temperature and vortex for 3–5 s. Spin the specimen tube briefly to collect the specimen in the base of the tube. Take care to avoid contaminating gloves when manipulating specimens.
4. Add 600 µL of Standard working lysis reagent to each of the labeled tubes and cap the tubes. Check that the working lysis reagent is pink to confirm that HIV-1 QS was added to the Standard lysis reagent.
5. Prepare Standard controls as follows:
   a. Vortex negative human plasma, HIV-1 (–) control, HIV-1 low (+) control, and HIV-1 high (+) control for 3–5 s.
   b. Add 200 µL of negative human plasma to each of the three control tubes. Cap the tubes and vortex for 3–5 s.
   c. Add 50 µL of HIV-1 (–) control to the tube labeled HIV-1 (–) C containing Standard working lysis reagent and negative human plasma. Cap the tube and vortex for 3–5 s.
   d. Add 50 µL of HIV-1 low (+) control to the tube labeled HIV-1 L(+)C containing Standard working lysis reagent and negative human plasma. Cap the tube and vortex for 3–5 s.
   e. Add 50 µL of HIV-1 high (+) control to the tube labeled HIV-1 H(+)C containing Standard working lysis reagent and negative human plasma. Cap the tube and vortex for 3–5 s.
6. Add 200 µL of each patient specimen to the appropriately labeled tubes containing Standard working lysis reagent. Cap the tubes and vortex for 3–5 s.
7. Incubate the specimen and control tubes for 10 min at room temperature.
8. For each specimen and control tube, remove the cap, add 800 µL of 100% isopropyl alcohol (at room temperature), recap the tube, and vortex vigorously for 3–5 s. Do not have more than one tube open at a time.

9. Put an orientation mark on each tube and place the tubes in the microcentrifuge with the orientation marks facing outward, so that the pellets will align with the orientation marks. Centrifuge the specimens and controls at maximum speed (12,500–16,000*g*) for 15 min at room temperature.
10. Using a new, fine-tip disposable transfer pipet for each tube carefully remove and discard the supernatant from each tube, being careful not to disrupt the pellet (which may not be visible). Remove as much liquid as possible without disturbing the pellet. Withdraw the supernatant slowly, allowing the liquid to drain completely off the sides of the tube. Do not use vacuum aspiration.
11. Add 1.0 mL of 70% ethanol (at room temperature) to each tube, recap and vortex for 3–5 s.
12. Place the tubes in a microcentrifuge with the orientation marks facing outward, and centrifuge the tubes for 5 minutes at maximum speed (12,500–16,000*g*) at room temperature.
13. Using a new, fine-tip disposable transfer pipet for each tube, carefully remove the supernatant without disturbing the pellet. The pellet should be clearly visible at this step. Remove as much of the supernatant as possible. (**Note:** Residual ethanol can inhibit amplification.)
14. Add 400 µL of HIV-1 diluent to each tube. Recap the tubes. Vortex vigorously for 10 s to resuspend the extracted RNA. Some insoluble material may remain. Start the reverse transcription/amplification procedure within 2 h of specimen and control preparation. If amplification cannot be undertaken within 2 h of preparation, the samples can be stored frozen at –20°C or colder for up to 1 wk, with no more than one freeze/thaw. More than one freeze/thaw cycle may result in loss of copy number. If processed specimens and controls were stored frozen prior to amplification, thaw at room temperature and vortex for 5 s before proceeding to **step 15**.
15. Add 50 µL of each processed specimen and control to appropriate reaction tubes or A-tubes containing Working master mix using a pipettor with an aerosol barrier or a positive displacement tip. Use a new tip for each specimen and control. Be careful to avoid transferring any precipitated material that may not have gone back into the solution. Cap the reaction tubes and seal the caps using the MicroAmp cap-installing tool or cap the A-tubes.
16. Record the positions of the controls and specimens. Reverse transcription/amplification must be started within 45 minutes of the time that the processed specimens and controls were added to the reaction tubes or A-tubes containing Working master mix. Move the prepared specimens and controls in the MicroAmp trays or A-rings to the amplification/detection area.

3.7. Reverse Transcription and PCR Amplification

The AMPLICOR HIV-1 Version 1.5 tests amplify and detect a 155-base target sequence located in a highly conserved region of the HIV-1 *gag* gene *(33)*, defined by the primers SK145 and SKCC1B. Each primer is biotinylated at its 5′ end.

The reverse transcription and amplification reaction are performed with the thermostable recombinant enzyme *Thermus thermophilus* DNA Polymerase (r*Tth* pol). In the presence of manganese and under the appropriate buffer conditions, r*Tth* pol has both RT and DNA polymerase activity ***(34)***. This allows both reverse transcription and PCR amplification to occur in the same reaction mixture.

3.7.1. Reverse Transcription

The reaction tubes are placed in a thermal cycler that automatically performs the heating and cooling steps required for reverse transcription and amplification. First, the reactions are heated to allow the downstream primer (SKCC1B) to anneal specifically to the HIV-1 and HIV-1 QS target RNA. In the presence of excess deoxynucleoside triphosphates, including deoxyadenosine, deoxyguanosine, deoxycytidine, thymidine, and dUTPs, r*Tth* pol extends the annealed primer, forming a complementary (cDNA) strand.

3.7.2. PCR Amplification

Following reverse transcription of the HIV-1 and HIV-1 QS target RNA, the reaction mixture is heated to denature the RNA:cDNA hybrid and expose the HIV-1 and HIV-1 QS target sequences. As the mixture cools, the upstream primer (SK145) anneals to the cDNA strand and the r*Tth* pol catalyzes the extension reaction, yielding a double-stranded DNA (dsDNA) copy of the target region of each HIV-1 and HIV-1 QS RNA. This completes the first cycle of PCR. The reaction mixture is heated again to separate the dsDNA and expose the primer target sequences. As the mixture cools, the primers anneal to the target DNA. In the presence of excess dNTPs, r*Tth* pol extends the annealed primers along the target templates to produce a 155-bp dsDNA molecule termed an *amplicon*. This process is automatically repeated for the appropriate number of cycles, each cycle effectively doubling the amount of amplicon DNA. Amplification occurs only in the region of the HIV-1 genome between the primers.

3.7.3. Performing Reverse Transcription/PCR Amplification (see **Notes 21–23**)

3.7.3.1. AMPLICOR HIV-1 MONITOR, VERSION 1.5 TEST

1. Place the tray/retainer assembly into the thermal cycler block.
2. Program the Perkin-Elmer GeneAmp PCR System 9600 or GeneAmp PCR System 2400 thermal cycler as follows:
   a. HOLD program: 2 min at 50°C.
   b. HOLD program: 30 min at 60°C.

c. CYCLE program (8 cycles): 10 s at 95°C, 10 s at 52°C, 10 s at 72°C.
d. CYCLE program (23 cycles): 10 s at 90°C, 10 s at 55°C, 10 s at 72°C.
e. HOLD program: 15 min at 72°C.

In the CYCLE programs, the ramp times should be left at the default setting (0:00), which is the maximum rate, and the allowed setpoint error at the default setting (2°C). Link the four programs together into a METHOD program.

3. Start the METHOD program. The program runs approx 1 h and 15 min.
4. After the thermal cycling is complete (i.e., during the final 15-min HOLD program), remove the caps from the tubes and immediately pipet 100 µL of denaturation solution into each reaction tube using a multichannel pipettor and mix by pipetting up and down five times. Do not allow the reaction tubes to remain in the thermal cycler beyond the end of the final HOLD program, and do not extend the final HOLD program beyond 15 min.
5. The denatured amplicon can be held at room temperature no more than 2 h before proceeding to the detection reaction. If the detection reaction cannot be performed within 2 h, recap the tubes and store the denatured amplicon at 2–8°C for up to 1 wk.

3.7.3.2. COBAS AMPLICOR HIV-1 MONITOR Test

The COBAS AMPLICOR Analyzer will automatically perform the correct thermal cycling program, as well as all subsequent assay procedures, after the user starts the instrument by performing the following operations:

1. Examine the quantities of reagents on board the COBAS AMPLICOR Analyzer. Prepare enough reagent cassettes to complete the workload.
2. Mix HIV probe suspension 1 (IM PS1, v1.5) well by vortexing. Add 2.5 mL of IM PS1, v1.5 to one cassette of probe suspension 2 (IM4, v1.5). Place the cassette on the test-specific reagent rack. Discard the used IM PS1, v1.5 vial. Record the date of reagent preparation on the IM4, v1.5 cassette.
3. Mix QS probe suspension 1 (IQ PS1, v1.5) well by vortexing. Add 2.5 mL of IQ PS1, v1.5 to one cassette of QS probe suspension 2 (IQ4, v1.5). Place the cassette on the test-specific rack. Discard the used IQ PS1, v1.5 vial. Record the date of reagent preparation on the IQ4, v1.5 cassette.
4. Prepare working substrate by pipetting 5 mL of substrate B (SB) into one cassette of substrate A (SB3). Pipet up and down to mix. Discard the open SB vial. Record the date of preparation on the SB3 cassette.
5. Place the working substrate in the generic reagent rack.
6. Place the cassette of Amplicon dilution reagent (AD3) in the test-specific reagent rack. Record the date on the AD3 cassette.
7. Place the cassettes of denaturation solution (DN4) and conjugate (CN4) in the generic reagent rack. Record on each cassette the date it was opened.
8. Identify the reagent racks as generic or test specific using the keypad, bar-code scanner, or AMPLILINK™ software as described in the operator's manual for the analyzer.

9. Configure the reagent racks by inputting reagent positions and lot numbers into the instrument using the keypad, bar-code scanner, or AMPLILINK software as described in the operator's manual.
10. Load the reagent rack onto the instrument using the keypad, bar-code scanner, or AMPLILINK software as described in the operator's manual. Make sure that each reagent cassette is in its assigned position and that each cassette fits tightly into its rack.
11. Place the D-cup rack on the D-cup platform. Six D-cups are required for each specimen or control and two D-cups are required for each cassette of working substrate to allow for blanking by the analyzer.
12. Place the A-ring(s) into the thermal cycler segment(s) of the analyzer.
13. Load the A-ring(s) into the analyzer using the keypad, bar-code scanner, or AMPLILINK software as described in the operator's manual.
14. Create an A-ring work list as described in the operator's manual. (**Note:** At this time the user will be required to enter the lot-specific Quantitation Standard copy number and the low [+] and high [+] control ranges provided on the COBAS AMPLICOR HIV-1 Test, v1.5 Data Cards. Enter appropriate control ranges based on specimen preparation utilized.)
15. Tightly close the cover of the thermal cycler segment(s).
16. Start the analyzer as described in the operator's manual.
17. Wait for the analyzer to indicate that the load check has passed.

3.8. Hybridization Reaction

Following PCR amplification, the HIV-1 and HIV-1 QS amplicons are chemically denatured to form single-stranded DNA by adding denaturation solution to the reaction tubes (*see* **Notes 22** and **23**). The denatured amplicon is serially diluted and aliquots of undiluted and diluted amplicon are hybridized to HIV-1-specific (SK102) and HIV-1 QS-specific (CP35) oligonucleotide probes that are bound to a solid phase. Microwell plates serve as the solid phase for the AMPLICOR test, and magnetic microparticles serve as the solid phase for the COBAS AMPLICOR test. In the manual AMPLICOR test, the microwell plates are incubated at 37°C for 60 min. The COBAS AMPLICOR Analyzer performs all these steps automatically without user intervention. The following specific instructions apply to the manual AMPLICOR test:

1. Allow the microwell plates to warm to room temperature before removing from the foil pouch. Add 100 µL of hybridization buffer to each well required for testing. Add 25 µL of the denatured amplicon to the HIV-1 wells in row A of the microwell plates, and mix up and down 10 times with a 12-channel pipettor with plugged tips (*see* **Note 24**). Make serial fivefold dilutions in the HIV-1 wells in rows B–F as follows. Transfer 25 µL from row A to B and mix as before. Continue through row F. Mix row F as before, and then remove and discard 25 µL. Discard the pipet tips. These operations may also be performed using the AMPLICOR Electronic Pipettor.

2. Add 25 µL of the denatured amplicon to the QS wells in row G of the microwell plates and mix up and down 10 times with a 12-channel pipettor with plugged tips. Transfer 25 µL from row G to H. Mix as before, and then remove 25 µL from row H and discard. These operations may also be performed using the AMPLICOR Electronic Pipettor (*see* **Note 25**).
3. Cover the microwell plates and incubate for 1 h at 37 ± 2°C.
4. Wash the microwell plates five times with the working wash solution using an automated microwell plate washer. Program the washer as follows:
   a. Aspirate the contents of the well.
   b. Fill each well to the top (400–450 µL). Soak for 30 s and aspirate dry.
   c. Repeat **step 4b** four more times.
   d. After automated washing is completed, tap the plate dry.

3.9. Detection of Reaction

Following the hybridization reaction, the microwell plates (or tubes of magnetic microparticles) are washed to remove any unbound material (*see* **Notes 26** and **27**). An avidin-horseradish peroxidase (Av-HRP) conjugate is added to each well of the microwell plates (or to tubes of magnetic microparticles) and incubated at 37°C for the appropriate amount of time. Av-HRP binds to the biotin-labeled amplicon captured by the plate-bound oligonucleotide probes. The microwell plates (or tubes of magnetic microparticles) are washed again to remove unbound Av-HRP, and a substrate solution containing hydrogen peroxide and 3,3′,5,5′-tetramethylbenzidine (TMB) is added to the microwell plates (or tubes of magnetic microparticles). In the presence of hydrogen peroxide, the bound Av-HRP catalyzes the oxidation of TMB to form a colored complex. In the AMPLICOR test, the reaction is stopped by addition of a weak acid, and the optical density (OD) at 450 nm is measured using an automated microwell plate reader. In the COBAS AMPLICOR test, the reaction is not stopped; after a precisely timed incubation, the OD of the reaction at 660 nm is measured by a spectrophotometer integrated in the COBAS AMPLICOR Analyzer. The COBAS AMPLICOR Analyzer performs all these steps automatically without user intervention. The following specific instructions apply to the manual AMPLICOR assays:

1. Add 100 µL Av-HRP conjugate to each well. Cover the microwell plates and incubate for 15 min at 37 ± 2°C.
2. Wash the microwell plates as described in **Subheading 3.8., step 4**.
3. Prepare working substrate solution. For each microwell plate, measure 12 mL of substrate A and 3 mL of substrate B. Mix together to prepare working substrate. Protect the working substrate from direct light. Working substrate must be at room temperature and used within 3 h of preparation (*see* **Notes 28** and **29**).
4. Pipet 100 µL of working substrate solution into each well.

5. Allow color to develop for 10 min at room temperature in the dark.
6. Add 100 µL of stop reagent to each well.
7. Measure the OD at 450 nm (single wavelength) within 10 min of adding the stop reagent (*see* **Notes 30** and **31**).

3.10. Calculation of HIV-1 RNA Concentration

Viral RNA load is quantitated by utilizing the HIV-1 QS, which is added to the test sample at a known concentration. For the AMPLICOR test, the following calculations are performed manually. The COBAS AMPLICOR Analyzer automatically performs these calculations and reports the viral titer, or the appropriate message when the viral titer cannot be calculated from the test results.

1. For each specimen or control, the wells in rows A, B, C, D, E, and F represent neat and 1:5, 1:25, 1:125, 1:625, and 1:3125 dilutions, respectively, of the HIV-1 amplicon. For each sample, select the well giving the lowest HIV-1 signal having an OD ≥0.20 and ≤2.0 absorbance units. The absorbance values should decrease with the serial dilutions, with the highest value for each specimen and control in well A and the lowest in well F.
   a. If all HIV-1 absorbance values are <0.2, do not proceed with **steps 2–7**. Report results as "HIV-1 RNA not detected (<400 copies/mL)" or "HIV-1 RNA not detected (<50 copies/mL)," depending on whether the Standard or UltraSensitive method was used.
   b. If all HIV-1 absorbance values are >2.0, the HIV-1 copy number is above the linear range of the assay. Do not proceed with **steps 2–7**. Report the result as "Not determined." If the Standard processing method was used, prepare a 1:50 dilution of the original specimen with HIV-1 negative human plasma and repeat the test. Calculate the HIV-1 concentration as described in **steps 2–7** and multiply the result by 50. If the UltraSensitive processing method was used, retest the original specimen using the Standard specimen-processing procedure.
   c. If HIV-1 absorbances do not follow the pattern of decreasing from well A to F, examine the data to determine whether an error in dilution occurred. If the out-of-sequence values and all more concentrated wells are >2.3, the signals are saturated: no error occurred. If the out-of-sequence values and all more diluted wells are <0.1, the signals are at background: no error occurred. In both cases, calculate the viral titer as described in **steps 2–7**. If the out-of-sequence values fall between 0.2 and 2.0, an error occurred. The result for that specimen is invalid, and the entire test procedure for that specimen (including specimen processing) must be repeated.
2. Subtract the background absorbance (0.07 for the AMPLICOR test) from the absorbance value of the selected well.
3. Calculate the HIV-1 total OD by multiplying the background-corrected HIV-1 absorbance by the dilution factor associated with the selected well.

4. For each specimen or control, the wells in rows G and H represent neat and 1:5 dilutions, respectively, of the HIV-1 amplicon. For each sample, select the well giving the lowest HIV-1 QS signal having an OD ≥0.30 and <2.0 absorbance units. For each specimen and control, the absorbance value for row G should be higher than the value for row H.
   a. If all HIV-1 QS absorbance values are <0.3, the result for that specimen is invalid. Either the processed specimen was inhibitory to amplification or the RNA was not recovered during specimen processing. Repeat the entire procedure (including specimen processing) for that specimen.
   b. If all HIV-1 QS absorbance values are >2.0, an error occurred and the result for that specimen is invalid. Repeat the entire procedure (including specimen processing) for that specimen.
   c. If HIV-1 QS absorbance of well H is greater than the absorbance for well G, an error occurred and the result for that specimen is invalid. Repeat the entire procedure (including specimen processing) for that specimen.
5. Subtract the background absorbance (0.07 for the AMPLICOR test) from the absorbance value for the selected well.
6. Calculate the HIV-1 QS total OD by multiplying the background-corrected QS absorbance by the dilution factor associated with the selected well.
7. Calculate the HIV-1 RNA copies/mL of plasma for each specimen using the following equation:

$$\text{HIV-1 RNA copies/mL} = (\text{Total HIV-1 OD/Total HIV-1 QS OD}) \times \text{Input HIV-1 QS copies/PCR} \times \text{sample volume factor}$$

   in which the sample volume factor is 4 for the UltraSensitive method or 40 for the Standard method (the equivalent of 250 or 25 µL of plasma is added to each amplification reaction, respectively).

3.11. Daily Maintenance of COBAS AMPLICOR Analyzer

1. Wipe the initialization post with a lint-free moist cloth and dry.
2. Wipe the D-cup handler tip with a lint-free moist cloth and dry.
3. Check the wash buffer reservoir and fill if necessary.
4. Prepare working wash buffer (1X) by adding 1 vol of 10X wash concentrate to 9 vol of distilled or deionized water. Mix well. Keep a minimum of 3–4 L of working wash buffer (1X) in the wash buffer reservoir of the system at all times.
5. Empty the waste container.
6. Prime the analyzer.
7. During the priming, check the syringes and tubing as well as the transfer tip.
8. Prior to each run, do the following:
   a. Check the waste container and empty if necessary.
   b. Check the wash buffer reservoir and add buffer if necessary.
   c. Replace used D-cup racks.
   d. Prime the analyzer.

3.12. Test Performance Characteristics

The AMPLICOR HIV-1 MONITOR, Version 1.5 and COBAS AMPLICOR HIV-1 MONITOR, Version 1.5 tests have a dynamic range of 50–75,000 copies of HIV RNA/mL of plasma for specimens processed by the UltraSensitive method *(26)*. The dynamic range for specimens processed by the Standard method is 400–750,000 copies of HIV-1 RNA/mL of plasma. For specimens that fell within the overlapping portion of the linear ranges, the UltraSensitive method yielded RNA concentrations that were only slightly lower (median = 22% lower) than those obtained by the Standard method *(26)*. This agreement means that laboratories can switch between the two specimen-processing methods, as dictated by the HIV-1 RNA titer, to obtain an overall dynamic range of 50–750,000 copies of HIV-1/mL of plasma.

The AMPLICOR HIV-1, Version 1.5 and COBAS AMPLICOR HIV-1 MONITOR, Version 1.5 tests amplified all group M subtypes with equal efficiency *(26)*. By contrast, the first-generation AMPLICOR HIV-1-MONITOR Test amplified subtypes A, E, F, and G less efficiently than the group B. The improved performance of the new tests was achieved by replacing the primer pair in the first-generation test with a single pair of consensus primers that recognize equally all group M subtypes.

4. Notes

1. Before work begins, all work surfaces used for PCR should be cleaned with 10% bleach followed by 70% alcohol (isopropanol or ethanol). This process will destroy bacteria and viruses, and will denature DNA or RNA. Rinsing surfaces with alcohol destroys any residual bleach, which could react with target nucleic acid and interfere with test performance. UV lighting should be used to irradiate DNA that may be on the work surface. It is good practice to turn on the UV light 20–30 min prior to beginning work.
2. Work flow in the laboratory must proceed in a unidirectional manner, beginning in the preamplification area and moving to the postamplification area. Preamplification activities must begin with reagent preparation and proceed to specimen preparation. Supplies and equipment must be dedicated to each preamplification activity and not used for other activities or moved between areas. Gloves must be worn in each area and must be changed before leaving that area. Equipment and supplies used for preparing reagents must not be used for preparing specimens or for processing amplified DNA or other sources of target DNA. Postamplification supplies and equipment must remain in the postamplification area at all times.
3. Separate sets of pipets and pipet tips must be dedicated for use in the reagent, specimen preparation, and detection procedures. Doing so will protect reagents from specimen or amplicon contamination.

4. Glove powder can nonspecifically inhibit each of the major steps in the PCR detection process. For this reason, all AMPLICOR PCRs should be performed with powder-free gloves.
5. For the AMPLICOR test, soak all Perkin-Elmer amplification trays, retainers, and bases in 10% bleach and rinse thoroughly with deionized water before reuse.
6. Use aerosol barrier tips for all liquid transfers to prevent reagent contamination. The use of aerosol barrier tips will also prevent RNases from being introduced into reaction tubes or A-tubes, which can destroy target RNA and lead to false-negative results.
7. Master mix should be inverted 10–15 times, not vortexed. Vortexing can inactivate the r*Tth* pol in the master mix.
8. Use aerosol barrier tips for all liquid transfers to prevent reagent contamination and cross contamination of nucleic acid from specimen to specimen. Aerosol barrier tips also prevent RNases from being introduced, which can destroy target RNA and lead to false-negative results.
9. Use only 70% ethanol; the 70% ethanol wash was found to be more reproducible during the development of this assay. Ethanol should be made fresh daily with deionized H_2O. Do not use diethylpyrocarbonate (DEPC)-treated water; various preparations of DEPC water have been reported to cause reduced signals.
10. Isopropanol and ethanol must be reagent-grade quality or better.
11. Dissolve the lysis reagent completely before adding the well-vortexed HIV-1 QS. Lysis buffer may be warmed at 37°C, but no warmer, for up to 30 min. Always bring warmed lysis reagent to room temperature before adding the HIV-1 QS.
12. The HIV-1 QS must never be heated to 37°C. The HIV-1 QS must be well vortexed before adding the lysis reagent. Original vials of all AMPLICOR controls and standards should be vortexed as follows: upright for 5 s, upside down for 5 s, upright for 10 s; finish by tapping the vial on the counter to remove any liquid inside the cap.
13. Use only sterile 2-mL screw-cap tubes for storing and preparing specimens. Flip-cap tubes can cause specimen aerosols when tubes are opened. They can also cause splashes that can result in cross contamination or a biosafety hazard.
14. To avoid cross contamination when transferring aliquots of specimen to labeled preparation tubes, uncap one specimen tube and one labeled preparation tube at a time. After transferring the specimen aliquot, recap both the specimen and the labeled preparation tubes before proceeding to the next specimen. Use a new aerosol barrier pipet tip for each specimen. Replace gloves immediately if they become contaminated with specimen.
15. When preparing controls, combine negative human plasma with the lysis buffer in the control tubes and vortex well before adding the control. This will destroy possible RNase activity in the negative human plasma that could degrade control RNA. It is best to add the control last and then start the 10-minute RT incubation.
16. Use fine-tip transfer pipets to aspirate all supernatants.
17. Arrange tubes of processed specimens, amplification tubes, and waste containers so that the pipet does not have to pass over open reaction tubes.

18. Uncap one tube of processed specimen at a time. After transferring an aliquot of specimen to the amplification tube, recap the tube before proceeding to the next specimen.
19. Use aerosol barrier tips when transferring aliquots of processed specimens to prevent pipettors from becoming contaminated with nucleic acid.
20. To avoid cross contamination between samples, cap each A-tube (for COBAS tests) or each column of MicroAmp tubes (for AMPLICOR tests) immediately after adding the processed specimens.
21. Use only Perkin-Elmer 9600 or 2400 thermal cyclers for performing manual AMPLICOR tests. The amplification parameters have been optimized for these systems and may yield suboptimal results when performed on other thermal cyclers.
22. Remove caps from amplification tubes slowly and with extreme care just prior to adding the denaturation solution. If the caps are opened too rapidly, droplets of reaction mixture may splash into neighboring tubes. Because reaction tubes may contain extremely high levels of amplicon, the introduction of a small amount of contaminating reaction mixture into a negative tube may be sufficient to produce a false-positive result.
23. Use plugged tips and a 12-channel multichannel pipettor (range 50–300 µL) or the AMPLICOR Electronic Pipettor to add denaturation solution to the wells. Change the tips for each row. Pipet up and down to mix well.
24. Use plugged tips and a 12-channel multichannel pipettor (range 5–50 µL) or the AMPLICOR Electronic Pipettor to transfer aliquots of reaction mixture to the microwell plates and perform the serial dilutions. Work carefully to avoid splashing, which could result in cross contamination of neighboring wells.
25. Recap reaction tubes with new caps immediately after transferring the reaction mixture to the microwell plates. This will help prevent accidental spillage, which could contaminate equipment and work surfaces with large amounts of amplicon.
26. Clean disposable reagent reservoirs should be used for detection reagents. If reagent reservoirs are reused they must be labeled for specific reagents and cleaned thoroughly between each use with deionized water. Do not reuse reagent reservoirs more than five times.
27. Working wash buffer must be prepared by measuring the 10X wash concentrate and then adding nine equal parts of deionized water. Owing to overfill, there may be up to 120 mL of wash buffer concentrate per bottle. Prepare wash buffer as follows: Mix well 100 mL of 10X wash concentrate + 900 mL of deionized water.
28. Substrates A and B must be measured when preparing the working substrate. All vials are overfilled so that the exact amount of reagents may be pipeted from the bottle. The overfill between substrates A and B might not be proportional.
29. Mix substrates A and B no more than 3 h before use. Store protected from light. Excessive storage or exposure to light may cause high background signals and false-positive results.

30. Microwell plates are measured at 450 nm without a reference filter. All AMPLICOR tests have been optimized for this measurement. Using a reference filter will falsely depress the sensitivity and results.
31. Measure the absorbance within 10 min of adding stop reagent to the microwell plates.

References

1. Lathey, J. L., Hughes, M. D., Fiscus, S. A., Pi, T., Jackson, J. B., Rasheed, S., Elbeik, T., Reichman, R., Japour, A., D'Aquila, R. T., Scott, W., Griffith, B. P., Hammer, S. M., and Katzenstein, D. A. for the AIDS Clinical Trials Group Protocol 175 Team. (1998) Variability and prognostic values of virologic and CD4 cell measures in human immunodeficiency virus type 1-infected patients with 200–500 CD4 cells/mm^3 (ACTG 175). *J. Infect. Dis.* **177,** 617–624.
2. Mellors, J. W., Kingsley, L. A., Rinaldo, C. R. Jr., Todd, J. A., Hoo, B. S., Kokka, R. P., and Gupta, P. (1995) Quantitation of HIV-1 RNA in plasma predicts outcome after seroconversion. *Ann. Intern. Med.* **122,** 573–579.
3. Mellors, J. W., Rinaldo, C. R. Jr., Gupta, P., White, R. M., Todd, J. A., and Kingsley, L. A. (1996) Prognosis in HIV-1 infection predicted by the quantity of virus in plasma. *Science* **272,** 1167–1170.
4. O'Brien, W. A., Hartigan, P. M., Martin, D., Esinhart, J., Hill, A., Benoit, S., Rubin, M., Simberkoff, M. S., and Hamilton, J. D. for the Veterans Affairs Cooperative Study Group on AIDS. (1996) Changes in plasma HIV-1 RNA and CD4$^+$ lymphocyte counts and the risk of progression to AIDS. *N. Engl. J. Med.* **334,** 426–431.
5. Saksela, K., Stevens, C. E., Rubinstein, P., Taylor, P. E., and Baltimore, D. (1995) HIV-1 messenger RNA in peripheral blood mononuclear cells as an early marker of risk for progression to AIDS. *Ann. Intern. Med.* **123,** 641–648.
6. Wong, M. T., Dolan, M. J., Kozlow, E., Doe, R., Melcher, G. P., Burke, D. S., Boswell, R. N., and Vahey, M. (1996) Patterns of virus burden and T cell phenotype are established early and are correlated with the rate of disease progression in human immunodeficiency virus type 1-infected persons. *J. Infect. Dis.* **173,** 877–887.
7. Mellors, J. W., Munoz, A., Giorgi, J. V., Margolick, J. B., Tassoni, C. J., Gupta, P., Kingsley, L. A., Todd, J. A., Saah, A. J., Detels, R., Phair, J. P., and Rinaldo, C. R. Jr. (1997) Plasma viral load and CD4+ lymphocytes as prognostic markers of HIV-1 infection. *Ann. Intern. Med.* **126,** 946–954.
8. Eron, J. J., Benoit, S. L., Jemsek, J., MacArthur, R. D., Santana J., Quinn, J. B., Kuritzkes, D. R., Fallon, M. A., and Rubin, M. for the North American HIV Working Party. (1995) Treatment with lamivudine, zidovudine, or both in HIV-positive patients with 200 to 500 CD4+ cells per cubic millimeter. *N. Engl. J. Med.* **333,** 1662–1669.
9. Fiscus, S. A., Hughes, M. D., Lathey, J. L., Pi, T., Jackson, B., Rasheed, S., Elbeik, T., Reichman, R., Japour, A., Byington, R., Scott, W., Griffith, B. P., Katzenstein,

D. A., and Hammer, S. M. for the AIDS Clinical Trials Group Protocol 175 Team. (1998) Changes in virologic markers as predictors of CD4 cell decline and progression of disease in human immunodeficiency virus type 1-infected adults treated with nucleosides. *J. Infect. Dis.* **177,** 625–633.

10. Gulick, R. M., Mellors, J. W., Havlir, D., Eron, J. J., Gonzalez, C., McMahon, D., Richman, D. D., Valentine, F. T., Jonas, L., Meibohm, A., Emini, E. A., and Chodakewitz, J. A. (1997) Treatment with indinavir, zidovudine, and lamivudine in adults with human immunodeficiency virus infection and prior antiretroviral therapy. *N. Engl. J. Med.* **337,** 734–739.
11. Hughes, M. D., Johnson, V. A., Hirsch, M. S., Bremer, J. W., Elbeik, T., Erice, A., Kuritzkes, D. R., Scott, W. A., Spector, S. A., Basgoz, N., Fischl, M. A., and D'Aquila, R. T. for the ACTG 241 Protocol Virology Substudy Team. (1997) Monitoring plasma HIV-1 RNA levels in addition to CD4+ lymphocyte count improves assessment of antiretroviral therapeutic response. *Ann. Intern. Med.* **126,** 929–938.
12. Myers, M. W., Montaner, J. G., and Group, T. I. S. (1996) A randomized, double-blinded comparative trial of the effects of zidovudine, didanosine and nevirapine combinations in antiviral naive, AIDS-free, HIV-infected patients with CD4 counts 200–600/mm^3, in *Program and Abstracts: XI International Conference on AIDS* (Vancouver, BC, Canada), XIth International Conference on AIDS Society, Vancouver, BC, Canada, p. 291.
13. O'Brien, W. A., Hartigan, P. M., Daar, E. S., Simberkoff, M. S., and Hamilton, J. D., for the VA Cooperative Study Group on AIDS. (1997) Changes in plasma HIV RNA levels and CD4+ lymphocyte counts predict both response to antiretroviral therapy and therapeutic failure. *Ann. Intern. Med.* **126,** 939–945.
14. Perelson, A. S., Essunger, P., Cao, Y., Vesanen, M., Hurley, A., Saksela, K., Markowitz, M., and Ho, D. D. (1997) Decay characteristics of HIV-1-infected compartments during combination therapy. *Nature* **387,** 188–191.
15. BHIVA Guidelines Co-ordinating Committee. (1997) British HIV Association guidelines for antiretroviral treatment of HIV seropositive individuals. *Lancet* **349,** 1086–1092.
16. Carpenter, C. C., Fischl, M. A., Hammer, S. M., et al. (1996) Antiretroviral therapy for HIV infection in 1996: recommendations of an international panel. International AIDS Society-USA. *JAMA* **276,** 146–154.
17. Centers for Disease Control and Prevention. (1998) Guidelines for the use of antiretroviral agents in HIV-infected adults and adolescents. *Morbid. Mortal. Weekly Rep.* **47(RR-5),** 43–82.
18. Centers for Disease Control and Prevention. (1998) Guidelines for the use of antiretroviral agents in pediatric HIV infection. *Morbid. Mortal. Weekly Rep.* **47(RR-4),** 1–43.
19. Centers for Disease Control and Prevention. (1998) Public Health Service Task Force recommendations for the use of antiretroviral drugs in pregnant women infected with HIV-1 for maternal health and for reducing perinatal HIV-1 transmission in the United States. *Morbid. Mortal. Weekly Rep.* **47(RR-2),** 1–30.

20. Volberding, P. A. (1996) HIV quantification: clinical applications. *Lancet* **347,** 71–73.
21. Saag, M. S., Holodniy, M., Kuritzkes, D. R., O'Brien, W. A., Coombs, R., Poscher, M. E., Jacobsen, D. M., Shaw, G. M., Richman, D. D., and Volberding, P. A. (1996) HIV viral load markers in clinical practice. *Nat. Med.* **2,** 625–629.
22. Mulder, J., McKinney, N., Christopherson, C., Sninsky, J., Greenfield, L., and Kwok, S. (1994) Rapid and simple PCR assay for quantitation of human immunodeficiency virus type 1 RNA in plasma: application to acute retroviral infection. *J. Clin. Microbiol.* **32,** 292–300.
23. Roche Diagnostic Systems. (1996) AMPLICOR HIV-1 MONITOR Test package insert. Roche Diagnostic Systems, Branchburg, NJ, pp. 8,9.
24. Segondy, M., Ly, T. D., Lapeyre, M., and Montes, B. (1998) Evaluation of the Nuclisens HIV-1 QT assay for quantitation of human immunodeficiency virus type 1 RNA levels in plasma. *J. Clin. Microbiol.* **36,** 3372–3374.
25. Lin, H. J., Pedneault, L., and Hollinger, F. B. (1998) Intra-assay performance characteristics of five assays for quantification of human immunodeficiency virus type 1 RNA in plasma. *J. Clin. Microbiol.* **36,** 835–839.
26. Nolte, F. S., Boysza, J., Thurmond, C., Clark, W. S., and Lennox, J. L. (1998) Clinical comparison of an enhanced-sensitivity branched-DNA assay and reverse transcription-PCR for quantitation of human immunodeficiency virus type 1 RNA in plasma. *J. Clin. Microbiol.* **36,** 716–720.
27. Mulder, J., Resnick, R., Saget, B., Scheibel, S., Herman, S., Payne, H., Harrigan, R., and Kwok, S. (1997) A rapid and simple method for extracting human immunodeficiency virus type 1 RNA from plasma: enhanced sensitivity. *J. Clin. Microbiol.* **35,** 1278–1280.
28. Schockmel, G. A., Yerly, S., and Perrin, L. (1997) Detection of low HIV-1 RNA levels in plasma. *J. Acquir. Immune Defic. Syndr. Hum. Retrovirol.* **14,** 179–183.
29. Sun, R., Ku, J., Jayakar, H., Kuo, J. C., Brambilla, D., Herman, S., Rosenstraus, M., and Spadoro, J. (1998) Ultrasensitive reverse transcription-PCR assay for quantitation of human immunodeficiency virus type 1 RNA in plasma. *J. Clin. Microbiol.* **36,** 2964–2969.
30. Triques, K., Coste, J., Petter, J. L., Segarra, C., Mpoudi, E., Reynes, J., Delaporte, E., Butcher, A., Dreyer, K., Herman, S., Spadoro, J., and Peeters, M. (1999) Efficiencies of four versions of the Amplicor HIV-1 Monitor test for quantification of different subtypes of human immunodeficiency virus type 1. *J. Clin. Microbiol.* **37,** 110–116.
31. DiDomenico, N., Link, H., Knobel, R., Caratsch, T., Weschler, W., Loewy, Z. G., and Rosenstraus, M. (1996) COBAS AMPLICOR: fully automated RNA and DNA amplification and detection system for routine diagnostic PCR. *Clin. Chem.* **42,** 1915–1923.
32. Longo, M. C., Berninger, M. S., and Hartley, J. L. (1990) Use of uracil DNA glycosylase to control carry-over contamination in polymerase chain reactions. *Gene* **93,** 125–128.

33. Kwok, S. and Sninsky, J. J. (1993) PCR detection of human immunodeficiency virus type 1 proviral DNA sequences, in *Diagnostic Molecular Microbiology Principles and Applications* (Persing, D. H., Smith, T. F., Tenover, F. C., and White, T. J., eds.), ASM, Washington, DC, pp. 309–315.
34. Myers, T. W. and Gelfand, D. H. (1991) Reverse transcription and DNA amplification by a *Thermus thermophilus* DNA polymerase. *Biochemistry* **30,** 7661–7666.

31

Molecular Diagnosis of Hereditary Thrombotic Disorders

James G. Donnelly

1. Introduction

Deep vein thrombosis (DVT) can be the result of coagulation pathway defects at the molecular level or damage to the vascular endothelium. Some of the acquired causes of DVT include malignancy, trauma, prolonged immobilization, and pregnancy *(1)*. Thrombophilia can be owing in part to both acquired and inherited defects. The relative risk for thrombosis is increased by estrogen replacement therapy *(2)* and homocysteinemia *(3)* Homocysteine metabolism is influenced by the use of alcohol, anticonvulsant drugs, cyclosporine, methotrexate, inadequate dietary vitamin B_{12}, folate and pyridoxine intake, organ transplantation, and reduced creatinine clearance *(4–8)*. Similar to venous thrombosis, homocysteinemia has genetic factors that influence susceptibility *(9–11)*.

Numerous defects within the coagulation pathway have been observed. Many mutations in the genes for protein C, protein S, and antithrombin III have been described, making it impractical to use molecular techniques to screen routinely for defects. Quantitative and functional assays are used instead.

Three genes with common missense mutations have been found to add to the relative risk of thrombosis *(9–11)*. Two of these gene mutations, *factor V* 1691A→G and *prothrombin* 20210G→A, have direct effects on the coagulation/anticoagulation pathways, and the enzyme expressed from the third gene, *methylenetetrahydrofolate reductase* 677C→T (*MTHFR C677T)*, influences the conversion of homocysteine to methionine.

From: *Methods in Molecular Medicine, vol. 49: Molecular Pathology Protocols*
Edited by: A. A. Killeen © Humana Press Inc., Totowa, NJ

The detection of a genetic defect in factor V has shed light on the mechanism of the major cause of activated protein C resistance (APCR) ***(9)***. A missense mutation in the exon 10 coding region for the A2 domain of *factor V* 1691A→G results in the substitution of arginine at residue 506 for glutamine. This mutation has a dominant phenotype that results in the loss of an antigen-presenting cell (APC)-specific proteolytic site on factor Va required for downregulation. This mutation is known as *factor* V_{Leiden} ***(9)*** and can be detected using restriction digestion with *Mnl*I. The frequency of *factor* V_{Leiden} is 5–7% in Western countries ***(9,12,13)***. Moreover, APCR has been identified in up to 40% of patients with DVT ***(9,13,14)***.

The missense mutation, *G20210A*, within the 3′ untranslated region (UTR) of the *prothrombin* gene also increases the risk of thrombosis ***(11)***. This mutation is not specific for known restriction enzymes, and, therefore, a mutagenic primer is used to create a *Hin*dIII site in the presence of the *20210A* allele. The frequency of this mutation is approx 1% in the general population ***(11)***, 18% in DVT patients with an established family history of venous thrombosis, and 6% in consecutive patients with DVT ***(11)***. Individuals inheriting a copy of the *A20210* allele of the prothrombin gene have significantly elevated levels of circulating prothrombin ***(11)***. The *G20210A* mutation occurs downstream from exon 14, the final coding region of the prothrombin gene. This mutation in the *prothrombin* UTR may affect transcriptional regulation.

The missense mutation of *MTHFR* 677C→T results in a thermolabile variant of this enzyme and reduced catalytic activity. Conversion of homocysteine to methionine is affected in individuals homozygous for the *677T* allele. The frequency for the *MTHFR 677T* allele is approx 0.38 in the Western Hemisphere ***(10)***. In one study, 10% of French-speaking Canadians were shown to be homozygous ***(10)***. The influence of this gene on homocysteine is related to folate concentration in plasma. Fasting homocysteine concentrations in plasma are increased significantly in *677T* homozygotes when plasma folate concentrations are <15.4 nmol/L ***(15)***. With this particular mutation, plasma homocysteine levels respond to increased dietary folate. Hyperhomocysteinemia has been shown to contribute a two- to threefold increase in risk for recurrent thrombosis ***(16)***. This mutation can be detected using the restriction enzyme *Hinf*I and amplified DNA.

Heritable factors for hypercoagulability such as underproduction of endogenous anticoagulant proteins or increased synthesis of coagulant proteins will result in increased risk of thrombosis. It is important to determine the heritable risk of thrombosis to properly treat, anticipate future risk, and identify other family members who may also be at risk. Identification of asymptomatic family members will permit these individuals to make informed decisions concerning choice of birth control method, estrogen therapy, and prophylactic anticoagulant therapy in high-risk situations such as pregnancy and surgery.

I present three polymerase chain reaction (PCR)-based genotyping assays that can be performed simultaneously using the same master mix, DNA preparation, and reaction conditions. Each assay can then be subjected to restriction digestion and separation using agarose gel electrophoresis with visualization using ethidium bromide (EtBr) staining. I also describe a second confirmatory assay for *factor* V_{Leiden}, using allele-specific oligonucleotide primers ***(17)***.

A rare mutation of *factor V* at 1692A→C has been reported ***(18)***. Although this missense mutation does not confer resistance to APC, it has the same digestion pattern as *factor* V_{Leiden}. This 1692C allele has been reported in only one individual and is likely a rare, isolated mutation. However, some laboratories may wish to confirm positive *factor* V_{Leiden} genotypes using the second method. I also present algorithms that can be used to assist in appropriate assay selection and, if followed, will minimize wasteful testing.

2. Materials

2.1. Isolation of Genomic DNA

1. Wizard™ Genomic DNA Purification Kit (Promega, Madison, WI).
2. Additional erythrocyte lysis fluid: 10 m*M* KCl, 10 m*M* NH_4Cl, 10 m*M* Tris-HCL, pH 7.5. Dissolve 0.75 g of KCl, 5.35 g of NH_4Cl, and 1.21 g of Tris base in 800 mL of deionized water. Adjust the pH to 7.50 with 1 *M* HCl. Adjust the volume to 1.0 L with deionized water.

2.2. PCR Amplification

1. Primers (Applied Biosystems) as follows:
   a. *Factor* V_{Leiden} A1691G:
      FV1 5′-ACCCACAGAAAATGATGCCCAG-3′.
      FV2 5′-TGCCCCATTATTTAGCCAGGAG-3′ ***(9)***.
   b. *MTHFR C677T:*
      MTHFR1 5′TGAAGGAGAAGGTGTCTGCGGGA3′.
      MTHFR2 5′AGGACGGTGCGGTGAGAGTG3′ ***(10)***.
   c. *Prothrombin G20210A:*
      UTPT1 5′TCTAGAAACAGTTGCCTGGC3′.
      UTPT2 5′ATAGCACTGGGAGCATTGAAGC3′ ***(11)***.
   d. *Factor* V_{Leiden} 1691G allele-specific confirmatory assay (optional):
      FVASO1 5′CTTTCAGGCAGGAACAACACC3′.
      FVASO2 5′TGGACAAAATACCTGTATACCTT3′ ***(17)***.
2. AmpliTaq™ DNA Polymerase Stoffel fragment 10X PCR buffer (Applied Biosystems).
3. 10X Stock $MgCl_2$ (25 m*M*) (Applied Biosystems).
4. AmpliTaq DNA Polymerase Stoffel fragment (10 U/µL) (Applied Biosystems).
5. GeneAmp™ dNTPs (10 m*M* stock solutions) (Applied Biosystems).
6. Perkin-Elmer 9600 Thermocycler (Applied Biosystems).

2.3. Restriction Enzyme Analysis

1. *Mnl*I restriction enzyme (10 U/μL) (MBI Fermantis) for *factor* V_{Leiden}.
2. *Hinf*I restriction enzyme (10 U/μL) (Promega) for *MTHFR C677T*.
3. *Hin*dIII restriction enzyme (10 U/μL) (Promega) for *prothrombin G20210A*.
4. *Eco*RI digested lambda phage DNA base pair marker for *Hin*dIII digest internal control (Roche).

2.4. High-Resolution Agarose Gel Electrophoresis

1. Metaphor™ high-resolution agarose (FMC Bioproducts).
2. Agarose (Gibco-BRL).
3. 1X Tris-borate EDTA (TBE) (Sigma, St. Louis, MO): 100 m*M* Tris, 90 m*M* boric acid, 1.0 m*M* EDTA, pH 8.33. Gel-Mix Running Mate™ TBE Buffer (Gibco-BRL) is used routinely in our laboratory rather than making this buffer from individual components.
4. Gel loading solution: 50% (v/v) glycerol and deionized water with a few grains of bromophenol blue stain.
5. EtBr solution (10 mg/mL).

3. Methods

Leukocyte (white blood cell [WBC]) nuclei serve as the source of DNA for thrombophilic genotyping assays. The PCR assays described herein require the sequential isolation of WBCs from red blood cells (RBCs). WBCs can be stored at –70°C for extended periods. When ready for analysis, DNA is then isolated from the WBC nuclei.

DNA is separated from the bulk of nuclear protein by differential precipitation of the proteins in a sodium dodecyl sulfate—ammonium acetate solution. The DNA is then precipitated from the supernatant solution using 2 vol of isopropanol. The pellet of DNA is washed with several volumes of 70% ethyl alcohol to remove salts and detergent. The DNA pellet is then rehydrated with DNA rehydration solution (TBE buffer). The method presented is modified from the Wizard Genomic DNA Purification Kit and is intended to maximize the quantity of DNA isolated. Using this procedure, enough DNA can be obtained from 2.5 mL of blood to perform between 20 and 50 separate PCRs. This is useful for banking DNA for future studies as new gene mutations are implicated in hereditary thrombosis.

3.1. Specimen Requirements

EDTA or citrate anticoagulated blood stored at room temperature for up to 4 d is suitable. Prepare the WBCs as soon as possible and store frozen. Heparinized whole blood has not been analyzed using these PCR genotyping methods, and heparin is known to inhibit PCRs.

3.2. Preparation of WBCs (*see* Note 1)

1. Centrifuge EDTA or citrate anticoagulated whole blood for 5 min at 1200*g*. The blood should be stored at room temperature. Do not store the blood at 4°C for prolonged periods. Glycolysis is inhibited in blood stored at 4°C and, therefore, WBC integrity is compromised and hemolysis is increased.
2. While the tube is being centrifuged, pipet 900 µL of RBC lysis solution to a labeled 1.5-mL microcentrifuge tube.
3. Using a disposable plastic pipet, remove the white cell layer (buffy coat) at the plasma-cell interface and add it to the tube. Some plasma and RBCs will also be transferred. Cap and mix.
4. Incubate the mixture at room temperature for 10 min. Invert two to three times while incubating. Centrifuge for 1 min in a microcentrifuge to pellet the WBC nuclei.
5. Remove the supernatant with a fine-tip disposable pipet. Remove as much of the liquid as possible without disturbing the pellet. Occasionally RBCs do not lyse completely. If this occurs, take the supernatant off and add RBC fresh lysis solution to a total volume of 1.2–1.4 mL. Mix and reincubate for 10 min, centrifuge, and remove the supernatant. Try to remove as much of the RBC stroma layer as possible. At this point, the WBC pellet should be almost completely free of hemoglobin. If it is not, **step 5** can be repeated.
6. If the DNA is not to be prepared immediately, freeze and store the WBC pellets at –70°C.

3.3. Preparation of DNA

1. Add 300 µL of the nuclei lysis solution to the tube containing the freshly thawed and resuspended WBCs. Vortex vigorously or rub across the top of a tube rack to ensure complete disruption of the pellet. The solution is very viscous at this point. There must be no clumps of WBCs in the tube; otherwise the yield will be reduced (*see* **Notes 2–4**).
2. Add 100 µL of protein precipitation solution to the nuclear lysate and vortex vigorously for 10–20 s. If the solution does not show signs of a precipitate, and instead has a viscous gel of nuclei, add another 100 µL of the protein precipitation solution and vortex again.
3. Centrifuge at 12,800*g* for 3 min at room temperature. A brown pellet should be visible.
4. Using a disposable pipet, transfer the supernatant to a clean 1.5-mL microcentrifuge tube containing 600 µL of isopropanol.
5. Gently mix the solution by inversion until white threads of DNA form. Should no precipitate be obvious, shake the tube three or four times.
6. Centrifuge for 1 min at 12,800*g* at room temperature. The DNA will be a visible white pellet. Using a permanent marker, place a line on the bottom of the tube prior to centrifugation. Orient the tube in the centrifuge with the line facing outward. After centrifugation, the DNA pellet will be visible against the mark on the tube.

7. Aspirate the supernatant and add 600 µL of 70% ethanol to the DNA. Invert the tube gently to wash the pellet and the walls of the tube. Do not attempt to resuspend the pellet. Centrifuge for 1 min at 12,800*g* at room temperature.
8. Aspirate the ethanol using a pipet. Repeat the ethanol wash once more. The DNA pellet is not firmly attached to the tube and care must be taken to avoid aspirating the pellet when removing the ethanol solution.
9. Air-dry the pellet to ensure that the ethanol is evaporated completely. Avoid overdrying the pellet.
10. Reconstitute DNA pellet by adding 50 µL of TBE, DNA hydration solution to the tube. Incubate at 65°C for 1 h on a heating block or at 4°C overnight. Genomic DNA will not come back into the solution readily. It is better to prepare the DNA the day before it is to be used. Mix well with a pipet before use, but do so gently to avoid shearing the DNA.
11. Store the rehydrated DNA at 2–8°C and use within 3 to 4 d; DNA stability is variable after 4 d. DNA is stable for several years when stored at –20°C.

3.4. Preparation of Working Primer Solutions

Deblocked primers are obtained from 40-nmol scale synthesis (*see* **Notes 5** and **6**).

1. Dilute primers in 200 µL of deionized water and further dilute a 5-µL aliquot of this stock into 500 µL (1/100 dilution).
2. Test the diluted primer at three or four volumes, typically 2, 4, 6, and 8 µL in PCR reactions. Then run out the reactions on a 2% agarose, 0.5X TBE (Gibco-BRL) gel.
3. Use the concentration that provides the optimal yield of PCR product to calculate the desired dilution of the stock primer. For method consistency, the volume of the primer is fixed at 2.5 µL in the PCR assays; therefore, the final dilution of the stock will depend on the optimal volume of primer determined in the test.

3.5. PCR Assays for Factor V_{Leiden}, MTHFR C677T, and Prothrombin G20210A

A master reaction mixture is prepared separately for each gene using reagents from Perkin-Elmer. **Table 1** lists the volumes of each reagent required for one tube. A Perkin-Elmer 9600 thermocycler is used for the reactions. The amplification conditions are as follows:

1. Initial 5-min denaturation step at 95°C: Place the rack in the thermocycler when the temperature is >85°C (*see* **Note 7**).
2. Thirty cycles of 94°C for 30 s, 50°C for 30 s, and 72°C for 1 min.
3. Final 5-min incubation at 72°C: This is particularly important for sharpening the prothrombin PCR product band.
4. The optional confirmatory PCR assay for specimens positive for *factor* V_{Leiden} uses the same master mix reagents (*see* **Subheading 3.4.**) with allele-specific primers (*see* **Subheading 2.2., step 1, part d**), under the same reaction conditions as in **steps 1–3** with 55°C used as the annealing temperature.

Table 1
Preparation of PCR Master Mix

Master mix	Volume (μL/tube)	Final concentration
Distilled/deionized water	23	—
10X Stoeffel buffer	5	1X
10X $MgCl_2$	5	2.5 m*M*
dNTPs	2 each	200 μ*M*
Stoeffel *Taq*	0.25	2.5 U
Primer 1	2.5	20 μ*M*
Primer 2	2.5	20 μ*M*

3.6. Verification of PCR Product (optional)

1. Use a 2% Gibco-BRL agarose gel with 0.5X TBE and 0.5 μg/mL of EtBr. Add 10 μL of PCR product and 5 μL of gel-loading solution per well in the gel.
2. To the left lane of each gel run, add a 50-bp marker (2.5 μL) (MBI Fermentas).
3. Run at 100 V, in the same TBE buffer strength used to make the gel, until the dye front has migrated approx 3 cm.

3.7. Restriction Digestion

1. Digest 10 μL of each of the specific PCR products with 1 U of *Mnl*I, *factor V*, and *Hinf*I for *MTHFR*, and 1 μ of *Hin*dIII for *prothrombin* (*see* **Note 8**).
2. As a restriction enzyme control, add *Eco*RI digested lambda phage (0.5 μg) to the prothrombin reaction prior to digestion. Allow digestion to proceed for a minimum of 2 h at room temperature (*see* **Note 9**).

3.8. 2.5% High-Resolution Gel for Digest Products

For two 50-mL gels, mix the following components: 100 mL of 1X cold TBE, 2.5 g of Metaphor agarose, 1.0 g of agarose. Before pouring the gel add 5 μL of EtBr (final concentration of 0.5 μg/mL from a 10 mg/mL stock).

1. Measure the buffer and transfer to a 500-mL Erlenmeyer flask. Weigh out the agarose and add to the buffer while swirling the flask. Mix well and loosely cap with a cotton gauze plug.
2. Microwave to melt the agarose. Periodically and carefully mix the solution to avoid boil-over of the agarose. Continue heating until the agarose is completely melted. Let the gel cool briefly and add 5 μL of EtBr stain. EtBr is considered mutagenic, and gloves must be worn when handling the solution, gels, and buffers. Swirl the molten agarose until the EtBr is completely dispersed. Then pour the gel into the casting stand.

3. One hundred milliliters of molten agarose is sufficient for two 5 × 8 cm mini gels. Place one 12-well comb in each gel and leave undisturbed until completely solidified. Refrigerate the gel for at least 30 min before using.
4. Cold 1X TBE should be used for the electrophoresis. Load a 50-bp DNA ladder into the left-most lane and then 20 μL of digested product in the adjacent lanes.
5. Electrophorese the DNA fragments at 100 V until the dye front has migrated two thirds to three fourths through the gel.

3.9. Separation of Restriction-Digested PCR Products

1. Separate the digested products using a gel consisting of 2.5% Metaphor agarose and 1% agarose prepared with 1X TBE (*see* **Note 10**).
2. Confirm positive *factor* V_{Leiden} in the optional allele-specific PCR assay by amplifying a DNA product of 234 bp in size observed on a 2% agarose gel electrophoresed with 0.5X TBE and stained with EtBr. Prepare the gels in advance. The gels may be stored in sealed plastic containers with a few milliliters of water to keep them from drying out.

3.10. Documentation of Results

After running the gel for a suitable length of time as judged by the bromophenol blue stain, visualize the bands under UV light and document. We use a Gel Doc™1000 (Bio-Rad, Hercules, CA) video capture system with Molecular Analyst™ (Bio-Rad) software for documentation of gels (*see* **Note 11**).

3.11. Interpretation of Results

Restriction isotyping yields specific band patterns for each allele. The base pair size of each fragment obtained after the restriction enzyme digestion is determined from its position relative to the base pair markers. **Figure 1** is representative of the typical digest separations using high-resolution agarose. **Table 2** lists the expected fragment size for each allele. **Table 3** shows suggested work flow for these assays.

The allele patterns are superimposed for heterozygotes. The *prothrombin 20210G* allele is not digested by *Hin*dIII. Therefore, *Eco*RI digested lambda phage virus DNA is added prior to digestion. A faint band at 564 bp indicates successful digestion in the absence of the 20210A allele. **Figure 2** illustrates the optional allele-specific confirmation assay for *factor* V_{Leiden} (*see* **Notes 12–15**).

MTHFR genotyping is useful for identifying hyperhomocysteinemic patients who would benefit from folate supplementation. Approximately 28% of our venous thrombotic patients are hyperhomocysteinemic ***(19)***. Therefore, homocysteine should be included in all initial patient assessments. Individuals homozygous for T677 MTHFR may have normal or elevated tissue folate

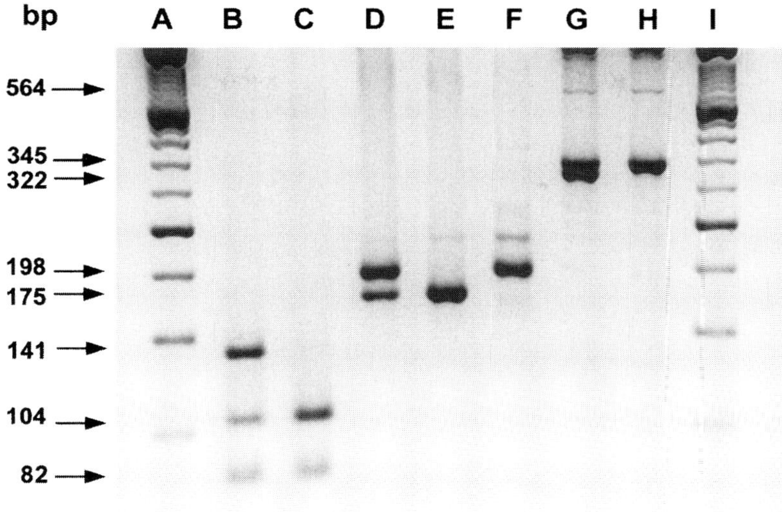

Fig. 1. Thrombophilia genotyping panel. Lanes A and I, 50-bp ladder; lane B, factor V 1691AG (heterozygous Leiden); lane C, factor V 1691AA (wild type); lane D, MTHFR 677CT; lane E, MTHFR 677TT (homozygous thermolabile variant); lane F, MTHFR 677CC (wild type); lane G, prothrombin 20210GA; lane H, prothrombin 20210GG (wild type). The band at 564 bp is the digestion control using *Eco*RI digested lambda DNA. Inverted image (positive–negative) of EtBr-stained gel.

pools. However plasma folate, part of which is derived from hepatic portal recirculation, is decreased. Jacques et al. ***(15)*** observed that homocysteine was reduced when plasma folate concentrations were >15.4 nmol/L.

Hyperhomocysteinemic patients who are not homozygous for the *677T* allele of *MTHFR*, and who have folate and vitamin B_{12} values within the reference interval and have no other acquired cause of impaired homocysteine metabolism, should be screened for cystathionine beta synthase (CBS) deficiency. An abbreviated 2-h methionine-loading assay is suitable for screening CBS deficiency ***(20)***. Although a small percentage of individuals can have a normal fasting homocysteine and be CBS deficient, we do not routinely perform the methionine-loading test in our institution.

4. Notes

1. Other preparations for DNA such as buccal scrapings may be suitable for DNA. However, most patients with DVT will be monitored for anticoagulant therapy or require homocysteine and B vitamin monitoring. Therefore, WBC DNA is available at some point in the normal course of treating these patients.

Table 2
Interpretation of Restriction Digest

Gene	Allele	DNA restriction fragments (bp)
Factor V	*1691 A*	104, 82, 37
	1691 G	141, 82
MTHFR	*677 C*	198
	677 T	175
Prothrombin	*20210 G*	345[a]
	20210 A	322

[a]Undigested PCR product. It requires an internal restriction enzyme control as outlined in **Subheading 3.**

2. Smaller volumes can be used for DNA isolation. This preparation is optimized for large yields of DNA. Banked DNA is useful for future studies concerning thrombophilia.
3. The RBC lysis solution is similar to that supplied by Promega. Following the procedure outlined, this reagent is limiting using the commercial kit, and therefore it is economical to prepare this component.
4. Should the occasional PCR not work, repeat using one half or two times the quantity of DNA. If this does not solve the problem, reprecipitate the DNA in isopropanol and wash the pellet again with 70% ethanol. We have not had this problem; however, contamination with detergents could occur if the pellet were not washed adequately.
5. Good quality primers from a reliable source are essential for successful PCR. The optimization step will ensure that the primers work before attempting to process patient specimens.
6. It is not necessary to purchase purified primers. Deblocked primers are adequate.
7. The rack is not loaded on the thermocycler until the temperature reaches 85°C. This is not a true hot-start technique. However, this does help prevent false priming and ensure a more specific start to the amplifications.
8. The digestion can take place in the parent tube of DNA to save an aliquoting step.
9. The tubes can be left overnight if required.
10. The restriction digest products are easily separated by the outlined procedure without the use of polyacrylamide gel electrophoresis. The use of agarose gels greatly reduces the analysis processing time.
11. Detection of small DNA fragments is difficult without optimal staining and a good photodocumentation system. Digital video capture is not required for detection of small DNA fragments. However, running the gels longer than necessary to visualize the bands is not recommended, because the longer the gels are electrophoresed the more the bands can diffuse through the gel.

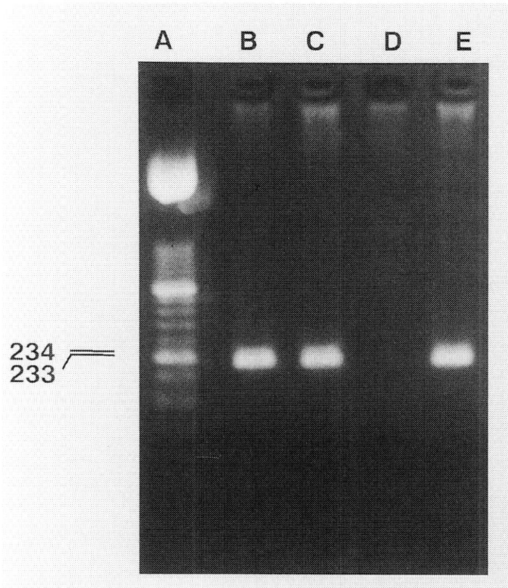

Fig. 2. Optional confirmation assay for *factor* V_{Leiden}. Lane A, 50-bp marker; lanes B and E, allele-specific primers for *factor V 1691A*; lanes C and D, allele-specific primers for *factor V 1691G*. Lanes B and C indicate 1691AG, and lanes D and E indicate 1691AA. Allele-specific primer for 1691A is 5′TGGACAAAATACCTGT-ATACCTT3′. This primer does not need to be used when the allele-specific oligonucleotide assays are used for confirmation.

12. The assays for heritable thrombophilia are expensive and utilization should be monitored closely. The prevalence in the patient population is one way to test for appropriate utilization. The prevalence of *factor* V_{Leiden}, *prothrombin A20210*, and *MTHFR TT677* in our patients is 21.5, 5.4, and 12.4%, respectively. The prevalence of APCR is 50.3% in our tested population. Approximately 6% of our patients cannot be tested for APCR because of anticoagulation or estrogen therapy.
13. Wasserman et al. ***(21)*** and Adcock et al. ***(22)*** have described approaches to the incorporation of *factor* V_{Leiden} genotyping into coagulation investigations. The normalized APCR ratio was more sensitive than the APCR ratio when used as a preliminary screen to eliminate unnecessary *factor* V_{Leiden} genotyping ***(21)***. The sensitivity and specificity of the normalized ratio using a cutoff value of <0.85 were 100 and 51%, respectively, in Wasserman et al.'s study ***(21)***. The APCR ratio cutoff of <1.57 was more specific (79%); however, sensitivity decreased to 94%. In the absence of preliminary screening for APCR, we found that approx 21.5% of our DVT patients were heterozygous for *factor* V_{Leiden}. APCR results

Table 3
Suggested Work Flow for Thrombophilia Genotyping

Day 1	Days 2 and 3
Prepare DNA from fresh and frozen leukocytes in the morning. Prepare master mix and run amplification in the afternoon.	Remove PCR tubes from thermocycler and aliquot for digest. Prepare digest working enzyme solution. Add *Eco*RI digested lambda to the prothrombin aliquots. Add working enzyme solution to the aliquots. Prepare high-resolution electrophoresis gels and refrigerate for a minimum of 30 min after the agarose has set. Load high-resolution agarose gels with 50-bp DNA ladder and digested PCR products. Separate at 100 V or less in cold 1X TBE. Record digest results.

are an economical screening tool for *factor* V_{Leiden} genotyping. Care must be taken to ensure that the patient history is accurate and communicated to the laboratory because the APCR assay will be abnormal irrespective of *factor V* genotype when a patient is anticoagulated, pregnant, or taking estrogens.

14. A mutation of *factor V A1692C* that destroys the *Mnl*I restriction site but does not confer APC resistance has been reported in one patient ***(18)***. It appears to be unlikely that this mutation is common. However, some laboratories may wish to confirm the results of restriction assay for *factor* V_{Leiden} until they are reasonably certain that the mutation is not present in their patient population.
15. We chose not to use the allele-specific oligonucleotide assay as our primary assay because of the uncertainty of amplification and the cost of running two assays per patient. As a primary assay, two sets of primers are required for *factor V*: the wild-type forward primer and the allele-specific reverse primer. **Figure 2** shows the results of both reactions. Additionally an internal control must be used in this assay to confirm the integrity of the PCR should this be selected as a stand-alone assay for *factor V* genotyping. However, even with the use of an internal control product, there is no guarantee that the allele-specific primers for *factor V* have amplified the target DNA. Moreover, this assay also is not cost-effective because two PCR tubes must be set up for each assay and two sets of primers; the *factor V* primers and the internal control primer must be used when this assay is run alone.

Acknowledgments

I am indebted to Ferne Shirley for her superior organizational skills and many contributions to the thrombophilia genotyping procedures.

References

1. Appleby, R. D. and Olds, R. J. (1997) The inherited basis of venous thrombosis. *Pathology* **29,** 341–347.
2. Helmerhorst, F. M., Bloemenkamp, K. W., Rosendaal, F. R., and Vandenbroucke, J. P. (1997) Oral contraceptives and thrombotic disease: risk of venous thromboembolism. *Thromb. Haemost.* **78,** 327–333.
3. D'Angelo, A., Mazzola, G., Crippa, L., Fermo, I., and Vigano, D. S. (1997) Hyperhomocysteinemia and venous thromboembolic disease. *Haematologica* **82,** 211–219.
4. Cravo, M. L., Gloria, L. M., Selhub, J., et al. (1996) Hyperhomocysteinemia in chronic alcoholism: correlation with folate, vitamin B-12, and vitamin B-6 status. *Am. J. Clin. Nutr.* **63,** 220–224.
5. Lucock, M. D., Wild, J., Schorah, C. J., Levene, M. I., and Hartley, R. (1994) The methylfolate axis in neural tube defects: in vitro characterisation and clinical investigation. *Biochem. Med. Metab. Biol.* **52,** 101–114.
6. Arnadottir, M., Hultberg, B., Vladov, V., Nilsson, E. P., and Thysell, H. (1996) Hyperhomocysteinemia in cyclosporine-treated renal transplant recipients. *Transplantation* **61,** 509–512.
7. Keuzenkamp, J. C., De, A. R., Blom, H. J., Bokkerink, J. P., Trijbels, J. M. (1996) Effects on transmethylation by high-dose 6-mercaptopurine and methotrexate infusions during consolidation treatment of acute lymphoblastic leukemia. *Biochem. Pharmacol.* **51,** 1165–1171.
8. Brattstrom, L., Lindgren, A., Israelsson, B., Andersson, A., and Hultberg, B. (1994) Homocysteine and cysteine: determinants of plasma levels in middle-aged and elderly subjects. *J. Intern. Med.* **236,** 633–641.
9. Bertina, M. R., Koeleman, B. P. C., Koster, T., et al. (1994) Mutation in blood coagulation factor V associated with resistance to activated protein C. *Nature* **369,** 64–67.
10. Frosst, P., Blom, H. J., Milos, R., et al. (1995) A candidate genetic risk factor for vascular disease: a common mutation in methylenetetrahydrofolate reductase. *Nat. Genet.* **10,** 111–113.
11. Poort, S. R., Rosendaal, F. R., Reitsma, P. H., and Bertina, R. M. (1996) A common genetic variation in the 3′-untranslated region of the prothrombin gene is associated with elevated plasma prothrombin levels and an increase in venous thrombosis. *Blood* **88,** 3698–3703.
12. Koster, T., Rosendaal, F. R., de Ronde, H., Briet, E., Vandenbroucke, J. P., and Bertina, R. M. (1993) Venous thrombosis due to poor anticoagulant response to activated protein C: Leiden Thrombophilia Study. *Lancet* **342,** 1503–1506.
13. Svensson, P. J. and Dalback, B. (1994) Resistance to activated protein C as a basis for venous thrombosis. *N. Engl. J. Med.* **330,** 517–522.

14. Griffin, J. H., Evatt, B., Wideman, C., and Fernandez, J. A. (1993) Anticoagulant protein C pathway defective in majority of thrombophilic patients. *Blood* **82,** 1908–1993.
15. Jacques, P. F., Bostom, A. G., Williams, R. R., et al. (1996) Relation between folate status, a common mutation in methylenetetrahydrofolate reductase, and plasma homocysteine concentrations. *Circulation* **93,** 7–9.
16. den Heiger, M., Blom, H. J., Gerrits, W. B., et al. (1995) Is hyperhomocysteinaemia a risk factor for recurrent venous thrombosis? *Lancet* **345,** 882–885.
17. Ridker, P. M., Hennekens, C. H., Lindpaintner, K., Stampfer, M. J., Eisenberg, P. R., and Miletich, J. P. (1995) Mutation in the gene coding for coagulation factor V and the risk of myocardial infarction, stroke, and venous thrombosis in apparently healthy men. *N. Engl. J. Med.* **332,** 912–917.
18. Liebman, H. A., Sutherland, D., Bacon, R., and McGehee, W. (1996) Evaluation of a tissue factor dependent factor V assay to detect factor V Leiden: demonstration of high sensitivity and specificity to a generally applicable assay for activated protein C resistance. *Br. J. Haematol.* **95,** 550–553.
19. Donnelly, J. G. (1998) Homocysteine and plasma folate relationship in patients with venous thrombosis, end-stage renal disease or atherosclerosis. *Clin. Chem.* **44(Suppl. 6),** A167,A168.
20. Bostom, A. G., Roubenoff, R., Dellaripa, P., et al. (1995)Validation of abbreviated oral methionine-loading test. *Clin. Chem.* **41,** 948,949.
21. Wasserman, L. M., Edson, J. R., Key, N. S., Chibbar, R., and McGlennen, R. C. (1997) Detection of the factor V Leiden mutation: development of a testing algorithm combining a coagulation assay and molecular diagnosis. *Am. J. Clin. Pathol.* **108,** 427–433.
22. Adcock, D. M., Fink, L., and Marlar, R. A. (1997) A laboratory approach to the evaluation of hereditary hypercoagulability. *Am. J. Clin. Pathol.* **108,** 434–449.

32

Prenatal Genotyping of the *RhD* Locus to Identify Fetuses at Risk for Hemolytic Disease of the Newborn

Martin J. Hessner and Daniel B. Bellissimo

1. Introduction

Hemolytic disease of the newborn (HDN) can occur when there are fetomaternal incompatibilities within any number of different erythrocyte antigen systems, including the RhD, Cc, Ee, Kidd and Duffy, and Kell antigen systems. In these disorders, maternal antibodies are developed by alloimmunization of the mother to fetal red blood cells during pregnancy when the fetal cells carry an alloantigen inherited from the father. The maternal antibodies result in the destruction of fetal erythrocytes leading to severe hemolytic anemia and hyperbilirubinemia. Permanent neurologic damage can result from HDN, and in extreme cases loss of the fetus or death of the neonate may occur. In subsequent pregnancies, it is important to determine the status of the incompatible allele in the fetus. If the father is heterozygous or homozygous for the allele, the chance of the fetus inheriting the paternal alloallele to which the mother is immunologically sensitized is 50 or 100%, respectively. Fetuses that do not inherit the alloallele will not be at risk for HDN.

Investigative and therapeutic measures used for alloimmunized pregnant women involve some risk to the fetus. Currently, women who present with alloantibody titers to red cell antigens are monitored by amniotic fluid spectrophotometric analysis to detect deviation from linearity at 450 nm, the wavelength at which bilirubin absorbs *(1)*. Accurate determination of fetal risk is achieved through serial analysis, generally weekly for several weeks. Although

From: *Methods in Molecular Medicine, vol. 49: Molecular Pathology Protocols*
Edited by: A. A. Killeen © Humana Press Inc., Totowa, NJ

the risk of placental trauma during amniocentesis has been greatly reduced since the introduction of ultrasound imaging techniques, there is still a 2% risk of placental trauma ***(2)***. Alternatively, percutaneous umbilical blood sampling allows direct measurements of all fetal blood parameters including blood groups. However, the procedure is technically more difficult and because of the risk of fetomaternal hemorrhage and further sensitization of the mother, its use is limited. The molecular characterization of many blood antigen systems has enabled the development of molecular diagnostic assays that are useful in identifying fetuses at risk for HDN. Prenatal identification of the relevant genotypes for fetuses potentially at risk for HDN requires fetal DNA isolated from a single amniocentesis. When fetuses are shown to be compatible with sensitized mothers, and therefore not at risk for HDN, the need for expensive and invasive monitoring throughout the pregnancy can be obviated.

The characterization of the *RhD* and *RhCcEe* genes has provided the molecular basis for prenatal testing for RhD. The *Rh* locus on chromosome 1 contains two distinct but highly homologous genes: *RhD* and *RhCcEe* ***(3,4)***. Generally, RhD-positive individuals possess one or two copies of the *RhD* gene and two copies of the *RhCcEe* gene, whereas RhD-negative individuals retain two copies of the *RhCcEe* gene but typically lack the *RhD* gene ***(4)***. The *RhD* and *RhCcEe* genes are arranged tandemly and are believed to have arisen through duplication of a single ancestral gene. The *Rh* genes, which are >95% homologous at the nucleotide sequence level, both consist of 10 exons spanning more than 75 kb, and both encode peptides of 417 amino acid residues with a predicted molecular mass of 30–35 kDa ***(5–8)***.

A number of sequence differences between the *RhCcEe* and *RhD* genes can be utilized in genotyping assays to identify the presence or absence of the *RhD* gene. Polymerase chain reaction (PCR)-based RhD typing assays, utilizing sequence differences in intron 4, exon 3, exon 7, and the untranslated region within exon 10, have been previously described ***(7,9–12)***. However, discrepancies between serotyping and genotyping have been observed. These discrepancies are largely owing to the existence of allelic variants, the molecular basis of which is often the result of recombination between the *RhD* and *RhCeEe* genes. In these hybrid genes, some *RhD* sequences are replaced with the corresponding sequences from the *RhCcEe* gene ***(9,13)***. For other variants, all that is known is that the sequences targeted by PCR primers or restriction enzymes are altered or deleted. These variants can potentially cause the misdiagnosis of the fetal RhD status during prenatal genotyping. To develop a reliable technique for prenatal RhD typing of fetuses at risk for HDN, we have evaluated the suitability of four different regions of the *RhD* gene for genotyping and compared these results to those obtained by serology.

The first RhD genotyping method is based on multiplexing the oligonucleotide primers of Arce et al. ***(7)*** with oligonucleotide primers derived from those described by Bennett et al. ***(10)***. The RhD genotyping strategy described by Arce et al. ***(7)*** detects a 600-bp deletion within intron 4 of the *RhD* gene that is not present within intron 4 of the *RhCcEe* gene ***(10)***. Amplification with a primer pair that targets exons 4 and 5 of the *RhD* and the *RhCcEe* genes results in a 1200-bp RhCcEe product and a 600-bp product in RhD-positive individuals. The RhD-specific oligonucleotide primers derived from those described by Bennett et al. ***(10)*** specifically amplify a 193-bp product of the 3′ untranslated region of exon 10. The second RhD genotyping method evaluated involves specific amplification of a 96-bp product from exon 7 of the *RhD* gene, previously described by Simsek et al. ***(12)***. Finally, the third method involves specific amplification of a 111-bp product from exon 3 of the *RhD* gene as previously described by Beckers et al. ***(9)***.

To evaluate these genotyping methods and their possible discrepancies with serologic typing, 50 Rh-phenotyped individuals (38 RhD positive and 12 Rh negative) were selected. The RhD-positive samples were chosen for their unusual serotyping results suggesting the samples were RhD variants. DNA was isolated from the peripheral blood, and these samples were genotyped using the aforementioned methods. **Figure 1** shows examples of genotyping from RhD-positive, RhD-negative, and variant samples. **Table 1** summarizes the discrepancies observed between serotyping and genotyping. Two serologically RhD-positive samples (95-0724-11 and 95-0718-3) gave false-negative results when amplifying exons 3 and 7 of the *RhD* gene. Three of five serologically weak RhD-positive samples yielded discrepant results with genotyping: sample 95-0622-1 lacked the exon 3 *RhD* product (**Fig. 1**), sample 95-0913-4 (**Fig. 1**) lacked the intron 4 *RhD* product; and sample 96-0110-10 lacked the exon 3, intron 4, and exon 7 products. Amplification of the 3′ untranslated region of exon 10 resulted in the best overall detection (38 of 38) of serologically typed RhD-positive and RhD-weak-positive samples in our laboratory. Okuda et al. ***(14)*** observed a similar result. However, other laboratories observed discordance between serology and genotyping when using this amplicon ***(12,15)***.

Twelve RhD-negative samples were evaluated. One sample, from an RhD-sensitized, serologically RhD-negative, pregnant African American woman with a history of HDN in previous pregnancies, was RhD positive in all four genotyping assays (**Fig. 1**, 96-0610-1) suggesting that a complete inactive *RhD* gene was present. This made the RhD-positive genotyping result of her fetus inconclusive, because it was possible that her fetus may have inherited this "nonfunctional" *RhD* allele. After birth, the child was typed RhD positive by

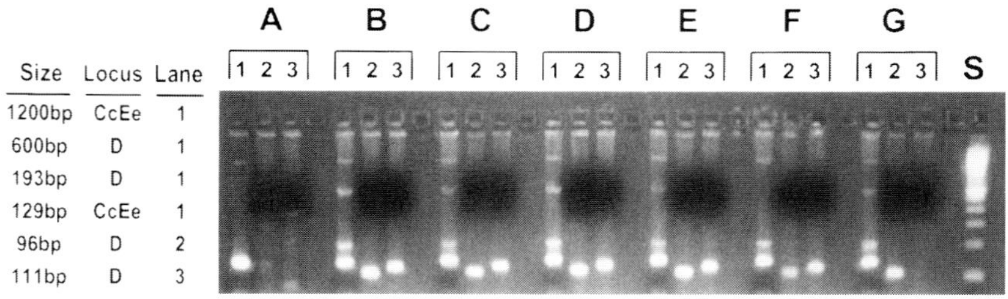

Fig. 1. RhD genotyping. A–G, RhD analysis by three different PCR amplifications. Lane 1, multiplex amplification of RhD intron 4 (600 bp) and exon 10 (193 bp); lane 2, amplification of RhD exon 7 (96 bp); lane 3, amplification of RhD exon 3 (111 bp). S, 100-bp DNA ladder size standard. A, RhD-negative control; B, RhD-positive control; C–E, prenatal RhD genotyping cases for a fetus at risk for RhD-related HDN in which C is a serologically RhD-positive father, D is a serologically RhD-negative mother (96-0610-1), and E is a fetus (amniotic fluid); F, RhD variant (95-0913-4); G, RhD variant (95-0622-1).

both serology and genotyping. A high incidence of false positives has been observed in non-Caucasian groups. In one study, 10 of 20 seronegative African Americans were typed as RhD positive with four different genotyping assays ***(15)***. In Asian populations, this observation may also be quite common because the *RhD* gene has been detected at a frequency of 27.7% among RhD-negative Japanese donors ***(14)***. When conducting prenatal *RhD* genotyping, it is clearly necessary to identify discrepancies between parental serotypes and genotypes to reduce the risk of false-negative and false-positive results. Even this precaution may not be sufficient when allelic variants such as 96-0110-10, which was negative in three of four different genotyping assays, can be masked in paternal samples by a "normal" *RhD* allele. In this scenario, the masked variant allele could be passed on to the fetus, where it may be undetected without a thorough analysis of the fetal *RhD* gene.

These results, as well as those generated in other laboratories, illustrate how the variability of the RhD system makes it necessary to use these assays in combination. The multiplex *RhD* genotyping method developed in our laboratory detects the sequence differences between *RhD* and *RhCcEe* in exon 10 and intron 4. By serotying and genotyping the parents, there is a high probability that genetic variants will be identified. For this reason, blood samples are requested from both parents along with 10–15 mL of amniotic fluid. A portion of the blood samples are serotyped in our immunohematology reference laboratory. DNA is isolated from the blood and amniocyte samples and genotyped using DNA-based molecular testing (*see* **Note 1**).

Table 1
Discrepancies between RhD Serotyping and RhD Genotyping

Sample	Serotype	Exon 3	Intron 4	Exon 7	Exon 10
95-1724-11	RhD positive	(–)	(+)	(–)	(+)
95-0718-3	RhD positive	(–)	(+)	(–)	(+)
95-0622-1	Weak RhD positive	(–)	(+)	(+)	(+)
95-0913-4	Weak RhD positive	(+)	(–)	(+)	(+)
96-0110-10	Weak RhD positive	(–)	(–)	(–)	(+)
96-0610-1	RhD negative	(+)	(+)	(+)	(+)

2. Materials

2.1. Preparation of Samples

1. Phenol/0.1% hydroxyquinoline (saturated with 10 m*M* Tris-HCl, 1 m*M* EDTA, pH 8.0).
2. Phenol/chloroform/isoamyl alcohol (25:24:1).
3. Chloroform.
4. Proteinase K (20 mg/mL).
5. Phosphate-buffered saline (PBS).
6. 2X Lysis buffer: 20 m*M* EDTA, 20 m*M* Tris-HCl, pH 8.0, 300 m*M* NaCl, 0.4% sodium dodecyl sulfate).
7. 3 *M* Sodium acetate, pH 5.2.
8. Ethanol/70% ethanol.

2.2. Polymerase Chain Reaction

1. DNA from samples, RhD-positive and RhD-negative controls.
2. 10X PCR buffer: 200 m*M* Tris-HCl, pH 8.3, 500 m*M* KCl, 15 m*M* MgCl, 0.01% gelatin.
3. dNTP mix: 25 m*M* dATP, 25 m*M* dCTP, 25 m*M* dGTP, 25 m*M* dTTP.
4. *Taq* polymerase (5 U/µL).
5. Nanopure/MilliQ water.
6. Mineral oil.
7. Ultrapure formamide, 10% solution.
8. Oligonucleotide primers: **Table 2** lists the primers, their sequences, and the appropriate stock concentration (*see* **Note 2**).

2.3. Reagents for Agarose Electrophoresis

1. Agarose, low EEO.
2. Tris-borate EDTA (TBE) buffer.
3. Loading dye.
4. Molecular weight marker, 100-bp ladder.

Table 2
RhD Assay PCR Primers

Primer	Gene/position	Sequence	Stock conc. (μ*M*)	nmol/ OD[a]	μg/ OD[a]	Tm[b] (°C)
A1	RhCcEe exon 7, 5′ primer	5′-TGT GTT GTA ACC GAG TGC TG-3′	10	5.27	33.0	61.7
A2	RhCcEe exon 7, 3′ primer	5′-ATT GCC GTT CCA GAC AGT AT-3′	10	5.17	31.9	61.2
A3	RhD exon 10, 5′ primer	5′-TTA AGC AAA AGC ATC CAA GA-3′	15	4.77	29.6	60.7
A4	RhD exon 10, 3′ primer	5′-AAT AAA TGG TGA GAT TCT CCT C-3′	15	4.59	31.3	59.0
A9	RhD exon 4, 5′ primer	5′-ACG ATA CCC AGT TTG TCT-3′	10	5.88	32.5	53.1
A6	RhD exon 5, 3′ primer	5′-TGA CCC TGA GAT GGC TGT-3′	10	5.93	33.3	60.1

[a]The nmol/OD and μg/OD were generated by the OLIGO program. These numbers enable one to calculate the molar and microgram concentrations from the A_{260} reading. The nmol/OD × Corrected A_{260}/mL = μmol/liter.

[b]Tm is the calculated melting temperature.

2.4. Equipment

1. Centrifuge for 15- and 50-mL conical tubes.
2. Microcentrifuge.
3. Thermocylcer.
4. Agarose gel electrophoresis apparatus.

3. Methods

3.1. Preparation of DNA from Amniotic Fluid

Many kits are commercially available that allow one to successfully isolate DNA from amniotic fluid and cultured amniocytes. By growing the cells in culture, one can ensure that a reasonable number of cells is available before proceeding with the DNA isolation. However, the number of cells present in the amniotic fluid varies depending on gestation age of the fetus and the amount of fluid received. To ensure that the DNA yield and the final concentration from uncultured amniocytes is acceptable, we have opted for a manual method that maximizes recovery from preparations with a limiting number of cells (*see* **Note 3**).

1. Transfer the amniotic fluid to a sterile 15-mL conical tube and centrifuge for 30 min at 500*g* in a tabletop centrifuge. Pour the supernatant back into the original container and store at 4°C until testing is complete (*see* **Note 4**).
2. Resuspend the cell pellet in 250 µL of PBS, then add 250 µL of 2X lysis buffer, and mix well.
3. Add 2.5 µL of proteinase K solution (20 mg/mL) for a final concentration of 100 µg/mL. Mix and incubate at 70°C for 15–60 min.
4. Add 500 µL of Tris-saturated phenol/0.1% hydroxyquinoline and vortex. Centrifuge for 5–10 min in a microfuge at 12,800*g*. Transfer the top (aqueous) phase to a new tube. If necessary, the organic phase can be back-extracted with 100 µL of TE.
5. Add 500 µL of TE-saturated phenol/chloroform/isoamyl alcohol (25:24:1) and vortex. Centrifuge for 5–10 min in a microfuge at 12,800*g*. Transfer the top (aqueous) phase to a new tube.
6. Repeat **step 5**.
7. Add 500 µL of chloroform and vortex. Centrifuge for 5–10 min in a microfuge at 12,800*g*. Transfer the top (aqueous) phase to a new tube.
8. Add 1/10 vol of 3 *M* sodium acetate, pH 5.2 (~50 µL), and 2 vol of cold 95–100% ethanol. Mix and store at –20°C for >2 h.
9. Recover the nucleic acid by centrifugation at 12,800*g* for 10–15 min. Carefully pour off the ethanol.
10. Add 1 mL of cold 70% ethanol and vortex. Centrifuge at 12,800*g* for 10–15 min. Carefully pour off the ethanol. Dry the nucleic acid pellet briefly in a Speed Vac for 1 to 2 min or allow the ethanol to evaporate.
11. Resuspend the pellet in 50 µL of TE or water. Make sure the DNA is completely resuspended before determining the DNA concentration by absorbance at 260 nm.

3.2. PCR Setup

The PCR procedure selectively amplifies the *RhD* gene using two sets of sequence-specific primers. This multiplex procedure uses the difference between *RhD* and *RhCcEe* genes in the 3′ coding region of exon 10 of RhD ***(10)*** and a difference in size of intron 4 ***(7)***. Primer set A1–A4 is essentially as described by Bennett et al. ***(10)*** except the length of the primers has been increased in order to increase the melting temperature of the primers. Primers A3/A4 produce a 193-bp product that is specific for exon 10 of the *RhD* gene. Primers A1/A2 are specific for the *RhCcEe* gene and serve as the positive control for the assay. The primers produce a 129-bp product that is present in both RhD-positive and RhD-negative individuals. Primers A9/A6 amplify a 600-bp product from intron 4 of the *RhD* gene and a 1200-bp product from the *RhCcEe* gene. The RhD type is assigned based on the presence or absence of two PCR products (193 and 600 bp) that are detected by agarose gel electrophoresis and ethidium bromide staining. A variant allele can be identified by samples that have one of two PCR products or when the serotype does not match the genotype. It is preferable to genotype and serotype both parents of the fetus. This ensures that the paternal allele in the fetus is detectable in the assay and that the maternal seronegative allele is not positive in the assay.

1. Determine the number of samples (*n*) to be analyzed. The samples should include a negative control, an RhD-positive control, and an RhD-negative control (*see* **Note 5**).
2. Prepare a master mix in a microfuge tube. Multiply the volumes of each solution by (*n* + 1). For each sample, add 10 µL of 10X PCR buffer, 0.8 µL of dNTP mix, 2 µL of A1, 2 µL of A2, 10 µL of A3, 10 µL of A4, 10 µL of A6, 10 µL of A9, 10 µL of 10% formamide, and 0.5 µL of *Taq* polymerase (5 U/µL).
3. Add 66 µL of premix to each reaction tube. The remaining 34 µL of the 100-µL reaction volume is distilled H_2O (dH_2O) and DNA.
4. Add the 250–500 ng of DNA to each reaction tube. Add dH_2O to a final volume of 100 µL.
5. Overlay each tube with two drops of mineral oil and close the cap.
6. Load the samples into a Perkin-Elmer Thermal Cycler and denature at 94°C for 5 min followed by 35 cycles of 94°C for 1 min, 55°C for 1 min and 30 s, 72°C for 2 min and 30 s, and then a final extension of 72°C for 10 min (*see* **Note 6**).

3.3. Agarose Gel Electrophoretic Analysis of RhD PCR Products

1. Prepare a 2.0% TBE agarose gel containing 0.5 µg/mL of ethidium bromide. Add 3 µL of 6X loading buffer to 15 µL of each PCR product, mix, and load the total volume on the gel. Include a suitable molecular weight marker (100-bp ladder) on the gel.
2. Subject PCR products to electrophoresis for 30 min at 8 V/cm. Visualize the results by placing the gel on a UV transilluminator and document by photography.

3.4. Analysis of Results

Evaluate for the presence and size of the amplification products associated with each sample. Examples of positive and negative samples are shown in **Fig. 1** (lane 1 of each sample). The negative control should have no PCR products present. If bands are present, PCR contamination may have compromised the assay.

The 129- and the 1200-bp *RhCcEe* bands should be present in every sample except the negative control. In some samples, the 1200-bp *RhCcEe* band may be light or difficult to detect. Its presence is not necessary as long as the 129-bp *RhCcEe* positive control band is present. Variant *RhCcEe* alleles may also lack one or both of these products. Both the 600- and the 193-bp bands should be present in RhD-positive samples. However, some variant *RhD* alleles may have only one of the bands. For this reason, it is important to genotype and serotype the parents to sort out the importance of these variant alleles. The presence and absence of these specific bands should be confirmed by the RhD-negative and RhD-positive controls (*see* **Note 7**).

4. Notes

1. It is important to note that this test cannot determine zygosity of the *RhD* allele. It would be useful to know whether the father is heterozygous or homozygous for *RhD* because it would enable one to predict the probability of the fetus being RhD positive. If the father is homozygous, every fetus would be potentially at risk for HDN related to anti-D. Although it may be possible to develop a quantitative PCR assay to determine RhD zygosity, the testing and interpretation would be technically more difficult, and the presence of *RhD* allelic variants would complicate the assessment of the results.
2. Primers should be stored in Tris-buffered solutions (pH 8.0–9.0) and aliquoted to prevent repeated freeze/thaw cycles and potential PCR contamination.
3. This method can also be used to isolate DNA from blood. White cells are isolated by lysing 0.5–2.0 mL of blood with a red cell lysis buffer. The cell pellet is recovered, washed with red cell lysis buffer, and then resuspended in 250 µL of PBS. Many procedures and kits will yield high-quality DNA from blood that is suitable for this assay. Our laboratory uses the QIAamp Blood Kit.
4. The amniotic fluid should not be grossly contaminated with blood because there is a possibility that the sample will be contaminated with maternal cells. Studies in our laboratory have demonstrated that this RhD typing assay can tolerate >90% contaminating RhD-negative DNA without a false-negative fetal result ***(16)***. The extreme sensitivity of PCR-based assays is beneficial because even extensive maternal contamination of an amniotic sample, which has been shown to be infrequent, is unlikely to interfere with the detection of an incompatible allele in the fetus. Variable number tandem repeat (VNTR) analysis can be used to determine the extent of the maternal contamination. Alternatively, amniocytes cultured from the amniotic fluid should provide a source of DNA free of maternal contamination.

5. All procedures for amplification of DNA must be carried out using precautions to avoid contamination with previously amplified DNA. Isolation of DNA and PCR setup should be done in an area free of PCR products. Negative controls and extraction blanks should be used to monitor PCR contamination. Reagents should be aliquoted, and filtered plugged tips should be used to pipet DNA-containing materials.
6. Variation between PCR machines and manufacturers may require that the annealing temperature be adjusted appropriately. The A9 primer Tm of 53°C is close to the annealing of 55°C, so it may be sensitive to temperature variations.
7. It is advisable to confirm the fetal origin of DNA used for genotyping by VNTR analysis before withdrawing further monitoring or therapy in fetuses identified as being not at risk, especially if the amniotic fluid sample is bloodstained ***(16,17)***.

References

1. Liley, A. W. (1961) Liquor amnii analysis in management of pregnancy complicated by rhesus immunization. *Am. J. Obstet. Gynecol.* **82,** 1359–1371.
2. Bowman, J. M. and Pollock, J. M. (1985) Transplacental fetal hemorrhage after amniocentesis. *Obstet. Gynecol.* **66,** 749–754.
3. Cherif-Zahar, B., Mattei, M. G., Le Van Kim, C., Bailly, P., Cartron, J. P., and Colin, Y. (1991) Localization of the human Rh blood group gene structure to chromosome region 1p34.3–1p36.1 by in situ hybridization. *Hum. Genet.* **86,** 398–400.
4. Colin, Y., Cherif-Zahar, B., Le Van Kim, C., Taynal, V., Cherrier, C., and Cartron, J. P. (1991) Genetic basis of the RhD-positive and RhD-negative blood group polymorphism as determined by Southern analysis. *Blood* **78,** 2747–2752.
5. Cherif-Zahar, B., Bloy, C., Le Van Kim, C., Blanchar, D., Bailly, P., Hermand, P., Salmon, C., Cartron, J. P., and Colin, Y. (1990) Molecular cloning and primary structure of a human blood group Rh polypeptide. *Proc. Natl. Acad. Sci. USA* **87,** 6243–6247.
6. Le Van Kim, C., Mouro, I., Cherif-Zahar, B., Raynal, V., Cherrier, C., Cartron, J. P., Colin, Y. (1992) Molecular cloning and primary structure of the human blood group RhD polypeptide. *Proc. Natl. Acad. Sci. USA* **89,** 10,925–10,929.
7. Arce, M. A., Thomson, E. S., Wagner, S., Coyne, K. E., Ferdman, B. A., and Lublin, D. M. (1993) Molecular cloning of RhD cDNA derived from a gene in RhD positive, but not RhD-negative individuals. *Blood* **82,** 651–655.
8. Mouro, I., Colin, Y., Cherif-Zahar, B., Cartron, J. P., and Le Van Kim, C. (1993) Molecular genetic basis of the human Rhesus blood group system. *Nat. Genet.* **5,** 62–65.
9. Beckers, E. A. M., Faas, B. H. W., Simsek, S, Overbeeke, M. A. M., van Rhenen, D. J., Wallace, M., von dem Borne, A. E., and van der Schoot, C. E. (1996) The genetic basis of a new partial D antigen: D^{DBT}. *Br. J. Haematol.* **93,** 720–727.

10. Bennett, P. R., Le Van Kim, C., Colin, Y., Warwick, R. M., Cherif-Zahar, B., Fisk, N. M., and Cartron, J. P. (1993) Prenatal determination of RhD type by DNA amplification. *N. Engl. J. Med.* **329,** 607–610.
11. Wolter, L. C., Hyland, C. A., and Saul, A. (1993) Rhesus D genotyping using the polymerase chain reaction. *Blood* **85,** 1682.
12. Simsek, S., Faas, R. H. W., Bleeker, P. M. M, Overbeeke, M. A. M., Cuijpers, H. T. M., van der Schoot, C. E., and von dem Borne, A. E. (1995) Rapid RhD genotyping by polymerase chain reaction-based amplification of DNA. *Blood* **85,** 2975–2980.
13. Mouro, I., Le Van Kim, C., Rouillac, C., van Rhenen, D. J., Le Pennec, P. Y., Bailly, P., Cartron, J. P., and Colin, Y. (1994) Rearrangements of the blood group *RhD* gene associated with the D(VI) category phenotype. *Blood* **83,** 1129–1135.
14. Okuda, H., Kawano, M., Iwamoto, S., Tanaka, M., Seno, T., Okubo, Y., and Kajii, E. (1997) The *RHD* gene is highly detectable in RhD-negative Japanese donors. *J. Clin. Invest.* **100,** 373–379.
15. Aubin, J.-T., Le Van Kim, C., Mouro, I., Colin, Y., Bignozzi, C., Brossard, Y., and Cartron, J.-P. (1997) Specificity and sensitivity of RHD genotyping methods by PCR-based DNA amplification. *Br. J. Haematol.* **98,** 356–364.
16. Hessner, M. J., Agostini, T. A., Bellissimo, D. B., Endean, D. J., Pircon, R. A., and Kirschbaum, N. E. (1997) The sensitivity of allele-specific polymerase chain reaction can obviate concern of maternal contamination when fetal samples are genotyped for immune cytopenic disorders. *Am. J. Obstet. Gynecol.* **176,** 327–333.
17. Denomme, G. A., Waye, J., Burrows, R. F., Hayward, C. P. M., Warkentin, T. E., Horsewood, P., Smith, J. W., Jelsema, R. D., Zuidema, L. J., and Kelton, J. G. (1995) The prenatal identification of fetal compatibility in neonatal alloimmune thrombocytopenia using amniotic fluid and variable number of tandem repeat (VNTR) analysis. *Br. J. Haematol.* **91,** 742–746.

33

Molecular Diagnosis of Hereditary Hemochromatosis

Suzanne Huber and Karl V. Voelkerding

1. Introduction

Hereditary hemochromatosis (HH) is an autosomal recessive disorder of iron metabolism with a frequency of homozygosity in the Caucasian population of 1 in 200–400. The pathophysiologic hallmark of HH is chronic, increased absorption of dietary iron beyond that required for normal iron homeostasis. The excess absorption leads to progressive iron accumulation in parenchymal cells that can manifest in adulthood as multiple end-organ damage *(1)*. In 1996, the gene responsible for the majority of cases of HH was identified. Designated *HFE*, the HH gene resides on the short arm of chromosome 6 telomeric of the major histocompatibility complex (MHC) and encodes a 343 amino acid protein (HFE) that shares sequence and structural homology to class I MHC proteins. Approximately 85% of unrelated HH patients are homozygous for a point mutation involving a G to A change at nucleotide 845 in the *HFE* cDNA sequence (G845A) that converts cysteine, at amino acid position 282, to tyrosine (Cys282Tyr or C282Y) *(2)*.

It is now known that the HFE protein is transported to the cell surface in association with β_2-microglobulin (β_2M) *(3,4)*. At the cell surface, HFE binds to transferrin receptors (TfRs) and appears to decrease TfR affinity for circulating iron-bound transferrin *(5–8)*. The Cys282Tyr mutation disrupts a disulfide bond in the α-3 domain of the HFE protein that is critical for proper protein folding and association with β_2M. HFE protein harboring Cys282Tyr has a reduced ability to associate with β_2M and undergoes accelerated intracellular degradation with a concomitant loss in cell surface expression *(4)*. While fur-

From: *Methods in Molecular Medicine, vol. 49: Molecular Pathology Protocols*
Edited by: A. A. Killeen © Humana Press Inc., Totowa, NJ

ther investigations are needed to more fully elucidate HFE function, confirmation of HFE's participation in iron metabolism has come from the demonstration that homozygous deletion of the *HFE* homolog in mice results in iron overload ***(9)***. Most recently, a mouse model of homozygous Cys282Tyr mutation has been shown to exhibit iron overload, albeit not as severe as that observed in mice with homozygous *HFE* deletion ***(10)***.

In the original report on the identification of *HFE*, a second mutation in *HFE*, involving a C to G change at nucleotide 187 of the cDNA sequence (C187G), was described ***(2)***. C187G results in the substitution of histidine, at amino acid position 63, with aspartic acid (His63Asp or H63D). A subset of patients with iron overload exists who are either compound heterozygotes (Cys282Tyr/His63Asp) or homozygous for His63Asp. The contribution of His63Asp to HH remains, in part, controversial. The His63Asp mutation does not affect HFE association with β_2M, cell surface expression, or binding to TfR ***(4)***. However, functional evidence supporting a pathologic role for His63Asp in HH comes from the observation that HFE protein harboring His63Asp has a reduced ability to decrease TfR affinity for iron-bound transferrin ***(6)***. A third mutation in *HFE* has been reported in a single patient with iron overload who is a compound heterozygote for Cys282Tyr and a novel splice site mutation (IVS3 + 1G→T). The location of this mutation predicts that mRNA splicing would be altered, resulting in the skipping of exon 3 in *HFE* ***(11)***.

Mutation analysis in *HFE* is increasingly being employed in the diagnostic evaluation of patients with iron overload. A variety of technical approaches are being utilized, and in the following sections, we present polymerase chain reaction (PCR)-based methodology for the detection of Cys282Tyr and His63Asp. The principle of this diagnostic approach is based on PCR amplification of two regions of the *HFE* genomic sequence that contain the nucleotides G845 and C187 of the corresponding cDNA. The G845A (Cys282Tyr) mutation creates an *Rsa*I restriction endonuclease recognition site, and the C187G (His63Asp) mutation results in loss of an *Mbo*I restriction endonuclease recognition site. Amplification followed by restriction endonuclease digestion and gel electrophoresis allows assignment of genotype by restriction fragment length polymorphism (RFLP).

2. Materials (*see* Note 1)

2.1. Preparation of DNA

1. ACE shocking buffer: 0.15 *M* NH_4Cl, 2.8 m*M* EDTA trisodium salt, 0.7 m*M* KH_2PO_2. Store at 4°C for up to 6 mo.
2. Phosphate-buffered saline (PBS) without Ca^{2+} and Mg^{2+}. (Gibco-BRL, Grand Island, NY). Store at 4°C for up to 6 mo.

3. Cell lysis buffer: 10 m*M* Tris-HCl, pH 8.0, 10 m*M* EDTA, pH 8.0, 50 m*M* NaCl. Store at 4°C for up to 6 mo.
4. Proteinase K (20 mg/mL) (Sigma, St. Louis, MO). Aliquot in small volumes and store at –20°C for up to 1 yr.
5. 20% Sodium dodecyl sulfate (SDS).
6. NaCl, saturated (6 *M*).
7. 100% Ethanol.
8. MilliQ purified and autoclaved water (dH_2O).

2.2. PCR Amplification

1. 10X Gene Amp Buffer II (Perkin-Elmer, Branchburg, NJ): 500 m*M* KCl, 100 m*M* Tris-HCl, pH 8.3. Store at –20°C.
2. Gene Amp 25 m*M* $MgCl_2$. Store at –20°C.
3. 100X dNTP mix (Promega, Madison, WI): 20 m*M* dATP, 20 m*M* dCTP, 20 m*M* dGTP, 20 m*M* dTTP in dH_2O. Aliquot in small volumes, store at –20°C for up to 6 mo, and avoid multiple freeze/thaws.
4. Ampli*Taq* Gold™ DNA polymerase (5 U/μL) (Perkin-Elmer). Store at –20°C.
5. Primers for detection of Cys282Tyr mutation (*see* **Note 2** and **Note 10**):
   a. Forward primer (A): 5′-TGG CAA GGG TAA ACA GAT CC-3′.
   b. Reverse primer (B): 5′-CTC AGG CAC TCC TCT CAA CC-3′.

   Primers for detection of His63Asp mutation (*see* **Note 3**):
   a. Forward primer (C): 5′-ACA TGG TTA AGG CCT GTT GC-3′.
   b. Reverse primer (D): 5′-GCC ACA TCT GGC TTG AAA TT-3′.

   Dilute all primers to a concentration of 60 μ*M* in dH_20. Aliquot in small volumes, store at –20°C for up to 1 yr, and avoid multiple freeze/thaws. Lyophilized or concentrated stocks of primers can be stored indefinitely.
6. MilliQ purified and autoclaved water (dH_2O).

2.3. Restriction Endonuclease Digestion

1. *Rsa*I restriction endonuclease and its accompanying buffer (Promega).
2. *Mbo*I restriction endonuclease and its accompanying buffer (Promega).

2.4. Polyacrylamide Gel Electrophoresis

1. 40% acrylamide stock (Bio-Rad, Hercules, CA): 19:1 acrylamide: *N,N′* methylene *bis*-acrylamide in 1X Tris-borate EDTA (TBE). This solution is light sensitive and has a shelf life of 6 mo. Store at 4°C. Acrylamide is a neurotoxin, and therefore, gloves and masks should be worn during preparation and handling. Unused acrylamide should be polymerized prior to disposal.
2. 10% (w/v) ammonium persulfate in dH_2O. Store ammonium persulfate powder (Bio-Rad) at 4°C in a desiccator. Make 10% (w/v) solution in dH_2O just prior to use.
3. TEMED (Bio-Rad). This solution is light sensitive. Store in desiccator at room temperature.
4. 5X TBE: 0.89 *M* Tris-base, 0.89 *M* boric acid, 0.02 *M* EDTA. Store at room temperature for up to 1 yr.

5. Ethidium bromide (EtBr): 1X solution of 10,000X stock (10 mg/mL) in TBE. Store protected from light at room temperature for up to 1 wk.
6. 6X Loading and tracking dye: 0.25% bromophenol blue, 30% glycerol in dH_2O. Store at 4°C for up to 24 mo.
7. Molecular weight markers (Research Genetics, Huntsville, AL): 50- to 1000-bp ladder with 6X tracking and loading dye. Store at 4°C for up to 1 yr.

3. Methods

The following procedure describes the techniques required to detect both the Cys282Tyr and the His63Asp mutations in the *HFE* gene. Briefly, DNA is prepared from buffy coat, regions of exon 2 and exon 4 are amplified using PCR, amplicons are subjected to restriction endonuclease digestion and the products of digestion are separated by polyacrylamide gel electrophoresis.

3.1. Preparation of DNA from Buffy Coat (see Note 4*)*

1. Collect 3–5 mL of whole blood in EDTA anticoagulant. One milliliter is the minimum volume.
2. Spin blood at 1000*g* for 15 min to obtain the buffy coat. Remove the buffy coat to 15 mL conical and suspend in 10 mL of ACE shocking buffer to achieve red blood cell lysis. Gently mix on a rocker for 10 min at room temperature.
3. Spin at 1000*g* to pellet leukocytes. Discard the supernatant, resuspend the cells, and wash with 10 mL of PBS without Ca^{2+} and Mg^{2+}.
4. Lyse the cell pellet by resuspending with 3 mL of lysis buffer followed by 20% SDS to a final concentration of 0.2% (30 µL of 20% SDS in 3 mL of lysis buffer). Mix well.
5. Add proteinase K (20 mg/mL) to a final concentration of 450 µg/mL (67.5 µL). Mix well and incubate at 60°C for 2 h or overnight at 42°C .
6. Add saturated NaCl to the sample at a ratio of 1:3 (1 mL of saturated NaCl to 3 mL of digested sample).
7. Shake the capped sample vigorously for 30 s; the sample will foam. Allow to sit at room temperature for 5 min.
8. Spin at 1500*g* at room temperature for 20 min. Immediately remove the supernatant to a clean 15-mL conical tube. Do not disturb the precipitate.
9. Add 2 vol of 100% ethanol to the supernatant and invert gently to precipitate the DNA. Using a pipet tip, spool out the DNA and transfer to a 1.5-mL microcentrifuge tube. Pulse spin at 14,000*g* and draw off the residual alcohol with a pipet. Allow the DNA pellet to air-dry at room temperature.
10. Resolubilize the DNA in 400 µL dH_2O. Incubate at 42°C for 2 h to overnight.
11. Quantitate the DNA by spectrophotometry or fluorimetry.

3.2. Polymerase Chain Reaction (see Note 5*)*

1. Prepare two separate mixes, i.e., one for detection of the Cys282Tyr mutation and one for the detection of the His63Asp mutation (*see* **Figs. 1–3**). Primer pairs are the only difference in the two mixes.

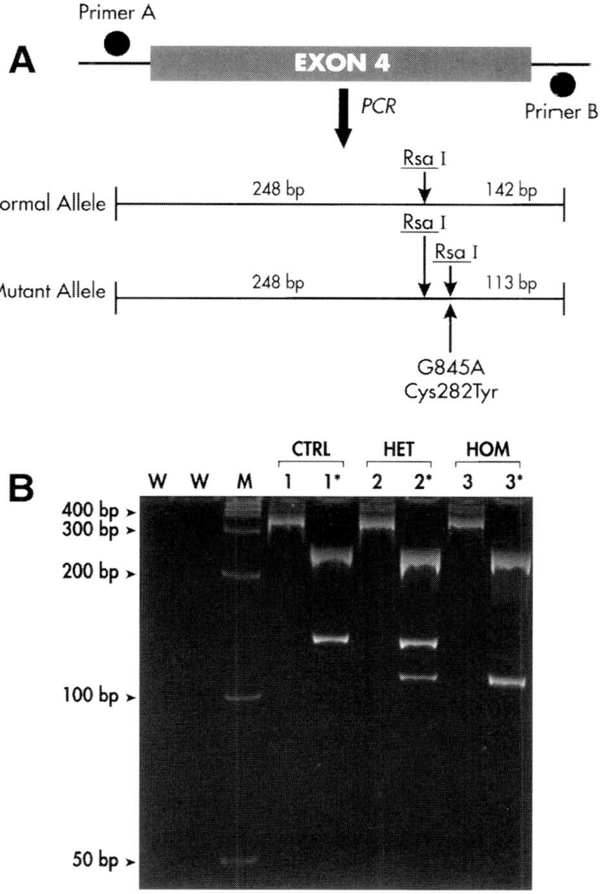

Fig. 1. PCR RFLP detection of Cys282Tyr in *HFE*. **(A)** Schematic of the 390-bp amplicon of *HFE* encompassing exon 4 and nucleotide 845 (cDNA sequence). Primers A and B are located in flanking intron sequences. The G845A mutation generates a new *Rsa*I recognition site as shown in the mutant allele. **(B)** Photograph of EtBr-stained 12.5% polyacrylamide gel demonstrating PCR RFLP analyis for Cys282Tyr in *HFE*. W, water (reagent) controls; M, molecular weight markers. Lanes 1, 2, and 3 show undigested 390-bp amplicons from wild-type (CTRL), heterozygous mutant (HET), and homozygous mutant (HOM) individuals. Lanes 1*, 2*, and 3* show*Rsa*I digestion products from the 390-bp amplicons shown in lanes 1, 2, and 3, respectively. *Rsa*I digestion of a wild-type allele yields fragments of 248 and 142 bp. *Rsa*I digestion of a mutant allele yields fragments of 248, 113, and 29 bp (the 29-bp fragment is not shown).

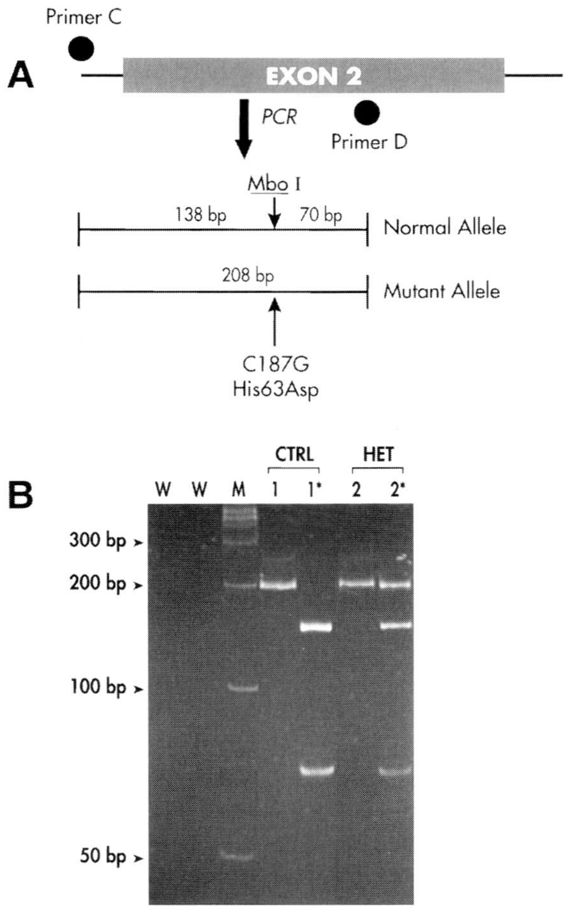

Fig. 2. PCR RFLP detection of His63Asp in *HFE*. **(A)** Schematic of the 208-bp amplicon of *HFE* encompassing a portion of exon 2 and nucleotide 187 (cDNA sequence). Primer C is located in intron 1 and primer D is located in exon 2. The C187G mutation results in loss of an *Mbo*I recognition site, as shown in the mutant allele. **(B)** Photograph of EtBr-stained 12.5% polyacrylamide gel demonstrating PCR RFLP analyis for His63Asp in *HFE*. W, water (reagent) controls; M, molecular weight markers. Lanes 1 and 2 show undigested 208-bp amplicons from wild-type (CTRL) and heterozygous mutant (HET) individuals. Lanes 1* and 2* show *Mbo*I digestion products from the 208-bp amplicons shown in lanes 1 and 2, respectively. *Mbo*I digestion of a wild-type allele yields fragments of 138 and 70 bp. *Mbo*I digestion of a mutant allele yields a 208-bp fragment.

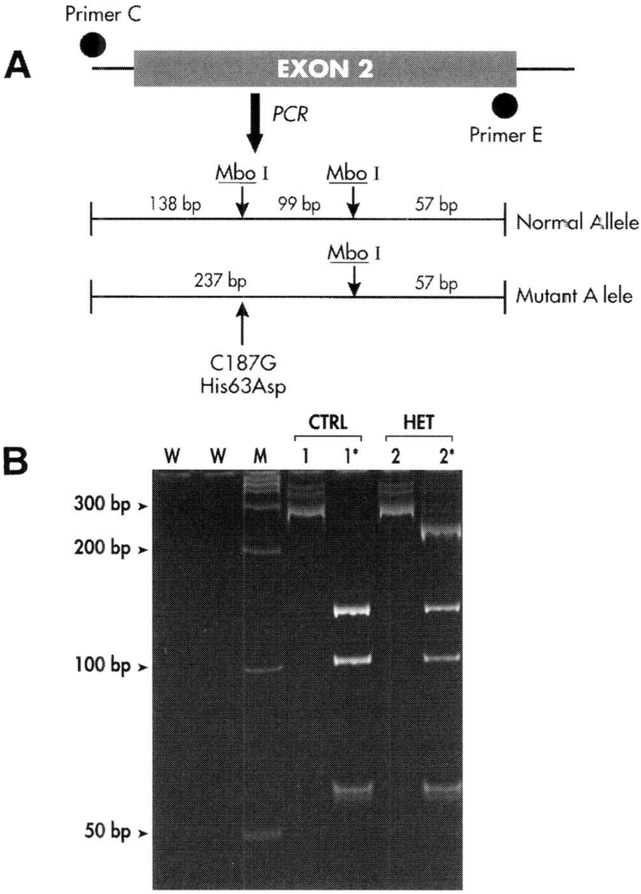

Fig. 3. Modified PCR RFLP detection of His63Asp in *HFE*. **(A)** Schematic of the 294-bp amplicon of *HFE* encompassing the majority of exon 2 and nucleotide 187 (cDNA sequence). Primer C is located in intron 1 and primer E is located in exon 2. The 294-bp amplicon contains two *Mbo*I sites, one of which serves as an internal control for digestion, and the other is lost as a result of C187G mutation, as shown in the mutant allele. **(B)** Photograph of EtBr-stained 12.5% polyacrylamide gel demonstrating the modified PCR RFLP analysis for His63Asp in *HFE*. W, water (reagent) controls; M, molecular weight markers. Lanes 1 and 2 show undigested 294-bp amplicons from wild-type (CTRL) and heterozygous mutant (HET) individuals. Lanes 1* and 2* show *Mbo*I digestion products from the 294-bp amplicons shown in lanes 1 and 2, respectively. *Mbo*I digestion of a wild-type allele yields fragments of 138, 99, and 57 bp. *Mbo*I digestion of a mutant allele yields fragments of 237 and 57 bp.

2. Prepare sufficient reaction mixes to include all test samples, two genotype controls—wild type and heterozygote (*see* **Note 6**)—and water controls. Prepare mix as described in **Table 1**. Multiply the volume/reaction by the number of reactions needed + 1 (n + 1).
3. Program the thermocycler to carry out a 10-min enzyme activation step at 95°C followed by 35 cycles of 94°C for 1 min, 53°C for 1 min, and 72°C for 1 min. Cool the reaction to 4°C.

3.3. Restriction Endonuclease Digestion (*see* Note 7)

1. Two separate digestion mixes (an *Rsa*I and an *Mbo*I) are required for each specimen. Prepare digestion mixes as follows: 26 µL of PCR products, 3 µL of 10X enzyme buffer, 1 µL of restriction enzyme (10 U/µL).
2. Incubate at 37°C for a minimum of 2 h. Digests can be incubated overnight.

3.4. Polyacrylamide Gel Electrophoresis (*see* Note 8)

1. Digested and undigested PCR products are analyzed on a 14 cm × 16 cm × 1.5 mm, 12.5% polyacrylamide gel containing 19:1 acrylamide: *N,N′*methylene *bis*-acrylamide. Prepare the gel by mixing 14 mL of 40% acrylamide:*bis*-acrylamide (19:1) and 31 mL of 1X TBE. To catalyze polymerization, add 315 µL of freshly prepared 10% (w/v) ammonium persulfate and 16 µL TEMED and swirl to mix well. A 15- or 20-tooth comb can be used and is inserted immediately after pouring the gel. Allow 45 min for the gel to polymerize.
2. Fill the electrophoresis tank with 1X TBE and position the gels firmly in the apparatus. Rinse each well completely with 1X TBE to remove traces of unpolymerized acrylamide.
3. Load two lanes for each sample. In the first lane, load 15 µL of undigested product mixed with 3 µL of 6X tracking dye. In the second lane, load 25 µL of digest mixed with 4 µL of 6X tracking dye. Load a molecular weight marker containing fragments ranging from 50 to 1000 bp and tracking dye (bromophenol blue). Run the gel for 550 V-h. At the end of the run, bromophenol blue will have run off the gel (*see* **Note 9**).
4. When the run is completed, stain the gel in a 1X solution of EtBr in TBE for 15 min. Rinse in distilled water for 10 min. The gel can then be analyzed using UV transillumination.

3.5. Interpretation of Results

Specimens are determined to be wild type, heterozygous mutant, or homozygous mutant based on amplicon fragment sizes following restriction enzyme digestion. **Figures 1–3** contain schematics that illustrate the locations and sizes of restriction fragments in normal and mutant alleles. Photographs in **Figs. 1–3** of EtBr-stained, 12.5% polyacrylamide gels show those fragments necessary for assignment of genotypes.

Table 1
Reaction Mix Preparation

Reagent	Volume/Reaction (µL)	Final Concentration
10X PCR Buffer II	10	1X
100X dNTPs	1	0.2 m*M*
Forward primer (60 pmol/µL)	1	0.6 µ*M*
Reverse primer (60 pmol/µL)	1	0.6 µ*M*
$MgCl_2$ (25 m*M*)	6	1.5 m*M*
Ampli*Taq* Gold (5 U/µL)	0.5	2.5 U
H_2O	70.5	—
DNA (20 ng/µL)	10	200 ng

4. Notes

1. Temperatures and expiration dates critical to reagent performance are listed in **Subheading 2.** Other reagents are stored at room temperature for up to 1 yr or according to the manufacturer's instructions.
2. All primer sequences can be found in GenBank (www.ncbi.nlm.nih.gov/entrez/nucleotide.html) using the accession Z92910, *HFE* gene (Albig et al., GenBank). Primer locations: Cys262Tyr primers to amplify a 390-bp fragment are nucleotides 6443–6462 (forward primer A) and 6813–6832 (reverse primer B). His63Asp primers to amplify a 208-bp fragment are nucleotides 4521–4640 (forward primer C) and 4809–4828 (reverse primer D).
3. The primer pair for the detection of His63Asp mutation generates a fragment that in the wild-type allele contains a single *Mbo*I recognition site at nucleotides 4759–4762. The mutant allele lacks this site. Failed or incomplete digestion by *Mbo*I could lead to a false-positive result. To address this limitation Merryweather-Clarke et al. ***(12)*** redesigned the reverse His63Asp primer to amplify a 294-bp fragment rather than a 208-bp fragment. The primer pair is as follows:
   a. Forward (C): 5′-ACA TGG TTA AGG CCT GTT GC-3′.
   b. Reverse (E): 5′-CTT GCT GTG GTT GTG ATT TTC C-3′.

   The additional 86-bp fragment contains a second *Mbo*I site that serves as an internal control for digestion preventing misdiagnosis owing to incomplete or failed digestion. Primers can be found in GenBank Z92910. Forward primer C corresponds to nucleotides 4621–4640 and reverse primer E corresponds to nucleotides 4893–4914.
4. Blood collected in sodium citrate anticoagulant is an acceptable sample, but heparinized blood should be avoided because it may inhibit PCR. Several DNA preparation kits are available commercially and can be used to recover DNA for use in PCR. Two that have performed well and with consistency are the QIAamp

Blood Kit (Qiagen, Santa Clarita, CA) and the MasterPure™ Genomic DNA Purification Kit (Epicentre Technologies, Madison WI). Purified DNA should have a 260:280 ratio of 1.7 or greater with a minimal recovery of 5 μg of DNA.

5. The following precautions should be taken to prevent contamination of the PCR:
   a. Provide physically separate areas for PCR setup (clean) and product analysis.
   b. Place dedicated equipment in each area.
   c. Wear gloves and change them frequently.
   d. Aliquot and store PCR reagents in small volumes in a clean area, isolated from patient and control samples.
   e. Use aerosol barrier tips for pipeting.
   f. Use disposable tubes and containers when possible.
   g. Wipe all surfaces with 10% bleach after use.
   h. Before and after use, illuminate surfaces with UV light for 15 min when possible.
6. Cell lines have been developed from known HFE genotype patients (Voelkerding, K. V., Borcherding, W., and Huber, S., unpublished data). DNA is extracted from these cells and used as wild-type and heterozygote controls. Alternatively, samples that have been validated by interlaboratory testing can be used as controls.
7. Wang et al. ***(13)*** have described the use of *Dpn*II, an isoschizomer of *Mbo*I, in the analysis of H63D. *Dpn*II yields a robust and reproducible digestion of the PCR product using 1 U of enzyme for only 20–30 min. The cost of *Dpn*II is as low as one fifth that of *Mbo*I ***(13)***.
8. Products of digestion can be analyzed using a 20 cm × 12.5 cm × 8 mm 2.5% NuSieve (3:1) agarose gel run for 325 V-h. These gels are more costly to run than polyacrylamide gels, and difficulty may be encountered in interpreting the heterozygous mutant in which fragments may appear more faint.
9. A single, empty lane on each gel can be loaded with tracking dye made of bromophenol blue and xylene cyanol (0.25% bromophenol blue, 0.25% xylene cyanol, 30% glycerol in dH_2O) to follow the gel run. When the 12.5% polyacrylamide gel has run for 550 V-h, the bromophenol blue will have run off the gel and xylene cyanol will have migrated 13 cm into the gel.
10. During the publication of this manuscript, a single nucleotide polymorphism in intron 4 of HFE was identified located in the binding region of the reverse primer ***(14)***. Under some PCR conditions, the polymorphism may result in a loss of allele amplification. To avoid this complication, a new reverse primer is recommended with the sequence 5′-TACCTCCTCAGGCACTCCTC-3′. Use of the new reverse primer generates different amplicon and Rsa1 digestion products as described ***(14)***.

References

1. Bonkovsky, H. L., Ponka, P., Bacon, B. R., Drysdale, J., Grace, N. D., and Tavill, A. S. (1996) An update on iron metabolism: summary of the fifth international conference on disorders of iron metabolism. *Hepatology* **24,** 718–729.

2. Feder, J.N., Gnirke, A., Thomas, W., et al. (1996) A novel MHC class I–like gene is mutated in patients with hereditary hemochromatosis. *Nat. Genetics* **13,** 399–408.
3. Feder, J. N., Tsuchihashi, Z., Irrinki, A., Lee, V. K., Mapa, F. A., Morikang, E., Prass, C. E., Starnes, S. M., Wolff, R. K., Parkkila, S., Sly, W. S., and Schatzman, R. C. (1997) The hemochromatosis founder mutation in HLA-H disrupts β_2-microglobulin interaction and cell surface expression. *J. Biol. Chem.* **272,** 14,025–14,028.
4. Waheed, A., Parkkila, S., Zhou, X. Y., Tomatsu, S., Tsuchihashi, Z., Feder, J. N., Schatzman, R. C., Britton, R. S., Bacon, B. R., and Sly, W. S. (1997) Hereditary hemochromatosis: effects of C282Y and H63D mutations on association with β_2-microglobulin, intracellular processing, and cell surface expression of the HFE protein in COS-7 cells. *Proc. Natl. Acad. Sci. USA* **94,** 12,384–12,389.
5. Parkilla, S., Waheed, A., Britton, R. S., Bacon, B. R., Zhou, X. Y., Tomatsu, S., Fleming, R. E., and Sly, W. S. (1997) Association of the transferrin receptor in human placenta with HFE, the protein defective in hereditary hemochromatosis. *Proc. Natl. Acad. Sci. USA* **94,** 13,198–13,202.
6. Feder, J. N., Penny, D. M., Irrinki, A., Lee, V. K., Lebron, J. A., Watson, N., Tsuchihashi, Z., Sigal, E., Bjorkman, P. J., and Schatzman, R. C. (1998) The hemochromatosis gene product complexes with the transferrin receptor and lowers its affinity for ligand binding. *Proc. Natl. Acad. Sci. USA* **95,** 1472–1477.
7. Gross, C. N., Irrinki, A., Feder, J. N., and Enns, C. A. (1998) Co-trafficking of HFE, a nonclassical major histocompatibility complex class I protein, with the transferrin receptor implies a role in intracellular iron regulation *J. Biol. Chem.* **273,** 22,068–22,074.
8. Lebron, J. A., Bennet, M. J., Vaughn, D. E., Chirino, A. J., Snow, P. M., Mintier, G. A., Feder, J. N., and Bjorkman, P. J. (1998) Crystal structure of the hemochromatosis protein HFE and characterization of its interaction with transferrin receptor. *Cell* **93,** 111–123.
9. Zhou, X. Y., Tomatsu, S., Fleming, R. E., Parkilla, S., Waheed, A., Jiang, J., Fei, Y., Brunt, E. M., Ruddy, D. A., Prass, C. E., Schatzman, R. C., O'Neill, R., Britton, R. S., Bacon, B. R., and Sly, W. S. (1998) HFE gene knockout produces a model of hereditary hemochromatosis. *Proc. Natl. Acad. Sci. USA* **95,** 2492–2497.
10. Levy, J. E., Montross, L. K., Cohen, D. E., and Andrews, N. C. (1999) The C282Y mutation causing hereditary hemochromatosis does not produce a null allele. *Blood* **94,** 9–11.
11. Wallace, D. F., Partridge, J., Dooley, J. S., and Walker, A. P., (1998) Classical phenotype of genetic haemochromatosis in a Cys282Tyr heterozygote due to compound heterozygosity with a novel splice site mutation. *Hepatology* **28(4)(Suppl. Pt. 2),** 526A.
12. Merryweather-Clarke, A. T., Shearman, J. D., Robson, K. J. H., Pointon, J. J., Liu, Y. T., Bomford, A., Dooley, J., Walker, A. P., and Worwood, M. (1998) Hemochromatosis related mutation detection. *Blood* **91,** 2620–2621.

13. Wang, Y. L., Chen, Z., Urmacher, J., and Kant, J. A. (1998) Enhanced detection of HFE H63D using restriction enzyme *Dpn* II. *Am. J. Pathol.* **153(5),** 1649 (abstract G9).
14. Jeffrey, G. P., Chakrabarti, S., Hegele, R. A., and Adams, P. C. (1999) Polymorphism in intron 4 of HFE may cause overestimation of C282Y homozygous prevalence in haemochromatosis. *Nat. Genet.* **22,** 325,326.

34

Genotyping of Apolipoprotein E

I. Cetin Ozturk, Nahida Akel, and Anthony A. Killeen

1. Introduction

Apolipoprotein E (apo E) is a 299-amino acid plasma protein involved in cholesterol transport and is found in chylomicrons, very low density lipoprotein, intermediate-density lipoprotein, and high-density lipoprotein *(1,2)*.

Apo E plays an important role in the metabolism of these lipoproteins by binding to the low-density lipoprotein (LDL) receptor in hepatic and extrahepatic tissues and a putative apo E receptor or LDL receptor-related protein. Apo E is synthesized predominantly in the liver and intestine but is also expressed in significant amounts in the brain, where apo E is the major mediator of cholesterol and lipid transport and plays an important role in membrane maintenance and repair. Apo E is the primary apolipoprotein in the brain, produced by astrocytes and oligodendrocytes. It is also produced in the adrenal gland and kidney.

The apolipoprotein is encoded by a 4 exon gene located on the long arm of chromosome 19 *(3)*. The *APOE* gene spans approx 3.7 kb and has been cloned and sequenced *(3,4)*. Like other apolipoprotein genes, it consists of four exons separated by three introns, with most of the protein-coding sequence contained in exon 4. The length of the mRNA is approx 1100 nucleotides. The expression of the *APOE* gene is regulated by multiple positive and negative elements within its promoter region *(3,5)*.

The polymorphic nature of *APOE* was first described 20 yr ago, and three common isoforms—E2, E3, and E4—are recognized. These are encoded by three common alleles—ε2, ε3, and ε4—that are expressed codominantly, generating six possible phenotypes—E2/2, E2/3, E2/4, E3/3, E3/4, and E4/4 *(2,6,7)*. E3 is the most common form in all populations studied. In typical

From: *Methods in Molecular Medicine, vol. 49: Molecular Pathology Protocols*
Edited by: A. A. Killeen © Humana Press Inc., Totowa, NJ

Table 1
Amino Acids Found at Residues 112 and 158

	Codon	
Isoform	112	158
E2	Cys	Cys
E3	Cys	Arg
E4	Arg	Arg

Caucasian populations, ε3 is the most common allele, occurring in more than 75% of chromosomes. The average frequencies of ε2 and ε4 are 8 and 15%, respectively *(2)*.

The ε4 allele is a dose-dependent risk factor for Alzheimer's disease. It is also associated with higher total serum cholesterol and LDL cholesterol levels and with increased risks of atherosclerosis and ischemic heart disease *(7)*. One to two percent of E2/E2 individuals develop a particular form of hyperlipidemia called type III hyperlipidemia. In addition to the common E2 variant, several other rare variants of apo E that bind defectively to the LDL receptor have been identified that are associated with type III hyperlipoproteinemia. The prevalence of type III hyperlipoproteinemia in the general population is approx 1 in 10,000. Therefore, genetic and environmental secondary factors are required for the full expression of the phenotype in susceptible persons with the E2/E2 genotype *(3,7)*.

The three isoforms can be distinguished by their charge by isoelectric focusing in polyacrylamide gels in a pH gradient. E4 is the most positively charged and E2 is the most negatively charged isoform. These three isoforms differ by amino acid substitution at 2 codons, 118 and 158 *(8)*. **Table 1** gives the amino acids found at these positions.

Because of the ease and accessibility of polymerase chain reaction (PCR)-based methods for genotyping *APOE*, these methods have largely replaced isoelectric focusing. It should be borne in mind, however, that most genotyping methods that involve PCR and restriction enzyme digestion test only the two polymorphic codons, and any other restriction sites for the enzyme within the PCR product. Thus, rare variants that might be recognized by protein isoelectric focusing may be misclassified. We use the method described in **ref.** ***9*** with minor modifications.

2. Materials

2.1. DNA Isolation

Any isolation method that yields DNA in suitable quantity and quality for PCR amplification is acceptable. Our laboratory uses the Puregene kit from

Gentra Systems (Minneapolis, MN), which is a method that does not involve the use of phenol/chloroform. These kits contain proprietary reagents as follows ***(1–4)***:

1. Red blood cell lysis solution.
2. Cell lysis solution.
3. Protein precipitation solution.
4. DNA hydration solution.
5. Isopropanol (not a component of the Puregene kit).

2.2. Polymerase Chain Reaction

1. 10X PCR Buffer (200 m*M* Tris-HCl, pH 8.4, 500 m*M* KCl).
2. *Taq* Polymerase (5 U/µL) (Perkin-Elmer).
3. 25 m*M* $MgCl_2$.
4. 10 µ*M* apo E-5′ primer: 5′ TAA-GCT-TGG-CAC-GGC-TGT-CCA-AGG-A 3′.
5. 10 µ*M* apo E-AT3′ primer: 5′ ATA-AAT-ATA-AAA-TAT-AAA-TAA-CAG-AAT-TCG-CCC-CGG-CCT-GGT-ACA-C 3′.
6. 10 m*M* dNTPs.
7. 100% Dimethyl sulfoxide (DMSO).
8. Double-distilled H_2O (ddH2O).

2.3. Restriction Enzyme Digestion

1. *Cfo*I (10 U/µL (Gibco-BRL).
2. Manufacturer's restriction buffer (50 m*M* Tris-HCl, pH 8.0, 10 m*M* $MgCl_2$).

2.4. Analysis of Digested PCR Products (Detection of Restriction Fragments)

1. 3% MetaPhor agarose (FMC Products, Rockland, ME) in 0.5X Tris-borate EDTA (TBE) buffer.
2. 0.5X TBE electrophoresis buffer: 0.05 *M* Tris, 0.045 *M* boric acid, 0.0005 *M* EDTA, pH 8.4 (prepared from 10X stock solution from Life Technologies, Gaithersburg, MD).
3. 10X Loading buffer: 25 g of Ficoll and 0.42 g of bromophenol blue in 100 mL of sterile water.
4. Phi X 174/ *Hae*III molecular weight markers (Life Technologies or equivalent).
5. Ethidium bromide (10 mg/mL).

2.5. Equipment

1. Thermocycler.
2. Spectrophotometer, with UV capability.
3. Agarose gel-running apparatus.
4. Centrifuge.

3. Methods

3.1. DNA Isolation from Whole Blood and Quantitation of DNA Yield

This protocol is for the Puregene kit from Gentra Systems.

3.1.1. Cell Lysis

1. Collect 300 µL of whole blood samples in EDTA anticoagulant tubes (*see* **Note 1**).
2. Add 300 µL of whole blood to a 1.5-mL microfuge tube containing 900 µL of red cell lysis solution. Incubate for 1 min at ambient temperature; invert gently 10 times during the incubation.
3. Centrifuge for 20 s at 13,000–16,000*g*. Remove as much supernatant as possible with a pipet, leaving behind the visible white cell pellet and about 10–20 µL of residual liquid.
4. Vortex the tube vigorously for 10 s to resuspend the white cells in the residual liquid.
5. Add 300 µL of cell lysis solution to the resuspended cells and pipet up and down to lyse the cells. Samples are stable in cell lysis solution for at least 18 mo at room temperature.

3.1.2. Protein Precipitation

1. Add 100 µL of protein precipitation solution to the cell lysate.
2. Vortex vigorously at high speed for 20 s to mix the protein precipitation solution uniformly with the cell lysate.
3. Centrifuge at 13,000–16,000*g* for 1 min. The precipitated proteins should form a tight, dark brown pellet. If the protein pellet is not tight, repeat **step 2**, followed by incubation on ice for 5 min and then repeat **step 3**.

3.1.3. DNA Precipitation

1. Pour the supernatant containing the DNA into a clean 1.5-mL microfuge tube containing 300 µL of 100% isopropanol.
2. Mix the sample by inverting gently 50 times.
3. Centrifuge at 13,000–16,000*g* for 1 min; the DNA will be visible as a small white pellet.
4. Pour off the supernatant and drain the tube onto clean absorbent paper. Add 300 µL of 70% ethanol and invert the tube several times to wash the DNA pellet.
5. Centrifuge at 13,000–16,000*g* for 1 min. Pour off the ethanol carefully. The pellet may be loose, so the ethanol should be poured slowly to avoid disturbing the pellet. If it becomes dislodged from the wall of the tube, recentrifuge and carefully aspirate and discard the supernatant.
6. Invert the tube and drain the tube onto clean absorbent paper and air-dry for 10–15 min.

3.1.4. DNA Hydration

1. Add 100 μL of DNA hydration solution.
2. Rehydrate the DNA by incubating the sample for 1 h at 65°C and/or overnight at room temperature. If possible, tap the tube periodically to aid in dispersing the DNA.
3. Store the DNA at 4°C. For long-term storage, store at –20 or –80°C.

3.1.5. Quantitation of DNA Yield

1. Make a 1:200 dilution of DNA preparation.
2. Read the sample on a spectrophotometer at 260 and 280 nm. (To blank the spectrophotometer use water.)
3. Calculate the DNA concentration (in micrograms/milliliter) using the following formula (*see* **Note 2**):

$$[\text{DNA}]\ (\text{ng}/\mu\text{L}) = A_{260} \times 200\ (\text{dilution factor}) \times 50$$

3.2. PCR on APOE

The oligonucleotide primers listed in **Subheading 2.2.** are used to amplify *APOE* gene by using PCR. It is very important to prevent contamination by using dedicated equipment in the dedicated areas (*see* **Note 3**).

1. In a microfuge tube, pipet and mix the following components per reaction to prepare a master mix. For convenience, multiply the amount of solutions used by the number of samples (n) to be analyzed plus one ($n + 1$). Per sample, pipet and mix the following components: 11.5 μL of ddH_2O, 2 μL of 10X PCR buffer, 1.2 μL of 25 m*M* $MgCl_2$, 1 μL of apo E-AT3′ primer, 1 μL of apo E-5′ primer, 0.2 μL of dNTP, 2 μL of 100% DMSO, and 0.1 μL of *Taq* polymerase (5 U/μL).
2. Take 1 μL of DNA sample and add to 19 μL of master mix solution.
3. Perform PCR in a thermocycler starting with a denaturation step at 94°C.
4. For *APOE* gene amplification, apply 30 cycles of 94°C for 30 s, 60°C for 60 s, and 72°C for 60 s.
5. After the last cycle, perform an additional extension phase of 3 min at 72°C. Subsequently the samples can be cooled to 4°C.

3.3. Restriction Enzyme Digestion of Amplified DNA

1. Prepare the enzyme digestion cocktail (*see* **Note 4**). Calculate the total volume needed by multiplying the volume of components per reaction by the number of samples to be digested plus one extra for pipeting loss. In a microfuge tube, pipet and mix the following components per digestion reaction: 7.5 μL of ddH_2O, 2 μL of 10X restriction buffer for *Cfo*I enzyme, and 0.5 μL of 10 U/μL *Cfo*I restriction enzyme.
2. Add 10 μL of restriction enzyme cocktail to labeled sample tubes and take these tubes to the post-PCR area. Take the amplified DNA to the post-PCR area.
3. Add 10 μL of each amplified DNA sample to the appropriately labeled tubes (*see* **Note 5**).
4. Place the tubes in a heat block at 37°C for 1.5 h.

Table 2
Restriction Fragment Sizes Seen on *Cfo*I Digestion of PCR Products

Genotype	Fragment sizes (bp)
E2/E2	104, 91
E2/E3	104, 91, 56, 48
E2/E4	104, 91, 72, 56, 48
E3/E3	91, 56, 48
E3/E4	91, 72, 56, 48
E4/E4	72, 56, 48

3.4. Detection of Restriction Fragments

1. Prepare a 3% TBE, MetaPhor agarose gel (*see* **Note 6**). Add the buffer to an Erlenmeyer flask, gradually add the agarose, and gently swirl to mix. Heat the flask to dissolve the agarose.
2. When the agarose has slightly cooled, add 5 μL of ethidium bromide (10 mg/mL), pour the molten agarose into the gel tray, insert combs, and let it sit until it solidifies. Place it in at 4°C for 30 min. Place the agarose gel into the electrophoresis apparatus and pour 0.5X TBE buffer to cover the gel. Remove the combs.
3. Place 2 μL of 10X loading buffer into the tubes containing the digested DNA samples and controls (samples, E2/E4 control, digested blank), molecular weight marker, undigested blank control, and undigested E2/E4 positive control tubes.
4. Load the marker and samples as follows:
   a. Phi X 174/ *Hae*III molecular weight marker.
   b. Blank control undigested.
   c. E2/E4 control digested.
   d. Patient samples digested.
   e. E2/E4 control digested.
   f. Blank control digested.
5. Connect the leads on the gel box. Run the gels at 150 V for approx 1–1.5 h.
6. Transfer the gel to a UV light box and take a photograph.

3.5. Interpretation of Results

1. Verify that the size of the uncut DNA is 267 bp in length and that all the fragments are detected for the E2/E4 control and are of the correct sizes: 104, 91, 78, 56, and 48 bp.
2. Record the band sizes seen with the control and patient samples that have been digested with *Cfo*I.
3. Identify the genotype by comparing to the expected fragment lengths seen with each genotype (*see* **Table 2**).

4. Notes

1. The preferred anticoagulant for whole blood collection is EDTA; acid citrate dextrose is also acceptable. Heparin is not preferred but can be used.
2. Setup of the PCR reaction can be performed without quantifying the DNA. If a problem was suspected with the extraction, then a quantitation is recommended to ensure the presence of DNA.
3. To prevent contamination, aliquot all the solutions used for PCR and use aerosol-resistant pipet tips. Perform PCR preparations and analysis of PCR products in separate areas (pre-PCR and post-PCR areas, respectively).
4. The enzyme digestion cocktail should be prepared in the pre-PCR area. To set up the digestion, tubes should be opened in the post-PCR area because this involves handling amplified DNA.
5. Always add patient DNA first, followed by positive then negative controls.
6. Gel boxes and assorted equipment should be designated for only post-PCR use and used exclusively in the post-PCR room.

References

1. Mahley, R. W. (1988) Apolipoprotein E: cholesterol transport protein with expanding role in cell biology. *Science* **240,** 622–630.
2. Walden, C. C. and Hegele, R. A. (1994) Apolipoprotein E in hyperlipidemia. *Ann. Intern. Med.* **120,** 1026–1036.
3. Das, H. K., McPherson, J., Bruns, G. A., Karathanasis, S. K., and Breslow, J. L. (1985) Isolation, characterization, and mapping to chromosome 19 of the human apolipoprotein E gene. *J. Biol. Chem.* **260,** 6240–6247.
4. Paik, Y. K., Chang, D. J., Reardon, C. A., Davies, G. E., Mahley, R. W., and Taylor, J. M. (1985) Nucleotide sequence and structure of the human apolipoprotein E gene. *Proc. Natl. Acad. Sci. USA* **82,** 3445–3449.
5. Smith, J. D., Melian, A., Leff, T., and Breslow, J. L. (1988) Expression of the human apolipoprotein E gene is regulated by multiple positive and negative elements. *J. Biol. Chem.* **263,** 8300–8308.
6. McCarron, M. O., Muir, K. W., Weir, C. J., Dyker, A. G., Bone, I., Nicoll, J. A. R., and Lees, K. R. (1998) The apolipoprotein E epsilon 4 allele and outcome in cerebrovascular disease. *Stroke* **29,** 1882–1887.
7. Farrer, L. A., Cupples, L. A., Haines, J. L., Hyman, B., Kukull, W. A., Mayeux, R., Myers, R. H., Pericak-Vance, M. A., Risch, N., and van Duijn, C. M. (1997) Effects of age, sex, and ethnicity on the association between apolipoprotein E genotype and Alzheimer disease: a meta-analysis. *JAMA* **278,** 1349–1356.
8. Wang, X. L., McCredie, R. M., and Wilcken, D. E. L. (1995) Polymorphisms of the apolipoprotein E gene and severity of coronary artery disease defined by angiography. *Arterioscl. Thromb.Vasc. Biol.* **15,** 1030–1034.
9. Reymer, W. A., Groenemeyer, B. E., van de Burg, R., and Kastelein, J. J. P. (1995) Apolipoprotein E genotyping on agarose gels. *Clin. Chem.* **41,** 1046,1047.

35

Genotyping for Functionally Important Human CYP2D6*4 (B) Mutation Using TaqMan Probes

Michael M. Shi, Scott P. Myrand, Michael R. Bleavins, and Felix A. de la Iglesia

1. Introduction

The microsomal enzyme cytochrome P450 2D6 (CYP2D6), also known as debrisoquine 4-hydroxylase, is involved in the oxidative metabolism of many widely used drugs, including neuroleptics, tricyclic antidepressants, antiarrhythmics, and β-adrenergic blocking agents *(1)*. Polymorphisms of CYP2D6 are the best characterized examples of genetically mediated effects on a drug-metabolizing enzyme of clinical importance *(2)*. When a drug that is a CYP2D6 substrate is taken by different individuals, it is not uncommon to observe large differences in plasma concentrations at steady state. This is explained, in part, by the three clinically distinct phenotypes associated with the CYP2D6 gene, normal metabolizers, poor metabolizers, and rapid metabolizers. In normal metabolizers, steady-state plasma drug concentrations fall within the desired therapeutic range and toxic effects are nonexistent or minimal. In fast-metabolizer individuals, desired concentrations are below therapeutic, and these patients generally do not respond at the recommended dosing regimen. In poor-metabolizer individuals, drug concentrations are above therapeutic level and undesired toxicity can be evoked.

This genetic impact on drug concentration is of particular concern for compounds, which are metabolized by CYP2D6 because many have narrow therapeutic windows. In addition, the poor-metabolizer phenotype occurs with a frequency of 7–10% in Caucasians *(1)*. The most common poor-metabolizer genotype for CYP2D6 is CYP2D6*4, or the "B" mutant, and in the Caucasian population, it constitutes about 75% of all mutant alleles *(1)*. This mutation involves a G-to-A transition at the intron 3 and exon 4 junction (nucleotide

From: *Methods in Molecular Medicine, vol. 49: Molecular Pathology Protocols*
Edited by: A. A. Killeen © Humana Press Inc., Totowa, NJ

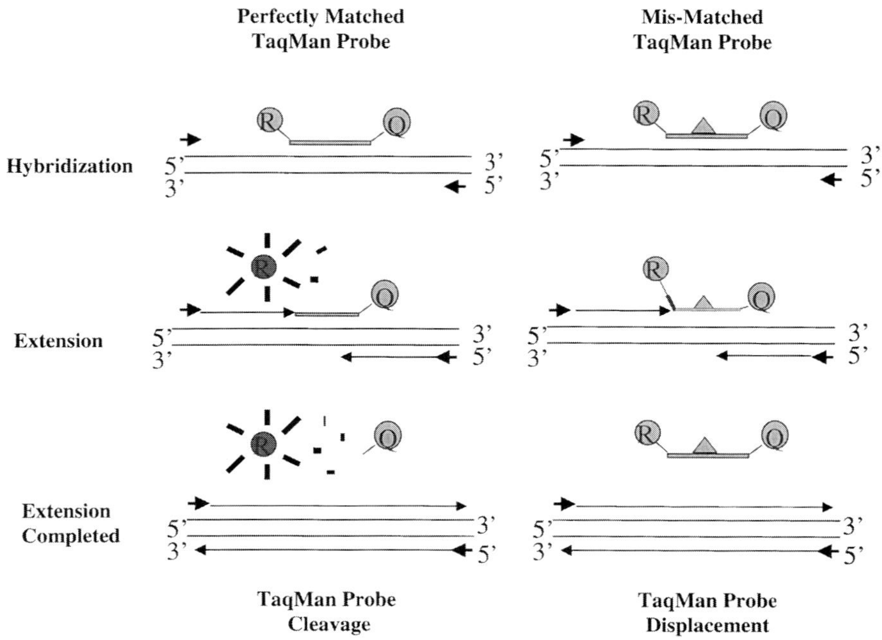

Fig. 1. Schematic representation of the TaqMan genotyping assay. Two TaqMan probes are targeted at the polymorphic site and are labeled with different reporter dyes FAM or TET. Only the perfectly hybridized probe will be cleaved by the *Taq* polymerase during the extension phase of the PCR reaction. A mismatched probe will not be recognized by the *Taq* polymerase. At the end of the genotyping reaction, the PCR product is analyzed for changes in fluorescence intensities of the reporter dyes FAM and TET. The ratio of FAM:TET will determine the sample's genotype.

3465, Genbank accession no. M33388), leading to a missplicing of the premature transcript that abolishes enzymatic activity in homozygous mutants *(3)*. The standard procedure to evaluate the metabolic consequence of this genotype involves phenotyping by administration of a probe drug such as debrisoquine and measuring the ratio of parent drug and its hydroxyl metabolite (4-hydroxydebrisoquine) in urine. Alternatively, molecular genotyping has become popular because of its simplicity, higher throughput capacity, and fast turnaround time. Genotyping to detect CYP2D6*4 defects generally involves polymerase chain reaction restriction fragment length polymorphism (PCR-RFLP) analysis. This approach, however, is time-consuming and labor-intensive. The required procedures are difficult to automate and require skilled staff to conduct the tests and evaluate the results. In this protocol, we describe a simple, robust, high-throughput genotyping method to detect the CYP2D6*4 polymorphism using TaqMan probes (*see* **Fig. 1**).

The TaqMan allelic discrimination employs the 5′-nuclease activity of AmpliTaq DNA polymerase to allow direct detection of the PCR product by the release of a fluorescent reporter *(4)*. Two TaqMan probes are used in this assay, one probe for each allele. Each probe consists of an oligonucleotide with 5′ reporter dye 6-carboxyfluorescein (FAM) or 6-carboxy-4,7,2′,7′-tetrachlorofluorescein (TET) and 3′-quencher dye 6-carboxy-*N*,*N*,*N*′,*N*′-tetrachlorofluorescein (TAMRA). When the probe is intact, the reporter dye's fluorescence is quenched owing to the physical proximity of the two dyes *(5)*. During the annealing phase of PCR reaction, forward and reverse primers anneal to the flanking regions of the polymorphic site, and the TaqMan probes hybridize to the polymorphic site. During the extension phase of the PCR reaction, the reporter dye is cleaved by *Taq* polymerase, resulting in increased dye fluorescence. By measuring the intensities of TET and FAM signal, the specific genotype of one allele can be discriminated *(6)*. Thus, genotyping of TaqMan allelic discrimination offers high-sample throughput and accurate detection of single-nucleotide polymorphisms. This fluorescent-based genotyping procedure significantly reduces the complexity of the assay protocol by eliminating the need for restriction enzyme digestion, gel electrophoresis, resolution of PCR products, and visual assessment of bands. In addition, the 96-well plate format and closed-tube PCR reactions eliminate subsequent processing, reducing the potential for contamination. Fluorescent reporter dye signals can be captured minutes after allelic discriminating reactions are performed, and genotypes can be automatically identified by the sequence detection software used. The ability to automate data handling further enhances accuracy by eliminating operator bias. We have integrated the PCR setup with a robotic liquid-handling station, such that one individual can comfortably handle the genotyping of 500–1000 samples in an 8-h working day.

2. Materials

2.1. Equipment

1. ABI 7200 or 7700 sequence detector (Perkin-Elmer/Applied Biosystems, Foster City, CA).
2. Thermocycler.
3. Microcentrifuge.
4. Incubators at 70 and 95°C for DNA extraction.
5. Spectrophotometer for DNA quantitation.
6. TaqMan allelic discrimination demonstration kit (Perkin-Elmer/Applied Biosystems).

2.2. Extraction of Genomic DNA

We use a Qiagen (Chatsworth, CA) QIAamp blood kit: cat. no. 29104 (50 preparations) or cat. no. 29106 (250 preparations). The method from these kits is described in this protocol. Equivalent DNA extraction methods are acceptable.

1. Prepare QIAGEN protease stock solution: Add 1.4 mL of distilled water to 25 mg of lyophilized protease in the QIAamp 50-preparation kit, or add 7 mL of water to 125 mg of protease in the 250-preparation kit. Solution is stable at 4°C for up to 3 mo. For longer-term storage, aliquot and store at –20°C for up to 1 yr. Avoid repeated freezing and thawing.
2. Prepare buffer AL by decanting all of reagent AL1 into buffer AL (Reagent AL2). Mix thoroughly by shaking. Buffer AL is stable for a least 1 yr when stored in the dark at room temperature.
3. Prepare buffer AW: Add 42 mL of ethanol (96–100%) to buffer AW concentrate (50-preparation kit) or 196 mL (250-preparation kit) before using the kit for the first time. Buffer AW is stable for at least 1 yr when stored closed at room temperature.

2.3. TaqMan Probes and PCR Reagents

1. TaqMan PCR Universal Mastermix (part no. 4304447; Perkin-Elmer).
2. Design and order high-performance liquid chromatography grade forward and reverse primers from Gibco-BRL (Gaithersburg, MD) or equivalent supplier on request. The forward primer sequence for CYP2D6 is 5′-CGC CTT CGC CAA CCA CT-3′ and the reverse primer is: 5′-CTT TGT CCA AGA GAC CGT TGG-3′.
3. Allele-specific TaqMan probes are custom ordered from the Applied Biosystems division of Perkin-Elmer. The following can be ordered: 50 n*M* scale (part no. 450025, screens 1–8 plates), 0.2 μ*M* scale (part no. 450024, screens 8–40 plates), and 1 μ*M* scale (part no. 450003, screens more than 40 plates). TaqMan probes for CYP2D6*4 genotyping are as follows: Allele 1 probe = mutant = TET – CAC CCC CA<u>A</u> GAC GCC CCT TT-TAMRA, and Allele 2 probe = wild type = 6FAM – CAC CCC CA<u>G</u> GAC GCC CCT-TAMRA.
4. Perkin-Elmer PCR plates (part no. N801-0560) and MicroAmp optical caps (part no. N801-0935) or equivalent.

3. Methods

3.1. Preparation of DNA

Fresh or frozen whole blood, collected into tubes containing citrate, heparin, or EDTA, is normally used. Buffy coats, leukocytes, or cultured cells also may be used.

1. Equilibrate the sample to room temperature.
2. Pipet 400 μL of sample into a 1.5-mL centrifuge tube.

3. Add 50 µL of QIAGEN protease stock solution and 400 µL of buffer AL.
4. Mix the contents of the tube immediately by vortexing until the pellet is completely dissolved.
5. Incubate the sample at 70°C for 10 min.
6. Inactivate potential infectious agents by incubating at 95°C for 15 min.
7. Add 420 µL of isopropanol for blood samples.
8. Add 420 µL of ethanol for buffy coat, lymphocytes, or cultured cells.
9. Mix the contents of the tube by vortexing.
10. Place a QIAamp spin column in a 2-mL collection tube.
11. Transfer up to 650 µL of the lysate from **step 9** into the spin column carefully without moistening the rim.
12. Close the cap and centrifuge at 6500*g* for 1 min. If the sample consists of buffy coat or lymphocytes, centrifuge at 15,800*g*.
13. Place the QIAamp spin column in a clean 2 mL tube and discard the tube containing the filtrate.
14. Repeat **steps 11–13** until the whole lysate is loaded onto the column. A maximum of 5 × 650 µL can be loaded onto the QIAamp spin column.
15. Carefully open the QIAamp spin column and add 500 µL of buffer AW.
16. Centrifuge at 6500*g* for 1 min or at 15,800*g* for buffy coats.
17. Remove the spin column from the collection tube and discard the filtrate.
18. Replace the QIAamp spin column in a fresh microcentrifuge tube.
19. Repeat **steps 15–18**.
20. Repeat **steps 15** and **16**. Then centrifuge for 2 min at full speed (15,800*g*).
21. Remove the spin column from the collection tube and discard the filtrate.
22. Place the QIAamp spin column in a clean 1.5 mL centrifuge tube.
23. Preheat buffer AE to 70°C.
24. Add 200 µL of preheated buffer AE to the spin column and incubate the tube at 70°C for 5 min.
25. Elute the DNA by spinning as in **step 16**.
26. Quantitate the DNA at 260 nm using a spectrophotomer.
27. Store the DNA at –20°C.

3.2. TaqMan Allelic Discrimination Assay

1. Dilute an aliquot of TaqMan probes to a final concentration of 10 µ*M*. Quantitate forward and reverse primers, and dilute an aliquot of each oligonucleotide to a final concentration of 20 µ*M*.
2. In a 96-well PCR plate (8 × 12 template or A1–H12), set up 8 No Template Control wells (NTC, A1–A8), 8 Allele 1 standard wells (AL1, A9–B4), 8 Allele 2 standard wells (AL2, B5–B12), and up to 72 genomic DNA samples (UNKN, C1–H12) (*see* **Notes 1** and **2**).
3. Prepare PCR master mix as directed (*see* **Table 1**). Vortex the master mix thoroughly. Aliquot 15 µL of PCR master mix up to 96 wells in the 96-well plate with the DNA samples to be screened (*see* **Note 3**).

Table 1
TaqMan PCR Master Mix Setup Sheet for CYP2D6*4

Reagent	Volume (μL) for each 20-μL reaction	Final concentration in each 20-μL reaction
2X Universal PCR master 2X mix	10.00	1X
20 μ*M* forward primer	0.45	450 n*M*
20 μ*M* reverse primer	0.45	450 n*M*
10 μ*M* FAM probe	0.10	50 n*M*
10 μ*M* TET probe	0.40	200 n*M*
Deionized water	3.60	—
Total volume	15.00	

4. Add 8 replicates of H_2O (wells A1–A8), AL1 control (wells A9–B4), AL2 control (wells B5–B12), and up to 72 samples of unknown DNA (C1–H12) into the 96-well PCR plate. Use 20–50 ng of genomic DNA in 5 μL of total volume.
5. Close the plate with MicroAmp optical caps; make sure the caps are tightly sealed.
6. Centrifuge the plate to collect the liquid at the bottom of the tubes and remove the air bubbles. Visually check that all volumes appear to be approximately the same before starting the PCR cycling program.
7. Place 96 well plates into a thermocycler and run the appropriate PCR program. PCR conditions are as follows:
   a. Step 1: 50°C for 2 min for 1 cycle.
   b. Step 2: 95°C for 10 min (95°C for 10 min is required to activate TaqGold.
   c. Step 3: 95°C for 15 s for 40 cycles.
   d. Step 4: 65°C for 1 min.
   e. Step 5: 4°C indefinitely.
8. Remove the 96-well plates from the thermocycler and read the results on the ABI 7200 sequence detector.

3.3. Reading Plate Results on Sequence Detector

1. Turn on both the ABI 7200 sequence detector and the computer.
2. Open the "Sequence Detector 1.6" program.
3. When the program begins, close out of the default plate by choosing *Close* under the *File* menu.
4. Under the *File* menu now choose *New Plate*.
5. A window will appear that shows the settings being used for the plate reading. Change the *Plate Type* setting to *Allelic Discrimination*, and *7200 Sequence Detector* under the instrument pop-up menu.
6. A new plate is brought up. Make sure that the top right corner reads *7200 Allelic Discrimination*.
7. Under comments, record the experiment name: match the reading on the 7200. Add any additional comments that may be useful for future reference of the cur-

rent experiment such as samples tested, study name, thermocycler, and initials of the person completing the assay.

8. Use the mouse to highlight all cells that need to be read as NTC (wells A1–A8) and across from *Sample Type* choose *NTC—No Template Control*. Do the same for those samples that are AL1 controls (wells A9–B4) and choose *AL1—Allele 1*. Also complete this for those samples that are AL2 controls (wells B5–B12) and choose *AL2—Allele 2*. Now highlight all cells that need to be read as unknown (wells C1–H12), and choose the *UNKN—Unknown* setting across from *Sample Type*.
9. Click on the *Show Analysis* box located above cell A1.
10. Place the plate in the 7200 sequence detector.
11. Click on *Post-PCR Read*.
12. On completion of reading, choose *Save as* under the *File* menu and save the plate.
13. Now choose *Analyze* under the *Analysis* menu.
14. Now under the *Analysis* window, again choose *Allelic Discrimination*. There should be four well-separated groups corresponding to the no amplification, Allele-1, Allele-2, and Allele 1 and 2.
15. Using the arrow, make a square and highlight those points that are clearly miscalls by the normalized calling and change their genotyping designation to the appropriate genotype. Any stray points not tightly grouped with controls and heterozyotes should be called no amplification.
16. From the *Export . . .* submenu under the *File* menu, choose *Results . . . Export the Results* file.

3.4. Interpretation of Results

Based on the fluorescent signals of the reporter dyes FAM and TET in the Sequence Detection Software, four distinct populations will be identified (**Fig. 2**). According to the FAM : TET ratio, the four populations could be categorized as no amplification (low reading in both FAM and TET), Allele-1 (mut/mut, homozygous mutant; FAM << TET), Allele-2 (wt/wt, homozygous wild type; FAM >> TET), and Allele 1/2 (wt/mut, heterozygous; FAM ≈ TET) (**Fig. 2**). Any stray points should be called "no amplification" (*see* **Notes 4** and **5**).

Subheadings 3.5.–3.9. are designed for standard TaqMan genotyping optimization. These steps are not required for genotyping the CYP2D6*4 polymorphism unless the ABI 7700 sequence detector is being used. Please also see the ABI handbook (in the TaqMan allelic discrimination demonstration kit) for additional reference (*see* **Note 6**).

3.5. Optimization of Primer Concentration

1. Dilute TaqMan probes to an aliquot to a final concentration of 10 µ*M*. Quantitate the forward and reverse primers, and dilute an aliquot of each oligonucleotide to a final concentration of 20 µ*M*.

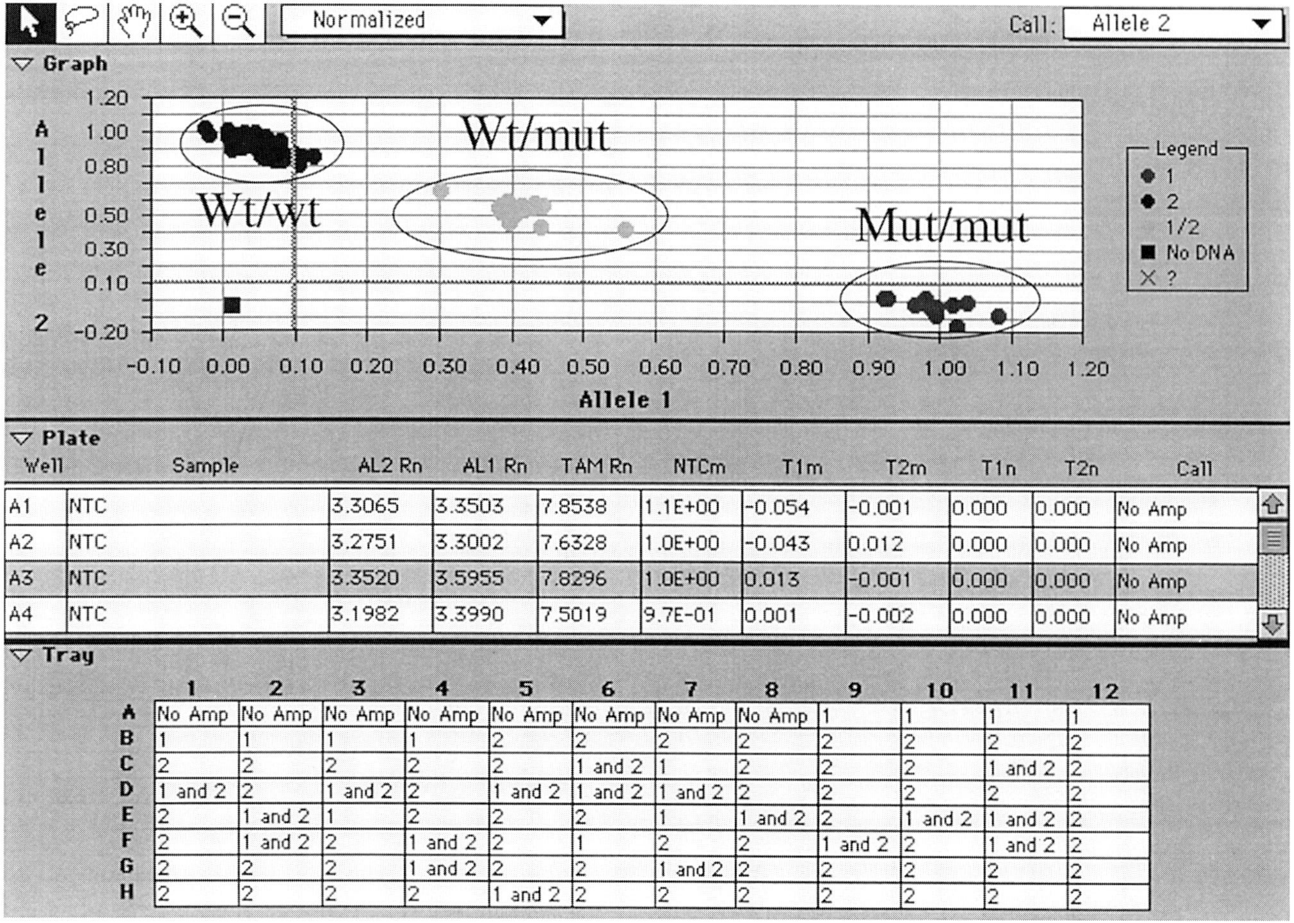
Normalized
Call: Allele 2
Graph
Allele 2
1.20
1.00
0.80
0.50
0.30
0.10
-0.20
-0.10 0.00 0.10 0.20 0.30 0.40 0.50 0.60 0.70 0.80 0.90 1.00 1.10 1.20
Allele 1
Wt/wt
Wt/mut
Mut/mut
Legend
1
2
1/2
No DNA
?
Plate
Well Sample AL2 Rn AL1 Rn TAM Rn NTCm T1m T2m T1n T2n Call
A1 NTC 3.3065 3.3503 7.8538 1.1E+00 -0.054 -0.001 0.000 0.000 No Amp
A2 NTC 3.2751 3.3002 7.6328 1.0E+00 -0.043 0.012 0.000 0.000 No Amp
A3 NTC 3.3520 3.5955 7.8296 1.0E+00 0.013 -0.001 0.000 0.000 No Amp
A4 NTC 3.1982 3.3990 7.5019 9.7E-01 0.001 -0.002 0.000 0.000 No Amp
Tray
1 2 3 4 5 6 7 8 9 10 11 12
A No Amp No Amp No Amp No Amp No Amp No Amp No Amp No Amp 1 1 1 1
B 1 1 1 1 2 2 2 2 2 2 2 2
C 2 2 2 2 2 1 and 2 1 2 2 2 1 and 2 2
D 1 and 2 2 1 and 2 2 1 and 2 1 and 2 1 and 2 2 2 2 2 2
E 2 1 and 2 1 2 2 2 1 1 and 2 2 1 and 2 1 and 2 2
F 2 1 and 2 2 1 and 2 2 1 2 2 1 and 2 2 1 and 2 2
G 2 2 2 1 and 2 2 2 1 and 2 2 2 2 2 2
H 2 2 2 2 1 and 2 2 2 2 2 2 2 2

2. Choose one normal human (NH) DNA control sample and add dilute DNA (4 ng/μL) to the wells (A1–C12, D5–D8) in the plate.
3. Set up the primer concentration optimization plate. This is a matrix of nine different primer concentrations done in quadruplicate for both NTC and an NH sample:

   9 different primer concentrations × (4) samples = 36 reactions

   4 NTCs and 4 no-amplification controls (NACs) = 8 reactions

   36 + 8 reactions = 44 total reactions

   Primer concentrations (n*M* forward primer; n*M* reverse primer) are as follows: 50:50, 50:300, 50:900, 300:50, 300:300, 300:900, 900:50, 900:300, and 900:900.
4. Prepare the primer concentration optimization master mix work sheet as shown in **Table 2**.
5. Put the samples in a thermocycler and program the machine for the following PCR conditions:
   a. Step 1: 50°C for 2 min for 1 cycle.
   b. Step 2: 95°C for 10 min.
   c. Step 3: 95°C for 15 s for 40 cycles.
   d. Step 4: 62°C for 1 min.
   e. Step 5: 4°C indefinitely.
6. After the cycling program is complete, allow the samples to return to room temperature for at least 5 min and read the samples on the ABI 7200 sequence detector.

3.6. Reading Results of Optimization of Primer Concentration

1. Turn on both the ABI 7200 (or 7700) sequence detector and the computer.
2. Open the "Sequence Detector 1.6" program.
3. When the program begins, close out of the default plate by choosing *Close* under the *File* menu.
4. Under the *File* menu now choose *New Plate*.
5. A window will appear that shows the settings being used for the plate reading. Change the *Plate Type* setting to *Single Reporter*, and *7200 Sequence Detector* under the instrument pop-up menu.

Fig. 2. *(see opposite page)* Scatter plot of the CYP2D6 genotype using standard TaqMan allelic discrimination assays with automatic allele calling. Each reaction plate contains 8 no template control, 8 homozygous allele 1, 8 homozygous allele 2, and 72 unrelated individuals with respect to the polymorphic CYP2D6*4 genotype. The CYP2D6 genotypes were automatically assigned by the sequence detection software according to the ratio of FAM:TET signal. Allele 1 = 3465 A/A (mut/mut, FAM << TET); allele 2 = 3465 G/G (wt/wt, FAM >> TET); alleles 1 and 2 = 3465 G/A (wt/mut, FAM (TET).

Table 2
Primer Concentration Optimization Setup Work Sheet

Wells	Universal PCR master 2X mix (μL)	10 μ*M* wild-type probe (μL)	NH target DNA (μL)	20 μ*M* forward primer (μL)	20 μ*M* reverse primer (μL)	Deionized water (μL)	Forward/reverse primer concentration (n*M*)
A1–A4	25	0.5	5.0	0.125	0.125	19.25	50/50
A5–A8	25	0.5	5.0	0.125	0.75	18.625	50/300
A9–A12	25	0.5	5.0	0.125	2.25	17.125	50/900
B1–B4	25	0.5	5.0	0.75	0.125	18.625	300/50
B5–B8	25	0.5	5.0	0.75	0.75	18.0	300/300
B9–B12	25	0.5	5.0	0.75	2.25	16.5	300/900
C1–C4	25	0.5	5.0	2.25	0.125	17.125	900/50
C5–C8	25	0.5	5.0	2.25	0.75	16.5	900/300
C9–C12	25	0.5	5.0	2.25	2.25	15.0	900/900
D1–D4 (NTC)	25	0.5	0.0	2.25	2.25	20.0	900/900
D5–D8 (NAC)[a]	25	0.5	5.0	2.25	2.25	14.0 +1 μL of 0.5% SDS	900/900

[a]Add 1 μL of 0.5% SDS to inhibit enzyme activity. SDS = sodium dodecyl sulfate.

6. A new plate is brought up. Verify that the top right corner reads *7200 Single Reporter*.
7. To the right of the *Show Analysis* box there is another box called *Dye Layer*. Choose FAM as the dye layer.
8. Use the mouse to highlight the cells that need to be read as NTC (wells D1–D4) and across from *Sample Type* choose *NTC—No Template Control*. Similarly, set up those samples that are NAC (wells D5–D8) and choose *NAC—No Amplification Control*. Now highlight all the cells that need to be read as unknown (wells A1–C12) and choose the *UNKN—Unknown* setting across from *Sample Type*.
9. Click on *Show Analysis*. Under *Analysis* choose *Display* and then choose *Rn/ΔRn*.
10. Place the plate into the 7200 sequence detector, and make sure that the DNA plate is oriented correctly.
11. Click on *Post-PCR Read*. On completion of reading, choose *Save as* under the *File menu* and save the plate.
12. Once analysis is completed, each well will have a + or – sign and numbers in them. The numbers represent the intensity level of the probe that corresponds to the NH sample. Determine the group of four wells in the FAM dye layer that have the highest average intensity readings. Select these forward and reverse concentrations for all subsequent TaqMan reactions using these primers.

3.7. Probe Optimization

1. Prepare the plate using the indicated solution volumes in each well according to **Table 3**.
2. Open the "Sequence Detector 1.6" program.
3. Once the screen opens up, close out of the default plate by choosing *Close* under the *File* menu.
4. Under the *File* menu now choose *New Plate*.
5. A window will appear that shows the settings being used for the plate reading. Change the *Plate Type* setting to *Allelic Discrimination*, and *7200 Sequence Detector* under the instrument pop-up menu.
6. A new plate is brought up. Verify that the top right corner reads *7200 Allelic Discrimination*.
7. Use the mouse to highlight all the cells that need to be read as unknown (wells A1–C4) and choose the *UNKN—Unknown* setting across from *Sample Type*.
8. Place the plate into the 7200 sequence detector, and make sure that the DNA plate is oriented correctly.
9. Click on *Show Analysis*.
10. Click on *Post-PCR Read*. The software will perform the *Plate Read*.
11. From the *File* menu, choose *Save as . . .* to save the plate.
12. From the *Diagnostics* submenu under the *Instrument* menu, choose *Advanced Options . . . Under Miscellaneous Options*, and deselect the *Use Spectral Compensation for Endpoint* checkbox. If you change the option, a dialog box will appear telling you to stop the application. Stop and restart the program to use the changes.
13. From the *Analysis* menu, choose *Analyze*.

Table 3
Probe Optimization Setup Work Sheet

Wells	Universal PCR master 2X mix (μL)	1 μ*M* FAM probe (μL)	1 μ*M* TET probe (μL)	H_2O (μL)	Total volume per well (μL)	Final FAM probe concentration (n*M*)	Final TET probe concentration (n*M*)
A1–A4	25	2.5	f0.5	20.0	50	50	50
A5–A8	25	2.5	f5.0	17.5	50	50	100
A9–A12	25	2.5	f7.5	15.0	50	50	150
B1–B4	25	2.5	10.0	12.5	50	50	200
B5–B8	25	2.5	12.5	10.0	50	50	250
B9–B12	25	2.5	15.0	f7.5	50	50	300
C1–C4	25	2.5	17.5	f5.0	50	50	350

14. From the *Analysis* menu, choose *Allelic Discrimination*.
15. From the *Export* submenu under the *File* menu, choose *Multicomponent*. Export the *Multicomponent* file.
16. Stop the sequence detection software.
17. Open the *Multicomponent* file exported from the sequence detection software using the "Simpletext" program.
18. Identify the probe ratio where the FAM and TET multicomponent values are closest to each other. Use this probe ratio in the subsequent allelic discrimination assay.
19. If the probes are not well balanced at any ratio, use the TET probe at 350 n*M*.

3.8. Performing TaqMan Allelic Discrimination Assay

Set up the PCR and sequence detection according to **Subheading 3.2.**, using the appropriate primer concentrations (determined by **Subheading 3.6.**) and the FAM and TET probe concentrations (determined by **Subheading 3.7.**).

3.9. Temperature Optimization

If the allelic discrimination does not show a good separation, the same experiment should be repeated at a higher temperature (using increasing annealing temperatures from 63 to 65°C, but not higher than 65°C).

4. Notes

1. Control Allele 1 and Allele 2 were previously characterized using a PCR-RFLP method *(7)*.
2. Eight no-template control, 8 homozygous wild type, 8 homozygous mutants, and up to 72 genomic DNA samples were utilized for automatic genotype calling using sequence detection software per the manufacturer's recommendation (**Fig. 2**). These control sample numbers were chosen to achieve a 99.7% confidence level for automatic allele identification.
3. The TaqMan Universal PCR Master Mix is a premix of all the components, except primers and probe, necessary to perform a 5′-nuclease assay.
4. Although it is recommended that the plates be read soon after PCR reaction, the FAM and TET signals are stable for up to 3 d post-PCR if stored in the dark.
5. Sometimes the sequence detection software fails to automatically call the genotype. There could be several reasons for this. The most frequent is the high background amplification in No Amp controls. This can be checked under the *Multicomponent* section. By examining the TET and FAM signals of the eight NACs, the higher backgrounds could be eliminated by using the *Not in Use* function in the *Show Setup* manual. A minimum of four NACs have to be used to achieve automatic allele calling.
6. The TaqMan genotyping protocol for CYP2D6*4 was optimized using an ABI 7200 sequence detector. **Subheadings 3.4.–3.7.** could be used to optimize TaqMan genotyping conditions for detection of any single nucleotide polymorphisms.

References

1. Linder, M. W., Prough, R. A., and Valdes, R. Jr. (1997) Pharmacogenetics: a laboratory tool for optimizing therapeutic efficiency. *Clin. Chem.* **43,** 254–266.
2. Kimura, S., Umeno M., Skoda, R. C., Meyer, U. A., and Gonzalez, F. J. (1989) The human debrisoquine 4-hydroxylase (CYP2D) locus: sequence and identification of the polymorphic CYP2D6 gene, a related gene and a pseudogene. *Am. J. Hum. Genet.* **45,** 889–904.
3. Gough, A. C., Miles, J. S., Spurr, N. K., et al. (1990) Identification of the primary gene defect at the cytochrome P450 CYP2D locus. *Nature* **347,** 773–776.
4. Lyamichev, V., Brow, M. A. D., and Dahlberg, J. E. (1993) Structure-specific endonucleolytic cleavage of nucleic acids by eubacterial DNA polymerase. *Science* **260,** 778–783.
5. Lackowicz, J. R. (1983) Energy transfer, in *Principles of Fluorescent Spectroscopy* (Lackowicz, J. R., ed.), Plenum, New York, pp. 303–339.
6. Livak, K. J., Flood, S. J. A., Marmaro, J., Giusti, W., and Deetz, K. (1995) Oligonucleotides with fluorescent dyes at opposite ends provide a quenched probe system useful for detecting PCR product and nucleic acid hybridization. *PCR Methods Appl.* **4,** 357–362.
7. Wolf, C. R., Smith, C. A. D., Gough, A. C., et al. (1992) Relationship between the debrisoquine hydroxylase polymorphism and cancer susceptibility. *Carcinogenesis* **13,** 1035–1038.

Index

C